WORLD *of* MICROBIOLOGY AND IMMUNOLOGY

WORLD *of*

MICROBIOLOGY AND IMMUNOLOGY

K. Lee Lerner and Brenda Wilmoth Lerner, *Editors*

Volume 2

M-Z

General Index

GALE®

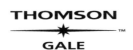

Detroit • New York • San Diego • San Francisco • Cleveland • New Haven, Conn. • Waterville, Maine • London • Munich

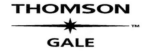

World of Microbiology and Immunology

K. Lee Lerner and Brenda Wilmoth Lerner, *Editors*

Project Editor
Brigham Narins

Editorial
Mark Springer

Permissions
Margaret Chamberlain, Jackie Jones

Imaging and Multimedia
Leitha Etheridge-Sims, Mary K. Grimes, Lezlie Light, Dan Newell, David G. Oblender, Christine O'Bryan, Robyn V. Young

Product Design
Michael Logusz

Manufacturing
Rhonda Williams

For permission to use material from this product, submit your request via Web at http://www.gale-edit.com/permissions, or you may download our Permissions Request form and submit your request by fax or mail to:

Permissions Department
The Gale Group, Inc.
27500 Drake Road
Farmington Hills, MI, 48331-3535
Permissions hotline:
248-699-8074 or 800-877-4253, ext. 8006
Fax: 248-699-8074 or 800-762-4058.

While every effort has been made to ensure the reliability of the information pre-sented in this publication, The Gale Group, Inc. does not guarantee the accuracy of the data contained herein. The Gale Group, Inc. accepts no payment for listing; and inclusion in the publication of any organization, agency, institution, publication, service, or individual does not imply endorsement of the editors or publisher. Errors brought to the attention of the publisher and verified to the satisfaction of the publisher will be corrected in future editions.

LIBRARY OF CONGRESS CATALOGING-IN-PUBLICATION DATA

World of microbiology and immunology / K. Lee Lerner and Brenda Wilmoth Lerner, editors.
    p. ; cm.
       Includes bibliographical references and index.
       ISBN 0-7876-6540-1 (set : alk. paper)—
       ISBN 0-7876-6541-X (v. 1 : alk. paper)—
       ISBN 0-7876-6542-8 (v. 2 : alk. paper)
       1. Microbiology—Encyclopedias. 2. Immunology—Encyclopedias.
       [DNLM: 1. Allergy and Immunology—Encyclopedias—English.
       2. Microbiology—Encyclopedias—English. QW 13 W927 2003]
       I. Lerner, K. Lee. II. Lerner, Brenda Wilmoth.
QR9 .W675 2003
579'.03—dc21   2002010181
ISBN: 0-7876-6541-X

Printed in the United States of America
10 9 8 7 6 5 4 3 2 1

CONTENTS

INTRODUCTION

Although microbiology and immunology are fundamentally separate areas of biology and medicine, they combine to provide a powerful understanding of human health and disease—especially with regard to infectious disease, disease prevention, and tragically, of the growing awareness that bioterrorism is a real and present worldwide danger.

World of Microbiology and Immunology is a collection of 600 entries on topics covering a range of interests—from biographies of the pioneers of microbiology and immunology to explanations of the fundamental scientific concepts and latest research developments. In many universities, students in the biological sciences are not exposed to microbiology or immunology courses until the later half of their undergraduate studies. In fact, many medical students do not receive their first formal training in these subjects until medical school. Despite the complexities of terminology and advanced knowledge of biochemistry and genetics needed to fully explore some of the topics in microbiology and immunology, every effort has been made to set forth entries in everyday language and to provide accurate and generous explanations of the most important terms. The editors intend *World of Microbiology and Immunology* for a wide range of readers. Accordingly, the articles are designed to instruct, challenge, and excite less experienced students, while providing a solid foundation and reference for more advanced students. The editors also intend that *World of Microbiology and Immunology* be a valuable resource to the general reader seeking information fundamental to understanding current events.

Throughout history, microorganisms have spread deadly diseases and caused widespread epidemics that threatened and altered human civilization. In the modern era, civic sanitation, water purification, immunization, and antibiotics have dramatically reduced the overall morbidity and the mortality of disease in advanced nations. Yet much of the world is still ravaged by disease and epidemics, and new threats constantly appear to challenge the most advanced medical and public health systems. For all our science and technology, we are far from mastering the microbial world.

During the early part of the twentieth century, the science of microbiology developed somewhat independently of other biological disciplines. Although for many years it did not exist as a separate discipline at all—being an "off-shoot" of chemistry (fermentation science) or medicine—with advances in techniques such as microscopy and pure culturing methodologies, as well as with the establishment of the germ theory of disease and the rudiments of vaccination, microbiology suddenly exploded as a separate discipline. Whereas other biological disciplines were concerned with such topics as cell structure and function, the ecology of plants and animals, the reproduction and development of organisms, the nature of heredity and the mechanisms of evolution, microbiology had a very different focus. It was concerned primarily with the agents of infectious disease, the immune response, the search for chemotherapeutic agents and bacterial metabolism. Thus, from the very beginning, microbiology as a science had social applications. A more detailed historical perspective of the development of the field may be found in the article "History of Microbiology" in this volume.

Microbiology established a closer relationship with other biological disciplines in the 1940s because of its association with genetics and biochemistry. This association also laid the foundations for the subsequent and still rapidly developing field of genetic engineering, which holds promise of profound impact on science and medicine.

Microorganisms are extremely useful experimental subjects because they are relatively simple, grow rapidly, and can be cultured in large quantities. George W. Beadle and Edward L. Tatum studied the relationship between genes and enzymes in 1941 using mutants of the bread mold *Neurospora*. In 1943 Salvador Luria and Max Delbrück used bacterial mutants to show that gene mutations were apparently spontaneous and not directed by the environment. Subsequently, Oswald Avery, Colin M. MacLeod, and Maclyn McCarty provided strong evidence that DNA was the genetic material and carried genetic information during transformation. The interactions between microbiology, genetics, and biochemistry soon led to the development of modern, molecularly oriented genetics.

Recently microbiology has been a major contributor to the rise of molecular biology, the branch of biology dealing with the physical and chemical bases of living matter and its function. Microbiologists have been deeply involved in studies of the genetic code and the mechanisms of DNA, RNA, and protein synthesis. Microorganisms were used in many of the early studies on the regulation of gene expression and the control of enzyme activity. In the 1970s new discoveries in microbiology led to the development of recombinant gene technology and genetic engineering. One indication of the importance of microbiology today is the number of Nobel Prizes awarded for work in physiology and medicine during the twentieth century; about a third of these were awarded to scientists working on microbiological problems.

Microorganisms are exceptionally diverse, are found almost everywhere, and affect human society in countless ways. The modern study of microbiology is very different from the chemically and medically oriented discipline pioneered by Louis Pasteur and Robert Koch. Today it is a large discipline with many specialities. It has impact on medicine, agricultural and food sciences, ecology, genetics, biochemistry, and many other fields. Today it clearly has both basic and applied aspects.

Many microbiologists are interested in the biology of the microorganisms themselves. They may focus on a specific group of microorganisms and be called virologists (scientists who study viruses), bacteriologists (scientists who study bacteria), phycologists or algologists (scientists who study algae), mycologists (scientists who study fungi), or protozoologists (scientists who study protozoa). Others may be interested in microbial morphology or particular functional processes and work in fields such as microbial cytology, physiology, ecology, genetics, taxonomy, and molecular biology. Some microbiologists may have a more applied orientation and work on problems in fields such as medical microbiology, food and dairy microbiology, or public health. Because the various fields of microbiology are interrelated, an applied microbiologist must always be familiar with basic microbiology. For example, a medical microbiologist must have a good understanding of microbial taxonomy, genetics, immunology, and physiology to identify and properly respond to the pathogen of concern.

It is clear that scientists study the microbial world in much the same way as they studied the world of multicellular organisms at the beginning of the twentieth century, when microbiology was a young discipline. This is in part due to the huge developments and refinements of techniques, which now allow scientists to more closely and fully investigate the world of bacteria and viruses.

One of the focuses of this book is the field of medical microbiology and its connection with immunology. Medical microbiology developed between the years 1875 and 1918, during which time many disease-causing bacteria were identified and the early work on viruses begun. Once people realized that these invisible agents could cause disease, efforts were

made to prevent their spread from sick to healthy people. The great successes that have taken place in the area of human health in the past 100 years have resulted largely from advances in the prevention and treatment of infectious disease. We can consider the eradication of smallpox, a viral disease, as a prime example. The agent that causes this disease is one of the greatest killers the world has ever known—and was probably the greatest single incentive towards the formalization of the specialized study of immunology. Research into the mechanism of Edward Jenner's "vaccination" discovery—he found that of a patient injected with cow-pox produces immunity to smallpox—laid the foundations for the understanding of the immune system and the possibility of dealing with other diseases in a similar way. Because of an active worldwide vaccination program, no cases of smallpox have been reported since 1977. (This does not mean, however, that the disease cannot reappear, whether by natural processes or bioterror.)

Another disease that had a huge social impact was bubonic plague, a bacterial disease. Its effects were devastating in the Middle Ages. Between 1346 and 1350, one third of the entire population of Europe died of bubonic plague. Now generally less than 100 people die each year from this disease. The discovery of antibiotics in the early twentieth century provided an increasingly important weapon against bacterial diseases, and they have been instrumental in preventing similar plague epidemics.

Although progress in the application of immunological research has been impressive, a great deal still remains to be done, especially in the treatment of viral diseases (which do not respond to antibiotics) and of the diseases prevalent in developing countries. Also, seemingly "new" diseases continue to arise. Indeed, there has been much media coverage in the past twenty years in the U.S. of several "new" diseases, including Legionnaires' disease, toxic shock syndrome, Lyme disease, and acquired immunodeficiency syndrome (AIDS). Three other diseases emerged in 1993. In the summer of that year a mysterious flu-like disease struck the Southwest, resulting in 33 deaths. The causative agent was identified as a virus, hantavirus, carried by deer mice and spread in their droppings. In the same year, more than 500 residents of the state of Washington became ill with a strain of *Escherichia coli* present in undercooked beef prepared at a fast-food restaurant. The organism synthesized a potent toxin and caused haemolytic-uremic syndrome. Three children died. In 1993, 400,000 people in Milwaukee became ill with a diarrheal disease, cryptosporidiosis, that resulted from the improper chlorination of the water supply.

It is a great credit to the biomedical research community that the causative agents for all these diseases were identified very soon after the outbreaks. The bacteria causing Legionnaires' disease and Lyme disease have only been isolated in the past few decades, as have the viruses that cause AIDS. A number of factors account for the fact that seemingly "new" diseases arise almost spontaneously, even in industrially advanced countries. As people live longer, their ability to ward off infectious agents is impaired and, as a result, the organisms that usually are unable to cause disease become potentially deadly agents. Also, lifestyles change and new opportunities arise for deadly agents. For example, the use of vaginal tampons by women has resulted in an environment in which the Staphylococcus bacterium can grow and produce a toxin causing toxic shock syndrome. New diseases can also emerge because some agents have the ability to change abruptly and thereby gain the opportunity to infect new hosts. It is possible that one of the agents that causes AIDS arose from a virus that at one time could only infect other animals.

Not only are new diseases appearing but many infectious diseases that were on the wane in the U.S. have started to increase again. One reason for this resurgence is that thousands of U.S. citizens and foreign visitors enter the country daily. About one in five visitors now come from a country where diseases such as malaria, cholera, plague, and yellow fever still exist. In developed countries these diseases have been largely eliminated through sanitation, vaccination, and quarantine. Ironically, another reason why certain diseases are on the rise is the very success of past vaccination programs: because many childhood diseases (including measles, mumps, whooping cough, and diphtheria) have been effectively controlled in both developed and developing countries, some parents now opt not to vaccinate their children. Thus if the disease suddenly appears, many more children are susceptible.

A third reason for the rise of infectious diseases is that the increasing use of medications that prolong the life of the elderly, and of treatments that lower the disease resistance of patients, generally weaken the ability of the immune system to fight diseases. People infected with human immunodeficiency virus (HIV), the virus responsible for AIDS, are a high-risk group for infections that their immune systems would normally resist. For this reason, tuberculosis (TB) has increased in the U.S. and worldwide. Nearly half the world's population is infected with the bacterium causing TB, though for most people the infection is inactive. However, many thousands of new cases of TB are reported in the U.S. alone, primarily among the elderly, minority groups, and people infected with HIV. Furthermore, the organism causing these new cases of TB is resistant to the antibiotics that were once effective in treating the disease. This phenomenon is the result of the uncontrolled overuse of antibiotics over the last 70 years.

Until a few years ago, it seemed possible that the terrible loss of life associated with the plagues of the Middle Ages or with the pandemic influenza outbreak of 1918 and 1919 would never recur. However, the emergence of AIDS dramatizes the fact that microorganisms can still cause serious, incurable, life-threatening diseases. With respect to disease control, there is still much microbiological research to be done, especially in relation to the fields of immunology and chemotherapy.

Recent advances in laboratory equipment and techniques have allowed rapid progress in the articulation and understanding of the human immune system and of the elegance of the immune response. In addition, rapidly developing knowledge of the human genome offers hope for treatments designed to effectively fight disease and debilitation both by directly attacking the causative pathogens, and by strengthening the body's own immune response.

Because information in immunology often moves rapidly from the laboratory to the clinical setting, it is increasingly important that scientifically literate citizens—those able to participate in making critical decisions regarding their own health care—hold a fundamental understanding of the essential concepts in both microbiology and immunology.

Alas, as if the challenges of nature were not sufficient, the evolution of political realities in the last half of the twentieth century clearly points toward the probability that, within the first half of the twenty-first century, biological weapons will surpass nuclear and chemical weapons as a threat to civilization. Accordingly, informed public policy debates on issues of biological warfare and bioterrorism can only take place when there is a fundamental understanding of the science underpinning competing arguments.

The editors hope that *World of Microbiology and Immunology* inspires a new generation of scientists who will join in the exciting worlds of microbiological and immunological research. It is also our modest wish that this book provide valuable information to students and readers regarding topics that play an increasingly prominent role in our civic debates, and an increasingly urgent part of our everyday lives.

K. Lee Lerner & Brenda Wilmoth Lerner, editors
St. Remy, France
June 2002

Editor's note: *World of Microbiology and Immunology* is not intended to be a guide to personal medical treatment or emergency procedures. Readers desiring information related to personal issues should always consult with their physician. The editors respectfully suggest and recommend that readers desiring current information related to emergency protocols—especially with regard to issues and incidents related to bioterrorism—consult the United States Centers for Disease Control and Prevention (CDC) website at http://www.cdc.gov/.

How to Use the Book

The articles in the book are meant to be understandable by anyone with a curiosity about topics in microbiology or immunology. Cross-references to related articles, definitions, and biographies in this collection are indicated by **bold-faced type**, and these cross-references will help explain and expand the individual entries. Although far from containing a comprehensive collection of topics related to genetics, *World of Microbiology and Immunology* carries specifically selected topical entries that directly impact topics in microbiology and immunology. For those readers interested in genetics, the editors recommend Gale's *World of Genetics* as an accompanying reference. For those readers interested in additional information regarding the human immune system, the editors recommend Gale's *World of Anatomy and Physiology*.

This first edition of *World of Microbiology and Immunology* has been designed with ready reference in mind:

- **Entries are arranged alphabetically** rather than chronologically or by scientific field. In addition to classical topics, *World of Microbiology and Immunology* contains many articles addressing the impact of advances in microbiology and immunology on history, ethics, and society.

- **Bold-faced terms** direct the reader to related entries.
- **"See also" references** at the end of entries alert the reader to related entries not specifically mentioned in the body of the text.
- A **Sources Consulted** section lists the most worthwhile print material and web sites we encountered in the compilation of this volume. It is there for the inspired reader who wants more information on the people and discoveries covered in this volume.
- The **Historical Chronology** includes many of the significant events in the advancement of microbiology and immunology. The most current entries date from just days before *World of Microbiology and Immunology* went to press.
- A **comprehensive General Index** guides the reader to topics and persons mentioned in the book. Bolded page references refer the reader to the term's full entry.

Although there is an important and fundamental link between the composition and shape of biological molecules and their functions in biological systems, a detailed understanding of biochemistry is neither assumed or required for *World of Microbiology and Immunology*. Accordingly, students and other readers should not be intimidated or deterred by the complex names of biochemical molecules (especially the names for particular proteins, enzymes, etc.). Where necessary, sufficient information regarding chemical structure is provided. If desired, more information can easily be obtained from any basic chemistry or biochemistry reference.

Advisory Board

In compiling this edition we have been fortunate in being able to rely upon the expertise and contributions of the following scholars who served as academic and contributing advisors for *World of Microbiology and Immunology*, and to them we would like to express our sincere appreciation for their efforts to ensure that *World of Microbiology and Immunology* contains the most accurate and timely information possible:

Robert G. Best, Ph.D.
Director, Division of Genetics, Department of Obstetrics and Gynecology
University of South Carolina School of Medicine
Columbia, South Carolina

Antonio Farina, M.D., Ph.D.
Visiting Professor, Department of Pathology and Laboratory Medicine
Brown University School of Medicine
Providence, Rhode Island
Professor, Department of Embryology, Obstetrics, and Gynecology
University of Bologna
Bologna, Italy

Brian D. Hoyle, Ph.D.
Microbiologist

Member, American Society for Microbiology and the Canadian Society of Microbiologists
Nova Scotia, Canada

Eric v.d. Luft, Ph.D., M.L.S.
Curator of Historical Collections
SUNY Upstate Medical University
Syracuse, New York

Danila Morano, M.D.
University of Bologna
Bologna, Italy

Judyth Sassoon, Ph.D., ARCS
Department of Biology & Biochemistry
University of Bath
Bath, England

Constance K. Stein, Ph.D.
Director of Cytogenetics, Assistant Director of Molecular Diagnostics
SUNY Upstate Medical University
Syracuse, New York

Acknowledgments

In addition to our academic and contributing advisors, it has been our privilege and honor to work with the following contributing writers, and scientists: Sherri Chasin Calvo; Sandra Galeotti, M.S.; Adrienne Wilmoth Lerner; Jill Liske, M.Ed.; and Susan Thorpe-Vargas, Ph.D.

Many of the advisors for *World of Microbiology and Immunology* authored specially commissioned articles within their field of expertise. The editors would like to specifically acknowledge the following contributing advisors for their special contributions:

Robert G. Best, Ph.D.
Immunodeficiency disease syndromes
Immunodeficiency diseases, genetic

Antonio Farina, M.D., Ph.D.
Reproductive immunology

Brian D. Hoyle, Ph.D.
Anthrax, terrorist use of as a biological weapon

Eric v.d. Luft, Ph.D., M.L.S.
The biography of Dr. Harry Alfred Feldman

Danila Morano, M.D.
Rh and Rh incompatibility

Judyth Sassoon, Ph.D.
BSE and CJD disease, ethical issues and socio-economic impact

Constance K. Stein, Ph.D.
Genetic identification of microorganisms

Susan Thorpe-Vargas, Ph.D
Immunology, nutritional aspects

The editors would like to extend special thanks Dr. Judyth Sassoon for her contributions to the introduction to *World of Microbiology and Immunology*. The editors also wish to acknowledge Dr. Eric v.d. Luft for his diligent and extensive research related to the preparation of many difficult biographies. The editors owe a great debt of thanks to Dr. Brian Hoyle for his fortitude and expertise in the preparation and review of a substantial number of articles appearing in *World of Microbiology and Immunology*.

The editors gratefully acknowledge the assistance of many at Gale for their help in preparing *World of Microbiology and Immunology*. The editors thank Ms. Christine Jeryan and Ms. Meggin Condino for their faith in this project. Special thanks are offered to Ms. Robyn Young and the Gale Imaging Team for their guidance through the complexities and difficulties related to graphics. Most directly, the editors wish to acknowledge and thank the Project Editor, Mr. Brigham Narins for his good nature, goods eyes, and intelligent sculptings of *World of Microbiology and Immunology*.

The editors dedicate this book to Leslie Moore, M.D., James T. Boyd, M.D., E.M. Toler, M.D., and to the memory of Robert Moore, M.D. Their professional skills and care provided a safe start in life for generations of children, including our own.

The editors and authors also dedicate this book to the countless scientists, physicians, and nurses who labor under the most dangerous and difficult of field conditions to bring both humanitarian assistance to those in need, and to advance the frontiers of microbiology and immunology.

ACKNOWLEDGMENTS

A group of seven exiled lepers, photograph. © Michael Maslan Historic Photographs/Corbis. Reproduced by permission.—A hand holds an oyster on the half-shell, photograph. © Philip Gould/Corbis. Reproduced by permission.—A magnified virus called alpha-plaque, photograph. © Lester V. Bergman/Corbis. Reproduced by permission.—A paramecium protozoan, photograph. © Lester V. Bergman/Corbis. Reproduced by permission.—A paramecium undergoing a sexual reproductive fission, photograph. © Lester V. Bergman/Corbis. Reproduced by permission.—A tubular hydrothermal, photograph. © Ralph White/Corbis. Reproduced by permission.—About 600 sheep from France and Great Britain, burning as precaution against spread of foot-and-mouth disease, photograph by Michel Spinger. AP/Wide World Photos. Reproduced by permission.—Aerial view shows the oil slick left behind by the Japanese fishing training vessel Ehime Maru, photograph. © AFP/Corbis. Reproduced by permission.—An employee of the American Media building carries literature and antibiotics after being tested for anthrax, photograph. © AFP/Corbis. Reproduced by permission.—An under-equipped system at the Detroit Municipal Sewage Water Treatment Plant, photograph. © Ted Spiegel/Corbis. Reproduced by permission.—Anthrax, photograph by Kent Wood. Photo Researcher, Inc. Reproduced by permission.—Arneson, Charlie, photograph. © Roger Ressmeyer/Corbis. Reproduced by permission.—Beer vats in brewery, Czechoslovakia, photograph by Liba Taylor. Corbis-Bettmann. Reproduced by permission.—Bellevue-Stratford Hotel, photograph. © Bettmann/Corbis. Reproduced by permission.—Bison grazing near Hot Springs, photograph. © Michael S. Lewis/Corbis. Reproduced by permission.—Boat collecting dead fish, photograph. AP/Wide World Photos. Reproduced by permission.—Bottles of the antibiotic Cipro, photograph. © FRI/Corbis Sygma. Reproduced by permission.—Bousset, Luc, photograph. © Vo Trung Dung/Corbis. Reproduced by permission.—Budding yeast cells, photograph. © Lester V. Bergman/Corbis. Reproduced by permission.—Chlorophyll, false-colour transmission electron micrograph of stacks of grana in a chloroplast, photograph by Dr. Kenneth R. Miller. Reproduced by permission.—Close-up of Ebola virus in the blood stream, photograph. © Institut Pasteur/Corbis Sygma. Reproduced by permission.—Close-up of Ebola virus, photograph. © Corbis Sygma/Corbis. Reproduced by permission.—Close-up of prion structure examined in 3-D, photograph. © CNRS/Corbis Sygma. Reproduced by permission.—Colonies of Penicillium Notatus, photograph. © Bettmann/Corbis. Reproduced by permission.—Colored fluids in chemical beakers, photograph. © Julie Houck/Corbis. Reproduced by permission.—Colored high resolution scanning electron micrograph of the nuclear membrane surface of a pancreatic acinar cell, photograph by P. Motta & T. Naguro/Science Photo Library/Photo Researchers, Inc. Reproduced by permission.—Composite image of three genetic researchers, photograph. Dr. Gopal Murti/Science Photo Library. Reproduced by permission.—Compost pile overflowing in community garden, photograph. © Joel W. Rogers/Corbis. Reproduced by permission.—Cosimi, Benedict, photograph. © Ted Spiegel/Corbis. Reproduced by permission.—Court In Open Air During 1918 Influenza Epidemic, photograph. © Bettmann/Corbis. Reproduced by permission.—Cringing girl getting vaccination injection against Hepatitis B, photograph. © Astier Frederik/Corbis Sygma. Reproduced by permission.—Crustose Lichen, photograph. © Richard P. Jacobs/JLM Visuals. Reproduced by permission.—Crying girl getting vaccination injection against Hepatitis B, photograph. © Astier Frederik/Corbis Sygma. Reproduced by permission.—Cultures of Photobacterium NZ-11 glowing in petri dishes, photograph. © Roger Ressmeyer/Corbis. Reproduced by permission.—Darwin, Charles, photograph. Popperfoto/Archive Photos. © Archive Photos, Inc. Reproduced by permission.—Detail view of an employee's hands using a pipette in a laboratory, photograph. © Bob Rowan; Progressive Image/Corbis. Reproduced by permission.—Diagram depicting DNA and RNA with an inset on the DNA side showing specific Base Pairing, diagram by Argosy Publishing. The Gale Group.—Diagram of DNA Replication I, inset showing Semiconservative Replication (DNA Replication II), diagram by Argosy Publishing. The Gale Group.—Diagram of the Central Dogma of Molecular Biology, DNA to RNA to Protein, diagram by Argosy Publishing. The Gale Group.—Diatom Plankton, circular, transparent organisms, photograph. Corbis/Douglas P. Wilson; Frank Lane Picture Agency. Reproduced by permission.—Dinoflagellate Peridinium sp., scanning electron micrograph. © Dr. Dennis Kunkel/Phototake. Reproduced by permission.—E. coli infection, photograph by Howard Sochurek. The Stock Market. Reproduced by permission.—Electron micrographs, hanta virus, and ebola virus, photograph. Delmar Publishers, Inc. Reproduced by permission.—Electron Microscope views Martian meteorite, photograph. © Reuters NewMedia Inc./Corbis. Reproduced by permission.—Elementary school student receiving a Vaccine, photograph. © Bob Krist/Corbis. Reproduced by permission.—Enzyme-lines immunoabsorbent assay (ELISA), photograph. © Lester V. Bergman/Corbis. Reproduced by permission.—False-color transmission electron micrograph of the aerobic soil bacterium, photograph by Dr. Tony Brain. Photo Researchers, Inc. Reproduced by permission.—Farmers feeding chickens, photograph. USDA—Firefighters preparing a decontamination chamber for FBI investigators, photograph. © Randall Mark/Corbis Sygma. Reproduced by permission.—First photographed view of the influenza virus, photograph. © Bettmann/Corbis. Reproduced by permission.—First sightings of actual antibody antigen docking seen on x-ray crystallography, photograph. © Ted Spiegel/Corbis. Reproduced by permission.—Fleming, Alexander, photograph. The Bettmann Archive/Corbis-Bettmann. Reproduced by permission.—Fleming, Sir Alexander, photograph. Corbis-Bettmann. Reproduced by permission.—Friend, Charlotte, photograph. The Library of Congress. Reproduced by permission.—Fungal skin infection causing Tinea, photograph. © Lester V. Bergman/Corbis. Reproduced by permission.—Fungus colony grown in a petri dish, photograph.© Lester V. Bergman/Corbis. Reproduced by permission.—Gambierdiscus toxicus, scanning electron micrograph by Dr. Dennis Kunkel. © Dr. Dennis Kunkel/Phototake. Reproduced by permission.—Genetic code related to models of amino acids inserting into a protein chart, diagram by Argosy Publishing. The Gale Group.—German firefighters remove suspicious looking packets from a post office distribution center, photograph. © Reuters NewMedia Inc./Corbis. Reproduced by permission.—Giardia, cells shown through a microscope, photograph by J. Paulin. Reproduced by permission.—Golden lichen, photograph. © Don Blegen/JLM Visuals. Reproduced by permission.—Hay fever allergy attack triggered by oilseed rape plants, photograph. © Niall Benvie/Corbis. Reproduced by permission.—Hemolytic Staphyloccoccus Streak Plate, photograph. © Lester V. Bergman/Corbis. Reproduced by permission.—Human Immunodeficiency Virus in color imaging, photograph. © Michael Freeman/Corbis. Reproduced by permission.—Industrial Breweries, man filling kegs, photograph. Getty Images. Reproduced by permission.—Investigators

wearing hazardous materials suits, U.S. Post Office in West Trenton, New Jersey, photograph. © AFP/Corbis. Reproduced by permission.—Iron lungs, photograph. UPI/Corbis-Bettmann. Reproduced by permission.—Jacob, Francois, photograph. The Library of Congress.—Jenner, Edward, photograph. Corbis-Bettmann. Reproduced by permission.—Kiefer, Sue, Dr., photograph. © James L. Amos/Corbis. Reproduced by permission.—Koch, Robert, studying Rinderpest in laboratory, photograph. © Bettmann/Corbis. Reproduced by permission.—Koch, Robert, photograph. The Library of Congress.—Laboratory technician doing medical research, photograph. © Bill Varie/Corbis. Reproduced by permission.—Laboratory technician performing a density test from urine samples, photograph. AP/Wide World Photos. Reproduced by permission.—Laboratory technician working with restriction enzymes, photograph. © Ted Spiegel/Corbis. Reproduced by permission.—Landsteiner, Karl, photograph. The Library of Congress.—Lederberg, Joshua and Esther, photograph, 1958. UPI-Corbis-Bettmann. Reproduced by permission.—Leeuwenhoek, Anton Van, photograph. Getty Images. Reproduced by permission.—Lightning strikes on Tucson horizon, photograph. Photo Researchers, Inc. Reproduced by permission.—Lister, Joseph, photograph. © Bettmann/Corbis. Reproduced by permission.—Magnification of a gram stain of pseudomonas aeruginosa, photograph. © Lester V. Bergman/Corbis. Reproduced by permission.—Magnification of bacillus, or rodlike bacteria, photograph. © Lester V. Bergman/Corbis. Reproduced by permission.—Magnification of human immunodeficiency virus (HIV), photograph. © Lester V. Bergman/Corbis. Reproduced by permission.—Magnification of klebsiella bacteria, photograph. © Lester V. Bergman/Corbis. Reproduced by permission.—Magnified fungi cells called Candida albicans sac, photograph. © Lester V. Bergman/Corbis. Reproduced by permission.—Making of a genetic marker, with an individual DNA sequence to indicate specific genes, photograph. © Richard T. Nowitz/Corbis. Reproduced by permission.—Mallon, Mary (Typhoid Mary), 1914, photograph. Corbis Corporation. Reproduced by permission.—Man carries stretcher with patient, dysentery epidemic amongst Hutu refugees, photograph. © Baci/Corbis. Reproduced by permission.—Man washing his hands, photograph. © Dick Clintsman/Corbis. Reproduced by permission.—Marine Plankton, green organisms with orange spots, photograph by Douglas P. Wilson. Corbis/Douglas P. Wilson; Frank Lane Picture Agency. Reproduced by permission.—Measles spots on child's back, photograph. © John Heselltine/Corbis. Reproduced by permission.—Medical Researcher, fills a sample with a pipette at the National Institute of Health Laboratory, photograph. © Paul A. Souders/Corbis. Reproduced by permission.—Medical researcher dills sample trays with a pipette in a laboratory, photograph. © Paul A. Souders/Corbis. Reproduced by permission.—Milstein, Cesar, photograph. Photo Researchers, Inc. Reproduced by permission.—Mitosis of an animal cell, immunofluorescence photomicrograph. © CNRI/Phototake. Reproduced by permission.—Mitosis telophase of an animal cell, photograph. © CNRI/Phototake. Reproduced by permission.—Montagnier, Luc, photograph by Gareth Watkins.

Reuters/Archive Photos, Inc. Reproduced by permission.—Mosquito after feeding on human, photograph by Rod Planck. National Audubon Society Collection/Photo Researchers, Inc. Reproduced by permission.—Novotny, Dr. Ergo, photograph. © Ted Spiegel/Corbis. Reproduced by permission.—Nucleus and perinuclear area-liver cell from rat, photograph by Dr. Dennis Kunkel. Phototake. Reproduced by permission.—Ocean wave curling to the left, photograph. Corbis. Reproduced by permission.—Oil slick on water, photograph. © James L. Amos/Corbis. Reproduced by permission.—Pasteur, Louis, photograph. The Library of Congress.—Patient getting vaccination injection against Hepatitis B, photograph. © Astier Frederik/Corbis Sygma. Reproduced by permission.—Patients at a Turkish Tuberculosis Hospital sit up in their beds, photograph. © Corbis. Reproduced by permission.—Petri dish culture of Klebsiella pneumoniae, photograph. © Lester V. Bergman/Corbis. Reproduced by permission.—Pharmaceutical technician, and scientist, discussing experiment results in laboratory, photograph. Martha Tabor/Working Images Photographs. Reproduced by permission.—Plague of 1665, photograph. Mary Evans Picture Library/Photo Researchers, Inc. Reproduced by permission.—Prusiner, Dr. Stanley B., photograph by Luc Novovitch. Reuters/Archive Photos, Inc. Reproduced by permission.—Raccoon in winter cottonwood, photograph by W. Perry Conway. Corbis Corporation. Reproduced by permission.—Researcher, in biochemistry laboratory using a transmission electron microscope, photograph by R. Maisonneuve. Photo Researchers, Inc. Reproduced by permission.—Resistant Staphyloccocus Bacteria, photograph. © Lester V. Bergman/Corbis. Reproduced by permission.—Sample in a Petri Dish, photograph. © Bob Krist/Corbis. Reproduced by permission.—Scientists test water samples from a canal, photograph. © Annie Griffiths Belt, Corbis. Reproduced by permission.—Scientists wearing masks hold up beaker in a laboratory of chemicals, photograph. © Steve Chenn/Corbis. Reproduced by permission.—Sheep grazing on field, photograph. © Richard Dibon-Smith, National Audubon Society Collection/Photo Researchers, Inc. Reproduced with permission.—Shelf Fungi on Nurse Log, photograph. © Darell Gulin/Corbis. Reproduced by permission.—Silvestri, Mike, and Neil Colosi, Anthrax, Decontamination Technicians, photograph. © Mike Stocke/Corbis. Reproduced by permission.—Single mammalian tissue culture cell, color transmission electron micrograph. Dr. Gopal Murti/Science Photo Library/Photo Researchers, Inc. Reproduced by permission.—Steam rises from the surface of Yellowstone's Grand Prismatic Spring, photograph. © Roger Ressmeyer/Corbis. Reproduced by permission.—Steam rising from Therman Pool, photograph. © Pat O'Hara/Corbis. Reproduced by permission.—Streptococcus pyogenes bacteria, colored transmission electron micrograph by Alfred Pasieka. © Alfred Pasieka/Science Photo Library, Photo Researchers, Inc. Reproduced by permission.—Streptococcus viridans Bacteria in petri dish, photograph. © Lester V. Bergman/Corbis. Reproduced by permission.—Surgeons operating in surgical gowns and masks, photograph. © ER Productions/Corbis. Reproduced by permission.—Technician at American type culture collection, photograph. © Ted Spiegel/Corbis. Reproduced by permission.—Technician places culture on agar plates in laboratory, photograph. © Ian Harwood; Ecoscene/Corbis. Reproduced by permission.—The parasitic bacteria Staphylococcus magnified 1000x, photograph. © Science Pictures Limited/Corbis. Reproduced by permission.—The Plague of Florence, photograph. Corbis-Bettmann. Reproduced by permission.—Three-dimensional computer model of a protein molecule of matrix porin found in the E. Coli bacteria, photograph. © Corbis. Reproduced by permission.—Three-dimensional computer model of a protein molecule of matrix porin found in the E. Coli bacteria, photograph. © Corbis. Reproduced by permission.—Three-dimensional computer model of the enzyme acetylcholinesterase, photograph. © Corbis. Reproduced by permission.—Three-dimensional computer model of the molecule dihydrofolate reducatase enzyme, photograph. © Corbis. Reproduced by permission.—Three-dimensional computer model of the protein Alzheimer Amyloid B, photograph. © Corbis. Reproduced by permission.—Twenty most common amino acids, illustration by Robert L. Wolke. Reproduced by permission—Two brown mountain sheep, photograph. © Yoav Levy/Phototake NYC. Reproduced by permission.—United States Coast Guard hazardous material workers wearing protective suits work inside the U.S. Senate's Hart Building, photograph. © AFP/Corbis. Reproduced by permission.—Urey, Harold, photograph. The Library of Congress.—Veterinarian technicians check the blood pressure of a dog, photograph. AP/Wide World Photos. Reproduced by permission.—View of aging wine in underground cellar, photograph. Getty Images. Reproduced by permission.—Virus Plaque in an E. Coli culture, photograph. © Lester V. Bergman/Corbis. Reproduced by permission.—Visual biography of monoclonal antibody development at the Wistar Institute, photograph. © Ted Spiegel/Corbis. Reproduced by permission.—Waksman, Selman Abraham, photograph. Getty Images. Reproduced by permission.—Watson, James and Crick, Francis, photograph. Getty Images. Reproduced by permission.—Watson, James Dewey, photograph. The Library of Congress.—Wind storm on the East Coast, Cape Cod, Massachusetts, photograph. Gordon S. Smith/Photo Researchers, Inc. Reproduced by permission.—Woman clerks wearing cloth masks to protect against influenza, photograph. © Bettmann/Corbis. Reproduced by permission.—Woman scientist mixes chemicals in beaker, photograph. © Julie Houck/Corbis. Reproduced by permission.—Woman sneezing, photograph. © Michael Keller/Corbis. Reproduced by permission.—Young Children lying on beds in tuberculosis camp, photograph. © Bettmann/Corbis. Reproduced by permission.

M

MacLeod, Colin Munro (1909-1972)

Canadian-born American microbiologist

Colin Munro MacLeod is recognized as one of the founders of **molecular biology** for his research concerning the role of **deoxyribonucleic acid** (**DNA**) in **bacteria**. Along with his colleagues Oswald Avery and **Maclyn McCarty**, MacLeod conducted experiments on bacterial **transformation** which indicated that DNA was the active agent in the genetic transformation of bacterial cells. His earlier research focused on the causes of **pneumonia** and the development of serums to treat it. MacLeod later became chairman of the department of microbiology at New York University; he also worked with a number of government agencies and served as White House science advisor to President John F. Kennedy.

MacLeod, the fourth of eight children, was born in Port Hastings, in the Canadian province of Nova Scotia. He was the son of John Charles MacLeod, a Scottish Presbyterian minister, and Lillian Munro MacLeod, a schoolteacher. During his childhood, MacLeod moved with his family first to Saskatchewan and then to Quebec. A bright youth, he skipped several grades in elementary school and graduated from St. Francis College, a secondary school in Richmond, Quebec, at the age of fifteen. MacLeod was granted a scholarship to McGill University in Montreal but was required to wait a year for admission because of his age; during that time he taught elementary school. After two years of undergraduate work in McGill's premedical program, during which he became managing editor of the student newspaper and a member of the varsity ice hockey team, MacLeod entered the McGill University Medical School, receiving his medical degree in 1932.

Following a two-year internship at the Montreal General Hospital, MacLeod moved to New York City and became a research assistant at the Rockefeller Institute for Medical Research. His research there, under the direction of Oswald Avery, focused on pneumonia and the Pneumococcal infections which cause it. He examined the use of animal antiserums (liquid substances that contain proteins that guard against antigens) in the treatment of the disease. MacLeod also studied the use of **sulfa drugs**, synthetic substances that counteract bacteria, in treating pneumonia, as well as how Pneumococci develop a resistance to sulfa drugs. He also worked on a mysterious substance then known as "C-reactive protein," which appeared in the blood of patients with acute infections.

MacLeod's principal research interest at the Rockefeller Institute was the phenomenon known as bacterial transformation. First discovered by Frederick Griffith in 1928, this was a phenomenon in which live bacteria assumed some of the characteristics of dead bacteria. Avery had been fascinated with transformation for many years and believed that the phenomenon had broad implications for the science of biology. Thus, he and his associates, including MacLeod, conducted studies to determine how the bacterial transformation worked in Pneumococcal cells.

The researchers' primary problem was determining the exact nature of the substance which would bring about a transformation. Previously, the transformation had been achieved only sporadically in the laboratory, and scientists were not able to collect enough of the transforming substance to determine its exact chemical nature. MacLeod made two essential contributions to this project: He isolated a strain of *Pneumococcus* which could be consistently reproduced, and he developed an improved nutrient **culture** in which adequate quantities of the transforming substance could be collected for study.

By the time MacLeod left the Rockefeller Institute in 1941, he and Avery suspected that the vital substance in these transformations was DNA. A third scientist, Maclyn McCarty, confirmed their hypothesis. In 1944, MacLeod, Avery, and McCarty published "Studies of the Chemical Nature of the Substance Inducing Transformation of Pneumococcal Types: Induction of Transformation by a Deoxyribonucleic Acid Fraction Isolated from *Pneumococcus* Type III" in the *Journal of Experimental Medicine*. The article proposed that DNA was the material which brought about genetic transformation. Though the scientific community was slow to recognize the article's significance, it was later hailed as the beginning of a revolution that led to the formation of molecular biology as a scientific discipline.

MacLeod married Elizabeth Randol in 1938; they eventually had one daughter. In 1941, MacLeod became a citizen of the United States, and was appointed professor and chairman of the department of microbiology at the New York University School of Medicine, a position he held until 1956. At New York University he was instrumental in creating a combined program in which research-oriented students could acquire both an M.D. and a Ph.D. In 1956, he became professor of research medicine at the Medical School of the University of Pennsylvania. MacLeod returned to New York University in 1960 as professor of medicine and remained in that position until 1966.

From the time the United States entered World War II until the end of his life, MacLeod was a scientific advisor to the federal government. In 1941, he became director of the Commission on Pneumonia of the United States Army Epidemiological Board. Following the unification of the military services in 1949, he became president of the Armed Forces Epidemiological Board and served in that post until 1955. In the late 1950s, MacLeod helped establish the Health Research Council for the City of New York and served as its chairman from 1960 to 1970. In 1963, President John F. Kennedy appointed him deputy director of the Office of Science and Technology in the Executive Office of the President; from this position he was responsible for many program and policy initiatives, most notably the United States/Japan Cooperative Program in the Medical Sciences.

In 1966, MacLeod became vice-president for Medical Affairs of the Commonwealth Fund, a philanthropic organization. He was honored by election to the National Academy of Sciences, the American Philosophical Society, and the American Academy of Arts and Sciences. MacLeod was en route from the United States to Dacca, Bangladesh, to visit a cholera laboratory when he died in his sleep in a hotel at the London airport in 1972. In the *Yearbook of the American Philosophical Society,* Maclyn McCarty wrote of MacLeod's influence on younger scientists, "His insistence on rigorous principles in scientific research was not enforced by stern discipline but was conveyed with such good nature and patience that it was simply part of the spirit of investigation in his laboratory."

See also Bacteria and bacterial infection; Microbial genetics; Pneumonia, bacterial and viral

MAD COW DISEASE · *see* BSE AND CJD DISEASE

MAGNETOTACTIC BACTERIA

Magnetotactic **bacteria** are bacteria that use the magnetic field of Earth to orient themselves. This phenomenon is known as magnetotaxis. Magnetotaxis is another means by which bacte-

ria can actively respond to their environment. Response to light (phototaxis) and chemical concentration (chemotaxis) exist in other species of bacteria.

The first magnetotactic bacterium, *Aquasprilla magnetotactum* was discovered in 1975 by Richard Blakemore. This organism, which is now called *Magnetospirillum magnetotacticum*, inhabits swampy water, where because of the decomposition of organic matter, the oxygen content in the water drops off sharply with increasing depth. The bacteria were shown to use the magnetic field to align themselves. By this behavior, they were able to position themselves at the region in the water where oxygen was almost depleted, the environment in which they grow best. For example, if the bacteria stray too far above or below the preferred zone of habitation, they reverse their direction and swim back down or up the lines of the magnetic field until they reach the preferred oxygen concentration. The bacteria have flagella, which enables them to actively move around in the water. Thus, the sensory system used to detect oxygen concentration is coordinated with the movement of the flagella.

Magnetic orientation is possible because the magnetic North Pole points downward in the Northern Hemisphere. So, magnetotactic bacteria that are aligned to the fields are also pointing down. In the Northern Hemisphere, the bacteria would move into oxygen-depleted water by moving north along the field. In the Southern Hemisphere, the magnetic North Pole points up and at an angle. So, in the Southern Hemisphere, magnetotactic bacteria are south-seeking and also point downward. At the equator, where the magnetic North Pole is not oriented up or down, magnetotactic bacteria from both hemispheres can be found.

Since the initial discovery in 1975, magnetotactic bacteria have been found in freshwater and salt water, and in oxygen rich as well oxygen poor zones at depths ranging from the near-surface to 2000 meters beneath the surface. Magnetotactic bacteria can be spiral-shaped, rods and spheres. In general, the majority of magnetotactic bacteria discovered so far gather at the so-called oxic-anoxic transition zone; the zone above which the oxygen content is high and below which the oxygen content is essentially zero.

Magnetotaxis is possible because the bacteria contain magnetically responsive particles inside. These particles are composed of an iron-rich compound called magnetite, or various iron and sulfur containing compounds (ferrimagnetite greigite, pyrrhotite, and pyrite). Typically, these compounds are present as small spheres arranged in a single chain or several chains (the maximum found so far is five) in the **cytoplasm** of each bacterium. The spheres are enclosed in a membrane. This structure is known as a magnetosome. Since many bacterial membranes selectively allow the movement of molecules across them, magnetosome membranes may function to create a unique environment within the bacterial cytoplasm in which the magnetosome crystal can form. The membranes may also be a means of extending the chain of magnetosome, with a new magnetosome forming at the end of the chain.

Magnetotactic bacteria may not inhabit just Earth. Examination of a 4.5 billion-year-old Martian meteorite in

2000 revealed the presence of magnetite crystals, which on Earth are produced only in magnetotactic bacteria. The magnetite crystals found in the meteorite are identical in shape, size and composition to those produced in *Magnetospirillum magnetotacticum*. Thus, magnetite is a "biomarker," indicating that life may have existed on Mars in the form of magnetotactic bacteria. The rationale for the use of magnetotaxis in Martian bacteria is still a point of controversy. The Martian atmosphere is essentially oxygen-free and the magnetic field is nearly one thousand times weaker than on Earth.

Magnetotactic bacteria are also of scientific and industrial interest because of the quality of their magnets. Bacterial magnets are much better in performance than magnets of comparable size that are produced by humans. Substitution of man-made micro-magnets with those from magnetotactic bacteria could be both feasible and useful.

See also Bacterial movement

MAJOR HISTOCOMPATIBILITY COMPLEX (MHC)

In humans, the proteins coded by the genes of the major **histocompatibility** complex (MHC) include human leukocyte antigens (**HLA**), as well as other proteins. HLA proteins are present on the surface of most of the body's cells and are important in helping the **immune system** distinguish "self" from "non-self" molecules, cells, and other objects.

The function and importance of MHC is best understood in the context of a basic understanding of the function of the immune system. The immune system is responsible for distinguishing foreign proteins and other antigens, primarily with the goal of eliminating foreign organisms and other invaders that can result in disease. There are several levels of defense characterized by the various stages and types of immune response.

Present on chromosome 6, the major histocompatibility complex consists of more than 70 genes, classified into class I, II, and III MHC. There are multiple alleles, or forms, of each HLA **gene**. These alleles are expressed as proteins on the surface of various cells in a co-dominant manner. This diversity is important in maintaining an effective system of specific **immunity**. Altogether, the MHC genes span a region that is four million base pairs in length. Although this is a large region, 99% of the time these closely linked genes are transmitted to the next generation as a unit of MHC alleles on each chromosome 6. This unit is called a haplotype.

Class I MHC genes include HLA-A, HLA-B, and HLA-C. Class I MHC are expressed on the surface of almost all cells. They are important for displaying **antigen** from **viruses** or **parasites** to killer T-cells in cellular immunity. Class I MHC is also particularly important in organ and tissue rejection following transplantation. In addition to the portion of class I MHC coded by the genes on chromosome 6, each class I MHC protein also contains a small, non-variable protein component called beta 2-microglobulin coded by a gene on chromosome

15. Class I HLA genes are highly polymorphic, meaning there are multiple forms, or alleles, of each gene. There are at least 57 HLA-A alleles, 111 HLA-B alleles, and 34 HLA-C alleles.

Class II MHC genes include HLA-DP, HLA-DQ, and HLA-DR. Class II MHC are particularly important in humoral immunity. They present foreign antigen to helper T-cells, which stimulate B-cells to elicit an **antibody** response. Class II MHC is only present on antigen presenting cells, including phagocytes and B-cells. Like Class I MHC, there are hundreds of alleles that make up the class II HLA gene pool.

Class III MHC genes include the **complement** system (i.e. C2, C4a, C4b, Bf). Complement proteins help to activate and maintain the inflammatory process of an immune response.

When a foreign organism enters the body, it is encountered by the components of the body's natural immunity. Natural immunity is the non-specific first-line of defense carried out by phagocytes, natural killer cells, and components of the complement system. Phagocytes are specialized white blood cells that are capable of engulfing and killing an organism. Natural killer cells are also specialized white blood cells that respond to cancer cells and certain viral infections. The complement system is a group of proteins called the class III MHC that attack antigens. Antigens consist of any molecule capable of triggering an immune response. Although this list is not exhaustive, antigens can be derived from toxins, protein, carbohydrates, **DNA**, or other molecules from viruses, **bacteria**, cellular parasites, or cancer cells.

The natural immune response will hold an infection at bay as the next line of defense mobilizes through acquired, or specific, immunity. This specialized type of immunity is usually what is needed to eliminate an infection and is dependent on the role of the proteins of the major histocompatibility complex. There are two types of acquired immunity. Humoral immunity is important in fighting infections outside the body's cells, such as those caused by bacteria and certain viruses. Other **types of viruses** and parasites that invade the cells are better fought by cellular immunity. The major players in acquired immunity are the antigen-presenting cells (APCs), B-cells, their secreted antibodies, and the T-cells. Their functions are described in detail below.

In humoral immunity, antigen-presenting cells, including some B-cells, engulf and break down foreign organisms. Antigens from these foreign organisms are then brought to the outside surface of the antigen-presenting cells and presented in conjunction with class II MHC proteins. The helper T-cells recognize the antigen presented in this way and release **cytokines**, proteins that signal B-cells to take further action. B-cells are specialized white blood cells that mature in the bone marrow. Through the process of maturation, each B-cell develops the ability to recognize and respond to a specific antigen. Helper T-cells aid in stimulating the few B-cells that can recognize a particular foreign antigen. B-cells that are stimulated in this way develop into plasma cells, which secrete antibodies specific to the recognized antigen. Antibodies are proteins that are present in the circulation, as well as being bound to the surface of B-cells. They can destroy the foreign organism from which the antigen came. Destruction occurs either directly, or by tagging the organism, which will then be more easily recognized and targeted by phagocytes and complement proteins. Some of the stimulated B-cells go on to become memory cells, which are able to mount an even faster response if the antigen is encountered a second time.

Another type of acquired immunity involves killer T-cells and is termed cellular immunity. T-cells go through a process of maturation in the organ called the thymus, in which T-cells that recognized self-antigens are eliminated. Each remaining T-cell has the ability to recognize a single, specific, non-self antigen that the body may encounter. Although the names are similar, killer T-cells are unlike the non-specific natural killer cells in that they are specific in their action. Some viruses and parasites quickly invade the body's cells, where they are hidden from antibodies. Small pieces of proteins from these invading viruses or parasites are presented on the surface of infected cells in conjunction with class I MHC proteins, which are present on the surface of most all of the body's cells. Killer T-cells can recognize antigen bound to class I MHC in this way, and they are prompted to release chemicals that act directly to kill the infected cell. There is also a role for helper T-cells and antigen-presenting cells in cellular immunity. Helper T-cells release cytokines, as in the humoral response, and the cytokines stimulate killer T-cells to multiply. Antigen-presenting cells carry foreign antigen to places in the body where additional killer T-cells can be alerted and recruited.

The major histocompatibility complex clearly performs an important role in functioning of the immune system. Related to this role in disease immunity, MHC is also important in organ and tissue transplantation, as well as playing a role in susceptibility to certain diseases. HLA typing can also provide important information in parentage, forensic, and anthropologic studies.

There is significant variability of the frequencies of HLA alleles among ethnic groups. This is reflected in anthropologic studies attempting to use HLA-types to determine patterns of migration and evolutionary relationships of peoples of various ethnicity. Ethnic variation is also reflected in studies of HLA-associated diseases. Generally, populations that have been subject to significant patterns of migration and assimilation with other populations tend to have a more diverse HLA gene pool. For example, it is unlikely that two unrelated individuals of African ancestry would have matched HLA types. Conversely, populations that have been isolated due to geography, cultural practices, and other historical influences may display a less diverse pool of HLA types, making it more likely for two unrelated individuals to be HLA-matched.

There is a role for HLA typing of individuals in various settings. Most commonly, HLA typing is used to establish if an organ or tissue donor is appropriately matched to the recipient for key HLA types, so as not to elicit a rejection reaction in which the recipient's immune system attacks the donor tissue. In the special case of bone marrow transplantation, the risk is for graft-versus-host disease (GVHD), as opposed to tissue rejection. Because the bone marrow contains the cells of the immune system, the recipient effectively receives the donor's immune system. If the donor immune system recognizes the recipient's tissues as foreign, it may begin to attack, causing the

inflammatory and other complications of GVHD. As advances occur in transplantation medicine, HLA typing for transplantation occurs with increasing frequency and in various settings.

There is an established relationship between the inheritance of certain HLA types and susceptibility to specific diseases. Most commonly, these are diseases that are thought to be autoimmune in nature. Autoimmune diseases are those characterized by inflammatory reactions that occur as a result of the immune system mistakenly attacking self tissues. The basis of the HLA association is not well understood, although there are some hypotheses. Most autoimmune diseases are characterized by the expression of class II MHC on cells of the body that do not normally express these proteins. This may confuse the killer T-cells, which respond inappropriately by attacking these cells. Molecular mimicry is another hypothesis. Certain HLA types may look like antigens from foreign organisms. If an individual is infected by such a foreign virus or bacteria, the immune system mounts a response against the invader. However, there may be a cross-reaction with cells displaying the HLA type that is mistaken for foreign antigen. Whatever the underlying mechanism, certain HLA-types are known factors that increase the relative risk for developing specific autoimmune diseases. For example, individuals who carry the HLA B-27 allele have a relative risk of 150 for developing ankylosing spondylitis—meaning such an individual has a 150-fold chance of developing this form of spinal and pelvic arthritis, as compared to someone in the general population. Selected associations are listed below (disease name is first, followed by MHC allele and then the approximate corresponding relative risk of disease).

- Type 1 diabetes, DR3, 5
- Type 1 diabetes, DR4, 5
- Type 1 diabetes, DR3 + DR4, 20-40
- Narcolepsy, DR2, 260-360
- Ankylosing spondylitis, B27, 80-150
- Reiter's disease, B27, 37
- Rheumatoid arthritis, DR4, 3-6
- Myasthenia gravis, B8, 4
- Lupus, DR3, 2
- Graves disease, DR3, 5
- Multiple sclerosis, DR2, 3
- Celiac disease, DR3 and DR7, 5-10
- Psoriasis vulgaris, Cw6, 8

In addition to autoimmune disease, HLA-type less commonly plays a role in susceptibility to other diseases, including cancer, certain infectious diseases, and metabolic diseases. Conversely, some HLA-types confer a protective advantage for certain types of infectious disease. In addition, there are rare immune deficiency diseases that result from inherited **mutations** of the genes of components of the major histocompatibility complex.

Among other tests, HLA typing can sometimes be used to determine parentage, most commonly paternity, of a child. This type of testing is not generally done for medical reasons, but rather for social or legal reasons.

HLA-typing can provide valuable DNA-based evidence contributing to the determination of identity in criminal cases. This technology has been used in domestic criminal trials. Additionally, it is a technology that has been applied internationally in the human-rights arena. For example, HLA-typing had an application in Argentina following a military dictatorship that ended in 1983. The period under the dictatorship was marked by the murder and disappearance of thousands who were known or suspected of opposing the regime's practices. Children of the disappeared were often adopted by military officials and others. HLA-typing was one tool used to determine non-parentage and return children of the disappeared to their biological families.

HLA-typing has proved to be an invaluable tool in the study of the evolutionary origins of human populations. This information, in turn, contributes to an understanding of cultural and linguistic relationships and practices among and within various ethnic groups.

See also Antibody and antigen; Immunity, cell mediated; Immunity, humoral regulation; Immunodeficiency disease syndromes; Immunodeficiency diseases; Immunogenetics; Immunological analysis techniques; Transplantation genetics and immunology

MALARIA AND THE PHYSIOLOGY OF PARASITIC INFECTIONS

Malaria is a disease caused by a unicellular parasite known as *Plasmodium*. Although more than 100 different species of *Plasmodium* exist, only four types are known to infect humans including, *Plasmodium falciparum, vivax, malariae,* and *ovale*. While each type has a distinct appearance under the **microscope**, they each can cause a different pattern of symptoms. *Plasmodium falciparum* is the major cause of death in Africa, while *Plasmodium vivax* is the most geographically widespread of the species and the cause of most malaria cases diagnosed in the United States. *Plasmodium malariae* infections produce typical malaria symptoms that persist in the blood for very long periods, sometimes without ever producing symptoms. *Plasmodium ovale* is rare, and is isolated to West Africa. Obtaining the complete sequence of the *Plasmodium* genome is currently under way.

The life cycle of *Plasmodium* relies on the insect host (for example, the Anopheles mosquito) and the carrier host (humans) for its propagation. In the insect host, the *Plasmodium* parasite undergoes sexual reproduction by uniting two sex cells producing what are called sporozoites. When an infected mosquito feeds on human blood, the sporozoites enter into the bloodstream. During a mosquito bite, the saliva containing the infectious sporozoite from the insect is injected into the bloodstream of the human host and the blood that the insect removes provides nourishment for her eggs. The parasite immediately is targeted for a human liver cell, where it can escape from being destroyed by the **immune system**. Unlike in the insect host, when the sporozoite infects a single liver cell

from the human host, it can undergo asexual reproduction (multiple rounds consisting of replication of the **nucleus** followed by budding to form copies of itself).

During the next 72 hours, a sporozoite develops into a schizont, a structure containing thousands of tiny rounded merozoites. Schizont comes from the Greek word *schizo,* meaning to tear apart. One infectious sporozoite can develop into 20,000 merozoites. Once the schizont matures, it ruptures the liver cells and leaks the merozoites into the bloodstream where they attack neighboring erythrocytes (red blood cells, RBC). It is in this stage of the parasite life cycle that disease and death can be caused if not treated. Once inside the **cytoplasm** of an erythrocyte, the parasite can break down hemoglobin (the primary oxygen transporter in the body) into amino acids (the building blocks that makeup protein). A byproduct of the degraded hemoglobin is hemozoin, or a pigment produced by the breakdown of hemoglobin. Golden-brown to black granules are produced from hemozoin and are considered to be a distinctive feature of a blood-stage parasitic infection. The blood-stage **parasites** produce schizonts, which rupture the infected erythrocytes, releasing many waste products, explaining the intermittent fever attacks that are associated with malaria.

The propagation of the parasite is ensured by a certain type of merozoite, that invades erythrocytes but does not asexually reproduce into schizonts. Instead, they develop into gametocytes (two different forms or sex cells that require the union of each other in order to reproduce itself). These gametocytes circulate in the human's blood stream and remain quiescent (dormant) until another mosquito bite, where the gametocytes are fertilized in the mosquito's stomach to become sporozoites. Gametocytes are not responsible for causing disease in the human host and will disappear from the circulation if not taken up by a mosquito. Likewise, the salivary sporozoites are not capable of re-infecting the salivary gland of another mosquito. The cycle is renewed upon the next feeding of human blood. In some types of *Plasmodium,* the sporozoites turn into hypnozoites, a stage in the life cycle that allows the parasite to survive but in a dormant phase. A relapse occurs when the hypnozoites are reverted back into sporozoites.

An infected erythrocyte has knobs on the surface of the cells that are formed by proteins that the parasite is producing during the schizont stage. These knobs are only found in the schizont stage of *Plasmodium falciparum* and are thought to be contacted points between the infected RBC and the lining of the blood vessels. The parasite also modifies the erythrocyte membrane itself with these knob-like structures protruding at the cell surface. These parasitic-derived proteins that provide contact points thereby avoid clearance from the blood stream by the spleen. Sequestration of schizont-infected erythrocytes to blood vessels that line vital organ such as the brain, lung, heart, and gut can cause many health-related problems.

A malaria-infected erythrocyte results in physiological alterations that involve the function and structure of the erythrocyte membrane. Novel parasite-induced permeation pathways (NPP) are produced along with an increase, in some cases, in the activity of specific transporters within the RBC. The NPP are thought to have evolved to provide the parasite with the appropriate nutrients, explaining the increased permeability of many solutes. However, the true nature of the NPP remains an enigma. Possible causes for the NPP include 1) the parasite activates native transporters, 2) proteins produced by the parasite cause structural defects, 3) **plasmodium** inserts itself into the channel thus affecting it's function, and 4) the parasite makes the membrane more 'leaky'. The properties of the transporters and channels on a normal RBC differ dramatically from that of a malaria-infected RBC. Additionally, the lipid composition in terms of its fatty acid pattern is significantly altered, possibly due to the nature in which the parasite interacts with the membrane of the RBC. The dynamics of the membranes, including how the fats that makeup the membrane are deposited, are also altered. The increase in transport of solutes is bidirectional and is a function of the developmental stage of the parasite. In other words, the alterations in erythrocyte membrane are proportional to the maturation of the parasite.

See also Parasites

MARGULIS, LYNN (1938-)
American biologist

Lynn Margulis is a theoretical biologist and professor of botany at the University of Massachusetts at Amherst. Her research on the evolutionary links between cells containing nuclei (**eukaryotes**) and cells without nuclei (prokaryotes) led her to formulate a symbiotic theory of **evolution** that was initially spurned in the scientific community but has become more widely accepted.

Margulis, the eldest of four daughters, was born in Chicago. Her father, Morris Alexander, was a lawyer who owned a company that developed and marketed a long-lasting thermoplastic material used to mark streets and highways. He also served as an assistant state's attorney for the state of Illinois. Her mother, Leone, operated a travel agency. When Margulis was fifteen, she completed her second year at Hyde Park High School and was accepted into an early entrant program at the University of Chicago.

Margulis was particularly inspired by her science courses, in large part because reading assignments consisted not of textbooks but of the original works of the world's great scientists. A course in natural science made an immediate impression and would influence her life, raising questions that she has pursued throughout her career: What is heredity? How do genetic components influence the development of offspring? What are the common bonds between generations? While at the University of Chicago she met Carl Sagan, then a graduate student in physics. At the age of nineteen, she married Sagan, received a B.A. in liberal arts, and moved to Madison, Wisconsin, to pursue a joint master's degree in zoology and genetics at the University of Wisconsin under the guidance of noted cell biologist Hans Ris. In 1960, Margulis and Sagan moved to the University of California at Berkeley, where she conducted genetic research for her doctoral dissertation.

The marriage to Sagan ended before she received her doctorate. She moved to Waltham, Massachusetts, with her two sons, Dorion and Jeremy, to accept a position as lecturer in the department of biology at Brandeis University. She was awarded her Ph.D. in 1965. The following year, Margulis became an adjunct assistant of biology at Boston University, leaving 22 years later as full professor. In 1967, Margulis married crystallographer Thomas N. Margulis. The couple had two children before they divorced in 1980. Since 1988, Margulis has been a distinguished university professor with the Department of Botany at the University of Massachusetts at Amherst.

Margulis' interest in genetics and the development of cells can be traced to her earliest days as a University of Chicago undergraduate. She always questioned the commonly accepted theories of genetics, but also challenged the traditionalists by presenting hypotheses that contradicted current beliefs. Margulis has been called the most gifted theoretical biologist of her generation by numerous colleagues. A profile of Margulis by Jeanne McDermott in the *Smithsonian* quotes Peter Raven, director of the Missouri Botanical Garden and a MacArthur fellow: "Her mind keeps shooting off sparks. Some critics say she's off in left field. To me she's one of the most exciting, original thinkers in the whole field of biology." Although few know more about cellular biology, Margulis considers herself a "microbial evolutionist," mapping out a field of study that doesn't in fact exist.

As a graduate student, Margulis became interested in cases of non-Mendelian inheritance, occurring when the genetic make-up of a cell's descendants cannot be traced solely to the genes in a cell's **nucleus**. For several years, she concentrated her research on a search for genes in the **cytoplasm** of cells, the area outside of the cell's nucleus. In the early 1960s, Margulis presented evidence for the existence of extranuclear genes. She and other researchers had found **DNA** in the cytoplasm of plant cells, indicating that heredity in higher organisms is not solely determined by genetic information carried in the cell nucleus. Her continued work in this field led her to formulate the serial endosymbiotic theory, or SET, which offered a new approach to evolution as well as an account of the origin of cells with nuclei.

Prokaryotes—bacteria and **blue-green algae** now commonly referred to as cyanobacteria—are single-celled organisms that carry genetic material in the cytoplasm. Margulis proposes that eukaryotes (cells with nuclei) evolved when different kinds of prokaryotes formed symbiotic systems to enhance their chances for survival. The first such symbiotic fusion would have taken place between fermenting **bacteria** and oxygen-using bacteria. All cells with nuclei, Margulis contends, are derived from bacteria that formed symbiotic relationships with other primordial bacteria some two billion years ago. It has now become widely accepted that mitochondria—those components of eukaryotic cells that process oxygen—are remnants of oxygen-using bacteria. Margulis' hypothesis that cell hairs, found in a vast array of eukaryotic cells, descend from another group of primordial bacteria much like the modern spirochaete still encounters resistance, however.

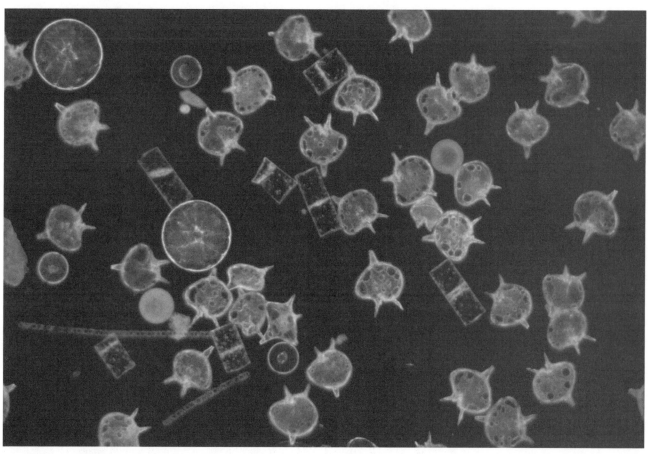

Light microscopic view of marine plankton.

The resistance to Margulis' work in microbiology may perhaps be explained by its implications for the more theoretical aspects of evolutionary theory. Evolutionary theorists, particularly in the English-speaking countries, have always put a particular emphasis on the notion that competition for scarce resources leads to the survival of the most well-adapted representatives of a species by natural **selection**, favoring adaptive genetic **mutations**. According to Margulis, natural selection as traditionally defined cannot account for the "creative novelty" to be found in evolutionary history. She argues instead that the primary mechanism driving biological change is symbiosis, while competition plays a secondary role.

Margulis doesn't limit her concept of symbiosis to the origin of plant and animal cells. She subscribes to the Gaia hypothesis first formulated by James E. Lovelock, British inventor and chemist. The Gaia theory (named for the Greek goddess of Earth) essentially states that all life, as well as the oceans, the atmosphere, and Earth itself are parts of a single, all-encompassing symbiosis and may fruitfully be considered as elements of a single organism.

Margulis has authored more than one hundred and thirty scientific articles and ten books, several of which are written with her son Dorion. She has also served on more than two dozen committees, including the American Association for the Advancement of Science, the MacArthur Foundation

Fellowship Nominating Committee, and the editorial boards of several scientific journals. Margulis is co-director of NASA's Planetary Biology Internship Program and, in 1983, was elected to the National Academy of Sciences.

See also Cell cycle (eukaryotic), genetic regulation of; Cell cycle (prokaryotic), genetic regulation of; Evolution and evolutionary mechanisms; Evolutionary origin of bacteria and viruses; Microbial genetics; Microbial symbiosis

MARINE MICROBIOLOGY

Marine microbiology refers to the study of the **microorganisms** that inhabit saltwater. Until the past two to three decades, the oceans were regarded as being almost devoid of microorganisms. Now, the importance of microorganisms such as **bacteria** to the ocean ecosystem and to life on Earth is increasingly being recognized.

Microorganisms such as bacteria that live in the ocean inhabit a harsh environment. Ocean temperatures are generally very cold—approximately 37.4° F (about 3° C) on average—and this temperature tends to remain the cold except in shallow areas. About 75% of the oceans of the world are below

3300 feet (1000 meters) in depth. The pressure on objects like bacteria at increasing depths is enormous.

Some marine bacteria have adapted to the pressure of the ocean depths and require the presence of the extreme pressure in order to function. Such bacteria are barophilic if their requirement for pressure is absolute or barotrophic if they can tolerate both extreme and near-atmospheric pressures. Similarly, many marine bacteria have adapted to the cold growth temperatures. Those which tolerate the temperatures are described as psychrotrophic, while those bacteria that require the cold temperatures are psychrophilic ("cold loving").

Marine waters are elevated in certain ions such as sodium. Not surprisingly, marine microbes like bacteria have an absolute requirement for sodium, as well as for potassium and magnesium ions. The bacteria have also adapted to grow on very low concentrations of nutrients. In the ocean, most of the organic material is located within 300 meters of the surface. Very small amounts of usable nutrients reach the deep ocean. The bacteria that inhabit these depths are in fact inhibited by high concentrations of organic material.

The bacterial communication system known as **quorum sensing** was first discovered in the marine bacterium *Vibrio fischeri*. An inhibitor of the quorum sensing mechanism has also been uncovered in a type of marine algae.

Marine microbiology has become the subject of much commercial interest. Compounds with commercial potential as nutritional additives and antimicrobials are being discovered from marine bacteria, actinomycetes and **fungi**. For example the burgeoning marine nutraceuticals market represents millions of dollars annually, and the industry is still in its infancy. As relatively little is still known of the marine microbial world, as compared to terrestrial microbiology, many more commercial and medically relevant compounds undoubtedly remain to be discovered.

See also Bacterial kingdoms; Bacterial movement; Biodegradable substances; Biogeochemical cycles

MARSHALL, BARRY J. (1951-   )
Australian physician

Barry Marshall was born in Perth, Australia. He is a physician with a clinical and research interest in gastroenterology. He is internationally recognized for his discovery that the bacterium *Helicobacter pylori* is the major cause of stomach ulcers.

Marshall studied medicine at the University of Western Australia from 1969 to 1974. While studying for his medical degree, Marshall decided to pursue medical research. He undertook research in the laboratory of Dr. Robin Warren, who had observations of a helical **bacteria** in the stomach of people suffering from ulcers.

Marshall and Warren succeeded in culturing the bacterium, which they named *Helicobacter pylori*. Despite their evidence that the organism was the cause of stomach ulceration, the medical community of the time was not convinced that a bacterium could survive the harsh acidic conditions of the stomach yet alone cause tissue damage in this environ-

ment. In order to illustrate the relevance of the bacterium to the disease, Marshall performed an experiment that has earned him international renown. In July of 1984, he swallowed a solution of the bacterium, developed the infection, including **inflammation** of the stomach, and cured himself of both the infection and the stomach inflammation by antibiotic therapy.

By 1994, Marshall's theory of Helicobacter involvement in stomach ulcers was accepted, when the United States National Institutes of Health endorsed **antibiotics** s the standard treatment for stomach ulcers.

Since Marshall's discovery, *Helicobacter pylori* has been shown to be the leading cause of stomach and intestinal ulcers, gastritis and stomach cancer. Many thousands of ulcer patients around the world have been successfully treated by strategies designed to attack **bacterial infection**. Marshall's finding was one of the first indications that human disease thought to be due to biochemical or genetic defects were in fact due to bacterial infections.

From Australia, Marshall spent a decade at the University of Virginia, where he founded and directed the Center for Study of Diseases due to *H. pylori*. While at Virginia, he developed an enzyme-based rapid test for the presence of the bacterium that tests patient's breath. The test is commercially available.

Currently, he is a clinician and researcher at the Sir Charles Gairdner Hospital in Perth, Australia.

Marshall's discovery has been recognized internationally. He has received the Warren Alpert Prize from the Harvard Medical School, which recognizes work that has most benefited clinical practice. Also, he has won the **Paul Ehrlich** Prize (Germany) and the Lasker Prize (United States).

See also Bacteria and bacterial infection; Helicobacteriosis

MASTIGOPHORA

Mastigophora is a division of single-celled protozoans. There are approximately 1,500 species of Mastigophora. Their habitat includes fresh and marine waters. Most of these species are capable of self-propelled movement through the motion of one or several flagella. The possession of flagella is a hallmark of the Mastigophora.

In addition to their flagella, some mastigophora are able to extend their interior contents (that is known as **cytoplasm**) outward in an arm-like protrusion. These protrusions, which are called pseudopodia, are temporary structures that serve to entrap and direct food into the microorganism. The cytoplasmic extensions are flexible and capable of collapsing back to form the bulk of the wall that bounds the microorganism.

Mastigophora replicate typically by the internal duplication of their contents flowed by a splitting of the microbes to form two daughter cells. This process, which is called binary fission, is analogous to the division process in **bacteria**. In addition to replicating by binary fission, some mastigophora can reproduce sexually, by the combining of genetic material from two mastigophora. This process is referred to as syngamy.

The mastigophora are noteworthy mainly because of the presence in the division of several disease-causing species. Some mastigophora are **parasites**, which depend on the infection of a host for the completion of their life cycle. These parasites cause disease in humans and other animals. One example is the Trypanosomes, which cause African **sleeping sickness** and Chaga's disease. Another example is *Giardia lamblia*. This microorganism is the agent that causes an intestinal malady called giardiasis. The condition has also been popularly dubbed "beaver fever," reflecting its presence in the natural habitat, where it is a resident of the intestinal tract of warm-blooded animals.

Giardia lamblia is an important contaminant of drinking water. The microorganism is resistant to the disinfectant action of chlorine, which is the most common chemical for the treatment of drinking water. In addition, a dormant form of the microorganism called a cyst is small enough that it can elude the filtration step in water treatment plants. The microbe is increasingly becoming a concern in drinking waters all over the world, even in industrialized countries with state of the art water treatment infrastructure.

See also Protozoa

MATIN, A. C. (1941-)
Indian American microbiologist

A. C. Matin is a Professor of Microbiology and **Immunology** at Stanford University in Stanford, California. He has made pioneering contributions to microbiology in a number of areas; these include his notable research into the ways in which **bacteria** like *Escherichia coli* adapt and survive periods of nutrient starvation. His studies have been important in combating infections and the remediation of wastes.

Matin was born in Delhi, India. He attended the University of Karachi, where he received his B.S. in microbiology and zoology in 1960 and his M.S. in microbiology in 1962. From 1962 until 1964 he was a lecturer in microbiology at St. Joseph's College for Women in Karachi. He then moved to the United States to attend the University of California at Los Angeles, from which he received a Ph.D. in microbiology (with distinction) in 1969. From 1969 until 1971 he was a postdoctoral research associate at the State University of The Netherlands. He then became a Scientific Officer, First Class, in the Department of Microbiology at the same institution, a post he held until 1975. That year Matin returned to the United States to accept a position at Stanford University, the institution with which he remains affiliated.

Matin has made fundamental contributions to the biochemical and molecular biological study of the bacterial stress response—that is, how bacteria adapt to stresses in parameters such as temperature, **pH** (a measure of the acidity and alkalinity of a solution), and food availability. Matin and his colleagues provided much of the early data on the behavior of bacteria when their nutrients begin to become exhausted and waste products accumulate. This phase of growth, termed the stationary phase, has since been shown to have great relevance to the growth conditions that disease-causing bacteria face in the body, and which bacteria can face in the natural environment.

Matin has also made important contributions to the study of multidrug resistance in the bacterium *Escherichia coli*, specifically the use of a protein pump to exclude a variety of antibacterial drugs, and to the **antibiotic resistance** of *Staphylococcus aureus*.

Matin has published over 70 major papers and over 30 book chapters and articles. He has consulted widely among industries concerned with bacterial drug resistance and bacterial behavior.

For his scientific contributions Matin has received numerous awards and honors. These include his appointment as a Fulbright Scholar from 1964 until 1971, election to the American Academy of Microbiology, and inclusion in publications such as *Who's Who in the Frontiers of Science* and *Outstanding People of the 20th Century*.

See also Antibiotic resistance, tests for; Bacterial adaptation

McCARTY, MACLYN (1911-)
American bacteriologist

Maclyn McCarty is a distinguished bacteriologist who has done important work on the biology of **Streptococci** and the origins of rheumatic fever, but he is best known for his involvement in early experiments which established the function of **DNA**. In collaboration with Oswald Avery and **Colin Munro MacLeod**, McCarty identified DNA as the substance which controls heredity in living cells. The three men published an article describing their experiment in 1944, and their work opened the way for further studies in bacteriological physiology, the most important of which was the demonstration of the chemical structure of DNA by James Watson and **Francis Crick** in 1953.

McCarty was born in South Bend, Indiana. His father worked for the Studebaker Corporation and the family moved often, with McCarty attending five schools in three different cities by the time he reached the sixth grade. In his autobiographical book, *The Transforming Principle,* McCarty recalled the experience as positive, believing that moving so often made him an inquisitive and alert child. He spent a year at Culver Academy in Indiana from 1925 to 1926, and he finished high school in Kenosha, Wisconsin. His family moved to Portland, Oregon, and McCarty attended Stanford University in California. He majored in **biochemistry** under James Murray Luck, who was then launching the *Annual Review of Biochemistry*. McCarty presented public seminars on topics derived from articles submitted to this publication, and he graduated with a B.A. in 1933.

Although Luck asked him to remain at Stanford, McCarty entered medical school at Johns Hopkins in Baltimore in 1933. He was married during medical school days, and he spent a summer of research at the Mayo Clinic in Minnesota. After graduation, McCarty spent three years working in pediatric medicine at the Johns Hopkins Hospital. Even in the decade before **penicillin**, new chemotherapeutic agents had begun to change infectious disease therapy. McCarty treated children suffering from Pneumococcal **pneumonia**, and he was able to save a child suffering from a Streptococcal infection, then almost uniformly fatal, by the use of the newly available sulfonamide antibacterials. Both of these groups of **bacteria**, *Streptococcus* and the *Pneumococcus*, would play important roles throughout the remainder of McCarty's career.

McCarty spent his first full year of medical research at New York University in 1940, in the laboratory of W. S. Tillett. In 1941, McCarty was awarded a National Research Council grant, and Tillett recommended him for a position with Oswald Avery at the Rockefeller Institute, which was one of the most important centers of biomedical research in the United States. For many years, Avery had been working with Colin Munro MacLeod on Pneumococci. In 1928, the British microbiologist Frederick Griffith had discovered what he called a "transforming principle" in Pneumococci. In a series of experiments now considered a turning point in the history of genetics, Griffith had established that living individuals of one strain or variety of Pneumococci could be changed into another, with different characteristics, by the application of material taken from dead individuals of a second strain. When McCarty joined Avery and MacLeod, the chemical nature of this transforming material was not known, and this was what their experiments were designed to discover.

In an effort to determine the chemical nature of Griffith's transforming principle, McCarty began as more of a lab assistant than an equal partner. Avery and MacLeod had decided that the material belonged to one of two classes of organic compounds: it was either a protein or a nucleic acid. They were predisposed to think it was a protein, or possibly **RNA**, and their experimental work was based on efforts to selectively disable the ability of this material to transform strains of Pneumococci. Evidence that came to light during 1942 indicated that the material was not a protein but a nucleic acid, and it began to seem increasingly possible that DNA was the molecule for which they were searching. McCarty's most important contribution was the preparation of a deoxyribonuclease which disabled the transforming power of the material and established that it was DNA. They achieved these results by May of 1943, but Avery remained cautious, and their work was not published until 1944.

In 1946, McCarty was named head of a laboratory at the Rockefeller Institute which was dedicated to the study of the Streptococci. A relative of Pneumococci, Streptococci is a cause of rheumatic fever. McCarty's research established the important role played by the outer cellular covering of this bacteria. Using some of the same techniques he had used in his work on DNA, McCarty was able to isolate the cell wall of the Streptococcus and analyze its structure.

McCarty became a member of the Rockefeller Institute in 1950; he served as vice president of the institution from 1965 to 1978, and as physician in chief from 1965 to 1974. For his work as co-discoverer of the nature of the transforming principle, he won the Eli Lilly Award in Microbiology and **Immunology** in 1946 and was elected to the National Academy of Sciences in 1963. He won the first Waterford Biomedical Science Award of the Scripps Clinic and Research Foundation

in 1977 and received honorary doctorates from Columbia University in 1976 and the University of Florida in 1977.

See also Microbial genetics; Microbiology, clinical; Streptococci and streptococcal infections

MEASLES

Measles is an infectious disease caused by a virus of the paramyxovirus group. It infects only man and the infection results in life-long **immunity** to the disease. It is one of several exanthematous (rash-producing) diseases of childhood, the others being rubella (German measles), chicken pox, and the now rare scarlet fever. The disease is particularly common in both pre-school and young school children.

The measles virus mainly infects mucous membranes of the respiratory tract and the skin. The symptoms include high fever, headache, hacking cough, conjunctivitis, and a rash that usually begins inside the mouth on the buccal mucosa as white spots, (called Koplik's spots) and progresses to a red rash that spreads to face, neck, trunk and extremities. The incubation period varies but is usually 10 to 12 days until symptoms appear. Four to five days before the onset of the rash, the child has fever or malaise and then may develop a sore throat and cough. The duration of the rash is usually five days. The child is infectious throughout the prodromal (early) period and for up to four days after the first appearance of the rash. The virus is highly contagious and is transmitted through respiratory droplets or though direct contact. Measles is also sometimes called rubeola or the nine-day measles.

Although certain complications can arise, in the vast majority of cases, children make a full recovery from measles. Acute local complications can occur if there is a secondary infection, for example **pneumonia** due to **bacteria** such as **staphylococci**, *Streptococcus pyogene*, pneumococci, or caused by the virus itself. Also, ear infections and secondary bacterial otitis media can seriously aggravate the disease. Central nervous system (CNS) complications include post-measles encephalitis, which occurs about 10 days after the illness with a significant mortality rate. Also, sub-acute sclerosing panencephalitis (SSPE), a rare fatal complication, presents several years after the original measles infection. Because hemorrhagic skin lesions, viraemia, and severe respiratory tract infection are particularly likely in malnourished infants, measles is still frequently a life-threatening infection in Africa and other underdeveloped regions of the world. The microbiological diagnosis of measles is not normally required because the symptoms are characteristic. However, if an acute CNS complication is suspected, paired sera are usually sent for the estimation of **complement** fixing antibodies to measles. If SSPE is suspected, the measles **antibody** titres in the CSF (determining the level of antibodies present) are also estimated.

Epidemiological studies have shown that there is a good correlation between the size of a population and the number of cases of measles. A population of at least 500,000 is required to provide sufficient susceptible individuals (i.e.

births) to maintain the virus within the population. Below that level, the virus will eventually die out unless it is re-introduced from an outside source. On the geological time-scale, man has evolved recently and has only existed in large populations in comparatively modern times. In the past, when human beings lived in small populations, it is concluded that the measles virus could not exist in its present form. It may have had another strategy of infection such as to persist in some form and infect the occasional susceptible passer-by, but this remains unproven. It has been suggested that the modern measles virus evolved from an ancestral animal virus, which is also common to the modern canine distemper and the cattle disease rinderpest. This theory is based on the similarities between these **viruses**, and on the fact that these animals have been commensal (living in close proximity) with man since his nomadic days. The ancestral virus is thought to have evolved into the modern measles virus when changes in the social behavior of man gave rise to populations large enough to maintain infection. This evolutionary event would have occurred within the last 6000 years when the river valley civilizations of the Tigris and Euphrates were established. To our knowledge, measles was first described as a disease in ninth century when a Persian physician, Rhazes, was the first to differentiate between measles and **smallpox**. The physician Rhazes also made the observation that the fever accompanying the disease is a bodily defense and not the disease itself. His writings on the subject were translated into English and published in 1847.

The measles virus itself was first discovered in 1930, and **John F. Enders** of the Children's Hospital in Boston successfully isolated the measles virus in 1954. Enders then began looking for an attenuated strain, which might be suitable for a live-virus **vaccine**. A successful **immunization** program for measles was begun soon after. Today measles is controlled in the United States with a **vaccination** that confers immunity against measles, **mumps**, and rubella and is commonly called the MMR vaccine. Following a series of measles **epidemics** occurring in the teenage population, a second MMR shot is now sometimes required by many school-age children as it was found that one vaccination appeared not to confer life-long immunity.

In October 1978, the Department of Health, Education, and Welfare announced their intention of eliminating the measles virus from the U.S.A. This idea was inspired by the apparently successful global elimination of smallpox by the **World Health Organization** vaccination program, which recorded its last smallpox case in 1977.

Death from measles due to respiratory or neurological causes occurs in about 1 out of every 1000 cases and encephalitis also occurs at this frequency, with survivors of the latter often having permanent brain damage. Measles virus meets all the currently held criteria for successful elimination. It only multiplies in man; there is a good live vaccine (95 % effective) and only one sero-type of the virus is known. Usually measles virus causes an acute infection but, rarely (1 out of every million cases), the virus persists and reappears some 2-6 years causing SSPE. However, measles virus can only be recovered with difficulty from infected tissue and

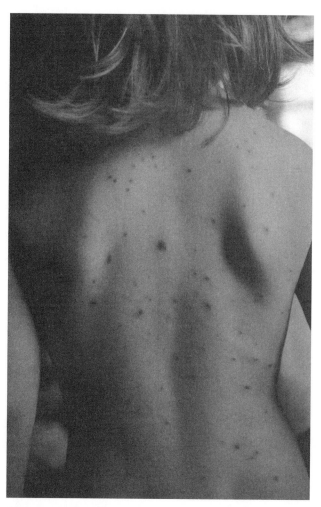

Measles rash on a child's back.

SSPE is a non-transmissible disease. To successfully eliminate measles, it would be necessary to achieve a high immunization level, especially in children.

See also Antibody-antigen, biochemical and molecular reactions; History of immunology; History of public health; Immunity, active, passive and delayed; Immunology; Varicella; Viruses and responses to viral infection

MEDAWAR, PETER BRIAN (1915-1987)
English biologist

Peter Brian Medawar made major contributions to the study of **immunology** and was awarded the Nobel Prize in physiology or medicine in 1960. Working extensively with skin grafts, he and his collaborators proved that the **immune system** learns to distinguish between "self" and "non-self." During his career, Medawar also became a prolific author, penning books such as *The Uniqueness of the Individual* and *Advice to a Young Scientist*.

Medawar was born on February 28, 1915, in Rio de Janeiro, Brazil, to Nicholas Medawar and the former Edith Muriel Dowling. When he was a young boy, his family moved to England, which he thereafter called home. Medawar attended secondary school at Marlborough College, where he first became interested in biology. The biology master encouraged Medawar to pursue the science under the tutelage of one of his former students, John Young, at Magdalen College. Medawar followed this advice and enrolled at Magdalen in 1932 as a zoology student.

Medawar earned his bachelor's degree from Magdalen in 1935, the same year he accepted an appointment as Christopher Welch Scholar and Senior Demonstrator at Magdalen College. He followed Young's recommendation that he work with pathologist Howard Florey, who was undertaking a study of **penicillin**, work for which he would later become well known. Medawar leaned toward experimental embryology and tissue cultures. While at Magdalen, he met and married a fellow zoology student. Medawar and his wife had four children.

In 1938, Medawar, by examination, became a fellow of Magdalen College and received the Edward Chapman Research Prize. A year later, he received his master's from Oxford. When World War II broke out in Europe, the Medical Research Council asked Medawar to concentrate his research on tissue transplants, primarily skin grafts. While this took him away from his initial research studies into embryology, his work with the military would come to drive his future research and eventually lead to a Nobel Prize.

During the war, Medawar developed a concentrated form of fibrinogen, a component of the blood. This substance acted as a glue to reattach severed nerves, and found a place in the treatment of skin grafts and in other operations. More importantly to Medawar's future research, however, were his studies at the Burns Unit of the Glasgow Royal Infirmary in Scotland. His task was to determine why patients rejected donor skin grafts. He observed that the rejection time for donor grafts was noticeably longer for initial grafts, compared to those grafts that were transplanted for a second time. Medawar noted the similarity between this reaction and the body's reaction to an invading virus or **bacteria**. He formed the opinion that the body's rejection of skin grafts was immunological in nature; the body built up an **immunity** to the first graft and then called on that already-built-up immunity to quickly reject a second graft.

Upon his return from the Burns Unit to Oxford, he began his studies of immunology in the laboratory. In 1944, he became a senior research fellow of St. John's College, Oxford, and university demonstrator in zoology and comparative anatomy. Although he qualified for and passed his examinations for a doctorate in philosophy while at Oxford, Medawar opted against accepting it because it would cost more than he could afford. In his autobiography, *Memoir of a Thinking Radish,* he wrote, "The degree served no useful purpose and cost, I learned, as much as it cost in those days to have an appendectomy. Having just had the latter as a matter of urgency, I thought that to have both would border on self-indulgence, so I remained a plain mister until I became a prof." He continued as researcher at Oxford University through 1947.

During that year Medawar accepted an appointment as Mason professor of zoology at the University of Birmingham. He brought with him one of his best graduate students at Oxford, Rupert Everett "Bill" Billingham. Another graduate student, Leslie Brent, soon joined them and the three began what was to become a very productive collaboration that spanned several years. Their research progressed through Medawar's appointment as dean of science, through his several-month-long trip to the Rockefeller Institute in New York in 1949—the same year he received the title of fellow from the Royal Society—and even a relocation to another college. In 1951, Medawar accepted a position as Jodrell Professor of Zoology and Comparative Anatomy at University College, London. Billingham and Brent followed him.

Their most important discovery had its experimental root in a promise Medawar made at the International Congress of Genetics at Stockholm in 1948. He told another investigator, Hugh Donald, that he could formulate a foolproof method for distinguishing identical from fraternal twin calves. He and Billingham felt they could easily tell the twins apart by transplanting a skin graft from one twin to the other. They reasoned that a calf of an identical pair would accept a skin graft from its twin because the two originated from the same egg, whereas a calf would reject a graft from its fraternal twin because they came from two separate eggs. The results did not bear this out, however. The calves accepted skin grafts from their twins regardless of their status as identical or fraternal. Puzzled, they repeated the experiment, but received the same results.

They found their error when they became aware of work done by Dr. **Frank Macfarlane Burnet** of the University of Melbourne, and Ray D. Owen of the California Institute of Technology. Owen found that blood transfuses between twin calves, both fraternal and identical. Burnet believed that an individual's immunological framework developed before birth, and felt Owen's finding demonstrated this by showing that the immune system tolerates those tissues that are made known to it before a certain age. In other words, the body does not recognize donated tissue as alien if it has had some exposure to it at an early age. Burnet predicted that this immunological tolerance for non-native tissue could be reproduced in a lab. Medawar, Billingham, and Brent set out to test Burnet's hypothesis.

The three-scientist team worked closely together, inoculating embryos from mice of one strain with tissue cells from donor mice of another strain. When the mice had matured, the trio grafted skin from the donor mice to the inoculated mice. Normally, mice reject skin grafts from other mice, but the inoculated mice in their experiment accepted the donor skin grafts. They did not develop an immunological reaction. The prenatal encounter had given the inoculated mice an acquired immunological tolerance. They had proven Burnet's hypothesis. They published their findings in a 1953 article in *Nature*. Although their research had no applications to transplants among humans, it showed that transplants were possible.

In the years following publication of the research, Medawar accepted several honors, including the Royal Medal from the Royal Society in 1959. A year later, he and Burnet accepted the Nobel Prize for Physiology or Medicine for their discovery of acquired immunological tolerance: Burnet developed the theory and Medawar proved it. Medawar shared the prize money with Billingham and Brent.

Medawar's scientific concerns extended beyond immunology, even during the years of his work toward acquired immunological tolerance. While at Birmingham, he and Billingham also investigated pigment spread, a phenomenon seen in some guinea pigs and cattle where the dark spots spread into the light areas of the skin. "Thus if a dark skin graft were transplanted into the middle of a pale area of skin it would soon come to be surrounded by a progressively widening ring of dark skin," Medawar asserted in his autobiography. The team conducted a variety of experiments, hoping to show that the dark pigment cells were somehow "infecting" the pale pigment cells. The tests never panned out.

Medawar also delved into animal behavior at Birmingham. He edited a book on the subject by noted scientist Nikolaas Tinbergen, who ultimately netted a Nobel Prize in 1973. In 1957, Medawar also became a book author with his first offering, *The Uniqueness of the Individual,* which was actually a collection of essays. In 1959, his second book, *The Future of Man,* was issued, containing a compilation of a series of broadcasts he read for British Broadcasting Corporation (BBC) radio. The series examined the impacts of **evolution** on man.

Medawar remained at University College until 1962 when he took the post of director of the National Institute for Medical Research in London, where he continued his study of transplants and immunology. While there, he continued writing with mainly philosophical themes. *The Art of the Soluble,* published in 1967, is an assembly of essays, while his 1969 book, *Induction and Intuition in Scientific Thought,* is a sequence of lectures examining the thought processes of scientists. In 1969 Medawar, then president of the British Association for the Advancement of Science, experienced the first of a series of strokes while speaking at the group's annual meeting. He finally retired from his position as director of the National Institute for Medical Research in 1971. In spite of his physical limitations, he went ahead with scientific research in his lab at the clinical research center of the Medical Research Council. There he began studying cancer.

Through the 1970s and 1980s, Medawar produced several other books—some with his wife as co-author—in addition to his many essays on growth, aging, immunity, and cellular transformations. In one of his most well-known books, *Advice to a Young Scientist,* Medawar asserted that for scientists, curiosity was more important that genius.

See also Antibody and antigen; Antibody-antigen, biochemical and molecular reactions; Antibody formation and kinetics; Antibody, monoclonal; Immunity, active, passive and delayed; Immunity, cell mediated; Immunity, humoral regulation; Immunochemistry; Immunogenetics; Major histocompatibility complex (MHC); Transplantation genetics and immunology

MEDICAL TRAINING AND CAREERS IN MICROBIOLOGY

The world of microbiology overlaps the world of medicine. As a result, trained microbiologists find a diversity of career paths and opportunity in medicine.

Research in medical microbiology can involve clinical or basic science. **Clinical microbiology** focuses on the microbiological basis of various diseases and how to alleviate the suffering caused by the infectious microorganism. Basic medical research is concerned more with the molecular events associated with infectious diseases or illnesses.

Both medical training and microbiology contain many different areas of study. Medical microbiology is likewise an area of many specialties. A medical bacteriologist can study how **bacteria** can infect humans and cause disease, and how these disease processes can be dealt with. A medical mycologist can study pathogenic (disease-causing) **fungi**, molds and **yeast** to find out how they cause disease. A parasitologist is concerned with how parasitic **microorganisms** (those that require a host in order to live) cause disease. A medical virologist can study the diseases attributed to infection by a virus, such as the hemorrhagic fever caused by the **Ebola virus**.

The paths to these varied disciplines of study are also varied. One route that a student can take to incorporate both research training and medical education is the combined M.D.-PhD. program. In several years of rigorous study, students become physician-scientists. Often, graduates develop a clinical practice combined with basic research. The experience gained at the bedside can provide research ideas. Conversely, laboratory techniques can be brought to bear on unraveling the basis of human disease. The M.D.–PhD. training exemplifies what is known as the transdisciplinary approach. Incorporating different approaches to an issue can suggest treatment or research strategies that might otherwise not be evident if an issue were addressed from only one perspective.

The training for a career in the area of medicine and medical microbiology begins in high school. Courses in the sciences lay the foundation for the more in-depth training that will follow in university or technical institution. With undergraduate level training, career paths can include research assistant, providing key technical support to a research team, quality assurance in the food, industrial or environmental microbiology areas, and medical technology.

Medical microbiology training at the undergraduate and graduate levels, in the absence of simultaneous medical training, can also lead to a career as a clinical microbiologist. Such scientists are employed in universities, hospitals and in the public sector. For example, the United Kingdom has an extensive Public Health Laboratory Service. The PHLS employs clinical microbiologists in reference laboratories, to develop or augment test methods, and as epidemiologists. The latter are involved in determining the underlying causes of disease outbreaks and in uncovering potential microbiological health threats. Training in medical microbiology can be at the Baccalaureate level, and in research that leads to a Masters or a Doctoral degree. The latter is usually undertaken if the aim

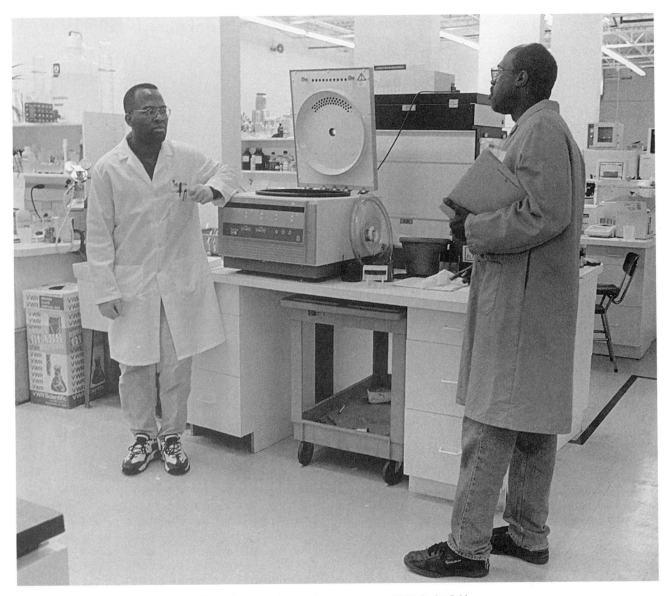

Working as a specialist in a medical microbiology laboratory is one of many careers available in the field.

is to do original and independent research, teach undergraduate and graduate students, or to assume an executive position.

Medical technologists are involved in carrying out the myriad of microbiological tests that are performed on samples such as urine, blood and other body fluids to distinguish pathogenic microorganisms from the normal flora of the body. This can be very much akin to detective work, involving the testing of samples by various means to resolve he identity of an organism based on the various biochemical behaviors. Increasingly, such work is done in conjunction with automated equipment. Medical technologists must be skilled at scheduling tests efficiently, independently and as part of a team. Training as a medical technologist is typically at a community college or technical institution and usually requires two years.

As in the other disciplines of medical microbiology, medical technology is a specialized field. Histopathology is

the examination of body cells or tissues to detect or rule out disease. This speciality involves knowledge of light and **electron microscopic examination** of samples. Cytology is the study of cells for abnormalities that might be indicative of infection or other malady, such as cancer. Medical **immunology** studies the response of the host to infection. A medical immunologist is skilled at identifying those immune cells that active in combating an infection. Medical technology also encompasses the area of clinical **biochemistry**, where cells and body fluids are analyzed for the presence of components related to disease. Of course the study of microorganism involvement in disease requires medical technologists who are specialized microbiologists and virologists, as two examples.

Medical microbiologists also can find a rewarding career path in industry. Specifically, the knowledge of the susceptibility or resistance of microorganisms to antimicrobial drugs is crucial to the development of new drugs. Work can be at the research and development level, in the manufacture of drugs, in the regulation and licensing of new antimicrobial agents, and even in the sale of drugs. For example, the sale of a product can be facilitated by the interaction of the sales associate and physician client on an equal footing in terms of knowledge of antimicrobial therapy or disease processes.

Following the acquisition of a graduate or medical degree, specialization in a chosen area can involve years of post-graduate or medical residence. The road to a university lab or the operating room requires dedication and over a decade of intensive study.

Careers in medical science and medical microbiology need not be focused at the patient bedside or at the lab bench. Increasingly, the medical and infectious disease fields are benefiting from the advice of consultants and those who are able to direct programs. Medical or microbiological training combined with experience or training in areas such as law or business administration present an attractive career combination.

See also Bioinformatics and computational biology; Food safety; History of public health; Hygiene; World Health Organization

MEMBRANE FLUIDITY

The membranes of **bacteria** function to give the bacterium its shape, allow the passage of molecules from the outside in and from the inside out, and to prevent the internal contents from leaking out. Gram-negative bacteria have two membranes that make up their cell wall, whereas Gram-positive bacteria have a single membrane as a component of their cell wall. Yeasts and **fungi** have another specialized nuclear membrane that compartmentalizes the genetic material of the cell.

For all these functions, the membrane must be fluid. For example, if the interior of a bacterial membrane was crystalline, the movement of molecules across the membrane would be extremely difficult and the bacterium would not survive.

Membrane fluidity is assured by the construction of a typical membrane. This construction can be described by the fluid mosaic model. The mosaic consists of objects, such as proteins, which are embedded in a supporting—but mobile—structure of lipid.

The fluid mosaic model for membrane construction was proposed in 1972 by S. J. Singer of the University of California at San Diego and G. L. Nicolson of the Salk Institute. Since that time, the evidence in support of a fluid membrane has become irrefutable.

In a fluid membrane, proteins may be exposed on the inner surface of the membrane, the outer surface, or at both surfaces. Depending on their association with neighbouring molecules, the proteins may be held in place or may capable of a slow drifting movement within the membrane. Some proteins associate together to form pores through which molecules can pass in a regulated fashion (such as by the charge or size of the molecule).

The fluid nature of the membrane rest with the supporting structure of the lipids. Membrane lipids of **microorganisms** tend to be a type of lipid termed phospholipid. A phospholipid consists of fatty acid chains that terminate at one end in a phosphate group. The fatty acid chains are not charged, and so do not tend to associate with water. In other words they are **hydrophobic**. On the other hand, the charged phosphate head group does tend to associate with water. In other words they are hydrophilic. The way to reconcile these chemistry differences in the membrane are to orient the **phospholipids** with the water-phobic tails pointing inside and the water-phyllic heads oriented to the watery external environment. This creates two so-called leaflets, or a bilayer, of phospholipid. Essentially the membrane is a two dimensional fluid that is made mostly of phospholipids. The consistency of the membrane is about that of olive oil.

Regions of the membrane will consist solely of the lipid bilayer. Molecules that are more hydrophobic will tend to dissolve into these regions, and so can move across the membrane passively. Additionally, some of the proteins embedded in the bilayer will have a transport function, to actively pump or move molecules across the membrane.

The fluidity of microbial membranes also allows the constituent proteins to adopt new configurations, as happens when molecules bind to receptor portions of the protein. These configurational changes are an important mechanism of signaling other proteins and initiating a response to, for example, the presence of a food source. For example, a protein that binds a molecule may rotate, carrying the molecule across the membrane and releasing the molecule on the other side. In bacteria, the membrane proteins tend to be located more in one leaflet of the membrane than the other. This asymmetric arrangement largely drives the various transport and other functions that the membrane can perform.

The phospholipids are capable of a drifting movement laterally on whatever side of the membrane they happen to be. Measurements of this movement have shown that the drifting can actually be quite rapid. A flip-flop motion across to the other side of the membrane is rare. The fluid motion of the phospholipids increases if the hydrophobic tail portion contains more double bonds, which cause the tail to be kinked instead of straight. Such alteration of the phospholipid tails can occur in response to temperature change. For example if the temperature decreases, a bacterium may alter the phospholipid chemistry so as to increase the fluidity of the membrane.

See also Bacterial membranes and cell wall

MEMBRANE TRANSPORT, EUKARYOTIC ·
see CELL MEMBRANE TRANSPORT

MEMBRANE TRANSPORT, PROKARYOTIC ·
see PROKARYOTIC MEMBRANE TRANSPORT

MENINGITIS, BACTERIAL AND VIRAL

Meningitis is a potentially fatal **inflammation** of the meninges, the thin, membranous covering of the brain and the spinal cord. Meningitis is most commonly caused by infection (by **bacteria**, **viruses**, or **fungi**), although it can also be caused by bleeding into the meninges, cancer, or diseases of the **immune system**.

The meninges are three separate membranes, layered together, which serve to encase the brain and spinal cord. The dura is the toughest, outermost layer, and is closely attached to the inside of the skull. The middle layer, the arachnoid, is important in the normal flow of the cerebrospinal fluid (CSF), a lubricating fluid that bathes both the brain and the spinal cord. The innermost layer, the pia, helps direct brain blood vessels into the brain. The space between the arachnoid and the pia contains CSF, which serves to help insulate the brain from trauma. Through this space course many blood vessels. CSF, produced within specialized chambers deep inside the brain, flows over the surface of the brain and spinal cord. This fluid serves to cushion these relatively delicate structures, as well as supplying important nutrients for brain cells. CSF is reabsorbed by blood vessels that are located within the meninges.

The cells lining the brain's capillaries (tiny blood vessels) are specifically designed to prevent many substances from passing into brain tissue. This is commonly referred to as the blood-brain barrier. The blood-brain barrier prevents various toxins (substances which could be poisonous to brain tissue), as well as many agents of infection, from crossing from the blood stream into the brain tissue. While this barrier obviously is an important protective feature for the brain, it also serves to complicate therapy in the case of an infection, by making it difficult for medications to pass out of the blood and into the brain tissue where the infection resides.

The most common infectious causes of meningitis vary according to an individual host's age, habits and living environment, and health status. In newborns, the most common agents of meningitis are those that are contracted from the newborn's mother, including Group B *Streptococci* (becoming an increasingly common infecting organism in the newborn period), *Escherichia coli*, and *Listeria monocytogenes*. Older children are more frequently infected by *Haemophilus influenzae*, *Neisseria meningitidis*, and *Streptococcus pneumoniae*, while adults are infected by *S. pneumoniae* and *N. meningitidis*. *N. meningitidis* is the only organism that can cause **epidemics** of meningitis. These have occurred in particular when a child in a crowded day-care situation, a college student in a dormitory, or a military recruit in a crowded training camp has fallen ill with *N. meningitidis* meningitis.

Viral causes of meningitis include the **herpes** simplex viruses, **mumps** and **measles** viruses (against which most children are protected due to mass **immunization** programs), the virus that causes chicken pox, the **rabies** virus, and a number of viruses that are acquired through the bite of infected mosquitoes. Patients with **AIDS** (Acquired Immune Deficiency Syndrome) are more susceptible to certain infectious causes of meningitis, including by certain fungal agents, as well as by

the agent that causes **tuberculosis**. Patients who have had their spleens removed, or whose spleens are no longer functional (as in the case of patients with sickle cell disease) are more susceptible to certain infections, including those caused by *N. meningitidis* and *S. pneumoniae*.

The majority of meningitis infections are acquired by blood-borne spread. An individual may have another type of infection (of the lungs, throat, or tissues of the heart) caused by an organism that can also cause meningitis. The organism multiplies, finds its way into the blood stream, and is delivered in sufficient quantities to invade past the blood-brain barrier.

Direct spread occurs when an already resident infectious agent spreads from infected tissue next to or very near the meninges, for example from an ear or sinus infection. Patients who suffer from skull fractures provide openings to the sinuses, nasal passages, and middle ears. Organisms that frequently live in the human respiratory system can then pass through these openings to reach the meninges and cause infection. Similarly, patients who undergo surgical procedures or who have had foreign bodies surgically placed within their skulls (such as tubes to drain abnormal amounts of accumulated CSF) have an increased risk of the organisms causing meningitis being introduced to the meninges.

The most classic symptoms of meningitis (particularly of bacterial meningitis) include fever, headache, vomiting, photophobia (sensitivity to light), irritability, lethargy (severe fatigue), and stiff neck. The disease progresses with seizures, confusion, and eventually coma.

Damage due to meningitis occurs from a variety of phenomena. The action of infectious agents on the brain tissue is one direct cause of damage. Other types of damage may be due to mechanical effects of swelling of brain tissue, and compression against the bony surface of the skull. Swelling of the meninges may interfere with the normal absorption of CSF by blood vessels, causing accumulation of CSF and damage due to resulting pressure on the brain. Interference with the brain's carefully regulated chemical environment may cause damaging amounts of normally present substances (carbon dioxide, potassium) to accumulate. Inflammation may cause the blood-brain barrier to become less effective at preventing the passage of toxic substances into brain tissue.

Antibiotic medications (forms of penicillins and cephalosporins, for example) are the most important element of treatment against bacterial agents of meningitis. Because of the effectiveness of the blood-brain barrier in preventing passage of substances into the brain, medications must be delivered directly into the patient's veins (intravenous or IV) at very high doses. Antiviral medications (acyclovir) may be helpful in the case of viral meningitis, and antifungal medications are available as well.

Other treatment for meningitis involves decreasing inflammation (with steroid preparations) and paying careful attention to the balance of fluids, glucose, sodium, potassium, oxygen, and carbon dioxide in the patient's system. Patients who develop seizures will require medications to halt the seizures and prevent their return.

A series of immunizations against *Haemophilus influenzae*, started at two months of age, has greatly reduced the incidence of that form of meningitis. Vaccines also exist against *Neisseria meningitidis* and *Streptococcus pneumoniae* bacteria, but these vaccines are only recommended for those people who have particular susceptibility to those organisms, due to certain immune deficiencies, lack of a spleen, or sickle cell anemia.

Because *N. meningitidis* is known to cause epidemics of disease, close contacts of patients with such meningitis are treated prophylactically, often with the antibiotic Rifampin. This measure generally prevents spread of the disease.

See also Bacteria and bacterial infection; Viruses and responses to viral infection

MESELSON, MATTHEW STANLEY

(1930-)

American molecular biologist

Matthew Meselson, in collaboration with biologist Franklin W. Stahl, showed experimentally that the replication of **deoxyribonucleic acid (DNA)** in **bacteria** is semiconservative. Semiconservative replication occurs in a double stranded DNA molecule when the two strands are separated and a new strand is copied from the parental strand to produce two new double stranded DNA molecules. The new double stranded DNA molecule is semiconservative because only one strand is conserved from the parent; the other strand is a new copy. (Conservative replication occurs when one offspring of a molecule contains both parent strands and the other molecule offspring contains newly replicated strands) The classical experiment revealing semiconservative replication in bacteria was central to the understanding of the living cell and to modern **molecular biology**.

Matthew Stanley Meselson was born May 24, 1930, in Denver, Colorado. After graduating in 1951 with a Ph.D. in liberal arts from the University of Chicago, he continued his education with graduate studies at the California Institute of Technology in the field of chemistry. Meselson graduated with a Ph.D. in 1957, and remained at Cal Tech as a research fellow. He acquired the position of assistant professor of chemistry at Cal Tech in 1958. In 1960, Meselson moved to Cambridge, Massachusetts to fill the position of associate professor of natural sciences at Harvard University. In 1964, he was awarded professor of biology, which he held until 1976. He was appointed the title of Thomas Dudley Cabot professor of natural sciences in 1976. From that time on, Meselson held a concurrent appointment on the council of the Smithsonian Institute in Washington, DC.

After graduating from the University of Chicago, Meselson continued his education in chemistry at the California Institute of Technology. It was during his final year at Cal Tech that Meselson collaborated with Franklin Stahl on the classical experiment of semiconservative replication of DNA. Meselson and Stahl wanted to design and perform an experiment that would show the nature of DNA replication from parent to offspring using the **bacteriophage** T4 (a virus

that destroys other cells, also called a phage). The idea was to use an isotope to mark the cells and centrifuge to separate particles that could be identified by their DNA and measure changes in the new generations of DNA. Meselson, Stahl, and Jerome Vinograd originally designed this technique of isolating phage samples. The phage samples isolated would contain various amounts of the isotope based on the rate of DNA replication. The amount of isotope incorporated in the new DNA strands, they hoped, would be large enough to determine quantitatively. The experiments, however, were not successful. After further contemplation, Meselson and Stahl decided to abandon the use of bacteriophage T4 and the isotope and use instead the bacteria ***Escherichia coli*** (*E. coli*) and the heavy nitrogen isotope 15N as the labeling substance. This time when the same experimental steps were repeated, the analysis showed three distinct types of bacterial DNA, two from the original parent strands and one from the offspring. Analysis of this offspring showed each strand of DNA came from a different parent. Thus the theory of semiconservative replication of DNA had been proven. With this notable start to his scientific career Meselson embarked on another collaboration, this time with biologists **Sydney Brenner**, from the Medical Research Council's Division of Molecular Biology in Cambridge, England, and **François Jacob** from the Pasteur Institute Laboratories in Paris, France. Together, Meselson, Brenner, and Jacob performed a series of experiments in which they showed that when the bacteriophage T4 enters a bacterial cell, the phage DNA incorporates into the cellular DNA and causes the release of messenger **RNA**. Messenger RNA instructs the cell to manufacture phage proteins instead of the bacterial cell proteins that are normally produced. These experiments led to the discovery of the role of messenger RNA as the instructions that the bacterial cell reads to produce the desired protein products. These experiments also showed that the bacterial cell could produce proteins from messenger RNA that are not native to the cell in which it occurs.

In his own laboratory at Harvard University, Meselson and a postdoctoral fellow, Robert Yuan, were developing and purifying one of the first of many known **restriction enzymes** commonly used in molecular biological analyses. Restriction **enzymes** are developed by cultivating bacterial strains with phages. Bacterial strains that have the ability to restrict foreign DNA produce a protein called an enzyme that actually chews up or degrades the foreign DNA. This enzyme is able to break up the foreign DNA sequences into a number of small segments by breaking the double stranded DNA at particular locations. Purification of these enzymes allowed mapping of various DNA sequences to be accomplished. The use of purified restriction enzymes became a common practice in the field of molecular biology to map and determine contents of many DNA sequences.

After many years working with the bacteria *E. coli*, Meselson decided to investigate the fundamentals of DNA replication and repair in other organisms. He chose to work on the fruit fly called *Drosophila melanogaster*. Meselson discovered that the fruit fly contained particular DNA sequences that would be transcribed only when induced by heat shock or stress conditions. These particular heat shock genes required a specific setup of DNA bases upstream of the initiation site in order for **transcription** to occur. If the number of bases was increased or reduced from what was required, the **gene** would not be transcribed. Meselson also found that there were particular DNA sequences that could be recombined or moved around within the entire chromosome of DNA. These moveable segments are termed **transposons**. Transposons, when inserted into particular sites within the sequence, can either turn on or turn off expression of the gene that is near it, causing **mutations** within the fly. These studies contributed to the identity of particular regulatory and structural features of the fruit fly as well as to the overall understanding of the properties of DNA.

Throughout his career as a scientist, Meselson has written over 50 papers published in major scientific journals and received many honors and awards for his contributions to the field of molecular biology. In 1963, Meselson received the National Academy of Science Prize for Molecular Biology, followed by the Eli Lilly Award for Microbiology and **Immunology** in 1964. He was awarded the Lehman Award in 1975 and the Presidential award in 1983, both from the New York Academy of Sciences. In 1990, Meselson received the Science Freedom and Responsibility Award from the American Association for the Advancement of Science. Meselson has also delved into political issues, particularly on government proposals for worldwide chemical and biological weapon disarmament.

See also Microbial genetics; Transposition

MESOPHILIC BACTERIA

Mesophiles are **microorganisms** such as some species of **Bacteria**, **Fungi**, and even some **Archaea** that are best active at median temperatures. For instance, bacterial species involved in biodegradation (i.e., digestion and decomposition of organic matter), which are more active in temperatures ranging from approximately 70° - 90°F (approx. 15°–40°C), are termed mesophilic bacteria. They take part in the web of micro-organic activity that form the humus layer in forests and other fertile soils, by decomposing both vegetable and animal matter.

At the beginning of the decomposition process, another group of bacteria, psychrophylic bacteria, start the process because they are active in lower temperatures up to 55°F (from below zero up to 20°C), and generate heat in the process. When the temperature inside the decomposing layer reaches 50–100°F, it attracts mesophilic bacteria to continue the biodegradation. The peak of reproductive and activity of mesophilic bacteria is reached between 86–99°F (30–37°C), and further increases the temperature in the soil environment. Between 104–170°F (40–85°C, or even higher), another group of bacteria (thermophyllic bacteria) takes up the process that will eventually result in organic soil, or humus. Several species of fungi also take part in each decomposing step.

Mesophilic bacteria are also involved in food **contamination** and degradation, such as in bread, grains, dairies, and meats. Examples of common mesophilic bacteria are *Listeria*

monocytogenes, Pesudomonas maltophilia, Thiobacillus novellus, Staphylococcus aureus, Streptococcus pyrogenes, Streptococcus pneumoniae, Escherichia coli, and *Clostridium kluyveri.* Bacterial infections in humans are mostly caused by mesophilic bacteria that find their optimum growth temperature around 37°C (98.6°F), the normal human body temperature. Beneficial bacteria found in human intestinal flora are also mesophiles, such as dietary *Lactobacillus acidophilus.*

See also Archaeobacteria; Bacteria and bacterial infection; Biodegradable substances; Composting, microbiological aspects; Extremophiles

METABOLISM

Metabolism is the sum total of chemical changes that occur in living organisms and which are fundamental to life. All prokaryotic and eukaryotic cells are metabolically active. The sole exception is **viruses**, but even viruses require a metabolically active host for their replication.

Metabolism involves the use of compounds. Nutrients from the environment are used in two ways by **microorganisms**. They can be the building blocks of various components of the microorganism (assimilation or anabolism). Or, nutrients can be degraded to yield energy (dissimilation or catabolism). Some so-called amphibolic biochemical pathways can serve both purposes. The continual processes of breakdown and re-synthesis are in a balance that is referred to as turnover. Metabolism is an open system. That is, there are constant inputs and outputs. A chain of metabolic reactions is said to be in a steady state when the concentration of all intermediates remains constant, despite the net flow of material through the system. That means the concentration of intermediates remains constant, while a product is formed at the expense of the substrate.

Primary metabolism comprises those metabolic processes that are basically similar in all living cells and are necessary for cellular maintenance and survival. They include the fundamental processes of growth (e.g., the synthesis of biopolymers and the macromolecular structures of cells and organelles), energy production (glycolysis and the tricarboxylic acid cycle) and the turnover of cell constituents. Secondary metabolism refers to the production of substances, such as bile pigments from porphyrins in humans, which only occur in certain eukaryotic tissues and are distinct from the primary metabolic pathways.

Metabolic control processes that occur inside cells include regulation of **gene** expression and metabolic feedback or feed-forward processes. The triggers of differential gene expression may be chemical, physical (e.g., bacterial cell density), or environmental (e.g., light). Differential gene expression is responsible for the regulation, at the molecular level, of differentiation and development, as well as the maintenance of numerous cellular "house-keeping" reactions, which are essential for the day-to-day functioning of a microorganism. In many metabolic pathways, the metabolites (substances produced or consumed by metabolism) themselves can act directly as signals in the control of their own breakdown and synthesis. Feedback control can be negative or positive. Negative feedback results in the inhibition by an end product, of the activity or synthesis of an enzyme or several **enzymes** in a reaction chain. The inhibition of the synthesis of enzymes is called enzyme repression. Inhibition of the activity of an enzyme by an end product is an allosteric effect and this type of feedback control is well known in many metabolic pathways (e.g., lactose **operon**). In positive feedback, an endproduct activates an enzyme responsible for its own production.

Many reactions in metabolism are cyclic. A metabolic cycle is a catalytic series of reactions, in which the product of one bimolecular (involving two molecules) reaction is regenerated as follows: A + B → C + A. Thus, A acts catalytically and is required only in small amounts and A can be regarded as carrier of B. The catalytic function of A and other members of the metabolic cycle ensure economic conversion of B to C. B is the substrate of the metabolic cycle and C is the product. If intermediates are withdrawn from the metabolic cycle, e.g., for biosynthesis, the stationary concentrations of the metabolic cycle intermediates must be maintained by synthesis. Replenishment of depleted metabolic cycle intermediates is called anaplerosis. Anaplerosis may be served by a single reaction, which converts a common metabolite into an intermediate of the metabolic cycle. An example of this is pyruvate to oxaloacetate reaction in the tricarboxylic acid cycle. Alternatively, it may involve a metabolic sequence of reactions, i.e., an anaplerotic sequence. An example of this is the glycerate pathway which provides phosphoenol pyruvate for anaplerosis of the tricarboxylic acid cycle.

Prokaryotes exhibit a great diversity of metabolic options, even in a single organism. For example, *Escherichia coli* can produce energy by **respiration** or **fermentation**. Respiration can be under aerobic conditions (e.g., using O_2 as the final electron acceptor) or anaerobically (e.g., using something other than oxygen as the final electron acceptor). Compounds like lactose or glucose can be used as the only source of carbon. Other **bacteria** have other metabolic capabilities including the use of sunlight for energy.

Some of these mechanisms are also utilized by eukaryotic cells. In addition, prokaryotes have a number of energy-generating mechanisms that do not exist in eukaryotic cells. Prokaryotic fermentation can be uniquely done via the phosphoketolase and Enter-Doudoroff pathways. Anaerobic respiration is unique to prokaryotes, as is the use of inorganic compounds as energy sources or as carbon sources during bacterial **photosynthesis**. Archaebacteria possess metabolic pathways that use H_2 as the energy source with the production of methane, and a nonphotosynthetic metabolism that can convert light energy into chemical energy.

In bacteria, metabolic processes are coupled to the synthesis of adenosine triphosphate (ATP), the principle fuel source of the cell, through a series of membrane-bound proteins that constituent the **electron transport system**. The movement of protons from the inside to the outside of the membrane during the operation of the electron transport system can be used to drive many processes in a bacterium, such as the movement of the flagella used to power the bacterium

along, and the synthesis of ATP in the process called oxidative phosphorylation.

The fermentative metabolism that is unique to some bacteria is evolutionarily ancient. This is consistent with the early appearance of bacteria on Earth, relative to eukaryotic organisms. But bacteria can also ferment sugars in the same way that brewing **yeast** (i.e., *Saccharomyces cerevesiae* ferment sugars to produce ethanol and carbon dioxide. This fermentation, via the so-called Embden Myerhoff pathway, can lead to different ends products in bacteria, such as lactic acid (e.g., *Lactobacillus*), a mixture of acids (*Enterobacteriaceae*, butanediol (e.g., *Klebsiella*, and propionic acid (e.g., *Propionibacterium*).

See also Bacterial growth and division; Biochemistry

METCHNIKOFF, ÉLIE (1845-1916)
Russian immunologist

Élie Metchnikoff was a pioneer in the field of **immunology** and won the 1908 Nobel Prize in physiology or medicine for his discoveries of how the body protects itself from disease-causing organisms. Later in life, he became interested in the effects of nutrition on aging and health, which led him to advocate some controversial diet practices.

Metchnikoff, the youngest of five children, was born in the Ukrainian village of Ivanovka on May 16, 1845, to Emilia Nevahovna, daughter of a wealthy writer, and Ilya Ivanovich, an officer of the Imperial Guard in St. Petersburg. He enrolled at the Kharkov Lycee in 1856, where he developed an especially strong interest in biology. At age 16, he published a paper in a Moscow journal criticizing a geology textbook. After graduating from secondary school in 1862, he entered the University of Kharkov, where he completed a four-year program in two years. He also became an advocate of the theory of **evolution** by natural **selection** after reading Charles Darwin's *On the Origin of Species by Means of Natural Selection*.

In 1864, Metchnikoff traveled to Germany to study, where his work with nematodes (a species of worm) led to the surprising conclusion that the organism alternates between sexual and asexual generations. His studies at Kharkov, coupled with his interest in Darwin's theory, convinced him that highly evolved animals should show structural similarities to more primitive animals. He pursued his studies of invertebrates in Naples, Italy, where he collaborated with Russian zoologist Alexander Kovalevsky. They demonstrated the homology (similarity of structure) between the germ layers—embryonic sheets of cells that give rise to specific tissue—in different multicellular animals. For this work, the scientists were awarded the Karl Ernst von Baer Prize.

Metchnikoff was only twenty-two when he received the prize and had a promising career ahead of himself. However, he soon developed severe eye strain, a condition that hampered his work and prevented him from using the **microscope** for the next fifteen years. Nevertheless, in 1867, he completed his doctorate at the University of St. Petersburg with a thesis on the embryonic development of fish and crustaceans. He taught at the university for the next six years before moving to the University of Odessa on the Black Sea where he studied marine animals.

During the summer of 1880, he spent a vacation on a farm where a beetle infection was destroying crops. In an attempt to curtail the devastation, Metchnikoff injected a fungus from a dead fly into a beetle to see if he could kill the pest. Metchnikoff carried this interest in infection with him when he left Odessa for Italy, following the assassination of Czar Alexander II in 1884. A zoologist up to that point, Metchnikoff began to focus more on pathology, or the study of diseases.

This **transformation** was due primarily to his study of the larva of the Bipinniara starfish. While studying this larva, which is transparent and can be easily observed under the microscope, Metchnikoff saw special cells surrounding and engulfing foreign bodies, similar to the actions of white blood cells in humans that were present in areas of **inflammation**. During a similar study of the water flea *Daphniae,* he observed white blood cells attacking needle-shaped spores that had invaded the insect's body. He called these cells phagocytes, from the Greek word *phagein,* meaning, to eat.

While scientists thought that human phagocytes merely transported foreign material throughout the body, and therefore spread disease, Metchnikoff realized they performed a protective function. He recognized that the human white blood cells and the starfish phagocytes were embryologically homologous, both being derived from the mesoderm layer of cells. He concluded that the human cells cleared the body of disease-causing organisms. In 1884, he injected infected blood under the skin of a frog and demonstrated that white blood cells in higher animals served a similar function as those in starfish larvae. The scientific community, however, still did not accept his idea that phagocytic cells fought off infections.

Metchnikoff returned to Odessa in 1886 and became the director of the Bacteriological Institute. He continued his research on phagocytes in animals and pursued vaccines for chicken cholera and sheep **anthrax**. Hounded by scientists and the press because of his lack of medical training, Metchnikoff fled Russia a year later. A chance meeting with French scientist **Louis Pasteur** led to a position as the director of a new laboratory at the Pasteur Institute in Paris. There, he continued his study of **phagocytosis** for the next twenty-eight years.

But conflict with his fellow scientists continued to follow him. Many scientists asserted that antibodies triggered the body's immune response to infection. Metchnikoff accepted the existence of antibodies but insisted that phagocytic cells represented another important arm of the **immune system**. His work at the Pasteur Institute led to many fundamental discoveries about the immune response, and one of his students, **Jules Bordet**, contributed important insights into the nature of **complement**, a system of antimicrobial **enzymes** triggered by antibodies. Metchnikoff received the Nobel Prize for physiology and medicine in 1908 jointly with **Paul Ehrlich** for their work in initiating the study of immunology and greatly influencing its development.

Metchnikoff's interest in **immunity** led to writings on aging and death. His book *The Nature of Man,* published in

1903, extolled the health virtues of "right living," which for him included consuming large amounts of fermented milk or yogurt made with a Bulgarian bacillus. In fact, his own name became associated with a popular commercial preparation of yogurt, although he received no royalties. With the exception of yogurt, Metchnikoff warned of eating uncooked foods, claiming that the **bacteria** present on them could cause cancer. Metchnikoff claimed he even plunged bananas into boiling water after unpeeling them and passed his silverware through flames before using it.

On July 15, 1916, after a series of heart attacks, Metchnikoff died in Paris at the age of 71. He was a member of the French Academy of Medicine, the Swedish Medical Society, and the Royal Society of London, from which he received the Copley Medal. He also received an honorary doctorate from Cambridge University.

See also Phagocyte and phagocytosis

METHANE OXIDIZING AND PRODUCING BACTERIA

Methane is a chemical compound that consists of a carbon atom to which are bound four hydrogen atoms. The gas is a major constituent of oxygen-free mud and water, marshes, the rumen of cattle and other animals, and the intestinal tract of mammals. In oxygen-free (anaerobic) environments, methane can be produced by a type of **bacteria** known as methanogenic bacteria. Methane can also be used as an energy source by other bacteria that grow in the presence of oxygen (aerobic bacteria), which break down the compound into carbon dioxide and water. These bacteria are known as methane oxidizing bacteria.

Bacteria from a number of genera are able to oxidize methane. These include *Methylosinus, Methylocystis, Methanomonas, Methylomonas, Methanobacter,* and *Methylococcus.* A characteristic feature of methane-oxidizing bacteria is the presence of an extensive system of membranes inside the bacterial cell. The membranes house the **enzymes** and other biochemical machinery needed to deal with the se of methane as an energy source.

The oxidation of methane by bacteria requires oxygen. The end result is the production of carbon dioxide and water. Methane oxidation is restricted to prokaryotes. Eukaryotic **microorganisms** such as algae and **fungi** do not oxidize methane.

The production of methane is a feature of anaerobic bacteria. Examples of methane producing genera are *Methanobacterium, Methanosarcina, Methanococcus,* and *Methanospirillum.* Methanogenic bacteria are widespread in nature, and are found in mud, sewage, and sludge and in the rumen of sheep and cattle. Some methanogenic bacteria have adapted to live in extreme environments. For example, *Methanococcus jannaschii* has an optimum growth temperature of 85° C (185° F), which is achieved in hot springs and thermal vents in the ocean. Such anaerobic bacteria are among the oldest life forms on Earth. They evolved long before the presence of photosynthetic green plants, and so existed in an oxygen-free world.

In the rumen, the methane-producing bacteria occupy a central role in regulating the anaerobic breakdown (**fermentation**) of food. The bacteria remove hydrogen gas through the se of the gas in the reduction of carbon dioxide to form methane. By producing methane, the concentration of hydrogen is kept at a low level that allows other bacterial species to grow. This microbial diversity makes fermentation more efficient.

The bacterial production of methane is of economic importance. "Biogas" obtained from digesters can be a commercial and domestic energy source, although more economic sources of energy currently limit this use. In large-scale livestock operations, the use of methane producing bacteria is being increasing popular as a means of odor-control.

As on Earth, methane producing bacteria may be one of the earliest forms of life on other planets. Experiments that duplicate the atmosphere of the planet Mars have been successful in growing methane producing bacteria. Aside from its fundamental scientific importance, the discovery might be exploited in future manned missions to Mars. Methane is described as being a greenhouse gas, which means it can warm the surface atmosphere. On a small-scale, methane production might create a more hospitable atmosphere on the surface of Mars. Additionally, the combustible nature of methane, utilized on Earth as a biogas, could someday provide rocket fuel for spacecraft.

See also Biogeochemical cycles; Chemoautotrophic and chemolithitrophic bacteria; Extremophiles

MICRO ARRAYS • *see* DNA CHIPS AND MICROARRAYS

MICROBIAL FLORA OF THE ORAL CAVITY, DENTAL CARIES

The microbial flora of the oral cavity are rich and extremely diverse. This reflects the abundant nutrients and moisture, and hospitable temperature, and the availability of surfaces on which bacterial populations can develop. The presence of a myriad of **microorganisms** is a natural part of proper oral health. However, an imbalance in the microbial flora can lead to the production of acidic compounds by some microorganisms that can damage the teeth and gums. Damage to the teeth is referred to a dental caries.

Microbes can adhere to surfaces throughout the oral cavity. These include the tongue, epithelial cells lining the roof of the mouth and the cheeks, and the hard enamel of the teeth. In particular, the microbial communities that exist on the surface of the teeth are known as dental **plaque**. The adherent communities also represent a biofilm. Oral biofilms develop over time into exceedingly complex communities. Hundreds of species of **bacteria** have been identified in such biofilms.

Development of the adherent populations of microorganisms in the oral cavity begins with the association and irreversible adhesion of certain bacteria to the tooth surface. Components of the host oral cavity, such as proteins and glycoproteins from the saliva, also adhere. This early coating is referred to as the conditioning film. The conditioning film alters the chemistry of the tooth surface, encouraging the adhesion of other microbial species. Over time, as the biofilm thickens, gradients develop within the biofilm. For example, oxygen may be relatively plentiful at the outer extremity of the biofilm, with the core of the biofilm being essentially oxygen-free. Such environmental alterations promote the development of different types of bacteria in different regions of the biofilm.

This changing pattern represents what is termed bacterial succession. Examples of some bacteria that are typically present as primary colonizers include *Streptococcus*, *Actinomyces*, *Neisseria*, and *Veillonella*. Examples of secondary colonizers include *Fusobacterium nucleatum*, *Prevotella intermedia*, and *Capnocytophaga* species. With further time, another group of bacteria can become associated with the adherent community. Examples of these bacteria include *Campylobacter rectus*, *Eikenella corrodens*, *Actinobacillus actinomycetemcomitans*, and the oral **spirochetes** of the genus *Treponema*.

Under normal circumstances, the microbial flora in the oral cavity reaches equilibrium, where the chemical by-products of growth of some microbes are utilized by other microbes for their growth. Furthermore, the metabolic activities of some bacteria can use up oxygen, creating conditions that are favorable for the growth of those bacteria that require oxygen-free conditions.

This equilibrium can break down. An example is when the diet is high in sugars that can be readily used by bacteria. The **pH** in the adherent community is lowered, which selects for the predominance of acid-loving bacteria, principally *Streptococcus mutans* and *Lactobacillus* species. These species can produce acidic products. The resulting condition is termed dental caries. Dental caries is the second most common of all maladies in humans, next only to the common **cold**. It is the most important cause of tooth loss in people under 10 years of age.

Dental caries typically proceeds in stages. Discoloration and loosening of the hard enamel covering of the tooth precedes the formation of a microscopic hole in the enamel. The hole subsequently widens and damage to the interior of the tooth usually results. If damage occurs to the core of the tooth, a region containing what is termed pulp, and the roots anchoring the tooth to the jaw, the tooth is usually beyond saving. Removal of the tooth is necessary to prevent accumulation of bacterial products that could pose further adverse health effects.

Dental caries can be lessened or even prevented by coating the surface of the tooth with a protective sealant. This is usually done as soon as a child acquires the second set of teeth. Another strategy to thwart the development of dental caries is the inclusion of a chemical called fluoride in drinking water. Evidence supports the use of fluoride to lessen the predominance of acid-producing bacteria in the oral cavity. Finally, good oral **hygiene** is of paramount importance in dental heath. Regular brushing of the teeth and the avoidance of excessive quantities of sugary foods are very prudent steps to maintaining the beneficial equilibrium microbial equilibrium in the oral cavity.

See also Bacteria and bacterial infection

MICROBIAL FLORA OF THE SKIN

The skin is the primary external coating of the human body. In adults, skin occupies approximately 2.4 square yards (approximately two square meters). Because it is exposed to the environment, the skin is inhabited by a number of **bacteria**. Over much of the body there are hundreds of bacteria per square inch of skin. In more moisture-laden regions, such as the armpit, groin, and in between the toes, bacteria can number upwards of one hundred thousand per square inch.

The majority of the skin microbes are found in the first few layers of the epidermis (the outermost layer of skin) and in the upper regions of the hair follicles. The bacteria found here are mostly *Staphylococcus epidermidis* and species of Corynebacteria, Micrococcus, Mycobacterium, and Pityrosporum. These species are described as being commensal; that is, the association is beneficial for one organism (in this case the microbe) and not harmful to the other organism (the human). They are part of the natural environment of the skin and as such are generally benign.

The skin microflora can also be a protective mechanism. By colonizing the skin, the commensal microbes can restrict the colonization by other, hostile **microorganisms**. This phenomenon is referred to as competitive exclusion. The environment of the skin also predisposes the skin to selective colonization. Glands of the skin secrete compounds called fatty acids. Many organisms will not tolerate these fatty acids. But, the normal microflora of the skin is able to tolerate and grow in the presence of the fatty acids. As well, sweat contains a natural antibiotic known as dermicidin. The normal flora seems to be more tolerant to dermicidin than are invading microbes. Thus, their presence of a normal population of microorganisms on the skin is encouraged by the normal physiological conditions of the body.

Newborn babies do not have established skin microorganisms. Colonization occurs within hours of birth, especially following contact with parents and siblings. The resulting competitive exclusion of more hostile microbes is especially important in the newborn, whose **immune system** is not yet fully developed.

In contrast to the protection they bestow, skin microorganisms can cause infections if they gain entry to other parts of the body, such as through cut or during a surgical procedure, or because of a malfunctioning immune system. Bacteria and other microbes that are normal residents of the skin cause some six to ten percent of common hospital-acquired infections. For example, the **yeast** *Candida albicans* can cause a urinary tract infection. In another example, if the sweat glands malfunction, the resident *Proprionibacterium acnes* can be encouraged to undergo explosive growth. The resulting block-

age of the sweat glands and **inflammation** can produce skin irritation and sores. As a final example, the Corynebacterium can cause infection of wounds and heart valve infections if they gain entry to deeper regions of the body.

Other microorganisms that are transient members of the skin population can be a problem. *Escherichia coli*, normally a resident of the intestinal tract, can be acquired due to poor personal **hygiene**. Another bacterial species, *Staphylococcus aureus*, can be picked up from infected patients in a hospital setting. One on the skin, these disease-causing bacteria can be passed on by touch to someone else directly or to a surface. Fortunately, these problematic bacteria can be easily removed by normal handwashing with ordinary soap. Unfortunately, this routine procedure is sometimes not as widely practiced as it should be. Organizations such as the American Society for Microbiology have mounted campaigns to increase awareness of the benefits of hand washing.

However, handwashing is not totally benign. Particularly harsh soaps, or very frequent hand washing (for example, 20–30 times a day) can increase the acidity of the skin, which can counteract some of the protective fatty acid secretions. Also the physical act of washing will shed skin cells. If washing is excessive, the protective microflora will be removed, leaving the newly exposed skin susceptible to colonization by another, potentially harmful microorganism. Health care workers, who scrub their hands frequently, are prone to **skin infections** and damage.

See also Acne, microbial basis of; Bacterial growth and division; Colony and colony formation; Fatty acids; structures and functions; Infection and resistance; Infection control; Microbial flora of the oral cavity, dental caries; Microbial flora of the stomach and gastrointestinal tract

MICROBIAL FLORA OF THE STOMACH AND GASTROINTESTINAL TRACT

The stomach and gastrointestinal tract are not sterile and are colonized by **microorganisms** that perform functions beneficial to the host, including the manufacture of essential vitamins, and the prevention of colonization by undesirable microbes.

The benefits of the close relationship between the microorganisms and the host also extends to the microbes. Microorganisms are provided with a protected place to live and their environment—rich in nutrients—and is relatively free from predators.

This mutually beneficial association is always present. At human birth, the stomach and gastrointestinal tract are usually sterile. But, with the first intake of food, colonization by **bacteria** commences. For example, in breast-fed babies, most of the intestinal flora consists of bacteria known as bifidobacteria. As breast milk gives way to bottled milk, the intestinal flora changes to include enteric bacteria, bacteroides, enterococci, lactobacilli, and clostridia.

The flora of the gastrointestinal tract in animals has been studied intensively. These studies have demonstrated that bacteria are the most numerous microbes present in the stomach and gastrointestinal tract. The composition of the bacterial populations varies from animal to animal, even within a species. Sometimes the diet of an animal can select for the dominance of one or a few bacteria over other species. The situation is similar in humans. Other factors that influence the bacterial make up of the human stomach and gastrointestinal tract include age, cultural conditions, and the use of **antibiotics**. In particular, the use of antibiotics can greatly change the composition of the gastrointestinal flora.

Despite the variation in bacterial flora, the following bacteria tend to be present in the gastrointestinal tract of humans and many animals: *Escherichia coli*, *Clostridium perfringens*, Enterococci, Lactobacilli, and *Bacteroides*.

The esophagus is considered to be part of the gastrointestinal tract. In this region, the bacteria present are usually those that have been swallowed with the food. These bacteria do not normally survive the journey through the highly acidic stomach. Only bacteria that can tolerate strongly acidic environments are able to survive in the stomach. One bacterium that has been shown to be present in the stomach of many people is *Helicobacter pylori*. This bacterium is now known to be the leading cause of stomach ulcers. In addition, very convincing evidence is mounting that links the bacterium to the development of stomach and intestinal cancers.

In humans, the small intestine contains low numbers of bacteria, some 100,000 to 10 million bacteria per milliliter of fluid. To put these numbers into perspective, a laboratory liquid **culture** that has attained maximum bacterial numbers will contain 100 million to one billion bacteria per milliliter. The bacterial flora of this region consists mostly of lactobacilli and *Enterococcus faecalis*. The lower regions of the small intestine contain more bacteria and a wider variety of species, including coliform bacteria such as *Escherichia coli*.

In the large intestine, the bacterial numbers can reach 100 billion per milliliter of fluid. The predominant species are anaerobic bacteria, which do not grow in the presence of oxygen. These include anaerobic **lactic acid bacteria**, *Bacteroides*, and *Bifidobacterium bifidum*. The bacteria numbers and composition in the large intestine is effectively that of fecal material.

The massive numbers of bacteria in the large intestine creates a great special variation in the flora. Sampling the intestinal wall at different locations will reveal differences in the species of bacteria present. As well, sampling any given point in the intestine will reveal differences in the bacterial population at various depths in the adherent growth on the intestinal wall.

Some bacteria specifically associate with certain cells in the gastrointestinal tract. Gram-positive bacteria such as **streptococci** and lactobacilli often adhere to cells by means of capsules surrounding the bacteria. Gram-negative bacteria such as *Escherichia coli* can adhere to receptors on the intestinal epithelial cells by means of the bacterial appendage called fimbriae.

The importance of the microbial flora of the stomach and gastrointestinal tract has been demonstrated by comparison of the structure and function of the digestive tracts of normal animals and notobiotic animals. The latter animals lack bacteria. The altered structure of the intestinal tract in the notobiotic animals is less efficient in terms of processing food and absorbing nutrients. Additionally, in animals like cows that consume cellulose, the **fermentation** activity of intestinal microorganisms is vital to digestion. Thus, the flora of the stomach and intestinal tract is very important to the health of animals including humans.

See also Enterobacteriaceae; Probiotics; Salmonella food poisoning

MICROBIAL GENETICS

Microbial genetics is a branch of genetics concerned with the transmission of hereditary characters in **microorganisms**. Within the usual definition, microorganisms include prokaryotes like **bacteria**, unicellular or mycelial **eukaryotes** e.g., yeasts and other **fungi**, and **viruses**, notably bacterial viruses (bacteriophages). Microbial genetics has played a unique role in developing the fields of molecular and cell biology and also has found applications in medicine, agriculture, and the food and pharmaceutical industries.

Because of their relative simplicity, microbes are ideally suited for combined biochemical and genetic studies, and have been successful in providing information on the **genetic code** and the regulation of **gene** activity. The **operon** model formulated by French biologists **François Jacob** (1920–) and **Jacques Monod** (1910–1976) in 1961, is one well known example. Based on studies on the induction of **enzymes** of lactose catabolism in the bacterium *Escherichia coli,* the operon has provided the groundwork for studies on gene expression and regulation, even up to the present day. The many applications of microbial genetics in medicine and the pharmaceutical industry emerge from the fact that microbes are both the causes of disease and the producers of **antibiotics**. Genetic studies have been used to understand variation in pathogenic microbes and also to increase the yield of antibiotics from other microbes.

Hereditary processes in microorganisms are analogous to those in multicellular organisms. In both prokaryotic and eukaryotic microbes, the genetic material is **DNA**; the only known exceptions to this rule are the **RNA** viruses. **Mutations**, heritable changes in the DNA, occur spontaneously and the rate of mutation can be increased by mutagenic agents. In practice, the susceptibility of bacteria to mutagenic agents has been used to identify potentially hazardous chemicals in the environment. For example, the Ames test was developed to evaluate the mutagenicity of a chemical in the following way. Plates containing a medium lacking in, for example, the nutrient histidine are inolculated with a histidine requiring strain of the bacterium *Salmonella typhimurium*. Thus, only cells that revert back to the wild type can grow on the medium. If plates are exposed to a mutagenic agent, the increase in the number of **mutants** compared with unexposed plates can be observed and a large number of revertants would indicate a strong mutagenic agent. For such studies, microorganisms offer the advantage that they have short mean generation times, are easily cultured in a small space under controlled conditions and have a relatively uncomplicated structure.

Microorganisms, and particularly bacteria, were generally ignored by the early geneticists because of their small in size and apparent lack of easily identifiable variable traits. Therefore, a method of identifying variation and mutation in microbes was fundamental for progress in microbial genetics. As many of the mutations manifest themselves as metabolic abnormalities, methods were developed by which microbial mutants could be detected by selecting or testing for altered phenotypes. Positive **selection** is defined as the detection of mutant cells and the rejection of unmutated cells. An example of this is the selection of **penicillin** resistant mutants, achieved by growing organisms in media containing penicillin such that only resistant colonies grow. In contrast, negative selection detects cells that cannot perform a certain function and is used to select mutants that require one or more extra growth factors. Replica plating is used for negative selection and involves two identical prints of **colony** distributions being made on plates with and without the required nutrients. Those microbes that do not grow on the plate lacking the nutrient can then be selected from the identical plate, which does contain the nutrient.

The first attempts to use microbes for genetic studies were made in the USA shortly before World War II, when George W. Beadle (1903–1989) and **Edward L. Tatum** (1909–1975) employed the fungus, *Neurospora,* to investigate the genetics of tryptophan **metabolism** and nicotinic acid synthesis. This work led to the development of the "one gene one enzyme" hypothesis. Work with bacterial genetics, however, was not really begun until the late 1940s. For a long time, bacteria were thought to lack sexual reproduction, which was believed to be necessary for mixing genes from different individual organisms—a process fundamental for useful genetic studies. However, in 1947, **Joshua Lederberg** (1925–) working with Edward Tatum demonstrated the exchange of genetic factors in the bacterium, *Escherichia coli.* This process of DNA transfer was termed **conjugation** and requires cell-to-cell contact between two bacteria. It is controlled by genes carried by **plasmids**, such as the fertility (F) factor, and typically involves the transfer of the plasmid from donor torecipient cell. Other genetic elements, however, including the donor cell chromosome, can sometimes also be mobilized and transferred. Transfer to the host chromosome is rarely complete, but can be used to map the order of genes on a bacterial genome.

Other means by which foreign genes can enter a bacterial cell include **transformation**, transfection, and **transduction**. Of the three processes, transformation is probably the most significant. Evidence of transformation in bacteria was first obtained by the British scientist, Fred Griffith (1881–1941) in the late 1920s working with *Streptococcus pneumoniae* and the process was later explained in the 1930s by **Oswald Avery** (1877–1955) and his associates at the Rockefeller Institute in New York. It was discovered that certain bacteria exhibit competence, a state in which cells are able to take up free DNA released by other bacteria. This is the process known as transformation, however, relatively few

microorganisms can be naturally transformed. Certain laboratory procedures were later developed that make it possible to introduce DNA into bacteria, for example electroporation, which modifies the bacterial membrane by treatment with an electric field to facilitate DNA uptake. The latter two processes, transfection and transduction, involve the participation of viruses for nucleic acid transfer. Transfection occurs when bacteria are transformed with DNA extracted from a bacterial virus rather than from another bacterium. Transduction involves the transfer of host genes from one bacterium to another by means of viruses. In generalized transduction, defective virus particles randomly incorporate fragments of the cell DNA; virtually any gene of the donor can be transferred, although the efficiency is low. In specialized transduction, the DNA of a temperate virus excises incorrectly and brings adjacent host genes along with it. Only genes close to the integration point of the virus are transduced, and the efficiency may be high.

After the discovery of DNA transfer in bacteria, bacteria became objects of great interest to geneticists because their rate of reproduction and mutation is higher than in larger organisms; i.e., a mutation occurs in a gene about one time in 10,000,000 gene duplications, and one bacterium may produce 10,000,000,000 offspring in 48 hours. Conjugation, transformation, and transduction have been important methods for mapping the genes on the **chromosomes** of bacteria. These techniques, coupled with restriction enzyme analysis, **cloning** DNA sequencing, have allowed for the detailed studies of the bacterial chromosome. Although there are few rules governing gene location, the genes encoding enzymes for many biochemical pathways are often found tightly linked in operons in prokaryotes. Large scale sequencing projects revealed the complete DNA sequence of the genomes of several prokaryotes, even before eukaryotic genomes were considered.

See also Bacterial growth and division; Bacteriophage and bacteriophage typing; Cell cycle (eukaryotic), genetic regulation of; Cell cycle (prokaryotic), genetic regulation of; Fungal genetics; Mutations and mutagenesis; Viral genetics; Viral vectors in gene therapy

MICROBIAL SYMBIOSIS

Symbiosis is generally defined as a condition where two dissimilar organisms live together in an intimate associate that sees both organisms benefit. Microbial symbiosis tends to be bit broader in definition, being defined as the co-existence of two **microorganisms**.

Microbial symbiosis can be evident as several different patterns of co-existence. One pattern is known as mutualism. In this relationship, both organisms benefit. Another type of relationship is called commensalism. Here the relationship is beneficial to one of the organisms and does no harm to the other.

Another relationship known as parasitism produces a benefit to one organism at the expense of the other organism. Parasitism is not considered to be a symbiosis between a microorganism and the host.

Microbial symbiosis has been a survival feature of **bacteria** since their origin. The best example of this is the presence of the energy factories known as mitochondria in eukaryotic cells. Mitochondria arose because of the symbiosis between an ancient bacterium and a eukaryote. Over evolutionary time the symbiosis became permanent, and the bacterium became part of the host. However, even to the present day the differences in constitution and arrangement of the genetic material of mitochondria and the host cell's **nucleus** attests to the symbiotic origin of mitochondria.

There are several well-known examples of bacterial mutualism. The first example is the presence of huge numbers of bacteria in the intestinal tract of warm-blooded animals such as humans. Fully 10 percent of the dry weight of a human consists of bacteria. The bacteria act to break down foodstuffs, and so directly participate in the digestive process. As well, some of the intestinal bacteria produce products that are crucial to the health of the host. For example. In humans, some of the gut bacteria manufacture vitamin K, vitamin B_{12}, biotin, and riboflavin. These vitamins are important to the host but are not made by the host. The bacteria benefit by inhabiting an extremely hospitable environment. The natural activities and numbers of the bacteria also serve to protect the host from colonization by disease-causing microorganisms. The importance of this type of symbiosis is exemplified by the adverse health effects to the host that can occur when the symbiotic balance is disturbed by antibiotic therapy.

A second example of symbiotic mutualism is the colonization of the nodules of leguminous plants by bacteria of the genus *Rhizobium*. The bacteria convert free nitrogen gas into a form of nitrogen called nitrate. This form of nitrogen can be readily utilized by the plant, which cannot otherwise use the gaseous form of nitrogen. The plant benefits by acquiring a readily available nitrogen source, and, as for the intestinal bacteria, *Rhizobium* benefits by virtue of the hospitable environment for growth.

The skin is colonized by a number of different types of bacteria, such as those from the genera *Staphylococcus* and *Streptococcus*. The bacteria are exposed to a read supply of nutrients, and their colonization of the skin helps protect that surface from colonization by less desirable microorganisms.

Microbial symbiosis can be exquisite. An example is the Gram-negative bacterium *Xenorhabdus nematophilus*. This bacterium lives in a nematode called *Steinernema carpocapsae*. Both organisms require the other for their survival. Thus the symbiosis is obligatory. The bacterium in fact supplies toxins that are used to kill insect that the nematode infects.

The scope of microbial symbiosis in nature is vast. In the 1970s the existence of thermal vents on the ocean floor was discovered. It has since been shown that the basis of the lush ecosystem surrounding these sources of heat is bacteria, and that a significant proportion of these bacteria live in symbiosis with the tubular worm-like creatures that thrives in this environment. In fact, the bacteria are absolutely required for the utilization of nutrients by the tube worms.

Numerous other examples of microbial symbiosis exist in nature. Animals, plants as exotic as coral, insects, fish, and birds all harbor microorganisms that assist them in their sur-vival. Indeed, the ancient roots of microbial symbiosis may be indicative of a more cooperative **evolution** of life on Earth than prior studies indicated.

See also Bacterial kingdoms; Microbial taxonomy

MICROBIAL TAXONOMY

Microbial taxonomy is a means by which **microorganisms** can be grouped together. Organisms having similarities with respect to the criteria used are in the same group, and are separated from the other groups of microorganisms that have different characteristics.

There are a number of taxonomic criteria that can be used. For example, numerical taxonomy differentiates microorganisms, typically **bacteria**, on their phenotypic characteristics. Phenotypes are the appearance of the microbes or the manifestation of the genetic character of the microbes. Examples of phenotypic characteristics include the Gram stain reaction, shape of the bacterium, size of the bacterium, where or not the bacterium can propel itself along, the capability of the microbes to grow in the presence or absence of oxygen, types of nutrients used, chemistry of the surface of the bacterium, and the reaction of the **immune system** to the bacterium.

Numerical taxonomy typically invokes a number of these criteria at once. The reason for this is that if only one criterion was invoked at a time there would be a huge number of taxonomic groups, each consisting of only one of a few microorganisms. The purpose of grouping would be lost. By invoking several criteria at a time, fewer groups consisting of larger number of microorganisms result.

The groupings result from the similarities of the members with respect to the various criteria. A so-called similarity coefficient can be calculated. At some imposed threshold value, microorganisms are placed in the same group.

A well-known example of taxonomic characterization is the kingdom, division, class, family, genus, species and strain divisions. Such a "classical" bacterial organization, which is typified by the Bergey's Manual of Determinative Bacteriology, is based on metabolic, immunological, and structural characteristics. Strains, for example, are all descended from the same organism, but differ in an aspect such as the antigenic character of a surface molecule.

Microbial taxonomy can create much order from the plethora of microorganisms. For example, the **American Type Culture Collection** maintains the following, which are based on taxonomic characterization (the numbers in brackets indicate the number of individual organisms in the particular category): algae (120), bacteria (14400), **fungi** (20200), **yeast** (4300), **protozoa** (1090), animal **viruses** (1350), **plant viruses** (590), and bacterial viruses (400). The actual number of microorganisms in each category will continue to change as new microbes are isolated and classified. The general structure, however, of this classical, so-called phenetic system will remain the same.

The separation of the microorganisms is typically represented by what is known as a dendrogram. Essentially, a dendrogram appears as a tree oriented on a horizontal axis. The dendrogram becomes increasingly specialized—that is, the similarity coefficient increases—as the dendrogram moves from the left to the right. The right hand side consists of the branches of the trees. Each branch contains a group of microorganisms.

The dendrogram depiction of relationships can also be used for another type of microbial taxonomy. In this second type of taxonomy, the criterion used is the shared evolutionary heritage. This heritage can be determined at the genetic level. This is termed molecular taxonomy.

Molecular microbial taxonomy relies upon the generation and inheritance of genetic **mutations** that is the replacement of a nucleotide building block of a **gene** by another nucleotide. Sometimes the mutation confers no advantage to the microorganism and so is not maintained in subsequent generations. Sometimes the mutation has an adverse effect, and so is actively suppressed or changed. But sometimes the mutation is advantageous for the microorganism. Such a mutation will be maintained in succeeding generations.

Because mutations occur randomly, the divergence of two initially genetically similar microorganisms will occur slowly over evolutionary time (millions of years). By sequencing a target region of genetic material, the relatedness or dissimilarity of microorganisms can be determined. When enough microorganisms have been sequenced, relationships can be established and a dendrogram constructed.

For a meaningful genetic categorization, the target of the comparative sequencing must be carefully chosen. Molecular microbial taxonomy of bacteria relies on the sequence of **ribonucleic acid** (**RNA**), dubbed 16S RNA, that is present in a subunit of prokaryotic **ribosomes**. Ribosomes are complexes that are involved in the manufacture of proteins using messenger RNA as the blueprint. Given the vital function of the 16S RNA, any mutation tends to have a meaningful, often deleterious, effect on the functioning of the RNA. Hence, the **evolution** (or change) in the 16S RNA has been very slow, making it a good molecule with which to compar microorganisms that are billions of years old.

Molecular microbial taxonomy has been possible because of the development of the technique of the **polymerase chain reaction**. In this technique a small amount of genetic material can be amplified to detectable quantities

The use of the chain reaction has produced a so-called bacterial phylogenetic tree. The structure of the tree is even now evolving. But the current view has the tree consisting of three main branches. One branch consists of the bacteria. There are some 11 distinct groups within the bacterial branch. Three examples are the green non-sulfur bacteria, Gram- positive bacteria, and cyanobacteria.

The second branch of the evolutionary tree consists of the Archae, which are thought to have been very ancient bacteria that diverged from both bacteria and eukaryotic organisms billions of years ago. Evidence to date places the Archae a bit closer on the tree to bacteria than to the final branch (the Eucarya). There are three main groups in the archae: halophiles (salt-loving), methanogens, and the extreme thermophiles (heat loving).

Finally, the third branch consists of the Eucarya, or the eukaryotic organisms. Eucarya includes organisms as diverse as fungi, plants, **slime molds** and animals (including humans).

See also Bacterial kingdoms; Genetic identification of microorganisms

MICROBIOLOGY, CLINICAL

Clinical microbiology is concerned with infectious **microorganisms**. Various **bacteria**, algae and **fungi** are capable of causing disease.

Disease causing microorganisms have been present for millennia. Examples include **anthrax**, **smallpox**, bacterial **tuberculosis**, plague, **diphtheria**, **typhoid fever**, bacterial diarrhea, and **pneumonia**. While modern technological advances, such as mass **vaccination**, have reduced the threat of some of these diseases, others remain a problem. Some illnesses are reemerging, due to acquisition of resistance to many **antibiotics**. Finally, other diseases, such as the often lethal hemorrhagic fever caused by the **Ebola virus**, have only been recognized within the past few decades.

Many bacterial diseases have only been recognized since the 1970s. These include **Legionnaires' disease**, Campylobacter infection of poultry, **toxic shock syndrome**, hemolytic uremic syndrome, **Lyme disease**, peptic ulcer disease, human ehrlichiosis, and a new strain of cholera. Clinical microbiology research and techniques were vital in identifying the cause of these maladies, and in seeking treatments and ultimately a cure for each malady.

Clinical microbiology involves both the detection and identification of disease-causing microorganisms, and research to find more effective means of treating the infection or preventing infections from occurring. The symptoms of the ailment, and the shape, **Gram stain** reaction (in the case of bacteria), and biochemical reactions of an unknown organism are used to diagnose the cause of an infection. Knowledge of the identity of the microbe suggests means of treatment, such as the application of antibiotics. Many clinical microbiologists are also researchers. In many cases, the molecular basis of an organism's disease-causing capability is not clear. Unraveling the reasons why a disease is produced can help find ways to prevent the disease.

There are several groups or categories of bacteria that are of medical importance. They are grouped into five categories based on their shape and reaction to the Gram stain. These criteria apply to the light **microscope**, as typically a first step in the identification of bacteria in an infection is the light microscope examination of material obtained from the infection or from a **culture**. The groups are Gram-positive bacilli (rod-shaped bacteria), Gram negative bacilli, Gram positive cocci (round bacteria), Gram negative cocci, and bacteria that react atypically to the Gram stain.

A group of spiral shaped bacteria called **spirochetes** are responsible for leptospirosis in dogs, and **syphilis** and Lyme disease in humans. These bacteria are easily identified under the light microscope because of their wavy shape and

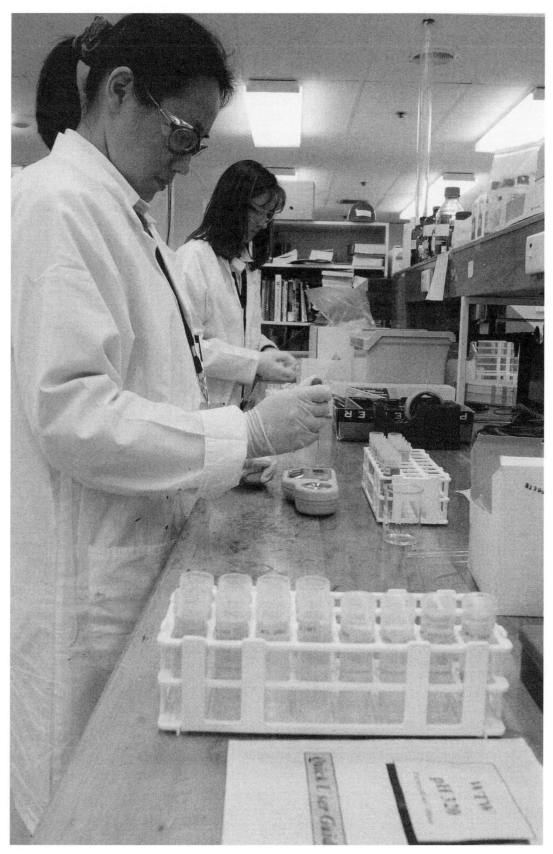

Laboratory technicians.

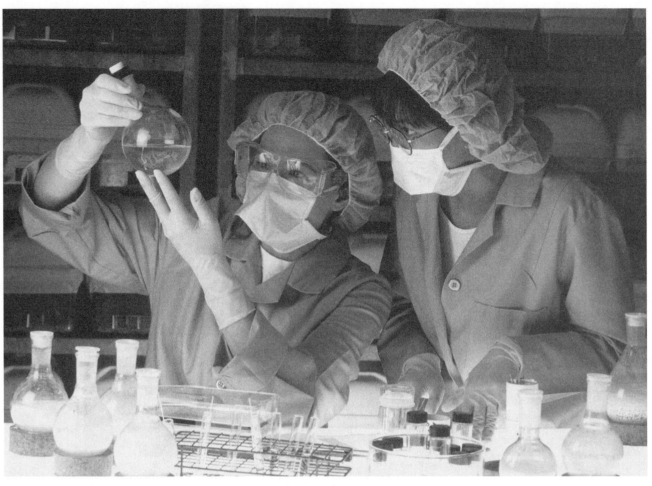

Laboratory technicians.

corkscrew movement (courtesy of rigid internal filaments that run the length of the bacterium). A related group (a genus) of spiral shaped bacteria is *Spirilla*. These bacteria move by means of external flagella, not by means of the internal filaments. Two members of *Spirilla* are important disease-causing bacteria. The first is *Campylobacter jejuni*, which frequently contaminates raw meat such as poultry and drinking water, and which is the cause of diarrhea, especially in children. The second bacterial type is *Helicobacter pylori*, which grows in the stomach and has been demonstrated to be the principle cause of stomach ulcers.

Another group of clinically relevant bacteria is termed pseudomonads. This group contains many different types of bacteria. They all are similar in shape and biochemical behavior to a species called *Pseudomonas aeruginosa*. Most pseudomonads, like *Pseudomonas aeruginosa* live in water and the soil. They cause a variety of ailments. *Bordetella pertussis* causes whooping cough, *Legionella pneumophila* causes Legionnaires' disease, *Neisseria gonorrhoeae* causes **gonorrhea**, and *Neisseria meningitides* causes bacterial **meningitis**. *Pseudomonas aeruginosa* is the quintessential so-called opportunitistic pathogen; a bacteria that does not normally cause an infection but can do so in a compromised host.

Examples of such infections are the chronic lung infections in those who have certain forms of cystic fibrosis, and infections in burn victims.

Yet another group of bacteria of medical importance live in the intestinal tracts of humans, other mammals and even in birds and reptiles. These are the enteric bacteria. The best-known enteric bacteria is ***Escherichia coli***, the cause of intestinal illness and sometimes even more severe damage to the urinary tract and kidneys from ingestion of contaminated water or food ("hamburger disease"). Other noteworthy enteric bacteria are *Shigella dysenteriae* (**dysentery**), *Salmonella* species **gastroenteritis** and typhoid fever), *Yersinia pestis* (**bubonic plague**), and *Vibrio cholerae* (cholera).

Bacteria including *Staphylococcus* and *Streptococcus,* which normally live on the skin, can cause infection when they gain entry to other pasts of the body. The illnesses they cause (such as **strep throat**, pneumonia, and blood infection, as examples), and the number of cases of these illnesses, make them the most clinically important disease-causing bacteria known to man. *Staphylococcus aureus* is the leading cause of hospital acquired infections of all the gram-positive bacteria. Ominously, a strain of this organism now exists that is resistant to many antibiotics. As this strain increases its worldwide distribution, *Staphylococcus* infections will become an increasing problem.

Bacteria that normally live in the mouth are responsible for the formation of dental **plaque** on the surface of teeth. Protected within the plaque, the bacteria produce acid that eats away tooth enamel, leading to the development of a cavity.

A few examples of other clinically important bacteria are *Bacillus anthracis* (anthrax), *Clostridium tetani* (**tetanus**), *Mycobacterium tuberculosis* (tuberculosis), *Corynebacterium diphtheriae* (diphtheria), various Rickettsias (Rocky Mountain Spotted Fever, **Q fever**), *Chlamydia trachomatis* (chlamydia).

Fungi and **yeast** are also capable of causing infection. For example, the fungal genus *Tinea* comprises species that cause conditions commonly described as "jock itch" and "athlete's foot." Scalp infections are also caused by some species of fungus.

Viruses are also the cause of a variety of infections. **Inflammation** of the coating of nerve cells (meningitis) and brain tissue (encephalitis), and infections of tissues in the mouth, bronchial tract, lungs and intestinal tract result from infection by various viruses.

See also Blood borne infections; Cold, viruses; Laboratory techniques in microbiology; Viruses and response to viral infection; Yeast, infectious

MICROBIOLOGY, HISTORY OF · *see* HISTORY OF MICROBIOLOGY

MICROORGANISMS

Microorganisms are minute organisms of microscopic dimensions, too small to be seen by the eye alone. To be viewed, microorganisms must be magnified by an optical or **electron microscope**. The most common types of microorganisms are **viruses**, **bacteria**, blue-green bacteria, some algae, some **fungi**, yeasts, and protozoans.

Viruses, bacteria, and blue-green bacteria are all prokaryotes, meaning that they do not have an organized cell **nucleus** separated from the protoplasm by a membrane-like envelope. Viruses are the simplest of the prokaryotic life forms. They are little more than simple genetic material, either **DNA (deoxyribonucleic acid)** or **RNA (ribonucleic acid)**, plus associated proteins of the viral shell (called a capsid) that together comprise an infectious agent of cells. Viruses are not capable of independent reproduction. They reproduce by penetrating a host cell and diverting much of its metabolic and reproductive physiology to the reproduction of copies of the virus.

The largest kingdom of prokaryotes is the Monera. In this group, the genetic material is organized as a single strand of DNA, neither meiosis nor mitosis occurs, and reproduction is by asexual cellular division. Bacteria (a major division of the Monera) are characterized by rigid or semi-rigid cell walls, propagation by binary division of the cell, and a lack of mito-

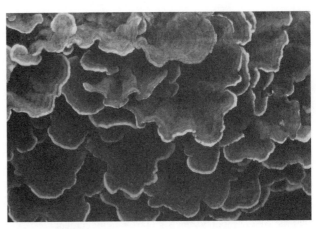

A lichen growing on wood.

sis. Blue-green bacteria or cyanobacteria (also in the Monera) use **chlorophyll** dispersed within the **cytoplasm** as the primary light-capturing pigment for their **photosynthesis**.

Many microorganisms are eukaryotic organisms, having their nuclear material organized within a nucleus bound by an envelope. **Eukaryotes** also have paired **chromosomes** of DNA, which can be seen microscopically during mitosis and meiosis. They also have a number of other discrete cellular organelles.

Protists are a major kingdom of eukaryotes that includes microscopic protozoans, some fungi, and some algae. Protists have flagellated spores, and mitochondria and plastids are often, but not always, present. Protozoans are single-celled microorganisms that reproduce by binary fission and are often motile, usually using cilia or flagellae for propulsion; some protozoans are colonial.

Fungi are heterotrophic organisms with chitinous cell walls, and they lack flagella. Some fungi are unicellular microorganisms, but others are larger and have thread-like **hyphae** that form a more complex **mycelium**, which take the form of mushrooms in the most highly developed species. Yeasts are a group of single-celled fungi that reproduce by budding or by cellular fission.

Algae are photosynthetic, non-vascular organisms, many of which are unicellular, or are found in colonies of several cells; these kinds of algae are microscopic.

In summary, microorganisms comprise a wide range of diverse but unrelated groups of tiny organisms, characterized only by their size. As a group, microorganisms are extremely important ecologically as primary producers, and as agents of decay of dead organisms and recycling of the nutrients contained in their biomass. Some species of microorganisms are also important as **parasites** and as other disease-causing agents in humans and other organisms.

See also Bacteria and bacterial infection; Genetic identification of microorganisms; Viruses and responses to viral infection; Microbial flora of the skin; Microbial genetics; Microbial symbiosis; Microbial taxonomy; Microscope and microscopy

MICROSCOPE AND MICROSCOPY

Microscopy is the science of producing and observing images of objects that cannot be seen by the unaided eye. A microscope is an instrument that produces the image. The primary function of a microscope is to resolve, that is distinguish, two closely spaced objects as separate. The secondary function of a microscope is to magnify. Microscopy has developed into an exciting field with numerous applications in biology, geology, chemistry, physics, and technology.

Since the time of the Romans, it was realized that certain shapes of glass had properties that could magnify objects. By the year 1300, these early crude lenses were being used as corrective eyeglasses. It wasn't until the late 1500s, however, that the first compound microscopes were developed.

Robert Hooke (1635–1703) was the first to publish results on the microscopy of plants and animals. Using a simple two-lens compound microscope, he was able to discern the cells in a thin section of cork. The most famous microbiologist was Antoni van Leeuwenhoek (1632–1723) who, using just a single lens microscope, was able to describe organisms and tissues, such as **bacteria** and red blood cells, which were previously not known to exist. In his lifetime, Leeuwenhoek built over 400 microscopes, each one specifically designed for one specimen only. The highest resolution he was able to achieve was about 2 micrometers.

By the mid-nineteenth century, significant improvements had been made in the light microscope design, mainly due to refinements in lens grinding techniques. However, most of these lens refinements were the result of trial and error rather than inspired through principles of physics. Ernst Abbé (1840–1905) was the first to apply physical principles to lens design. Combining glasses with different refracting powers into a single lens, he was able to reduce image distortion significantly. Despite these improvements, the ultimate resolution of the light microscope was still limited by the wavelength of light. To resolve finer detail, something with a smaller wavelength than light would have to be used.

In the mid-1920s, Louis de Broglie (1892–1966) suggested that electrons, as well as other particles, should exhibit wave like properties similar to light. Experiments on electron beams a few years later confirmed de Broglie's hypothesis. Electrons behave like waves. Of importance to microscopy was the fact that the wavelength of electrons is typically much smaller than the wavelength of light. Therefore, the limitation imposed on the light microscope of 0.4 micrometers could be significantly reduced by using a beam of electrons to illuminate the specimen. This fact was exploited in the 1930s in the development of the **electron microscope**.

There are two types of electron microscope, the transmission electron microscope (TEM) and the scanning electron microscope (SEM). The TEM transmits electrons through an extremely thin sample. The electrons scatter as they collide with the atoms in the sample and form an image on a photographic film below the sample. This process is similar to a medical x ray, where x rays (very short wavelength light) are transmitted through the body and form an image on photographic film behind the body. By contrast, the SEM reflects a narrow beam of electrons off the surface of a sample and detects the reflected electrons. To image a certain area of the sample, the electron beam is scanned in a back and forth motion parallel to the sample surface, similar to the process of mowing a square section of lawn. The chief differences between the two microscopes are that the TEM gives a two-dimensional picture of the interior of the sample while the SEM gives a three-dimensional picture of the surface of the sample. Images produced by SEM are familiar to the public, as in television commercials showing pollen grains or dust mites.

For the light microscope, light can be focused and bent using the refractive properties of glass lenses. To bend and focus beams of electrons, however, it is necessary to use magnetic fields. The magnetic lens, which focuses the electrons, works through the physical principle that a charged particle, such as an electron that has a negative charge, will experience a force when it is moving in a magnetic field. By positioning magnets properly along the electron beam, it is possible to bend the electrons in such a way as to produce a magnified image on a photographic film or a fluorescent screen. This same principle is used in a television set to focus electrons onto the television screen to give the appropriate images.

Electron microscopes are complex and expensive. To use them effectively requires extensive training. They are rarely found outside the research laboratory. Sample preparation can be extremely time consuming. For the TEM, the sample must be ground extremely thin, less than 0.1 micrometer, so that the electrons will make it through the sample. For the SEM, the sample is usually coated with a thin layer of gold to increase its ability to reflect electrons. Therefore, in electron microscopy, the specimen can't be living. Today, the best TEMs can produce images of the atoms in the interior of a sample. This is a factor of a 1,000 better than the best light microscopes. The SEM, on the other hand, can typically distinguish objects about 100 atoms in size.

In the early 1980s, a new technique in microscopy was developed which did not involve beams of electrons or light to produce an image. Instead, a small metal tip is scanned very close to the surface of a sample and a tiny electric current is measured as the tip passes over the atoms on the surface. The microscope that works in this manner is the scanning tunneling microscope (STM). When a metal tip is brought close to the sample surface, the electrons that surround the atoms on the surface can actually "tunnel through" the air gap and produce a current through the tip. This physical phenomenon is called tunneling and is one of the amazing results of quantum physics. If such phenomenon could occur with large objects, it would be possible for a baseball to tunnel through a brick wall with no damage to either. The current of electrons that tunnel through the air gap is very much dependent on the width of the gap and therefore the current will rise and fall in succession with the atoms on the surface. This current is then amplified and fed into a computer to produce a three dimensional image of the atoms on the surface.

Without the need for complicated magnetic lenses and electron beams, the STM is far less complex than the electron microscope. The tiny tunneling current can be simply amplified through electronic circuitry similar to circuitry that is

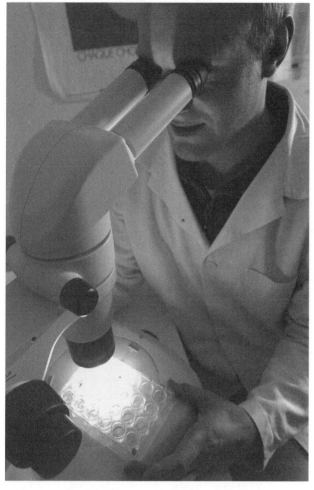

Researcher using light microscope to examine cell cultures.

used in other electronic equipment, such as a stereo. In addition, the sample preparation is usually less tedious. Many samples can be imaged in air with essentially no preparation. For more sensitive samples that react with air, imaging is done in vacuum. A requirement for the STM is that the samples be electrically conducting, such as a metal.

There have been numerous variations on the types of microscopy outlined so far. A sampling of these is: acoustic microscopy, which involves the reflection of sound waves off a specimen; x-ray microscopy, which involves the transmission of x rays through the specimen; near field optical microscopy, which involves shining light through a small opening smaller than the wavelength of light; and atomic force microscopy, which is similar to scanning tunneling microscopy but can be applied to materials that are not electrically conducting, such as quartz.

One of the most amazing recent developments in microscopy involves the manipulation of individual atoms. Through a novel application of the STM, scientists at IBM were able to arrange individual atoms on a surface and spell out the letters "IBM." This has opened up new directions in microscopy, where the microscope is both an instrument with

which to observe and to interact with microscopic objects. Future trends in microscopy will most likely probe features within the atom.

See also Electron microscope, transmission and scanning; Electron microscopic examination of microorganisms; Laboratory techniques in immunology; Laboratory techniques in microbiology

MILLER-UREY EXPERIMENT

A classic experiment in **molecular biology**, the Miller-Urey experiment, established that the conditions that existed in Earth's primitive atmosphere were sufficient to produce amino acids, the subunits of proteins comprising and required by living organisms. In essence, the Miller-Urey experiment fundamentally established that Earth's primitive atmosphere was capable of producing the building blocks of life from inorganic materials.

In 1953, University of Chicago researchers **Stanley L. Miller** and Harold C. Urey set up an experimental investigation into the molecular origins of life. Their innovative experimental design consisted of the introduction of the molecules thought to exist in early Earth's primitive atmosphere into a closed chamber. Methane (CH_4), hydrogen (H_2), and ammonia (NH_3) gases were introduced into a moist environment above a water-containing flask. To simulate primitive lightning discharges, Miller supplied the system with electrical current.

After a few days, Miller observed that the flask contained organic compounds and that some of these compounds were the amino acids that serve as the essential building blocks of protein. Using chromatological analysis, Miller continued his experimental observations and confirmed the ready formation of amino acids, hydroxy acids, and other organic compounds.

Although the discovery of amino acid formation was of tremendous significance in establishing that the raw materials of proteins were easily to obtain in a primitive Earth environment, there remained a larger question as to the nature of the origin of genetic materials mdash; in particular the origin of **DNA** and **RNA** molecules.

Continuing on the seminal work of Miller and Urey, in the early 1960s Juan Oro discovered that the nucleotide base adenine could also be synthesized under primitive Earth conditions. Oro used a mixture of ammonia and hydrogen cyanide (HCN) in a closed aqueous environment.

Oro's findings of adenine, one of the four nitrogenous bases that combine with a phosphate and a sugar (deoxyribose for DNA and ribose for RNA) to form the nucleotides represented by the **genetic code**: (adenine (A), thymine (T), guanine (G), and cytosine (C). In RNA molecules, the nitrogenous base uracil (U) substitutes for thymine. Adenine is also a fundamental component of adenosine triphosphate (ATP), a molecule important in many genetic and cellular functions.

Subsequent research provided evidence of the formation of the other essential nitrogenous bases needed to construct DNA and RNA.

The Miller-Urey experiment remains the subject of scientific debate. Scientist continue to explore the nature and composition of Earth's primitive atmosphere and thus, continue to debate the relative closeness of the conditions of the Miller-Urey experiment (e.g., whether or not Miller's application of electrical current supplied relatively more electrical energy than did lightning in the primitive atmosphere). Subsequent experiments using alternative stimuli (e.g., ultraviolet light) also confirm the formation of amino acids from the gases present in the Miller-Urey experiment. During the 1970s and 1980s, astrobiologists and astrophyicists, including American physicist Carl Sagan, asserted that ultraviolet light bombarding the primitive atmosphere was far more energetic that even continual lightning discharges. Amino acid formation is greatly enhanced by the presence of an absorber of ultraviolet radiation such as the hydrogen sulfide molecules (H_2S) also thought to exist in the early Earth atmosphere.

Although the establishment of the availability of the fundamental units of DNA, RNA and proteins was a critical component to the investigation of the origin of biological molecules and life on Earth, the simple presence of these molecules is a long step from functioning cells. Scientists and evolutionary biologists propose a number of methods by which these molecules could concentrate into a crude cell surrounded by a primitive membrane.

See also Biochemistry; DNA (Deoxyribonucleic acid); Evolution and evolutionary mechanisms; Evolutionary origin of bacteria and viruses; Mitochondrial inheritance

MILLER, STANLEY L. (1930-)
American chemist

Stanley Lloyd Miller is most noted for his experiments that attempted to replicate the chemical conditions that may have first given rise to life on Earth. In the early 1950s he demonstrated that amino acids could have been created under primordial conditions. Amino acids are the fundamental units of life; they join together to form proteins, and as they grow more complex they eventually become nucleic acids, which are capable of replicating. Miller has hypothesized that the oceans of primitive Earth were a mass of molecules, a prebiological "soup," which over the course of a billion years became a living system.

Miller was born in Oakland, California, the younger of two children. His father, Nathan Harry Miller, was an attorney and his mother, Edith Levy Miller, was a homemaker. Miller attended the University of California at Berkeley and received his B.S. degree in 1951. He began his graduate studies at the University of Chicago in 1951.

In an autobiographical sketch entitled "The First Laboratory Synthesis of Organic Compounds under Primitive Earth Conditions," Miller recalled the events that led to his famous experiment. Soon after arriving at the University of Chicago, he attended a seminar given by **Harold Urey** on the origin of the solar system. Urey postulated that the earth was reducing when it was first formed—in other words, there was

an excess of molecular hydrogen. Strong mixtures of methane and ammonia were also present, and the conditions in the atmosphere favored the synthesis of organic compounds. Miller wrote that when he heard Urey's explanation, he knew it made sense: "For the nonchemist the justification for this might be explained as follows: it is easier to synthesize an organic compound of biological interest from the reducing atmosphere constituents because less chemical bonds need to be broken and put together than is the case with the constituents of an oxidizing atmosphere."

After abandoning a different project for his doctoral thesis, Miller told Urey that he was willing to design an experiment to test his hypothesis. However, Urey expressed reluctance at the idea because he considered it too time consuming and risky for a doctoral candidate. But Miller persisted, and Urey gave him a year to get results; if he failed he would have to choose another thesis topic. With this strict deadline Miller set to work on his attempt to synthesize organic compounds under conditions simulating those of primitive earth.

Miller and Urey decided that ultraviolet light and electrical discharges would have been the most available sources of energy on Earth billions of years ago. Having done some reading into amino acids, Miller hypothesized that if he applied an electrical discharge to his primordial environment, he would probably get a deposit of hydrocarbons, organic compounds containing carbon and hydrogen. As he remembered in "The First Laboratory Synthesis of Organic Compounds": "We decided that amino acids were the best group of compounds to look for first, since they were the building blocks of proteins and since the analytical methods were at that time relatively well developed." Miller designed an apparatus in which he could simulate the conditions of prebiotic Earth and then measure what happened. A glass unit was made to represent a model ocean, atmosphere, and rain. For the first experiment, he filled the unit with the requisite "primitive atmosphere"—methane, hydrogen, water, and ammonia—and then submitted the mixture to a low-voltage spark over night. There was a layer of hydrocarbons the next morning, but no amino acids.

Miller then repeated the experiment with a spark at a higher voltage for a period of two days. This time he found no visible hydrocarbons, but his examination indicated that glycine, an amino acid, was present. Next, he let the spark run for a week and found what looked to him like seven spots. Three of these spots were easily identified as glycine, alpha-alanine, and beta-alanine. Two more corresponded to a-amino-n-butyric acid and aspartic acid, and the remaining pair he labeled A and B.

At Urey's suggestion, Miller published "A Production of Amino Acids under Possible Primitive Earth Conditions" in May of 1953 after only three-and-a-half months of research. Reactions to Miller's work were quick and startling. Articles evaluating his experiment appeared in major newspapers; when a Gallup poll asked people whether they thought it was possible to create life in a test tube; seventy-nine percent of the respondents said no.

After Miller finished his experiments at the University of Chicago, he continued his research as an F. B. Jewett Fellow at the California Institute of Technology from 1954 to 1955. Miller established the accuracy of his findings by performing further tests to identify specific amino acids. He also ruled out the possibility that **bacteria** might have produced the spots by heating the apparatus in an autoclave for eighteen hours (fifteen minutes is usually long enough to kill any bacteria). Subsequent tests conclusively identified four spots that had previously puzzled him. Although he correctly identified the a-amino-n-butyric acid, what he had thought was aspartic acid (commonly found in plants) was really iminodiacetic acid. Furthermore, the compound he had called A turned out to be sarcosine (N-methyl glycine), and compound B was N-methyl alanine. Other amino acids were present but not in quantities large enough to be evaluated.

Although other scientists repeated Miller's experiment, one major question remained: was Miller's apparatus a true representation of the primitive atmosphere? This question was finally answered by a study conducted on a meteorite that landed in Murchison, Australia, in September 1969. The amino acids found in the meteorite were analyzed and the data compared to Miller's findings. Most of the amino acids Miller had found were also found in the meteorite. On the state of scientific knowledge about the origins of human life, Miller wrote in "The First Laboratory Synthesis of Organic Compounds" that "the synthesis of organic compounds under primitive earth conditions is not, of course, the synthesis of a living organism. We are just beginning to understand how the simple organic compounds were converted to polymers on the primitive earth...nevertheless we are confident that the basic process is correct."

Miller's later research has continued to build on his famous experiment. He is looking for precursors to **ribonucleic acid (RNA)**. "It is a problem not much discussed because there is nothing to get your hands on," he told Marianne P. Fedunkiw in an interview. He is also examining the natural occurrence of clathrate hydrates, compounds of ice and gases that form under high pressures, on the earth and other parts of the solar system.

Miller has spent most of his career in California. After finishing his doctoral work in Chicago, he spent five years in the department of **biochemistry** at the College of Physicians and Surgeons at Columbia University. He then returned to California as an assistant professor in 1960 at the University of California, San Diego. He became an associate professor in 1962 and eventually full professor in the department of chemistry.

Miller served as president of the International Society for the Study of the Origin of Life (ISSOL) from 1986 to 1989. The organization awarded him the Oparin Medal in 1983 for his work in the field. Outside of the United States, he was recognized as an Honorary Councilor of the Higher Council for Scientific Research of Spain in 1973. In addition, Miller was elected to the National Academy of Sciences. Among Miller's other memberships are the American Chemical Society, the American Association for the Advancement of Science, and the American Society of Biological Chemists.

See also Evolution and evolutionary mechanisms; Evolutionary origin of bacteria and viruses; Miller-Urey experiment

MILSTEIN, CÉSAR (1927-2002)
Argentine English biochemist

César Milstein conducted one of the most important late twentieth century studies on antibodies. In 1984, Milstein received the Nobel Prize for physiology or medicine, shared with **Niels K. Jerne** and **Georges Köhler**, for his outstanding contributions to **immunology** and immunogenetics. Milstein's research on the structure of antibodies and their genes, through the investigation of **DNA (deoxyribonucleic acid)** and **ribonucleic acid (RNA)**, has been fundamental for a better understanding of how the human **immune system** works.

Milstein was born on October 8, 1927, in the eastern Argentine city of Bahía Blanca, one of three sons of Lázaro and Máxima Milstein. He studied **biochemistry** at the National University of Buenos Aires from 1945 to 1952, graduating with a degree in chemistry. Heavily involved in opposing the policies of President Juan Peron and working part-time as a chemical analyst for a laboratory, Milstein barely managed to pass with poor grades. Nonetheless, he pursued graduate studies at the Instituto de Biología Química of the University of Buenos Aires and completed his doctoral dissertation on the chemistry of aldehyde dehydrogenase, an alcohol enzyme used as a catalyst, in 1957.

With a British Council scholarship, he continued his studies at Cambridge University from 1958 to 1961 under the guidance of Frederick Sanger, a distinguished researcher in the field of **enzymes**. Sanger had determined that an enzyme's functions depend on the arrangement of amino acids inside it. In 1960, Milstein obtained a Ph.D. and joined the Department of Biochemistry at Cambridge, but in 1961, he decided to return to his native country to continue his investigations as head of a newly created Department of **Molecular Biology** at the National Institute of Microbiology in Buenos Aires.

A military coup in 1962 had a profound impact on the state of research and on academic life in Argentina. Milstein resigned his position in protest of the government's dismissal of the Institute's director, Ignacio Pirosky. In 1963, he returned to work with Sanger in Great Britain. During the 1960s and much of the 1970s, Milstein concentrated on the study of antibodies, the protein organisms generated by the immune system to combat and deactivate antigens. Milstein's efforts were aimed at analyzing myeloma proteins, and then DNA and RNA. Myeloma, which are tumors in cells that produce antibodies, had been the subject of previous studies by Rodney R. Porter, **MacFarlane Burnet**, and **Gerald M. Edelman**, among others.

Milstein's investigations in this field were fundamental for understanding how antibodies work. He searched for **mutations** in laboratory cells of myeloma but faced innumerable difficulties trying to find antigens to combine with their anti-

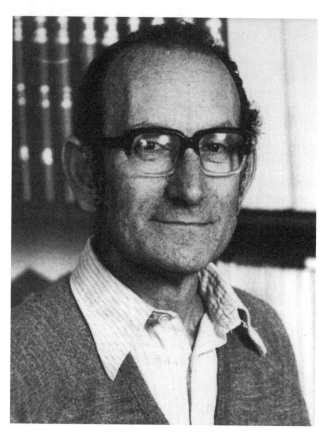

César Milstein

bodies. He and Köhler produced a hybrid myeloma called hybridoma in 1974. This cell had the capacity to produce antibodies but kept growing like the cancerous cell from which it had originated. The production of monoclonal antibodies from these cells was one of the most relevant conclusions from Milstein and his colleague's research. The Milstein-Köhler paper was first published in 1975 and indicated the possibility of using monoclonal antibodies for testing antigens. The two scientists predicted that since it was possible to hybridize antibody-producing cells from different origins, such cells could be produced in massive cultures. They were, and the technique consisted of a fusion of antibodies with cells of the myeloma to produce cells that could perpetuate themselves, generating uniform and pure antibodies.

In 1983, Milstein assumed leadership of the Protein and Nucleic Acid Chemistry Division at the Medical Research Council's laboratory. In 1984, he shared the Nobel Prize with Köhler and Jerne for developing the technique that had revolutionized many diagnostic procedures by producing exceptionally pure antibodies. Upon receiving the prize, Milstein heralded the beginning of what he called "a new era of immunobiochemistry," which included production of molecules based on antibodies. He stated that his method was a by-product of basic research and a clear example of how an investment in research that was not initially considered commercially viable had "an enormous practical impact." By 1984, a thriving business was being done with monoclonal

antibodies for diagnosis, and works on vaccines and cancer based on Milstein's breakthrough research were being rapidly developed.

In the early 1980s, Milstein received a number of other scientific awards, including the Wolf Prize in Medicine from the Karl Wolf Foundation of Israel in 1980, the Royal Medal from the Royal Society of London in 1982, and the Dale Medal from the Society for Endocrinology in London in 1984. He was a member of numerous international scientific organizations, among them the U.S. National Academy of Sciences and the Royal College of Physicians in London.

See also Antibody and antigen; Antibody formation and kinetics; Antibody, monoclonal; Antibody-antigen, biochemical and molecular reactions

MINIMUM INHIBITORY CONCENTRATION (MIC) • *see* ANTIBIOTICS

MITOCHONDRIA AND CELLULAR ENERGY

Mitochondria are cellular organelles found in the **cytoplasm** in round and elongated shapes, that produce adenosine tri-phosphate (ATP) near intra-cellular sites where energy is needed. Shape, amount, and intra-cellular position of mitochondria are not fixed, and their movements inside cells are influenced by the cytoskeleton, usually in close relationship with the energetic demands of each cell type. For instance, cells that have a high consumption of energy, such as muscular, neural, retinal, and gonadic cells present much greater amounts of mitochondria than those with a lower energetic demand, such as fibroblasts and lymphocytes. Their position in cells also varies, with larger concentrations of mitochondria near the intra-cellular areas of higher energy consumption. In cells of the ciliated epithelium for instance, a greater number of mitochondria is found next to the cilia, whereas in spermatozoids they are found in greater amounts next to the initial portion of the flagellum, where the flagellar movement starts.

Mitochondria have their own **DNA**, **RNA** (rRNA, mRNA and tRNA) and **ribosomes,** and are able to synthesize proteins independently from the cell **nucleus** and the cytoplasm. The internal mitochondrial membrane contains more than 60 proteins. Some of these are **enzymes** and other proteins that constitute the electron-transporting chain; others constitute the elementary corpuscle rich in ATP-synthetase, the enzyme that promotes the coupling of electron transport to the synthesis of ATP; and finally, the enzymes involved in the active transport of substances through the internal membrane.

The main ultimate result of **respiration** is the generation of cellular energy through oxidative phosphorilation, i.e., ATP formation through the transfer of electrons from nutrient molecules to molecular oxygen. Prokaryotes, such as **bacteria,** do not contain mitochondria, and the flow of electrons and the oxidative phosphorilation process are associated to the internal membrane of these unicellular organisms. In eukaryotic cells, the oxidative phosphorilation occurs in the mitochondria, through the chemiosmotic coupling, the process of transferring hydrogen protons (H+) from the space between the external and the internal membrane of mitochondria to the elementary corpuscles. H+ are produced in the mitochondrial matrix by the citric acid cycle and actively transported through the internal membrane to be stored in the inter-membrane space, thanks to the energy released by the electrons passing through the electron-transporting chain. The transport of H+ to the elementary corpuscles is mediated by enzymes of the ATPase family and causes two different effects. First, 50% of the transported H+ is dissipated as heat. Second, the remaining hydrogen cations are used to synthesize ATP from ADP (adenosine di-phosphate) and inorganic phosphate, which is the final step of the oxidative phosphorilation. ATP constitutes the main source of chemical energy used by the **metabolism** of eukaryotic cells in the activation of several multiple signal **transduction** pathways to the nucleus, intracellular enzymatic system activation, active transport of nutrients through the cell membrane, and nutrient metabolization.

See also Cell membrane transport; Krebs cycle; Mitochondrial DNA; Mitochondrial inheritance

MITOCHONDRIAL DNA

Mitochondria are cellular organelles that generate energy in the form of ATP through oxidative phosphorylation. Each cell contains hundreds of these important organelles. Mitochondria are inherited at conception from the mother through the **cytoplasm** of the egg. The mitochondria, present in all of the cells of the body, are copies of the ones present in at conception in the egg. When cells divide, the mitochondria that are present are randomly distributed to the daughter cells, and the mitochondria themselves then replicate as the cells grow.

Although many of the mitochondrial genes necessary for ATP production and other genes needed by the mitochondria are encoded in the **DNA** of the **chromosomes** in the **nucleus** of the cell, some of the genes expressed in mitochondria are encoded in a small circular chromosome which is contained within the mitochondrion itself. This includes 13 polypeptides, which are components of oxidative phosphorylation **enzymes**, 22 transfer **RNA** (t-RNA) genes, and two genes for ribosomal RNA (r-RNA). Several copies of the mitochondrial chromosome are found in each mitochondrion. These chromosomes are far smaller than the chromosomes found in the nucleus, contain far fewer genes than any of the autosomes, replicate without going through a mitotic cycle, and their morphological structure is more like a bacterial chromosome than it is like the chromosomes found in the nucleus of **eukaryotes**.

Genes which are transmitted through the mitochondrial DNA are inherited exclusively from the mother, since few if any mitochondria are passed along from the sperm. Genetic diseases involving these genes show a distinctive pattern of inheritance in which the trait is passed from an affected female to all of her children. Her daughters will likewise pass the trait on to all of her children, but her sons do not transmit the trait at all.

The types of disorders which are inherited through **mutations** of the mitochondrial DNA tend to involve disorders of nerve function, as neurons require large amounts of energy to function properly. The best known of the mitochondrial disorders is Leber hereditary optic neuropathy (LHON), which involves bilateral central vision loss, which quickly worsens as a result of the death of the optic nerves in early adulthood. Other mitochondrial diseases include Kearns-Sayre syndrome, myoclonus epilepsy with ragged red fibers (MERFF), and mitochondrial encephalomyopathy, lactic acidosis and stroke-like episodes (MELAS).

See also Mitochondria and cellular energy; Mitochondrial inheritance; Ribonucleic acid (RNA)

MITOCHONDRIAL INHERITANCE

Mitochondrial inheritance is the study of how mitochondrial genes are inherited. Mitochondria are cellular organelles that contain their own **DNA** and **RNA**, allowing them to grow and replicate independent of the cell. Each cell has 10,000 mitochondria each containing two to ten copies of its genome. Because mitochondria are organelles that contain their own genome, they follow an inheritance pattern different from simple Mendelian inheritance, known as extranuclear or cytoplasmic inheritance. Although they posses their own genetic material, mitochondria are semi-autonomous organelles because the nuclear genome of cells still codes for some components of mitochondria.

Mitochondria are double membrane-bound organelles that function as the energy source of eukaryotic cells. Within the inner membrane of mitochondria are folds called cristae that enclose the matrix of the organelle. The DNA of mitochondria, located within the matrix, is organized into circular duplex **chromosomes** that lack histones and code for proteins, rRNA, and tRNA. A nucleoid, rather than a nuclear envelope, surrounds the genetic material of the organelle. Unlike the DNA of nuclear genes, the genetic material of mitochondria does not contain introns or repetitive sequences resulting in a relatively simple structure. Because the chromosomes of mitochondria are similar to those of prokaryotic cells, scientists hold that mitochondria evolved from free-living, aerobic **bacteria** more than a billion years ago. It is hypothesized that mitochondria were engulfed by eukaryotic cells to establish a symbiotic relationship providing metabolic advantages to each.

Mitochondria are able to divide independently without the aid of the cell. The chromosomes of mitochondria are replicated continuously by the enzyme DNA polymerase, with each strand of DNA having different points of origin. Initially, one of the parental strands of DNA is displaced while the other parental strand is being replicated. When the copying of the first strand of DNA is complete, the second strand is replicated in the opposite direction. Mutation rates of mitochondria are much greater than that of nuclear DNA allowing mitochondria to evolve more rapidly than nuclear genes. The resulting **phe-**

notype (cell death, inability to generate energy, or a silent mutation that has no phenotypic effect) is dependent on the number and severity of **mutations** within tissues.

During fertilization, mitochondria within the sperm are excluded from the zygote, resulting in mitochondria that come only from the egg. Thus, mitochondrial DNA is inherited through the maternal lineage exclusively without any **recombination** of genetic material. Therefore, any trait coded for by mitochondrial genes will be inherited from mother to all of her offspring. From an evolutionary standpoint, Mitochondrial Eve represents a single female ancestor from who our mitochondrial genes, not our nuclear genes, were inherited 200,000 years ago. Other women living at that time did not succeed in passing on their mitochondria because their offspring were only male. Although the living descendants of those other females were able to pass on their nuclear genes, only Mitochondrial Eve succeeded in passing on her mitochondrial genes to humans alive today.

See also Mitochondria and cellular energy; Mitochondrial DNA; Molecular biology and molecular genetics; Molecular biology, central dogma of

MOLD

Mold is the general term given to a coating or discoloration found on the surface of certain materials; it is produced by the growth of a fungus. Mold also refers to the causative organism itself.

A mold is a microfungus (as opposed to the macrofungi, such as mushrooms and toadstools) that feeds on dead organic materials. Taxonomically, the molds belong to a group of true **fungi** known as the Ascomycotina. The characteristics of the Ascomycotina are that their spores, that is their reproductive propagules (the fungal equivalent of seeds), are produced inside a structure called an ascus (plural asci). The spores are usually developed eight per ascus, but there are many asci per fruiting body (structures used by the fungus to produce and disperse the spores). A fruiting body of the Ascomycotina is properly referred to as an ascomata. Another characteristic of molds is their rapid growth once suitable conditions are encountered. They can easily produce a patch visible to the naked eye within one day.

The visible appearance of the mold can be of a soft, velvety pad or cottony mass of fungal tissue. If closely observed, the mass can be seen to be made up of a dense aggregation of thread-like mycelia (singular, **mycelium**) of the fungus. Molds can be commonly found on dead and decaying organic material, including improperly stored food stuffs.

The type of mold can be identified by its color and the nature of the substrate on which it is growing. One common example is white bread mold, caused by various species of the genera *Mucor* and *Rhizobium*. Citrus fruits often have quite distinctive blue and green molds of *Penicillium*. Because of the damages this group can cause, they are an economically important group.

In common with the other fungi, the molds reproduce by means of microscopic spores. These tiny spores are easily spread by even weak air currents, and consequently very few places are free of spores due to the astronomical number of spores a single ascomata can produce. Once a spore has landed on a suitable food supply, it requires the correct atmospheric conditions, i.e., a damp atmosphere, to germinate and grow.

Some molds such as *Mucor* and its close relatives have a particularly effective method of a sexual reproduction. A stalked structure is produced, which is topped by a clear, spherical ball with a black disc, within which the spores are developed and held. The whole structure is known as a sporangium (plural, sporangia). Upon maturity, the disc cracks open and releases the spores, which are spread far and wide by the wind. Some other molds, such as *Pilobolus,* fire their spores off like a gun and they land as a sticky mass up to 3 ft (1 m) away. Most of these never grow at all, but due to the vast number produced, up to 100,000 in some cases, this is not a problem for the fungus. As has already been mentioned, these fungi will grow on organic materials, including organic matter found within soil, so many types of molds are present in most places.

When sexual reproduction is carried out, each of the molds require a partner, as they are not capable of self-fertilization. This sexual process is carried out when two different breeding types grow together, and then swap haploid nuclei (containing only half the normal number of **chromosomes**), which then fuse to produce diploid zygospores (a thick-walled cell with a full number of chromosomes). These then germinate and grow into new colonies.

The *Mucor* mold, when grown within a closed environment, has mycelia that are thickly covered with small droplets of water. These are, in fact, diluted solutions of secondary metabolites. Some of the products of mold **metabolism** have great importance.

Rhizopus produces fumaric acid, which can be used in the production of the drug cortisone. Other molds can produce alcohol, citric acid, oxalic acid, or a wide range of other chemicals. Some molds can cause fatal neural diseases in humans and other animals.

Moldy bread is nonpoisonous. Nevertheless, approximately one hundred million loaves of moldy bread are discarded annually in the United States. The molds typically cause spoilage rather than rendering the bread poisonous. Some molds growing on food are believed to cause cancer, particularly of the liver. Another curious effect of mold is related to old, green wallpaper. In the nineteenth century, wallpaper of this color was prepared using compounds of arsenic, and when molds grow on this substrate, they have been known to release arsenic gas.

The first poison to be isolated from a mold is aflatoxin. This and other poisonous substances produced by molds and other fungi are referred to as mycotoxins. Some mycotoxins are deadly to humans in tiny doses, others will only affect certain animals. Aflatoxin was first isolated in 1960 in Great Britain. It was produced by *Aspergillus flavus* that had been growing on peanuts. In that year, aflatoxin had been responsible for the death of 100,000 turkeys—a massive financial loss that led to the research that discovered aflatoxin. From the beginning of the twentieth century, scientists had tentatively linked a number of diseases with molds, but had not been able to isolate the compounds responsible. With the discovery of aflatoxin, scientists were able to provide proof of the undesirable effects of a mold.

Just because a particular mold can produce a mycotoxin does not mean it always will. For example, *Aspergillus flavus* has been safely used for many centuries in China in the production of various cheeses and soy sauce. *Aspergillus flavus* and related species are relatively common, and will grow on a wide variety of substrates, including various food-stuffs and animal feeds. However, the optimum conditions for vegetative growth are different from those required for the production of aflatoxin. The mycotoxin in this species is produced in largest quantities at high moisture levels and moderate temperatures on certain substrates. For a damaging amount of the toxin to accumulate, about ten days at these conditions may be required. Aflatoxin can be produced by *A. flavus* growing on peanuts. However, *A. flavus* will grow on cereal grains (such as wheat, corn, barley, etc.), but the mycotoxin is not produced on these growth media. Aflatoxin production is best prevented by using appropriate storage techniques.

Other molds can produce other mycotoxins, which can be just as problematical as aflatoxin. The term mycotoxin can also include substances responsible for the death of **bacteria**, although these compounds are normally referred to as **antibiotics**.

The molds do not only present humans with problems. Certain types of cheeses are ripened by mold fungi. Indeed, the molds responsible for this action have taken their names from the cheeses they affect. Camembert is ripened by *Penicillium camemberti,* and Roquefort is by *P. roqueforti.*

The *Pencillium* mold have another important use—the production of antibiotics. Two species have been used for the production of **penicillin**, the first antibiotic to be discovered: *Penicillium notatum* and *P. chrysogenum.* The *Penicillium* species can grow on different substrates, such as plants, cloth, leather, paper, wood, tree bark, cork, animal dung, carcasses, ink, syrup, seeds, and virtually any other item that is organic.

A characteristic that this mold does not share with many other species is its capacity to survive at low temperatures. Its growth rate is greatly reduced, but not to the extent of its competition, so as the temperature rises the *Penicillium* is able to rapidly grow over new areas. However, this period of initial growth can be slowed by the presence of other, competing **microorganisms**. Most molds will have been killed by the cold, but various bacteria may still be present. By releasing a chemical into the environment capable of destroying these bacteria, the competition is removed and growth of the *Penicillium* can carry on. This bacteria killing chemical is now recognized as penicillin.

The anti-bacterial qualities of penicillin were originally discovered by Sanford Fleming in 1929. By careful **selection** of the *Penicillium* cultures used, the yield of antibiotic has been increased many hundred fold since the first attempts of commercial scale production during the 1930s.

Other molds are used in various industrial processes. *Aspergillus* terreus is used to manufacture icatonic acid, which

is used in plastics production. Other molds are used in the production of alcohol, a process that utilizes *Rhizopus,* which can metabolize starch into glucose. The *Rhizopus* species can then directly ferment the glucose to give alcohol, but they are not efficient in this process, and at this point brewers **yeast** *(Saccharomyces cerevisiae)* is usually added to ferment the glucose much quicker. Other molds are used in the manufacture of flavorings and chemical additives for food stuffs.

Cheese production has already been mentioned. It is interesting to note that in previous times cheese was merely left in a place where mold production was likely to occur. However, in modern production cheeses are inoculated with a pure **culture** of the mold (some past techniques involved adding a previously infected bit of cheese). Some of the mold varieties used in cheese production are domesticated, and are not found in the wild. In cheese production, the cultures are frequently checked to ensure that no **mutants** have arisen, which could produce unpalatable flavors.

Some molds are important crop **parasites** of species such as corn and millet. A number of toxic molds grow on straw and are responsible for diseases of livestock, including facial eczema in sheep, and slobber syndrome in various grazing animals. Some of the highly toxic chemicals are easy to identify and detect; others are not. Appropriate and sensible storage conditions, i.e., those not favoring the growth of fungi, are an adequate control measure in most cases. If mold is suspected then the use of anti fungal agents (**fungicides**) or destruction of the infected straw are the best options.

See also Fermentation; Food preservation; Food safety; Mycology; Yeast genetics; Yeast, infectious

MOLECULAR BIOLOGY AND MOLECULAR GENETICS

At its most fundamental level, molecular biology is the study of biological molecules and the molecular basis of structure and function in living organisms.

Molecular biology is an interdisciplinary approach to understanding biological functions and regulation at the level of molecules such as nucleic acids, proteins, and carbohydrates. Following the rapid advances in biological science brought about by the development and advancement of the Watson-Crick model of **DNA (deoxyribonucleic acid)** during the 1950s and 1960s, molecular biologists studied **gene** structure and function in increasing detail. In addition to advances in understanding genetic machinery and its regulation, molecular biologists continue to make fundamental and powerful discoveries regarding the structure and function of cells and of the mechanisms of genetic transmission. The continued study of these processes by molecular biologists and the advancement of molecular biological techniques requires integration of knowledge derived from physics, microbiology, mathematics, genetics, **biochemistry**, cell biology and other scientific fields.

Molecular biology also involves organic chemistry, physics, and biophysical chemistry as it deals with the physic-

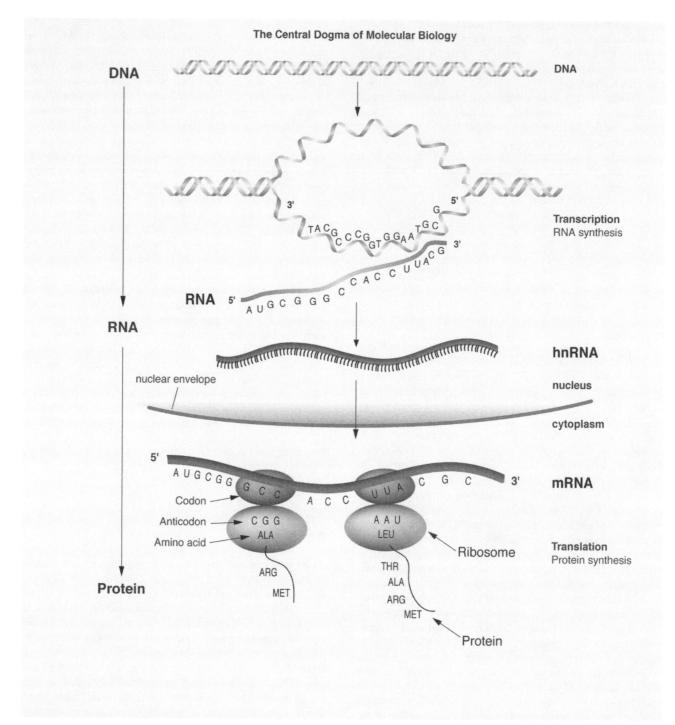

The central dogma of molecular biology, DNA to RNA to protein.

ochemical structure of macromolecules (nucleic acids, proteins, lipids, and carbohydrates) and their interactions. Genetic materials including DNA in most of the living forms or **RNA** (**ribonucleic acid**) in all **plant viruses** and in some animal **viruses** remain the subjects of intense study.

The complete set of genes containing the genetic instructions for making an organism is called its genome. It contains the master blueprint for all cellular structures and activities for the lifetime of the cell or organism. The human genome consists of tightly coiled threads of deoxyribonucleic acid (DNA) and associated protein molecules organized into structures called **chromosomes**. In humans, as in other higher organisms, a DNA molecule consists of two strands that wrap around each other to resemble a twisted ladder whose sides, made of sugar and phosphate molecules are connected by rungs of nitrogen-containing chemicals called bases (nitrogenous bases). Each strand is a linear arrangement of repeating similar units called nucleotides, which are each composed of one sugar, one phosphate, and a nitrogenous base. Four different bases are present in DNA adenine (A), thymine (T), cytosine (C), and guanine (G). The particular order of the bases arranged along the sugar-phosphate backbone is called the DNA sequence; the sequence specifies the exact genetic instructions required to create a particular organism with its own unique traits.

Each time a cell divides into two daughter cells, its full genome is duplicated; for humans and other complex organisms, this duplication occurs in the **nucleus**. During cell division the DNA molecule unwinds and the weak bonds between the base pairs break, allowing the strands to separate. Each strand directs the synthesis of a complementary new strand, with free nucleotides matching up with their complementary bases on each of the separated strands. Nucleotides match up according to strict base-pairing rules. Adenine will pair only with thymine (an A-T pair) and cytosine with guanine (a C-G pair). Each daughter cell receives one old and one new DNA strand. The cell's adherence to these base-pairing rules ensures that the new strand is an exact copy of the old one. This minimizes the incidence of errors (**mutations**) that may greatly affect the resulting organism or its offspring.

Each DNA molecule contains many genes, the basic physical and functional units of heredity. A gene is a specific sequence of nucleotide bases, whose sequences carry the information required for constructing proteins, which provide the structural components of cells and as well as **enzymes** for essential biochemical reactions.

The chromosomes of prokaryotic **microorganisms** differ from eukaryotic microorganisms, in terms of shape and organization of genes. Prokaryotic genes are more closely packed and are usually is arranged along one circular chromosome.

The central dogma of molecular biology states that DNA is copied to make mRNA (messenger RNA), and mRNA is used as the template to make proteins. Formation of RNA is called **transcription** and formation of protein is called **translation**. Transcription and translation processes are regulated at various stages and the regulation steps are unique to prokaryotes and **eukaryotes**. DNA regulation determines what type and amount of mRNA should be transcribed, and this subsequently determines the type and amount of protein. This process is the fundamental control mechanism for growth and development (morphogenesis).

All living organisms are composed largely of proteins, the end product of genes. Proteins are large, complex molecules made up of long chains of subunits called amino acids. The protein-coding instructions from the genes are transmitted indirectly through messenger ribonucleic acid (mRNA), a transient intermediary molecule similar to a single strand of DNA. For the information within a gene to be expressed, a complementary RNA strand is produced (a process called transcription) from the DNA template. In eukaryotes, messenger RNA (mRNA) moves from the nucleus to the cellular **cyto-**

plasm, but in both eukaryotes and prokaryotes mRNA serves as the template for **protein synthesis**.

Twenty different kinds of amino acids are usually found in proteins. Within the gene, sequences of three DNA bases serve as the template for the construction of mRNA with sequence complimentary codons that serve as the language to direct the cell's protein-synthesizing machinery. Cordons specify the insertion of specific amino acids during the synthesis of protein. For example, the base sequence ATG codes for the amino acid methionine. Because more than one codon sequence can specify the same amino acid, the **genetic code** is termed a degenerate code (i.e., there is not a unique codon sequence for every amino acid).

Areas of intense study by molecular biology include the processes of DNA replication, repair, and mutation (alterations in base sequence of DNA). Other areas of study include the identification of agents that cause mutations (e.g., ultra-violet rays, chemicals) and the mechanisms of rearrangement and exchange of genetic materials (e.g. the function and control of small segments of DNA such as **plasmids**, transposable elements, **insertion sequences**, and **transposons** to obtain recombinant DNA).

Recombinant DNA technologies and genetic engineering are an increasingly important part of molecular biology. Advances in **biotechnology** and molecular medicine also carry profound clinical and social significance. Advances in molecular biology have led to significant discoveries concerning the mechanisms of the embryonic development, disease, immunologic response, and **evolution**.

See also Immunogenetics; Microbial genetics

MONOCLONAL ANTIBODY · *see* ANTIBODY, MONOCLONAL

MONOD, JACQUES LUCIEN (1910-1976)
French biologist

French biologist Jacques Lucien Monod and his colleagues demonstrated the process by which messenger **ribonucleic acid** (mRNA) carries instructions for **protein synthesis** from **deoxyribonucleic acid** (**DNA**) in the cell **nucleus** out to the **ribosomes** in the **cytoplasm**, where the instructions are carried out.

Jacques Monod was born in Paris. In 1928, Monod began his study of the natural sciences at the University of Paris, Sorbonne where he went on to receive a B.S. from the *Faculte des Sciences* in 1931. Although he stayed on at the university for further studies, Monod developed further scientific grounding during excursions to the nearby Roscoff marine biology station.

While working at the Roscoff station, Monod met André Lwoff, who introduced him to the potentials of microbiology and microbial nutrition that became the focus of Monod's early research. Two other scientists working at Roscoff station, Boris Ephrussi and Louis Rapkine, taught Monod the importance of physiological and biochemical genetics and the relevance of learning the chemical and molecular aspects of living organisms, respectively.

During the autumn of 1931, Monod took up a fellowship at the University of Strasbourg in the laboratory of Edouard Chatton, France's leading protistologist. In October 1932, he won a Commercy Scholarship that called him back to Paris to work at the Sorbonne once again. This time he was an assistant in the Laboratory of the **Evolution** of Organic Life, which was directed by the French biologist Maurice Caullery. Moving to the zoology department in 1934, Monod became an assistant professor of zoology in less than a year. That summer, Monod also embarked on a natural history expedition to Greenland aboard the *Pourquoi pas?* In 1936, Monod left for the United States with Ephrussi, where he spent time at the California Institute of Technology on a Rockefeller grant. His research centered on studying the fruit fly (*Drosophila melanogaster*) under the direction of Thomas Hunt Morgan, an American geneticist. Here Monod not only encountered new opinions, but he also had his first look at a new way of studying science, a research style based on collective effort and a free passage of critical discussion. Returning to France, Monod completed his studies at the Institute of Physiochemical Biology. In this time he also worked with Georges Teissier, a scientist at the Roscoff station who influenced Monod's interest in the study of **bacterial growth**. This later became the subject of Monod's doctoral thesis at the Sorbonne where he obtained his Ph.D. in 1941.

Monod's work comprised four separate but interrelated phases beginning with his practical education at the Sorbonne. In the early years of his education, he concentrated on the kinetic aspects of biological systems, discovering that the growth rate of **bacteria** could be described in a simple, quantitative way. The size of the **colony** was solely dependent on the food supply; the more sugar Monod gave the bacteria to feed on, the more they grew. Although there was a direct correlation between the amounts of food Monod fed the bacteria and their rate of growth, he also observed that in some colonies of bacteria, growth spread over two phases, sometimes with a period of slow or no growth in between. Monod termed this phenomenon *diauxy* (double growth), and guessed that the bacteria had to employ different **enzymes** to metabolize different kinds of sugars.

When Monod brought the finding to Lwoff's attention in the winter of 1940, Lwoff suggested that Monod investigate the possibility that he had discovered a form of enzyme adaptation, in that the latency period represents a hiatus during which the colony is switching between enzymes. In the previous decade, the Finnish scientist, Henning Karstroem, while working with protein synthesis had recorded a similar phenomenon. Although the outbreak of war and a conflict with his director took Monod away from his lab at the Sorbonne, Lwoff offered him a position in his laboratory at the Pasteur Institute where Monod would remain until 1976. Here he began working with Alice Audureau to investigate the genetic consequences of his kinetic findings, thus beginning the second phase of his work.

To explain his findings with bacteria, Monod shifted his focus to the study of **enzyme induction**. He theorized that cer-

tain colonies of bacteria spent time adapting and producing enzymes capable of processing new kinds of sugars. Although this slowed down the growth of the colony, Monod realized that it was a necessary process because the bacteria needed to adapt to varying environments and foods to survive. Therefore, in devising a mechanism that could be used to sense a change in the environment, and thereby enable the colony to take advantage of the new food, a valuable evolutionary step was taking place. In Darwinian terms, this colony of bacteria would now have a very good chance of surviving, by passing these changes on to future generations. Monod summarized his research and views on relationship between the roles of random chance and adaptation in evolution in his 1970 book *Chance and Necessity*.

Between 1943 and 1945, working with Melvin Cohn, a specialist in **immunology**, Monod hit upon the theory that an inducer acted as an internal signal of the need to produce the required digestive enzyme. This hypothesis challenged the German biochemist Rudolf Schoenheimer's theory of the dynamic state of protein production that stated it was the mix of proteins that resulted in a large number of random combinations. Monod's theory, in contrast, projected a fairly stable and efficient process of protein production that seemed to be controlled by a master plan. In 1953, Monod and Cohn published their findings on the generalized theory of induction.

That year Monod also became the director of the department of cellular biology at the Pasteur Institute and began his collaboration with **François Jacob**. In 1955, working with Jacob, he began the third phase of his work by investigating the relationship between the roles of heredity and environment in enzyme synthesis, that is, how the organism creates these vital elements in its metabolic pathway and how it knows when to create them.

It was this research that led Monod and Jacob to formulate their model of protein synthesis. They identified a **gene** cluster they called the **operon**, at the beginning of a strand of bacterial DNA. These genes, they postulated, send out messages signaling the beginning and end of the production of a specific protein in the cell, depending on what proteins are needed by the cell in its current environment. Within the operons, Monod and Jacob discovered two key genes, which they named the operator and structural genes. The scientists discovered that during protein synthesis, the operator gene sends the signal to begin building the protein. A large molecule then attaches itself to the structural gene to form a strand of mRNA. In addition to the operon, the regulator gene codes for a repressor protein. The repressor protein either attaches to the operator gene and inactivates it, in turn, halting structural gene activity and protein synthesis; or the repressor protein binds to the regulator gene instead of the operator gene, thereby freeing the operator and permitting protein synthesis to occur. As a result of this process, the mRNA, when complete, acts as a template for the creation of a specific protein encoded by the DNA, carrying instructions for protein synthesis from the DNA in the cell's nucleus, to the ribosomes outside the nucleus, where proteins are manufactured. With such a system, a cell can adapt to changing environmental conditions, and produce the proteins it needs when it needs them.

Word of the importance of Monod's work began to spread, and in 1958 he was invited to become professor of **biochemistry** at the Sorbonne, a position he accepted conditional to his retaining his post at the Pasteur Institute. At the Sorbonne, Monod was the chair of chemistry of **metabolism**, but in April 1966, his position was renamed the chair of **molecular biology** in recognition of his research in creating the new science. Monod, Jacob, Lwoff won the 1965 Nobel Prize for physiology or medicine for their discovery of how genes regulate cell metabolism.

See also Bacterial growth and division; Microbial genetics; Molecular biology and molecular genetics

MONONUCLEOSIS, INFECTIOUS

Infectious mononucleosis is an illness caused by the **Epstein-Barr virus**. The symptoms of "mono," as the disease is colloquially called, include extreme fatigue, fever, sore throat, enlargement of the lymph nodes in the neck, armpit, and throat, sore muscles, loss of appetite, and an enlarged spleen. More infrequently, an individual will experience nausea, **hepatitis**, jaundice (which indicates malfunction of the liver), severe headache, chest pain, and difficulty breathing. Children may display only a few or none of these symptoms, while all can be present in adolescents.

The illness can be passed from person to person via the saliva. In adolescents, mononucleosis was once known as "the kissing disease" since kissing is a route of transmission of the Epstein-Barr virus. Given the relative ease of transmissions, epidemic outbreaks of mononucleosis can occur in environments such as schools, hospitals and the workplace.

Infectious mononucleosis is usually self-limiting. Recovery occurs with time and rest, and is usually complete with no after effects. Analgesics can help relieve the symptoms of pain and fever in adults. However, children should avoid taking aspirin, as use of the drug in viral illnesses is associated with the development of Reye syndrome, which can cause liver failure and even death.

Recovery from mononucleosis is not always complete. In some people there can be a decrease in the number of red and white blood cells, due either to damage to the bone marrow (where the blood cells are produced) or to enhanced destruction of the red blood cells (a condition known as hemolytic anemia). Another temporary complication of the illness is weakened or paralyzed facial muscles on one side of the face. The condition, which is called Bell's palsy, leaves the individual with a drooping look to one side of the face. Much more rarely, very severe medical complications can arise. These include rupture of the spleen, swelling of the heart (myocarditis), malfunction of the central nervous system, and Guillain-Barré syndrome. The latter condition is a paralysis resulting from disruption of nervous system function.

The illness is diagnosed in a number of ways. Clinically, the presence of fever, and **inflammation** of the pharynx and the lymph nodes are hallmarks of the illness. Secondly, the so-called "mono spot" test will demonstrate an elevated amount

of **antibody** to the virus in the bloodstream. A third diagnostic feature of the illness is an increase in the number of white blood cells. These cells, which are also called lymphocytes, help fight viral infections.

Antibodies to the Epstein-Barr virus persist for a long time. Therefore, one bout of the illness usually bestows long-lasting **immunity** in an individual. Testing has demonstrated that most people have antibodies to the Epstein-Barr virus. Thus, most people have been infected with the virus at some point in their lives, but have displayed only a few minor symptoms or no symptoms at all. Many children are infected with the virus and either display no symptoms or become transiently ill with one of the retinue of infections acquired during the first few years of life. When the initial infection occurs during adolescence, the development of mononucleosis results 35–50% of the time. Understanding of the reasons for this failure to infect could lead to a **vaccine** to prevent infectious mononucleosis. As of 2002, there is no vaccine available.

The Epstein-Barr virus that is responsible for the illness is a member of the herpesvirus family. The virus is found all over the world and is one of the most common human **viruses**. In infectious mononucleosis, the virus infects and makes new copies of itself in the epithelial cells of the oropharynx. Also, the virus invades the **B cells** of the **immune system**.

For most patients, the infection abates after two to four weeks. Several more weeks may pass before the spleen resumes its normal size. A period of low activity is usually prescribed after a bout of mononucleosis, to protect the spleen and to help energy levels return to normal.

Epstein-Barr virus is usually still present after an infection has ended. The virus becomes dormant in some cells of the throat, in the blood, and in some cells of the immune system. Very rarely in some individuals, the latent virus may be linked to the appearance years later of two types of cancers; Burkitt's lymphoma and nasopharyngeal carcinoma.

See also Viruses and responses to viral infection

MONTAGNIER, LUC (1932-)
French virologist

Luc Montagnier, Distinguished Professor at Queens College in New York and the Institut Pasteur in Paris, has devoted his career to the study of **viruses**. He is perhaps best known for his 1983 discovery of the **human immunodeficiency virus (HIV)**, which has been identified as the cause of acquired **immunodeficiency** syndrome (**AIDS**). However, in the twenty years before the onset of the AIDS epidemic, Montagnier made many significant discoveries concerning the nature of viruses. He made major contributions to the understanding of how viruses can alter the genetic information of host organisms, and significantly advanced cancer research. His investigation of interferon, one of the body's defenses against viruses, also opened avenues for medical cures for viral diseases. Montagnier's ongoing research focuses on the search for an AIDS **vaccine** or cure.

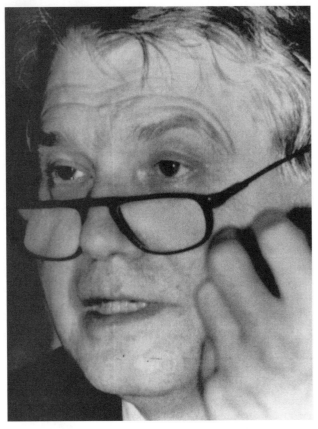

Luc Montagnier

Montagnier was born in Chabris (near Tours), France, the only child of Antoine Montagnier and Marianne Rousselet. He became interested in science in his early childhood through his father, an accountant by profession, who carried out experiments on Sundays in a makeshift laboratory in the basement of the family home. At age fourteen, Montagnier himself conducted nitroglycerine experiments in the basement laboratory. His desire to contribute to medical knowledge was also kindled by his grandfather's long illness and death from colon cancer.

Montagnier attended the Collège de Châtellerault, and then the University of Poitiers, where he received the equivalent of a bachelor's degree in the natural sciences in 1953. Continuing his studies at Poitiers and then at the University of Paris, he received his licence ès sciences in 1955. As an assistant to the science faculty at Paris, he taught physiology at the Sorbonne and in 1960, qualified there for his doctorate in medicine. He was appointed a researcher at the Centre National de la Recherche Scientifique (C.N.R.S.) in 1960, but then went to London for three and a half years to do research at the Medical Research Council at Carshalton.

Viruses are agents that consist of genetic material surrounded by a protective protein shell. They are completely dependent on the cells of a host animal or plant to multiply, a process that begins with the shedding of their own protein shell. The virus research group at Carshalton was investigating **ribonucleic acid** (**RNA**), a form of nucleic acid that normally is involved in taking genetic information from **deoxyribonucleic acid** (**DNA**) (the main carrier of genetic information) and translating it into proteins. Montagnier and F. K. Sanders, investigating viral RNA (a virus that carries its genetic material in RNA rather than DNA), discovered a double-stranded RNA virus that had been made by the replication of a single-stranded RNA. The double-stranded RNA could transfer its genetic information to DNA, allowing the virus to encode itself in the genetic make-up of the host organism. This discovery represented a significant advance in knowledge concerning viruses.

From 1963 to 1965, Montagnier did research at the Institute of **Virology** in Glasgow, Scotland. Working with Ian MacPherson, he discovered in 1964 that **agar**, a gelatinous extractive of a red alga, was an excellent substance for culturing cancer cells. Their technique became standard in laboratories investigating oncogenes (genes that have the potential to make normal cells turn cancerous) and cell transformations. Montagnier himself used the new technique to look for cancer-causing viruses in humans after his return to France in 1965.

From 1965 to 1972, Montagnier worked as laboratory director of the Institut de Radium (later called Institut Curie) at Orsay. In 1972, he founded and became director of the viral oncology unit of the Institut Pasteur. Motivated by his findings at Carshalton and the belief that some cancers are caused by viruses, Montagnier's basic research interest during those years was in **retroviruses** as a potential cause of cancer. Retroviruses possess an enzyme called reverse transcriptase. Montagnier established that reverse transcriptase translates the genetic instructions of the virus from the viral (RNA) form to DNA, allowing the genes of the virus to become permanently established in the cells of the host organism. Once established, the virus can begin to multiply, but it can do so only by multiplying cells of the host organism, forming malignant tumors. In addition, collaborating with Edward De Mayer and Jacqueline De Mayer, Montagnier isolated the messenger RNA of interferon, the cell's first defense against a virus. Ultimately, this research allowed the **cloning** of interferon genes in a quantity sufficient for research. However, despite widespread hopes for interferon as a broadly effective anti-cancer drug, it was initially found to be effective in only a few rare kinds of malignancies.

AIDS (acquired immunodeficiency syndrome), an epidemic that emerged in the early 1980s, was first adequately characterized around 1982. Its chief feature is that it disables the **immune system** by which the body defends itself against numerous diseases. It is eventually fatal. By 1993, more than three million people had developed AIDS. Montagnier considered that a retrovirus might be responsible for AIDS. Researchers had noted that one pre-AIDS condition involved a persistent enlargement of the lymph nodes, called lymphadenopathy. Obtaining some tissue **culture** from the lymph nodes of an infected patient in 1983, Montagnier and two colleagues, Françoise Barré-Sinoussi and Jean-Claude Chermann, searched for and found reverse transcriptase, which constitutes evidence of a retrovirus. They isolated a virus they called LAV (lymphadenopathy-associated virus). Later, by international agreement, it was renamed HIV, human immunodeficiency virus. After the virus had been isolated, it was possible to develop a test for antibodies that had developed against it—the HIV test. Montagnier and his group also discovered that HIV attacks T4 cells, which are crucial in the immune system. A second similar but not identical HIV virus called HIV–2 was discovered by Montagnier and colleagues in April 1986.

A controversy developed over the patent on the HIV test in the mid–1980s. **Robert C. Gallo** of the National Cancer Institute in Bethesda, Maryland, announced his own discovery of the HIV virus in April 1984 and received the patent on the test. The Institut Pasteur claimed the patent (and the profits) based on Montagnier's earlier discovery of HIV. Despite the controversy, Montagnier continued research and attended numerous scientific meetings with Gallo to share information. Intense mediation efforts by **Jonas Salk** (the scientist who developed the first polio vaccine) led to an international agreement signed by the scientists and their respective countries in 1987. Montagnier and Gallo agreed to be recognized as co-discoverers of the virus, and the two governments agreed that the profits of the HIV test be shared most going to a foundation for AIDS research).

The scientific dispute continued to resurface, however. Most HIV viruses from different patients differ by six to twenty percent because of the remarkable ability of the virus to mutate. However, Gallo's virus was less than two percent different from Montagnier's, leading to the suspicion that both viruses were from the same source. The laboratories had exchanged samples in the early 1980s, which strengthened the suspicion. Charges of scientific misconduct on Gallo's part led to an investigation by the National Institutes of Health in 1991, which initially cleared Gallo. In 1992, the investigation was reviewed by the newly created Office of Research Integrity. The ORI report, issued in March of 1993, confirmed that Gallo had in fact "discovered" the virus sent to him by Montagnier. Whether Gallo had been aware of this fact in 1983 could not be established, but it was found that he had been guilty of misrepresentations in reporting his research and that his supervision of his research lab had been desultory. The Institut Pasteur immediately revived its claim to the exclusive right to the patent on the HIV test. Gallo objected to the decision by the ORI, however, and took his case before an appeals board at the Department of Health and Human Services. The board in December of 1993 cleared Gallo of all charges, and the ORI subsequently withdrew their charges for lack of proof.

More than a decade after setting the personal considerations aside, in May of 2002, the two scientists announced a partnership in the effort to speed the development of a vaccine against AIDS. Gallo will oversee research from the Institute of Human Virology, while Montagnier pursues concurrent research as head of the World Foundation for AIDS Research and Prevention in New York, Rome, and Paris.

Montagnier's continuing work includes investigation of the envelope proteins of the virus that link it to the T-cell. He is also extensively involved in research of possible drugs to combat AIDS. In 1990, Montagnier hypothesized that a second organism, called a mycoplasma, must be present with the HIV virus for the latter to become deadly. This suggestion,

which has proved controversial among most AIDS researchers, is the subject of ongoing research.

Montagnier married Dorothea Ackerman in 1961. The couple has three children. He has described himself as an aggressive researcher who spends much time in either the laboratory or traveling to scientific meetings. Montagnier enjoys swimming and classical music, and loves to play the piano, especially Mozart sonatas.

See also AIDS, recent advances in research and treatment; Immunodeficiency diseases; Viruses and responses to viral infection

MONTAGUE, MARY WORTLEY
(1689-1762)
English smallpox vaccination advocate

Lady Mary Wortley Montague contributed to microbiology and **immunology** by virtue of her powers of observation and her passion for letter writing. As the wife of the British Ambassador Extraordinary to the Turkish court, Montague and her family lived in Istanbul. While there she observed and was convinced of the protective power of inoculation against the disease **smallpox**. She wrote to friends in England describing inoculation and later, upon their return to England, she worked to popularize the practice of inoculation in that country.

Montague's interest in smallpox stemmed from her brush with the disease in 1715, which left her with a scarred face and lacking eyebrows, and also from the death of her brother from the disease. While posted in Istanbul, she was introduced to the practice of inoculation. Material picked from a smallpox scab on the surface of the skin was rubbed into an open cut of another person. The recipient would usually develop a mild case of smallpox but would never be ravaged by the full severity of the disease caused by more virulent strains of the smallpox virus. Lady Montague was so enthused by the protection offered against smallpox that she insisted on having her children inoculated. In 1718, her three-year-old son was inoculated. In 1721, having returned to England, she insisted that her English doctor inoculate her five-year-old daughter.

Upon her return to England following the expiration of her husband's posting, Montague used her standing in the high society of the day to promote the benefits of smallpox inoculation. Her passion convinced a number of English physicians and even the reigning Queen, who decreed that the royal children and future heirs to the crown would be inoculated against the disease. In a short time, it became fashionable to be one of those who had received an inoculation, partly perhaps because it was a benefit available only to the wealthy. Inoculation became a sign of status.

Smallpox outbreaks of the eighteenth century in England demonstrated the effectiveness of inoculation. The death rate among those who had been inoculated against smallpox was far less than among the uninoculated.

A few decades later, **Edward Jenner** refined the inoculation process by devising a **vaccine** for smallpox. History has tended to credit Jenner with the discovery of a cure for small-pox. This is likely a reflection of the lack of credence given by the mostly male medical profession to the opinions of women. But there is no doubt that Jenner was aware of, and built upon, the inoculation strategy popularized by Lady Montague.

The receptiveness toward smallpox **vaccination** initially, and subsequently to a variety of vaccination strategies, stemmed from the efforts of Lady Montague. The acceptance of inoculation among the rich, powerful and influential of Europe led to the general acceptance of the practice among all sectors of society. With time, smallpox vaccination grew in worldwide popularity. So much so that in 1979, the United Nations **World Health Organization** declared that smallpox had been essentially eradicated. The pioneering efforts of Lady Montague have saved hundreds of millions of lives over the last 284 years.

See also Immunity, active, passive and delayed

MOORE, RUTH ELLA (1903-1994)
American bacteriologist

Ruth Ella Moore achieved distinction when she became the first African American woman to earn a Ph.D. in bacteriology from Ohio State in 1933. Her entire teaching career was spent at Howard University in Washington, D.C., where she remained an associate professor emeritus of microbiology until 1990.

Moore was born in Columbus, Ohio, on May 19, 1903. After receiving her B.S. from Ohio State in 1926, she continued at that university and received her M.A. the following year. In 1933 she earned her Ph.D. in bacteriology from Ohio State, becoming the first African American woman to do so. Her achievement was doubly significant considering that her minority status was combined with that era's social prejudices against women in professional fields. During her graduate school years (1927–1930), Moore was an instructor of both **hygiene** and English at Tennessee State College. Upon completing her dissertation at Ohio State—where she focused on the bacteriological aspects of **tuberculosis** (a major national health problem in the 1930s—she received her Ph.D.

Moore accepted a position at the Howard University College of Medicine as an instructor of bacteriology. In 1939 she became an assistant professor of bacteriology, and in 1948 she was named acting head of the university's department of bacteriology, preventive medicine, and **public health**. In 1955, she became head of the department of bacteriology and remained in that position until 1960 when she became an associate professor of microbiology at Howard. She remained in that department until her retirement in 1973, whereupon she became an associate professor emeritus of microbiology.

Throughout her career, Moore remained concerned with public health issues, and remained a member of the American Public Health Association and the American Society of Microbiologists.

See also History of microbiology; History of public health; Medical training and careers in microbiology

MOST PROBABLE NUMBER (MPN) · *see*
LABORATORY TECHNIQUES IN MICROBIOLOGY

MUMPS

Mumps is a contagious viral disease that causes painful enlargement of the salivary glands, most commonly the parotids. Mumps is sometimes known as epidemic parotitis and occurs most often in children between the ages of 4 and 14.

Mumps was first described by Hippocrates (c.460–c.370 B.C.), who observed that the diseases occurred most commonly in young men, a fact that he attributed to their congregating at sports grounds. Women, who were inclined to be isolated in their own homes, were seldom taken ill with the disease. Over the centuries, medical writers paid little attention to mumps. Occasionally, mention was made of a local epidemic of the disease, as recorded in Paris, France, in the sixteenth century by Guillaume de Baillou (1538–1616). Most physicians believed that the disease was contagious, but no studies were made to confirm this suspicion. The first detailed scientific description of mumps was provided by the British physician Robert Hamilton (1721–1793) in 1790. Hamilton's paper in the Transactions of the Royal Society of Edinburgh finally made the disease well known among physicians. Efforts to prove the contagious nature of mumps date around 1913. In that year, two French physicians, Charles-Jean-Henri Nicolle (1866–1936) and Ernest Alfred Conseil, attempted to transmit mumps from humans to monkeys, but were unable to obtain conclusive results. Eight years later, Martha Wollstein injected **viruses** taken from the saliva of a mumps patient into cats, producing **inflammation** of the parotid, testes, and brain tissue in the cats. Conclusive proof that mumps is transmitted by a filterable virus was finally obtained by two American researchers, Claude D. Johnson and **Ernest William Goodpasture** (1886–1960), in 1934.

The mumps virus has an incubation period of 12-28 days with an average of 18 days. Pain and swelling in the region of one parotid gland, accompanied by some fever, is the characteristic initial presenting feature. About five days later, the other parotid gland may become affected while the swelling in the first gland has mainly subsided. In most children, the infection is mild and the swelling in the salivary glands usually disappears within two weeks. Occasionally, there is no obvious swelling of the glands during the infection. Children with mumps are infectious from days one to three before the parotid glands begin to swell, and remain so until about seven days after the swelling has disappeared. The disease can be transmitted through respiratory droplets. There are occasional complications in children with mumps. In the central nervous system (CNS), a rare complication is aseptic **meningitis** or encephalitis. This usually has an excellent prognosis. In about 20% of post-pubertal males, orchitis may arise as a complication and, rarely, can lead to sterility. A very rare additional complication is pancreatitis, which may require treatment and hospitalization.

The diagnosis of mumps in children is usually made on the basis of its very characteristic symptoms. The virus can be cultured, however, and can be isolated from a patient by taking a swab from the buccal (mouth) outlet of the parotid gland duct. The swab is then broken off into viral transport medium. **Culture** of the virus is rarely necessary in a straightforward case of mumps parotitis. Occasionally, it is necessary to isolate the virus from the cerebro-spinal fluid (CSF) of patients with CNS complications such as mumps meningitis. Also, serological investigations may be useful in aseptic meningitis and encephalitis.

A **vaccine** for mumps was developed by the American microbiologist, John Enders, in 1948. During World War II, Enders had developed a vaccine using a killed virus, but it was only moderately and temporarily successful. After the war, he began to investigate ways of growing mumps virus in a suspension of minced chick embryo and ox blood. The technique was successful and Enders' live virus vaccine is now routinely used to vaccinate children. In the U.S.A., the live attenuated mumps vaccine is sometimes given alone or together with **measles** and/or rubella vaccine. The MMR vaccine came under investigation with regard to a possible link to autism in children. The United States **Centers for Disease Control** concludes that current scientific evidence does not support any hypothesis that the MMR vaccine causes any form of autism. The hypothetical relationship, however, did discourage and continues to discourage some parents from allowing their children to receive the triple vaccine.

See also Antibody-antigen, biochemical and molecular reactions; History of immunology; History of public health; Immunity, active, passive and delayed; Immunology; Varicella; Viruses and responses to viral infection

MURCHISON METEORITE

The Murchison meteorite was a meteorite that entered Earth's atmosphere in September, 1969. The meteor fragmented before impact and remnants were recovered near Murchison, Australia (located about 60 miles north of Melbourne). The fragments recovered dated to nearly five billion years ago—to the time greater than the estimated age of Earth. In addition to interest generated by the age of the meteorite, analysis of fragments revealed evidence of carbon based compounds. The finds have fueled research into whether the organic compounds were formed from inorganic processes or are proof of extraterrestrial life dating to the time of Earth's creation.

In particular, it was the discovery of amino acids—and the percentages of the differing types of amino acids found (e.g., the number of left handed amino acids vs. right handed amino acids—that made plausible the apparent evidence of extraterrestrial organic processes, as opposed to biological **contamination** by terrestrial sources.

If the compounds prove to be from extraterrestrial life, this would constitute a profound discovery that would have far reaching global scientific and social impact concerning pre-

vailing hypotheses concerning the **origin of life**. For example, some scientists, notably one of the discoverers of the structure of **DNA**, Sir **Francis Crick**, assert that in the period from the formation of Earth to the time of the deposition of the earliest discovered fossilized remains, there was insufficient time for evolutionary process to bring forth life in the abundance and variety demonstrated in the fossil record. Crick and others propose that a form of organic molecular "seeding" by meteorites exemplified by the Murchison meteorite (meteorites rich in complex carbon compounds) greatly reduced the time needed to develop life on Earth.

In fact, the proportions of the amino acids found in the Murchison meteorite approximated the proportions proposed to exist in the primitive atmosphere modeled in the **Miller-Urey experiment**. First conducted in 1953, University of Chicago researchers **Stanley L. Miller** and Harold C. Urey developed an experiment to test possible mechanisms in Earth's primitive atmosphere that could have produced organic molecules from inorganic processes. Methane (CH_4), hydrogen (H_2), and ammonia (NH_3) gases were introduced into a moist environment above a water-containing flask. To simulate primitive lightning discharges, Miller supplied the system with electrical current. Within days, organic compounds formed—including some amino acids. A classic experiment in **molecular biology**, the Miller-Urey experiment established that the conditions that existed in Earth's primitive atmosphere were sufficient to produce amino acids, the subunits of proteins comprising and required by living organisms. It is possible, however, that extraterrestrial organic molecules could have accelerated the formation of terrestrial organic molecules by serving as molecular templates.

In 1997, NASA scientists announced evidence that the Murchison meteorite contained microfossils that resemble **microorganisms**. The microfossils were discovered in fresh breaks of meteorite material. The potential finding remains the subject of intense scientific study and debate.

University of Texas scientists Robert Folk and F. Leo Lynch also announced the observation of fossils of terrestrial nanobacteria in another carbonaceous chondrite meteorite named the Allende meteorite. Other research has demonstrated that the Murchison and Murray meteorites (a carbonaceous chondrite meteorite found in Kentucky) contain sugars critical for the development of life.

See also Evolution and evolutionary mechanisms; Evolutionary origin of bacteria and viruses; Life, origin of

MUREIN • *see* PEPTIDOGLYCAN

MURRAY, ROBERT (1919-)
British bacteriologist

Robert George Everitt Murray is professor emeritus and former department chair of the Department of Microbiology and **Immunology** at the University of Western Ontario in London. His numerous accomplishments in bacterial taxonomy, ultrastructure, and education have been recognized by his investiture as an officer of the Order of Canada in 1998.

Murray received his early education in Britain, but moved to Montreal in 1930 where his father was Professor of Bacteriology and Immunology at McGill University. He attended McGill from 1936 to 1938,then returned to England to study at Cambridge University (B.A. in Pathology and Bacteriology in 1941 and with a M.A. in the same discipline in 1945). In 1943 he also received a M.D. degree from McGill.

In 1945, Murray joined the faculty of the Department of Bacteriology and Immunology at the University of Western Ontario in London as a Lecturer. He remained at Western for the remainder of his career. He was appointed Professor and Head of the department in 1949 and served as head until 1974. Since his retirement in 1984 he has been Professor Emeritus.

Murray has served as President of the American Society for Microbiology in 1972–1973 and was one of the founders of the Canadian Society for Microbiologists in 1951. In 1954, he became the founding editor of the Canadian Journal of Microbiology, which continues to publish to this day.

His interest in taxonomy continued a family tradition begun by his father, E.G.D. Murray, who was a trustee of the Bergey's Manual of determinative Bacteriology from 1936 until his death in 1964. Robert Murray succeeded his late family on the Board of Trustees of the Manual. He chaired the Board from 1976 to 1990.

In addition to these responsibilities, Murray has served the microbiology community by his editorial guidance of various journals of the American Society for Microbiology and other international societies.

During his tenure at the University of Western Ontario, Murray and his colleagues and students conducted research that has greatly advanced the understanding of how **bacteria** are constructed and function. For example, the use of light and electron microscopy and techniques such as x-ray diffraction revealed the presence and some of the structural details of the so-called regularly structured (or RS) layer that overlays some bacteria. In another area, Murray discovered and revealed many structural and behavior aspects of a bacterium called *Deinococcus radiodurans*. This bacterium displays resistance to levels of radiation that are typically lethal to bacteria.

Such research has been acknowledged with a number of awards and honorary degrees. Murray's contribution to Canadian microbiology continues. He is a member of the Board of Directors of the Canadian Bacterial Diseases Network of Centres of Excellence.

See also Bacterial ultrastructure; Radiation resistant bacteria

MUTANTS: ENHANCED TOLERANCE OR SENSITIVITY TO TEMPERATURE AND pH RANGES

Microorganisms have optimal environmental conditions under which they grow best. Classification of microorganisms in terms of growth rate dependence on temperature includes the thermopiles, the mesophiles and psychrophiles. Similarly, while most organisms grow well in neutral **pH** conditions, some organisms grow well under acidic conditions, while others can grow under alkaline conditions. The mechanism by which such control exists is being studied in detail. This will overcome the need to obtain mutants by a slow and unsure process of acclimatization.

When some organisms are subjected to high temperatures, they respond by synthesizing a group of proteins that help to stabilize the internal cellular environment. These, called heat shock proteins, are present in both prokaryotes and **eukaryotes**. Heat stress specifically induces the **transcription** of genes encoding these proteins. Comparisons of amino acid sequences of these proteins from the **bacteria** *Escherichia coli* and the fruit fly *Drosophila* show that they are 40%–50% identical. This is remarkable considering the length of evolutionary time separating the two organisms.

Fungi are able to sense extracellular pH and alter the expression of genes. Some fungi secrete acids during growth making their environment particularly acidic. A strain of *Asperigillus nidulans* encodes a regulatory protein that activates transcription of genes during growth under alkaline conditions and prevents transcription of genes expressed in acidic conditions. A number of other genes originally found by analysis of mutants have been identified as mediating pH regulation, and some of these have been cloned. Improved understanding of pH sensing and regulation of **gene** expression will play an important role in gene manipulation for **biotechnology**.

The pH of the external growth medium has been shown to regulate gene expression in several enteric bacteria like *Vibrio cholerae*. Some of the acid-shock genes in *Salmonella* may turn out to assist its growth, possibly by preventing lysosomal acidification. Interestingly, acid also induces virulence in the plant pathogen (harmful microorganism) *Agrobacterium tumefaciens*.

Study of pH-regulated genes is slowly leading to knowledge about pH homeostasis, an important capability of many enteric bacteria by which they maintain intracellular pH. Furthermore, it is felt that pH interacts in important ways with other environmental and metabolic pathways involving anaerobiosis, sodium (Na^+) and potassium (K^+) levels, **DNA** repair, and amino acid degradation. Two different kinds of inducible pH homeostasis mechanisms that have been demonstrated are acid tolerance and the sodium-proton antiporter NhaA. Both cases are complex, involving several different stimuli and gene loci.

Salmonella typhimurium(the bacteria responsible for **typhoid fever**) that grows in moderately acid medium (pH 5.5–6.0) induces genes whose products enable cells to retain viability (ability to live) under more extreme acid conditions (below pH 4) where growth is not possible. Close to 100% of acid-tolerant (or acid-adapted) cells can recover from extreme-acid exposure and grow at neutral pH. The inducible survival mechanism is called acid tolerance response. The retention of viability by acid-tolerant cells correlates with improved pH homeostasis at low external pH represents inducible pH homeostasis.

Cells detect external alkalization with the help of a mechanism known as the alkaline signal **transduction** system. Under such environmental conditions, an inducible system for internal pH homeostasis works in *E. coli*. The so-called sodium-proton antiporter gene NhaA is induced at high external pH in the presence of high sodium. The NhaA antiporter acts to acidify the **cytoplasm** through proton/sodium exchange. This allows the microorganism to survive above its normal pH range. As *B. alkalophilus* may have as many as three sodium-proton antiporters, it is felt that the number of antiporters may relate to the alkalophilicity of a species.

The search for **extremophiles** has intensified recently. Standard **enzymes** stop working when exposed to heat or other extreme conditions, so manufacturers that rely on them must often take special steps to protect (stabilize) the proteins during reactions or storage. By remaining active when other enzymes would fail, enzymes from extremophiles (extremozymes) can potentially eliminate the need for those added steps, thereby increasing efficiency and reducing costs in many applications.

Many routes are being followed to use the capacity that such extremophiles possess. First, the direct use of these natural mutants to grow and produce the useful products. Also, it is possible with recombinant DNA technology to isolate genes from such organisms that grow under unusual conditions and clone them on to a fast growing organism. For example, an enzyme alpha-amylase is required to function at high temperature for the hydrolysis of starch to glucose. The gene for the enzyme was isolated from *Bacillus stearothermophilus,* an organism that is grows naturally at 194°F (90°C), and cloned into another suitable organism. Finally, attempts are being made to stabilize the proteins themselves by adding some groups (e.g., disulfide bonds) that prevent its easy denaturation. This process is called protein engineering.

Conventional mutagenesis and **selection** schemes can be used in an attempt to create and perpetuate a mutant form of a gene that encodes a protein with the desired properties. However, the number of mutant proteins that are possible after alteration of individual nucleotides within a structural gene by this method is extremely large. This type of mutagenesis also could lead to significant decrease in the activity of the enzyme. By using set techniques that specifically change amino-acids encoded by a cloned gene, proteins with properties that are better than those obtained from the naturally occurring strain can be obtained. Unfortunately, it is not possible to know in advance which particular amino acid or short sequence of amino acids will contribute to particular changes in physical, chemical, or kinetic properties. A particular property of a protein, for example, will be influenced by amino acids quite far apart in the linear chain as a consequence of the folding of the protein, which may bring them into close proximity. The amino acid sequences that would bring about change in physical properties of the protein can be obtained after characterization of the three dimensional structure of purified and crystallized protein using x-ray crystallography and other analytical procedures. Many approaches are being tried to bring about this type of "directed mutagenesis" once the specific nucleotide that needs to be altered is known.

See also Bacterial adaptation; Evolutionary origin of bacteria and viruses; Microbial genetics; Mutations and mutagenesis

MUTATIONS

A mutation is any change in genetic material that is passed on to the next generation. The process of acquiring change in genetic material forms the fundamental underpinning of **evolution**. Mutation is a source of genetic variation in all life forms. Depending on the organism or the source of the mutation, the genetic alteration may be an alteration in the organized collection of genetic material, or a change in the composition of an individual **gene**.

Mutations may have little impact, or they may produce a significant positive or negative impact, on the health, competitiveness, or function of an individual, family, or population.

Mutations arise in different ways. An alteration in the sequence, but not in the number of nucleotides in a gene is a nucleotide substitution. Two types of nucleotide substitution mutations are missense and nonsense mutations. Missense mutations are single base changes that result in the substitution of one amino acid for another in the protein product of the gene. Nonsense mutations are also single base changes, but create a termination codon that stops the **transcription** of the gene. The result is a shortened, dysfunctional protein product.

Another mutation involves the alteration in the number of bases in a gene. This is an insertion or deletion mutation. The impact of an insertion or deletion is a frameshift, in which the normal sequence with which the genetic material is interpreted is altered. The alteration causes the gene to code for a different sequence of amino acids in the protein product than would normally be produced. The result is a protein that functions differently—or not all—as compared to the normally encoded version.

Genomes naturally contain areas in which a nucleotide repeats in a triplet. Trinucleotide repeat mutations, an increased number of triplets, are now known to be the cause of at least eight genetic disorders affecting the nervous or neuromuscular systems.

Mutations arise from a number of processes collectively termed mutagenesis. Frameshift mutations, specifically insertions, result from mutagenic events where **DNA** is inserted into the normally functioning gene. The genetic technique of insertional mutagenesis relies upon this behavior to locate target genes, to study gene expression, and to study protein structure-function relationships.

DNA mutagenesis also occurs because of breakage or base modification due to the application of radiation, chemicals, ultraviolet light, and random replication errors. Such mutagenic events occur frequently, and the cell has evolved repair mechanisms to deal with them. High exposure to DNA damaging agents, however, can overwhelm the repair machinery.

Genetic research relies upon the ability to induce mutations in the lab. Using purified DNA of a known restriction map, site-specific mutagenesis can be performed in a number of ways. Some **restriction enzymes** produce staggered nicks at the site of action in the target DNA. Short pieces of DNA (linkers) can subsequently be introduced at the staggered cut site, to alter the sequence of the DNA following its repair. Cassette mutagenesis can be used to introduce selectable genes at the specific site in the DNA. Typically, these are drug-resistance genes. The activity of the insert can then be monitored by the development of resistance in the transformed cell. In deletion formation, DNA can be cut at more than one restriction site and the cut regions can be induced to join, eliminating the region of intervening DNA. Thus, deletions of defined length and sequence can be created, generating tailor-made deletions. With site-directed mutagenesis, DNA of known sequence that differs from the target sequence of the original DNA, can be chemically synthesized and introduced at the target site. The insertion causes the production of a mutation of pre-determined sequence. Site-directed mutagenesis is an especially useful research tool in inducing changes in the shape of proteins, permitting precise structure-function relationships to be probed. Localized mutagenesis, also known as heavy mutagenesis, induces mutations in a small portion of DNA. In many cases, mutations are identified by the classical technique of phenotypic identification—looking for an alteration in appearance or behavior of the mutant.

Mutagenesis is exploited in **biotechnology** to create new **enzymes** with new specificity. Simple mutations will likely not have as drastic an effect as the simultaneous alteration of multiple amino acids. The combination of mutations that produce the desired three-dimensional change, and so change in enzyme specificity, is difficult to predict. The best progress is often made by creating all the different mutational combinations of DNA using different **plasmids**, and then using these **plasmids** as a mixture to transform *Escherichia coli* **bacteria**. The expression of the different proteins can be monitored and the desired protein resolved and used for further manipulations.

See also Cell cycle (eukaryotic), genetic regulation of; Cell cycle (prokaryotic), genetic regulation of; Chemical mutagenesis; Chromosomes, eukaryotic; Chromosomes, prokaryotic; DNA (Deoxyribonucleic acid); Laboratory techniques in immunology; Mitochondrial DNA; Mitochondrial inheritance; Molecular biology and molecular genetics

MYCELIUM

Mycelium (plural, mycelia) is an extension of the **hyphae** of **fungi**. A hyphae is a thread-like, branching structure formed by fungi. As the hyphae grows, it becomes longer and branches off, forming a mycelium network visually reminiscent of the branches of tree.

The mycelium is the most important and permanent part of a fungus. The mycelia network that emanates from a fungal spore can extend over and into the soil in search of nutrients. The ends of some mycelia terminate as mushrooms and toadstools.

Mycelium have been recognized as fungal structures for a long time. The author Beatrix Potter provided accurate sketches of mycelium over 100 years ago. At the time her

observations were considered irrelevant and the significance of mycelium was lost until some years after her work.

The growth of mycelia can be extensive. A form of honey fungus found in the forests of Michigan, which began from a single spore and grows mainly underground, now is estimated to cover 40 acres. The mycelia network is thought to be over 100 tons in weight and is at least 1,500 years old. More recently, another species of fungus discovered in Washington State was found to cover at least 1,500 acres

The initial hyphae produced by a fungus has only one copy of each of its **chromosomes**. Thus, it is haploid. The resulting mycelium will also be haploid. When one haploid mycelium meets another haploid mycelium of the same species, the two mycelia can fuse. The fused cells then contain two nuclei. In contrast to plants and animals, where the nuclei would fuse, forming a functional **nucleus** containing two copies of each chromosome (a diploid state), the two nuclei in the fugal cell remain autonomous and function separate from one another.

Fusion of the nuclei does occur as a prelude to spore formation. Several duplications and shuffling of the genetic material produces four spores, each with a unique genetic identity.

At any one time, part of a mycelia network may be actively growing while another region may be dormant, awaiting more suitable conditions for growth. Mycelium is able to seek out such suitable conditions by moving towards a particular food source, such as a root. Also mycelium can change their texture, for example from a fluffy state to a thin compressed state or to thicker cord-like growths. All these attributes enable the mycelium to ensure the continued growth of the fungus.

See also Armillaria ostoyae; Fungal genetics

MYCOBACTERIAL INFECTIONS, ATYPICAL

Atypical mycobacteria are species of mycobacteria that are similar to the mycobacteria that are the cause of **tuberculosis**. Like other mycobacteria, they are rod-like in shape and they are stained for observation by light microscopy using a specialized staining method called acid-fast staining. The need for this staining method reflects the unusual cell wall chemistry of mycobacteria, relative to other **bacteria**. In contrast to other mycobacteria, atypical mycobacteria do not cause tuberculosis. Accordingly, the group of bacteria is also described as nonpneumoniae mycobacteria. This group of bacteria is also designated as MOTT (mycobacteria other than tuberculosis). Examples of atypical mycobacteria include *Mycobacterium kansasii*, *Mycobacterium avium*, *Mycobacterium intracellulare*, *Mycobacterium marinum*, and *Mycobacterium ulcerans*.

The atypical mycobacteria are widely present in the environment. They inhabit fresh and salt water, milk, soil, and the feces of birds. Other environmental niches, which so far have not been determined, are possible. The nature of their habitats suggests that transmission to people via soiled or dirty hands, and the ingestion of contaminated water or milk would be typical. Yet, little is still known about how people become contaminated. One species, known as *Mycobacterium marinum*, is found in swimming pool water, and can cause a skin infection in fingers or toes upon contact with the skin of a swimmer. Additionally, some evidence supports the transmission of atypical mycobacteria in aerosols (that is, as part of tiny droplets that can drift through the air and become inhaled).

Contamination with atypical mycobacteria may be a natural part of life. For the majority of people, whose immune systems are functioning efficiently, the microbe does not establish an infection. However, for those who **immune system** is not operating well, the presence of the atypical mycobacteria is a problem. Indeed, for those afflicted with acquired **immunodeficiency** syndrome (**AIDS**), infection with atypical mycobacteria (typically with *Mycobacterium avium* and *Mycobacterium intracellulare*) is almost universal.

Atypical mycobacteria tend to first establish a foothold in the lungs. From there the bacteria can spread, via the bloodstream, throughout the body. Infections in almost every organ of the body can ensue. Examples of sites of infection include the brain, lymph nodes, spleen, liver, bone marrow, and gastrointestinal tract. The overwhelming nature of the infections can be fatal, especially to people already weakened by AIDS.

The spectrum of infection sites produces a wide range of symptoms, which include a feeling of malaise, nausea, worsening diarrhea, and, if the brain is affected, headaches, blurred vision, and loss of balance.

Infrequently, those with healthy immune systems can acquire an atypical mycobacterial infection. The result can be a bone infection (osteomyelitis), a form of arthritis known as septic arthritis, and localized infections known as abscesses.

The diagnosis of infection caused by atypical mycobacteria is complicated by the fact that the growth of the **microorganisms** on conventional laboratory **agar** is very difficult. Specialized growth medium is required, which may not be available or in stock in every clinical laboratory. The delay in diagnosis can result in the explosive development of multiorgan infections that are extremely difficult to treat.

Treatment of atypical mycobacteria is complicated by the unusual cell wall possessed by the bacterium, relative to other bacteria. The cell wall is made predominantly of lipids. Partially as a result of their wall construction, atypical mycobacteria are not particularly susceptible to antibiotic therapy. As well, aggressive therapy is often not possible, given the physical state of the AIDS patient being treated. A prudent strategy for AIDS is the use of certain drugs as a means of preventing infection, and to try to avoid those factors that place the individual at risk for acquiring atypical mycobacterial infections. Some risk factors that have been identified include the avoidance of unwashed raw fruit and vegetables. As well, contact with pigeons should be limited, since these birds are known to harbor atypical mycobacteria in their intestinal tracts.

See also Bacteria and bacterial infections; Immunodeficiency diseases

MYCOLOGY

Mycology is the study of **fungi**, including molds and yeasts. The study of mycology encompasses a huge number of **microorganisms**. Indeed, just considering molds, the estimates of the number of species ranges from the tens of thousands to over 300,000.

Fungi are eukaryotic microorganisms (**eukaryotes** have their nucleic material contained within a membrane), which can produce new daughter fungi by a process similar to **bacteria**, where the nuclear material replicates and then the cell splits to form two daughter cells, or via sexual reproduction, where nuclear material from two fungi are mixed together and the daughter cells inherit material from both parents. Growth of fungi can occur either by the budding off of the new daughter cells from the parent or by the extension of the branch (or **hyphae**) of a fungus.

The study of fungi can take varied forms. Discovery of new fungi and their grouping with the existing fungi is one aspect of mycology. Unraveling the chemical nature of the fungal survival and growth is another aspect of mycology. For example, some fungi produce **antibiotics** such as **penicillin** as part of their defensive strategies. This aspect of mycology has proved to be extremely important for human health. The adverse effects of fungi on human health and plants constitutes yet another aspect of mycology. Still another aspect of mycology, which can encompass some of the preceding, is concerned with the economic impact, beneficial or not, of fungi. For example, those fungi that are edible or which produce antibiotics have a tremendous positive economic impact, whereas fungi that cause damage to agricultural plants exact a negative economic toll.

Some mycologists (scientists who study fungi) conduct extensive research into the origin of fungi. The discovery of fossilized fungi that resemble those from the four major groups of modern fungi in rocks that date back 360–410 million years indicate that fungi were already well-established and diversifying even before other forms of life had made the transition from the sea to the land.

Mycology has resulted in the classification of fungi into four divisions. These divisions are the Chytridiomycota, Zygomycota (which include the bread molds such as Neurospora), Ascomycota (which include yeasts), and the Basidiomycota. **Lichens** do not fit this classification, as lichens are not single-celled fungi. Rather, they are a symbiotic association (an association that is beneficial for both participants) between a fungus and an alga.

The health-oriented aspect of mycology is important, particularly as the danger of fungal infections, especially to those whose **immune system** is compromised, has been recognized since the identification of acquired **immunodeficiency** syndrome in the 1970s.

For example, in those whose immune systems are functioning properly, an infection with the **mold** known as *Aspergillus* can produce a mild allergic type of reaction. However, in those people whose immune systems are not operating efficiently, the mold can grow in the lungs, and can produce a serious infection called bronchopulmonary aspergillosis. As well, a more invasive infection via the blood-stream can result in mold growth in the eye, heart, kidneys, and the skin. The invasive infection can be lethal.

Mycologists are becoming increasingly involved in the remediation of buildings. The so-called "sick building syndrome" is often due to the growth of fungi, particularly molds, in the insulation of buildings. The growth of the molds including *Cladosporium, Penicilium, Alternaria, Aspergillus,* and *Mucor* can produce allergic reactions ranging from inconvenient to debilitating to building users.

See also Candidiasis; Economic uses and benefits of microorganisms; Slime molds

MYCOPLASMA INFECTIONS

Mycoplasma are **bacteria** that lack a conventional cell wall. They are capable of replication. Mycoplasma cause various diseases in humans, animals, and plants.

There are seven species of mycoplasma that are known to cause disease in humans. *Mycoplasma pneumoniae* is an important cause of sore throat, **pneumonia**, and the **inflammation** of the channels in the lung that are known as the bronchi. Because of the atypical nature of the bacterium, mycoplasma-induced pneumonia is also referred to as atypical pneumonia. The pneumonia can affect children and adults. The symptoms tend to be more pronounced in adults. In fact, children may not exhibit any symptoms of infection. Symptoms of infection include a fever, general feeling of being unwell, sore throat, and sometimes an uncomfortable chest. These symptoms last a week to several months and usually fade without medical intervention.

Mycoplasma pneumoniae can also cause infections in areas of the body other than the lungs, including the central nervous system, liver, and the pancreas.

Another species, *Mycoplasma genitalium*, is associated with infections of the urethra, especially when the urethra has been infected by some other bacteria. The mycoplasma infection may occur due to the stress imposed on the **immune system** by the other infection.

A mycoplasma called *Ureaplasma urealyticum* is present in the genital tract of many sexually active women. The resulting chronic infection can contribute to premature delivery in pregnant women. As well, the mycoplasma can be transmitted from the mother to the infant. The infant can contract pneumonia, infection of the central nervous system, and lung malfunction.

A group of four mycoplasma species are considered to be human pathogens and may contribute to the development an **immunodeficiency** virus infection to the more problematic and debilitating symptoms of Acquired Immunodeficiency Syndrome (**AIDS**). The species of mycoplasma are *Mycoplasma fermentans, Mycoplasma pirum, Mycoplasma hominis,* and *Mycoplasma penetrans.*

Mycoplasma have also been observed in patients who exhibit other diseases. For example, studies using genetic probes and the **polymerase chain reaction** technique of detecting target **DNA** have found *Mycoplasma fermentans* in upwards of 35% of those afflicted with chronic fatigue syndrome. The bacterium is present in less than 5% of healthy populations. Similar percentages have been found in soldiers of the Persian Gulf War who are exhibiting chronic fatigue-like symptoms. While the exact relationship between mycoplasma and the chronic fatigue state is not fully clear, the current consensus is that the bacteria is playing a secondary role in the development of the symptoms.

Over 20 years ago, mycoplasma was suggested as a cause of rheumatoid arthritis. With the development of molecular techniques of bacterial detection, this suggestion could be tested. The polymerase chain reaction has indeed detected *Mycoplasma fermentans* in a significant number of those afflicted with the condition. But again, a direct causal relationship remains to be established.

The association of mycoplasma with diseases like arthritis and chronic fatigue syndrome, which has been implicated with a response of the body's immune system against its own components, is consistent with the growth and behavior of mycoplasma. The absence of a conventional cell wall allows mycobacteria to penetrate into the white blood cells of the immune system. Because some mycoplasma will exist free of the blood cells and because the bacteria are capable of slow growth in the body, the immune system will detect and respond to a mycobacterial infection. But this response is generally futile. The bacteria hidden inside the white blood cells will not be killed. The immune components instead might begin to attack other antigens of the host that are similar in three-dimensional structure to the mycobacterial antigens. Because mycoplasma infections can become chronic, damage to the body over an extended time and the stress produced on the immune system may allow other **microorganisms** to establish infections.

The polymerase chain reaction is presently the best means of detecting mycoplasma. The bacteria cannot be easily grown on laboratory media. Labs that test using the polymerase technique are still rare. Thus, a mycoplasma infection might escape detection for years.

Strategies to eliminate mycoplasma infections are now centering on the strengthening of the immune system, and long-term antibiotic use (e.g., months or years). Even so, it is still unclear whether **antibiotics** are truly effective on mycoplasma bacteria. Mycoplasma can alter the chemical composition of the surface each time a bacterium divides. Thus, there may be no constant target for an antibiotic.

See also Bacteria and bacterial infection; Bacterial membranes and cell wall

N

VAN NEIL, CORNELIUS B. (1897-1985)

Dutch microbiologist and teacher

Cornelius B. van Neil made pioneering contributions to the study of **photosynthesis** in the **bacteria** that are known as the purple and green sulfur bacteria. These rather exotic bacteria are plant-like in that they use specific wavelengths of sunlight as a source of energy, instead of the **metabolism** of carbon-containing compounds. In addition to his research contributions, van Neil is noteworthy because of his tremendous teaching contributions. He inspired many people to take up a career in research microbiology in the first half of the twentieth century. Several of his students went on to obtain the Nobel Prize for their scientific contributions.

Van Neil was born in Haarlem, The Netherlands. His interest in chemistry was sparked while he was still in high school. This interest led him to enroll in the Chemistry Division of the Technical University of The Netherlands. His education was interrupted by a brief stint in the Dutch army. But ultimately he received a degree in Chemical Engineering in 1923. He then became a laboratory assistant to **Albert Jan Kluyver**, a renowned microbial physiologist and taxonomist. van Neil was responsible for the **culture** collection of **yeast**, bacteria, and **fungi** that Kluyver has amassed. During this time, van Neil isolated *Chromatium spp.* and *Thiosarcina rosea* and demonstrated that their growth did not involve the production of oxygen.

van Neil received a Ph.D. from The Technical University in 1928 for his research on proprionic acid bacteria (now well-known as one of the causes of acne). Following this, he came to the United States to accept a position at the Hopkins Marine Station, a research institution of Stanford University located on the Monterey Peninsula. He remained at Hopkins until his retirement in 1962. From 1964 until 1968, he was a visiting Professor at the University of California at Santa Cruz. He then retired from teaching and research entirely.

During his tenure at the Hopkins Marine Station, van Neil produced his most fundamentally important work. He was able to demonstrate that the ability of purple and green sulfur bacteria to exist without oxygen depends on the presence of sunlight. The photosynthetic reaction causes carbon dioxide to become reduced, providing the building blocks needed by the bacteria for growth and division. van Neil went on to broaden his work to photosynthesis in general. His observations that radiant energy activates a hydrogen donating compound instead of carbon dioxide was seminal in the development of subsequent studies of photosynthetic reactions in nature.

Another area where van Neil made a fundamental contribution was the emerging field of bacterial classification. Through his efforts in identifying over 150 strains of bacteria, and consolidating these organisms into six species contained within the two genera of *Rhodopseudomonas* and *Rhodo-spirillum*, van Neil and Kluyver laid the groundwork for the use of bacterial physical and chemical characteristics as a means of classifying bacteria.

van Neil's teaching legacy is as important as his research contributions. He established the first course in general microbiology in the United States. He was a riveting lecturer, and his classes could last an entire day. He taught and mentored many students who went on to considerable achievements of their own.

See also Microbial taxonomy; Photosynthetic microorganisms

NEISSERIA • *see* GONORRHEA

NEOMYCIN • *see* ANTIBIOTICS

NEURAMINIDASE (NA) • *see* HEMAGGLUTININ (HA) AND NEURAMINIDASE (NA)

NEUROSPORA

The bread **mold** *Neurospora crassa* is a simple fungal eukaryote which has been used extensively as a model organism to elucidate many of the principles of genetics of higher organisms. It is relatively easy to cultivate in the laboratory. *Neurospora* are eukaryotic organisms; that is, they organize their genes onto **chromosomes**. They may exist as either diploid cells (two copies of **gene** and chromosome) or haploid (one copy of each gene and chromosome). *Neurospora* has both a sexual and an asexual reproductive cycle which allows exploration of genetic processes more complex than those found in **bacteria**.

The asexual cycle consists of a filamentous growth of haploid mycelia. This stage is the vegetative stage. While the nuclei in this stage are indeed haploid, the tubular filaments contain multiple nuclei often without the distinction of individual cells. Under conditions of sparse food resources, the filaments (called **hyphae**) become segmented producing bright orange colored macroconidia, asexual spores that can become detached and are more readily dispersed throughout the environment. Asexual spores can develop again into multicellular hyphae, completing the cycle. Asexual spores can also function as male gametes in the sexual reproductive cycle.

The sexual part of the life cycle begins with the mature fruiting body called the perithecium. These are sacs of sexual spores (ascospores) resulting from meiotic division. The sexual spores are discharged from the perithecium and can germinate into haploid cultures or fuse with conidia of complementary mating types. There are two genetically distinct mating types A and a. *Neurospora* cannot self fertilize, rather haploid sexual spores of opposite mating types must be joined at fertilization. Nuclear fusion of the male and female gametes occurs setting the stage for meiotic division to form ascospores. The diploid stage is brief as nuclear fusion quickly gives way to two meiotic divisions that produce eight ascospores. Ascospores are normally black and shaped like a football. The physical position of the ascospores is linear and corresponds to the physical position of the individual chromosomes during meiosis. In the absence of crossing over, the four a-mating type ascospores are next to each other followed by the four A-mating type ascospores.

The existence of a large collection of distinct mutant strains of *Neurospora* and the linear array of the products of meiosis makes *Neurospora* an ideal organism for studying mutation, chromosomal rearrangements, and **recombination**. As a relatively simple eukaryote, *Neurospora* has permitted study of the interactions of nuclear genes with mitochondrial genes. *Neurospora* also exhibits a normal circadian rhythm in response to light in the environment, and much of the fundamental genetics and biology of circadian clock cycles (chronobiology) have been elucidated through the careful study of mutant cells which exhibit altered circadian cycles.

See also Microbial genetics

NITROGEN CYCLE IN MICROORGANISMS

Nitrogen is a critically important nutrient for organisms, including **microorganisms**. This element is one of the most abundant elemental constituents of eukaryotic tissues and prokaryotic cell walls, and is an integral component of amino acids, proteins, and nucleic acids.

Most plants obtain their nitrogen by assimilating it from their environment, mostly as nitrate or ammonium dissolved in soil water that is taken up by roots, or as gaseous nitrogen oxides that are taken up by plant leaves from the atmosphere. However, some plants live in a symbiotic relationship with microorganisms that have the ability to fix atmospheric nitrogen (which can also be called dinitrogen) into ammonia. Such plants benefit from access to an increased supply of nitrogen.

As well, nitrogen-assimilating microorganisms are of benefit to animals. Typically animals obtain their needed nitrogen through the plants they ingest. The plant's organic forms of nitrogen are metabolized and used by the animal as building blocks for their own necessary biochemicals. However, some animals are able to utilize inorganic sources of nitrogen. For example, ruminants, such as the cow, can utilize urea or ammonia as a consequence of the metabolic action of the microorganisms that reside in their forestomachs. These microbes can assimilate nitrogen and urea and use them to synthesize the amino acids and proteins, which are subsequently utilized by the cow.

Nitrogen (N) can occur in many organic and inorganic forms in the environment. Organic nitrogen encompasses a diversity of nitrogen-containing organic molecules, ranging from simple amino acids, proteins, and nucleic acids to large and complex molecules such as the humic substances that are found in soil and water.

In the atmosphere, nitrogen exists as a diatomic gas (N_2). The strong bond between the two nitrogen atoms of this gas make the molecule nonreactive. Almost 80% of the volume of Earth's atmosphere consists of diatomic nitrogen, but because of its almost inert character, few organisms can directly use this gas in their nutrition. Diatomic nitrogen must be "fixed" into other forms by certain microorganisms before it can be assimilated by most organisms.

Another form of nitrogen is called nitrate (chemically displayed as NO_3-). Nitrate is a negatively charged ion (or anion), and as such is highly soluble in water.

Ammonia (NH_{3S}) usually occurs as a gas, vapor, or liquid. Addition of a hydrogen atom produces ammonium (NH_4+). Like nitrate, ammonium is soluble in water. Ammonium is also electrochemically attracted to negatively charged surfaces associated with clays and organic matter in soil, and is therefore not as mobile as nitrate.

These, and the other forms of nitrogen are capable of being transformed in what is known as the nitrogen cycle.

Nitrogen is both very abundant in the atmosphere and is relatively inert and nonreactive. To be of use to plants, dinitrogen must be "fixed" into inorganic forms that can be taken up by roots or leaves. While dinitrogen fixation can occur non-biologically, biological fixation of dinitrogen is more prevalent.

A bacterial enzyme called nitrogenase is capable of breaking the tenacious bond that holds the two nitrogen atoms together. Examples of nitrogen-fixing **bacteria** include *Azotobacter*, *Beijerinkia*, some species of *Klebsiella*, *Clostridium*, *Desulfovibrio*, purple sulfur bacteria, purple nonsulfur bacteria, and green sulfur bacteria.

Some species of plants live in an intimate and mutually beneficial symbiosis with microbes that have the capability of fixing dinitrogen. The plants benefit from the symbiosis by having access to a dependable source of fixed nitrogen, while the microorganisms benefit from energy and habitat provided by the plant. The best known symbioses involve many species in the legume family (Fabaceae) and strains of a bacterium known as *Rhizobium japonicum*. Some plants in other families also have dinitrogen-fixing symbioses, for example, red alder (*Alnus rubra*) and certain member of Actinomycetes. Bacteria from the genera *Frankia* and *Azospirillum* are also able to establish symbiotic relationships with non-leguminous plants. Many species of **lichens**, which consist of a symbiotic relationship between a fungus and a blue-green bacterium, can also fix dinitrogen.

Ammonification is a term for the process by which the organically bound nitrogen of microbial, plant, and animal biomass is recycled after their death. Ammonification is carried out by a diverse array of microorganisms that perform ecological decay services, and its product is ammonia or ammonium ion. Ammonium is a suitable source of nutrition for many species of plants, especially those living in acidic soils. However, most plants cannot utilize ammonium effectively, and they require nitrate as their essential source of nitrogen nutrition.

Nitrate is synthesized from ammonium by an important bacterial process known as nitrification. The first step in nitrification is the oxidation of ammonium to nitrite (NO_2^-), a function carried out by bacteria in the genus *Nitrosomonas*. Once formed, the nitrite is rapidly oxidized further to nitrate, by bacteria in the genus *Nitrobacter*. The bacteria responsible for nitrification are very sensitive to acidity, so this process does not occur at significant rates in acidic soil or water.

Denitrification is another bacterial process, carried out by a relatively wide range of species. In denitrification, nitrate is reduced to either nitrous oxide or dinitrogen, which is then emitted to the atmosphere. One of the best studies bacterial examples is *Pseudomonas stutzeri*. This bacterial species has almost 50 genes that are known to have a direct role in denitrification. The process of denitrification occurs under conditions where oxygen is not present, and its rate is largest when concentrations of nitrate are large. Consequently, fertilized agricultural fields that are wet or flooded can have quite large rates of denitrification. In some respects, denitrification can be considered to be an opposite process to dinitrogen fixation. In fact, the global rates of dinitrogen fixation and denitrification are in an approximate balance, meaning that the total quantity of fixed nitrogen in Earth's ecosystems is neither increasing nor decreasing substantially over time.

See also Biogeochemical cycles; Economic uses and benefits of microorganisms

NON-CULTURABLE BACTERIA • *see* VIABLE BUT NON-CULTURABLE BACTERIA

NON-SELECTIVE MEDIA • *see* GROWTH AND GROWTH MEDIA

NON-SPECIFIC IMMUNITY • *see* IMMUNITY, ACTIVE, PASSIVE, AND DELAYED

NOSOCOMIAL INFECTIONS

A nosocomial infection is an infection that is acquired in a hospital. More precisely, the **Centers for Disease Control** in Atlanta, Georgia, defines a nosocomial infection as a localized infection or one that is widely spread throughout the body that results from an adverse reaction to an infectious microorganism or toxin that was not present at the time of admission to the hospital.

The term nosocomial infection derives from the *nosos*, which is the Greek word for disease.

Nosocomial infections have been a part of hospital care as long as there have been hospitals. The connection between the high death rate of hospitalized patients and the exposure of patients to infectious **microorganisms** was first made in the mid-nineteenth century. Hungarian physician **Ignaz Semmelweis** (1818–1865) noted the high rate of death from puerperal fever in women who delivered babies at the Vienna General Hospital. Moreover, the high death rate was confined to a ward at which medical residents were present. Another ward, staffed only by midwives who did not interact with other areas of the hospital, had a much lower death rate. When the residents were made to wash their hands in a disinfectant solution prior to entering the ward, the death rate declined dramatically.

At about the same time, the British surgeon **Joseph Lister** (1827–1912) also recognized the importance of hygienic conditions in the operating theatre. His use of phenolic solutions as sprays over surgical wounds helped lessen the spread of microorganisms resident in the hospital to the patient. Lister also required surgeons to wear rubber gloves and freshly laundered operating gowns for surgery. He recognized that infections could be transferred from the surgeon to the patient. Lister's actions spurred a series of steps over the next century, which has culminated in today's observance of sterile or near-sterile conditions in the operating theatre.

Despite these improvements in hospital hygienic practices, the chance of acquiring a nosocomial infection still approaches about 10%. Certain hospital situations are even riskier. For example, the chance of acquiring a urinary tract infection increases by 10% for each day a patient is equipped with a urinary catheter. The catheter provides a ready route for the movement of **bacteria** from the outside environment to the urinary tract.

The most common microbiological cause of nosocomial infection is bacteria. The microbes often include both Gram-negative and Gram-positive bacteria. Of the Gram-negative bacteria, *Escherichia coli*, *Proteus mirabilis,* and other members of the family known as Enterobacteriacaea are predominant. These bacteria are residents of the intestinal tract. They are spread via fecal **contamination** of people, instruments or

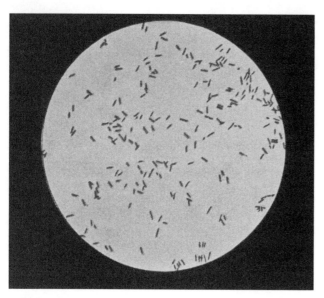

Pseudomonas aeruginosa, an important cause of nosocomial infections.

other surfaces. Other Gram-negative bacteria of consequence include members of the genera *Pseudomonas* and *Acinetobacter*.

Gram-positive bacteria, especially *Staphylococcus aureus*, frequently cause infections of wounds. This bacterium is part of the normal flora on the surface of the skin, and so can readily gain access to a wound or surgical incision.

One obvious cause of nosocomial infections is the state of the people who require the services of a hospital. Often people are ill with ailments that adversely affect the ability of their immune systems to recognize or combat infections. These people are more vulnerable to disease than they would otherwise be. A hospital is a place where, by its nature, infectious microorganisms are encountered more often than in other environments, such as the home or workplace. Simply by being in a hospital, a person is exposed to potentially disease-causing microorganisms.

A compounding factor, and one that is the cause of many nosocomial infections, is the developing resistance of bacteria to a number of **antibiotics** in common use in hospitals. For example, strains of *Staphylococcus aureus* that are resistant to all but a few conventional antibiotics are encountered in hospitals so frequently as to be almost routine. Indeed, many hospitals now have contingency plans to deal with outbreaks of these infections, which involve the isolation of patients, **disinfection** of affected wards, and monitoring of other areas of the hospital for the bacteria. As another example, a type of bacteria known as enterococci has developed resistance to virtually all antibiotics available. Ominously, the genetic determinant for the multiple **antibiotic resistance** in enterococci has been transferred to *Staphylococcus aureus* in the laboratory setting. Were such genetic transfer to occur in the hospital setting, conventional antibiotic therapy for *Staphylococcus aureus* infections would become virtually impossible.

See also Bacteria and bacterial infection; History of public health; History of the development of antibiotics

NOTOBIOTIC ANIMALS · *see* ANIMAL MODELS OF INFECTION

NUCLEUS

The nucleus is a membrane-bounded organelle found in eukaryotic cells that contains the **chromosomes** and nucleolus. Intact eukaryotic cells are comprised of a nucleus and **cytoplasm**. A nuclear envelope encloses chromatin, the nucleolus, and a matrix which fills the nuclear space.

The chromatin consists primarily of the genetic material, **DNA**, and histone proteins. Chromatin is often arranged in fiber like nucleofilaments.

The nucleolus is a globular cell organelle important to ribosome function and **protein synthesis**. The nucleolus is a small structure within the nucleus that is rich in ribosomal **RNA** and proteins. The nucleolus disappears and reorganizes during specific phases of cell division. A nucleus may contain from one to several nucleoli. Nucleoli are associated with protein synthesis and enlarged nucleoli are observed in rapidly growing embryonic tissue (other than cleavage nuclei), cells actively engaged in protein synthesis, and malignant cells. The nuclear matrix itself is also protein rich.

The genetic instructions for an organism are encoded in nuclear DNA that is organized into chromosomes. Eukaryotic chromosomes are composed of proteins and nucleic acids (nucleoprotein). Accordingly, cell division and reproduction require a process by which the DNA (or in some prokaryotes, RNA) can be duplicated and passed to the next generation of cells (daughter cells)

It is possible to obtain genetic replicates through process termed nuclear transplantation. Genetic replicas are cloned by nuclear transplantation. The first **cloning** program using nuclear transplantation was able, as early a 1952, to produce frogs by nuclear transplantation. Since that time, research programs have produced an number of different species that can be cloned. More recently, sheep (Dolly) and other creatures have been produced by cloning nuclei from adult animal donors.

The cloning procedures for frogs or mammals are similar. Both procedures require the insertion of a nucleus into an egg that has been deprived of its own genetic material. The reconstituted egg, with a new nucleus, develops in accordance with the genetic instructions of the nuclear donor.

There are, of course, cells which do not contain the usual nuclear structures. Embryonic cleavage nuclei (cells forming a blastula) do not have a nucleolus. Because the cells retain the genetic competence to produce nucleoli, gastrula and all later cells contain nucleoli. Another example is found upon examination of mature red blood cells, erythrocytes, that in most mammals are without (devoid) of nuclei. The loss of nuclear material, however, does not preclude the competence to carry oxygen.

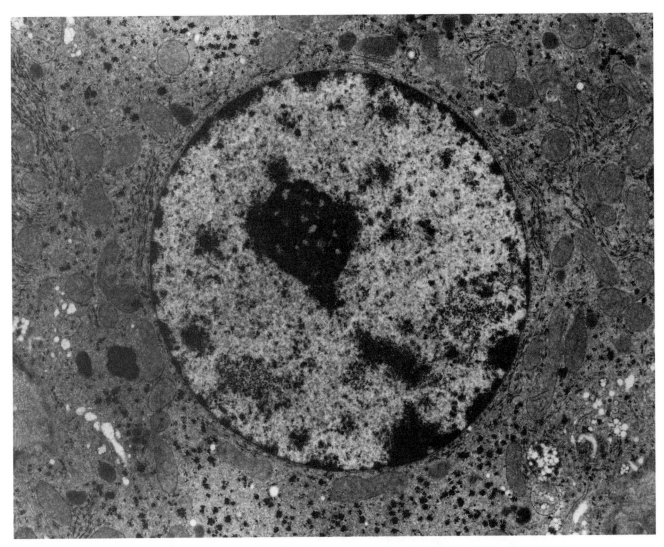

Thin section electron micrograph of a nucleus from a eukaryotic cell, showing the membrane that surrounds the nuclear contents.

See also Cell cycle (eukaryotic), genetic regulation of; DNA (deoxyribonucleic acid)

NUTTALL, GEORGE H. F. (1862-1937)

American bacteriologist

George Henry Falkiner Nuttall is noteworthy for his accomplishments while at Cambridge University in England; his research was concerned with **parasites** and of insect carriers of microbiological diseases. He was instrumental in establishing a diploma course in tropical medicine. In 1907, Nuttall moved into a new laboratory. There, he carried out research that clarified the disease of piroplasmosis, a still-serious disease of domesticated animals such as cattle. He showed that Trypan Blue could be used as a treatment. During this period, space limitations of the laboratory prompted him to seek funding to build and equip a new institute for parasitological research.

His efforts were successful, and he established the Molteno Institute for Research in Parasitology at Cambridge in 1921. The institute was named in honor of a South African farming family who were the principle financial backers of the initiative. He became the institute's first Director.

Nuttall's years at The Molteno Institute were spent in parasitological research and research on the cytochrome system of insects.

Nuttall was born in San Francisco. His early years were spent in Europe. He returned to America to train as a physician, receiving his M.D. from the University of California in 1884. He then undertook research on various microbiological and immunological projects in laboratories in North America and Europe. His burgeoning interest in parasitology and the role of insects and other agents of disease transmission led him to pursue further study. He received a Ph.D. in biology from the University of Göttingen in 1890. In 1899, at the age of 38, he moved to Cambridge, where he became a full Professor of biology in 1906.

Nuttall also contributed much the scientific literature. In 1901, he established and was founding editor of the *Journal of Hygiene*, and in 1908 founded and edited *Parasitology*. His writing includes *Blood Immunity and Blood Relationships* in 1904 and *The Bacteriology of Diphtheria* in 1908.

See also Parasites; Transmission of pathogens

O

O157:H7 INFECTION · *see* E. COLI O157:H7 INFECTION

ONCOGENE

An oncogene is a special type of **gene** that is capable of transforming host cells and triggering carcinogenesis. The name is derived from the Greek *onkos*, meaning bulk, or mass, because of the ability to cause tumor growth. Oncogenes were first discovered in **retroviruses** (**viruses** containing the enzyme reverse transcriptase, and **RNA**, rather than **DNA**) that were found to cause cancer in many animals (e.g., feline leukemia virus, simian sarcoma virus). Although this is a relatively common mechanism of oncogenesis in animals, very few oncogene-carrying viruses have been identified in man. The ones that are known include the papilloma virus HPV16 that is associated with cervical cancer, HTLV-1 and HTLV-2 associated with T-cell leukemia, and HIV-1 associated with Kaposi sarcoma.

Studies of humans led to the discovery of related genes called proto-oncogenes that exist naturally in the human genome. These genes have DNA sequences that are similar to oncogenes, but under normal conditions, the proto-oncogenes do not cause cancer. However, specific **mutations** in these genes can transform them to an oncogenic form that may lead to carcinogenesis. So, in humans, there are two unique ways in which oncogenesis occurs, by true viral infection and by mutation of proto-oncogenes that already exist in human cells.

See also Molecular biology and molecular genetics; Oncogenetic research; Viral genetics; Viral vectors in gene therapy; Virology; Virus replication; Viruses and responses to viral infection

ONCOGENE RESEARCH

Research into the structure and function of oncogenes has been a major endeavor for many years. The first chromosome rearrangement (Ph') involving a proto-oncogene to be directly associated with cancer induction was identified in 1960. Since then, over 50 proto-oncogenes have been mapped in the human genome, and many cancer-related **mutations** have been detected. Once the role of oncogenes and proto-oncogenes in cancer was understood, the task of elucidating the exact mutations, specific breakpoints for translocations, and how protein products are altered in the disease process was undertaken.

Karyotype analysis has been used for many years to identify chromosome abnormalities that are specifically associated with particular types of leukemia and lymphoma aiding in diagnosis and the understanding of prognosis. Now that many of the genes involved in the chromosome rearrangements have been cloned, newer, more effective detection techniques, have been discovered. **FISH, fluorescence** *in situ* **hybridization**, uses molecular probes to detect chromosome rearrangements. Probes are developed to detect deletions or to flank the breakpoints of a translocation. or example, using a dual color system for chronic myelogenous leukemia (CML), a green probe hybridizes just distal to the c-*abl* locus on chromosome 9 and a red probe hybridizes just proximal to the locus on chromosome 22. In the absence of a rearrangement, independent colored signals (two green and two red) are observed. When the rearrangement occurs, two of the fluorescent probes are moved adjacent to one another on one chromosome and their signals merge producing a new color (yellow) that can be easily detected (net result: one green, one red, and one yellow signal).

Other molecular techniques such as Southern blotting and **PCR** are also used for cancer detection and can identify point mutations as well as translocations. These systems are set up such that one series of **DNA** fragments indicate no mutation, and a different size fragment or series of fragments will be seen if a mutation is present. All of the newer techniques are more sensitive than cytogenetic analysis and can pick up abnormal cell lines occurring at very low frequencies. Clinically, it may be useful to detect the disease in an early stage when there are fewer cancer cells present so that treatment may begin before severe symptoms are experienced. In addition, these techniques aid in detection of minimal residual disease (the presence of low levels of disease after treatment) and may give warning that the disease is returning.

A major breakthrough has come in treatment of diseases caused by oncogenes. The current standard of care for cancer patients has been **chemotherapy** and radiation therapy. This is successful in limiting or eradicating the disease, but, because the whole body is affected by these treatments, there are usually multiple side effects such as hair loss, nausea, fatigue, etc. New drugs are designed to counteract the particular mutation associated with the patient's disease and thus are target specific. This is only possible if the mutation causing the disease is known and a treatment can be developed that inactivates the negative affect of that mutation. Because only one cellular component is affected, negative physical side effects may be reduced.

The most successful of these drugs to date is STI-571, or Gleevec, and was developed for use in patients with chronic myelogenous leukemia (CML). In CML, the proto-oncogene translocation results in overproduction of the enzyme tyrosine kinase. Gleevec is an inhibitor of tyrosine kinase and works at the cellular level to block excess enzyme activity. Although there are several different types of tyrosine kinase in humans, STI-571 is specific to the form produced by the CML mutation and does not affect other members of this enzyme family. The drug is therefore so specific, other cells and tissues in the body are not impacted, and there are few negative side effects resulting in a therapy that is much more tolerable to the patient. Early clinical trials showed such a high degree of success that the trails were terminated early and the drug was FDA approved and released for general use. There is now new evidence to suggest that this drug also may be effective for other diseases, including some types of solid tumors. This is clearly the way drug treatments will be designed in the future. By targeting only the defect and correcting that, a disease can be managed without impairing other aspects of a patient's health or quality of life.

Other types of ongoing research include further elucidation of normal proto-oncogene function and how the oncogenic mutations change cellular regulation. In particular, issues involving **oncogene** impact on apoptosis, programmed cell death, have become an important avenue of investigation. It has been shown that normal cells have a fixed life span but that cancer cells lose this characteristic and exhibit uncontrolled cell growth with aspects of immortality. A better understanding of the role oncogenes play in this process may give insight into additional ways to treat cancer.

See also Fluorescence *in situ* hybridization (FISH); Immunogenetics; Immunologic therapies; Mutations and mutagenesis

OPERON

An operon is a single unit of physically adjacent genes that function together under the control of a single operator **gene**. With respect to **transcription** and **translation**, the genes within an operon code for **enzymes** or proteins that are functionally related and are usually members of a single enzyme system. The operon is under the control of a single gene that is responsible for switching the entire operon "on" or "off." A repressor molecule that is capable of binding to the operator gene and switching it, and consequently the whole operon, off, controls the operator gene. A gene that is not part of the operon produces the repressor molecule. The repressor molecule is itself produced by a regulator gene. The repressor molecule is inactivated by a metabolite or signal substance (effector). In other words, the effector causes the operon to become active.

The *lac* operon in the bacterium *E. coli* was one of the first discovered and still remains one of the most studied and well known. The **deoxyribonucleic acid** (**DNA**) segment containing the *lac* operon is some 6,000 base pairs long. This length includes the operator gene and three structural genes (*lac* Z, *lac* Y, and *lac* A). The three structural genes and the operator are transcribed into a single piece of messenger **ribonucleic acid** (mRNA), which can then be translated. Transcription will not take place if a repressor protein is bound to the operator. The repressor protein is encoded by *lac* I, which is a gene located to the left of the *lac* promoter. The *lac* promoter is located immediately to the left of the *lac* operator gene and is outside the *lac* operon. The enzymes produced by this operon are responsible for the hydrolysis (a reaction that adds a water molecule to a reactant and splits the reactant into two molecules) of lactose into glucose and galactose. Once glucose and galactose have been produced, a side reaction occurs forming a compound called allolactose. Allolactose is the chemical responsible for switching on the *lac* operon by binding to the repressor and inactivating it.

Operons are generally encountered in lower organisms such as **bacteria**. They are commonly encountered for certain systems, suggesting that there is a strong evolutionary pressure for the genes to remain together as a unit. Operons have not yet been found in higher organisms, such as multicellular life forms.

A mutation in the operator gene that renders it non-functional would also render the whole operon inactive. As a direct result of inactivation, the coded pathway would no longer operate within the cell. Even though the genes are still separate individual units, they cannot function by themselves, without the control of the operator gene.

See also Genetic code; Microbial genetics

OPSONIZATION

Opsonization is a term that refers to an immune process where particles such as **bacteria** are targeted for destruction by an immune cell known as a **phagocyte**. The process of opsonization is a means of identifying the invading particle to the phagocyte. Without the opsonization process the recognition and destruction of invading agents such as bacteria would be inefficient.

The process of opsonization begins when the **immune system** recognizes a particle (e.g., a bacterium) as an invader. The recognition stimulates the production of antibodies that are specific for the antigenic target. Certain **antibody** molecules are stimulated to bind to the surface of the particle. Typically, the binding molecules are a type of antibody classified as IgG. As well, proteins involved in the complement-mediated clearance of foreign material, specifically a protein designated C3b, can bind to the surface of the foreign object. Proteins such as IgG and C3b, which can promote opsonization, are designated as opsonins.

When the IgG antibodies bind to the invading bacterium, the binding is in a specific orientation. An antibody is somewhat "Y" shaped. The binding of IgG to the bacterium is via the branching arms of the "Y." The stalk of the molecule, which is termed the Fc region, then protrudes from the surface. The Fc region is recognized by a receptor on the surface of an immune cell called a phagocyte. When the Fc region is bound to the phagocytic receptor the invading particle is taken into the phagocyte and enzymatically digested.

The Cb3 **complement** protein can bind in a nonspecific manner to an invading particle. Phagocytes also contain surface receptors that recognize and bind Cb3. As with IgG, the binding of Cb3 to the phagocytes triggers a process whereby the invading particle is engulfed, surrounded, and taken inside the phagocytic cell for destruction.

Examples of phagocytic cells that can participate in opsonization are neutrophils and monocytes.

Bacteria that are associated with the development of infections typically possess a capsule, which is a layer of carbohydrate material. The capsular material encases the bacterial cell. The carbohydrate is not recognized as readily by the immune machinery of the body as is protein. As well, the penetration of antibodies through the capsule network to the surface of the bacterium is impeded. Thus, possession of a capsule can dampen the opsonization response.

See also Complement; Immunoglobulins and immunoglobulin deficiency syndromes; Immunity, active, passive and delayed

OPTIC INFECTIONS, CHRONIC · *see* EYE INFECTIONS

OPTICAL DENSITY AND MEASUREMENTS OF · *see* LABORATORY TECHNIQUES IN MICROBIOLOGY

ORIGIN OF LIFE · *see* LIFE, ORIGIN OF

OTIC INFECTIONS, CHRONIC · *see* EAR INFECTIONS, CHRONIC

OXIDATION-REDUCTION REACTION

Oxidation-reduction reactions are significant to physiological reactions and biochemical pathways important to **microorganisms** and immune processes.

The term oxidation was originally used to describe reactions in which an element combines with oxygen. In contrast, reduction meant the removal of oxygen. By the turn of this century, it became apparent that oxidation always seemed to involve the loss of electrons and did not always involve oxygen. In general, oxidation- reduction reactions involve the exchange of electrons between two species.

An oxidation reaction is defined as the loss of electrons, while a reduction reaction is defined as the gain of electrons. The two reactions always occur together and in chemically equivalent quantities. Thus, the number of electrons lost by one species is always equal to the number of electrons gained by another species. The combination of the two reactions is known as a redox reaction. Species that participate in redox reactions are described as either reducing or oxidizing agents. An oxidizing agent is a species that causes the oxidation of another species. The oxidizing agent accomplishes this by accepting electrons in a reaction. A reducing agent causes the reduction of another species by donating electrons to the reaction.

In general, a strong oxidizing agent is a species that has an attraction for electrons and can oxidize another species. The standard voltage reduction of an oxidizing agent is a measure of the strength of the oxidizing agent. The more positive the species' standard reduction potential, the stronger the species is as an oxidizing agent.

In reactions where the reactants and products are not ionic, there is still a transfer of electrons between species. Chemists have devised a way to keep track of electrons during chemical reactions where the charge on the atoms is not readily apparent. Charges on atoms within compounds are assigned oxidation states (or oxidation numbers). An oxidation number is defined by a set of rules that describes how to divide up electrons shared within compounds. Oxidation is defined as an increase in oxidation state, while reduction is defined as a decrease in oxidation state. Because an oxidizing agent accepts electrons from another species, a component atom of the oxidizing agent will decrease in oxidation number during the redox reaction.

There are many examples of oxidation-reduction reactions in the world. Important processes that involve oxidation-reduction reactions include combustion reactions that convert energy stored in fuels into thermal energy, the corrosion of metals, and metabolic reactions.

Oxidation-reduction reaction occur in both physical and biological settings (where carbon-containing compounds such as carbohydrates are oxidized). The burning of natural gas is an oxidation-reduction reaction that releases energy [$CH_4(g) + 2O_2(g) \rightarrow CO_2(g) + 2H_2O(g)$ + energy]. Redox reactions burn carbohydrates that provide energy [$C_6H_{12}O_6(aq) + 6O_2(g) \rightarrow 6CO_2(g) + 6H_2O(l)$]. In both examples, the carbon-containing compound is oxidized, and the oxygen is reduced.

See also Biochemistry

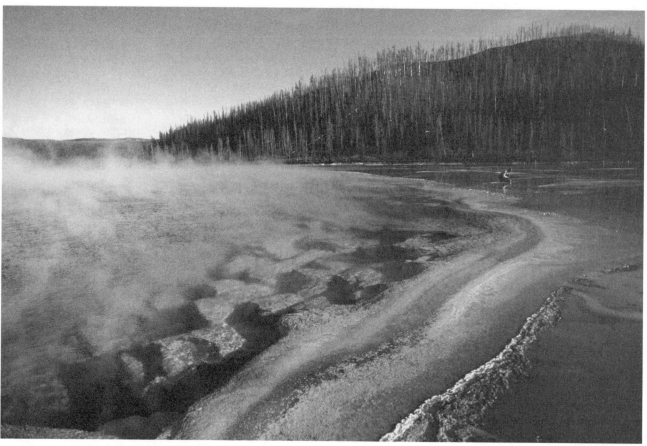

Life on Earth, made possible because of oxygen.

OXYGEN CYCLE IN MICROORGANISMS

The oxygen cycle is a global cycle of oxygen circulation between living organisms and the non-living environment. **Microorganisms** are an important facet of this cycle.

There is substantial evidence in the fossil record that the present atmosphere is due to the activity of **bacteria**, in particular to the bacteria known as cyanobacteria. Originally, the Earth's atmosphere was virtually oxygen-free. With the **evolution** of cyanobacteria, which derive their energy from **photosynthesis** with the subsequent release of oxygen, the oxygen level in the atmosphere increased. Over millions of years of bacterial (and later plant) activity, the oxygen content attained the present day level. Microorganisms such as the cyanobacteria are thus considered producers of atmospheric oxygen.

Microorganisms are also involved in the removal of oxygen from the atmosphere (i.e., they are consumers of oxygen) The process of **respiration** uses oxygen to produce energy. For example, the decay of organic material by microorganisms such as bacteria and **fungi** consumes oxygen. The microbial decomposition process involves numerous species of bacteria and fungi. Some of these release oxygen.

Microorganisms also contribute to the oxygen cycle in an indirect way. For example, the degradation of organic compounds (e.g., cellulose) by bacteria can make the compounds capable of being used as a food source by another organism. This subsequent utilization can both consume and produce oxygen at various stages of the digestive process.

The oxygen cycle in microorganisms also operates at a much smaller scale. The best example of this is the stratification of microbial life in water that occurs due to the oxygen concentration. Oxygen does not dissolve easily in water. Thus, oxygen from the atmosphere enters water very slowly. In a body of water—for example, a lake—the result is a higher concentration of oxygen in the uppermost region of the water. Those bacteria that produce oxygen (i.e., cyanobacteria) will also be located in this surface region of the water, because Sunlight is most available there. Food sources that are not consumed by these bacteria and other surface-dwelling life sink to deeper water. In the deeper water, bacteria and other microorganisms that can live in the presence of low oxygen levels then utilize the nutrients. At the greatest depths reside microorganisms that cannot tolerate oxygen. These anaerobic microorganisms degrade the nutrients that reach the bottom. This stratification of microbial life will affect the presence of other life in the water, as well as the cycling of other compounds (e.g., the carbon cycle).

The oxygen cycle in microorganisms in bodies of water such as lakes and rivers can have important consequences on the health of the water. For example, if mixing of the water in the lake does not readily occur, the body of water can become stagnant. In other words, the oxygen content of the water becomes depleted and, without mixing, insufficient surface level oxygen is available to replenish the supply. Fish life in the water can suffer. Another example is the depletion of oxygen from a lake by the explosive growth of algae. The algal "bloom" can essentially make the water body incapable of supporting life. Furthermore, if the algal species is a toxin producer, the water can become hazardous to health. A final example is the relationship between the oxygen cycle in microorganisms and **water pollution**. Polluted water is typi-

cally enriched in nutrients that will support the rapid growth of bacteria and other microbes. Their growth depletes the oxygen in the water. In grossly polluted water, this depletion can be so extensive that the water cannot support oxygen-dependent life.

Thus, the oxygen cycle in microorganisms, mainly bacteria, is very important in determining the quality of a water body and so of the ability of the water to be a productive source of life.

See also Carbon cycle in microorganisms; Composting, microbiological aspects; Life, origin of; Nitrogen cycle in microorganisms

P

PAEOPHYTA

Also known as brown algae, Paeophyta (or Phaeophyta) are photosynthetic **protists**, belonging to the Chromista Kingdom (i.e., "with color"), a kingdom closely related neither to plants nor to other algae. This kingdom includes microscopic life forms such as **diatoms**, colorless mildews, giant kelps, and sargassum. Most Chromista are photosynthetic, including Paeophyta, but they also make other pigments not found in plants, including a modified **chlorophyll** with a different molecular shape from that synthesized by plants. Paeophytes also make high levels of carotenoids, in special fucoxanthin, which give them their golden and brown colors. Unlike plants, they do not store energy as glucose and starch, but as laminarin, a polymer formed by glucose and a six-carbon sugar alkaloid termed mannitol. Most paeophytes reproduce through sexual alternation of generations, with some species presenting a dominant diploid phase (such as kelps) and others isomorphic phases (i.e., each generation being very similar to each other).

Paeophyta comprises several genera, including the largest species among the Chromista, although many species are microscopic brown algae, which grow on underwater rock or coral surfaces, or on vegetation, forming encrustations or filamentous networks, such as those commonly found in and around underwater giant kelp forests. Giant kelps form dense sea forests such as those found in the tidepools nearby Monterrey, California, with long and strong stalks up to 50–60 meters (197 feet) high, fixed at the sea bottom through brushy holdfasts. From the stalks grow flat blades termed lamina that capture sunlight and make **photosynthesis**. Some **kelp** have flotation bladders that sustain their photosynthetic blades near the water surface, for better exposition to solar energy. Paeophytes grow in coastal marine cold and temperate water, with a few species growing in freshwaters as well. Many are intertidal species, and are exposed to open air during low tide, such as Fucus (rockweed). Some Paeophytes, such as *Sargassum natans* and *Sargassum fluitans* are pelagic species (i.e., free-floating species), due to their gas-filled vesicles.

They form floating ecosystems in the western North Atlantic sea that support more than 50 different species of fish and several species of crabs, as well as invertebrates, such as gastropods, polychaetes, anemones, sea-spiders, etc.

See also Photosynthetic microorganisms

PANDEMICS · *see* EPIDEMICS AND PANDEMICS

PARAMECIUM

Paramecium are single celled **eukaryotes**, reminiscent of a football in shape, that belong to the group of **microorganisms** known as the **Protozoa**. The protozoan inhabits freshwater bodies such as ponds. The organism is useful as a teaching tool for light microscopy.

There are at least eight species of *Paramecium*. Two examples are *Paramecium caudatum* and *Paramecium bursaria*.

Paramecium are large enough to be visible to the unaided eye. However, the internal detail is resolved only by the use of a **microscope**. A student is best able to observe the complex internal organization of the organism by using what is termed the hanging drop technique. Here a drop of water is suspended upside-down on a cover slip that is positioned over a cavity on a microscope slide. The cover slip is sealed to prevent leakage.

Paramecium contain organized structures called vacuoles that are essentially a primitive mouth, stomach, and excretion system. As food enters the organism, it is stored in specialized vacuoles known as food vacuoles. These can circulate through the **cytoplasm** of the organism, in order to provide food where needed. Characteristic of eukaryotes, nuclear material is segregated by a nuclear membrane.

Another characteristic features of *Paramecium* is the so-called contractile vacuole. This vacuole is able to store water and then, by virtue of the compression of the side arms that radiate from the central vacuole, to expel the water out of the

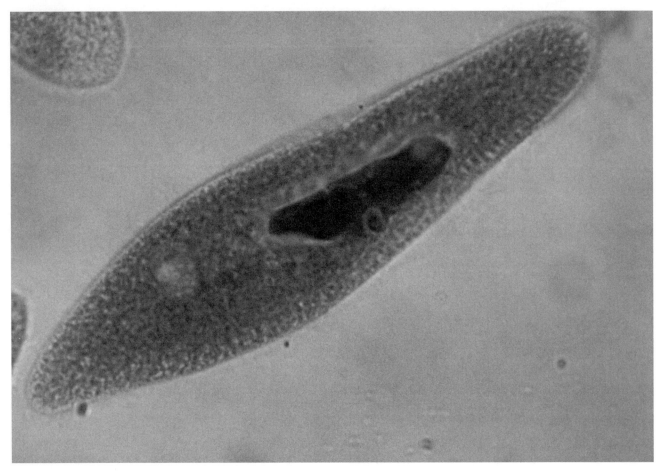

Light micrograph of a paramecium.

organism. In this way, the amount of water inside the paramecia can be controlled. The operation of the contractile vacuole is another feature that is visible by the light microscopic observation of living paramecia.

On the exterior lies a membrane that is called the pellicle. The pellicle is both stiff, to provide support and to maintain the shape of the organism, and is flexible, to allow some flexing of the surface. Also on the surface are hundreds of tiny hairs called cilia. The cilia wave back and forth, and act to sweep food particles (**bacteria** and smaller protozoa) towards the primitive mouth of the organism (the gullet). The cilia are also important in locomotion, acting analogous to the oars of a rowboat. The beating of the cilia is easily visible under light microscopic examination, especially if the movement of the organism has been retarded by the addition of a viscous compound such as glycerol to the sample.

See also Eukaryotes

PARASITES

A parasite is an organism that depends upon another organism, known as a host, for food and shelter. The parasite usually gains all the benefits of this relationship, while the host may suffer from various diseases and discomforts, or show no signs of the infection. The life cycle of a typical parasite usually includes several developmental stages and morphological changes as the parasite lives and moves through the environment and one or more hosts. Parasites that remain on a host's body surface to feed are called ectoparasites, while those that live inside a host's body are called endoparasites. Parasitism is a highly successful biological adaptation. There are more known parasitic species than nonparasitic ones, and parasites affect just about every form of life, including most all animals, plants, and even **bacteria**.

Parasitology is the study of parasites and their relationships with host organisms. Throughout history, people have coped with over 100 types of parasites affecting humans. Parasites have not, however, been systematically studied until the last few centuries. With his invention of the **microscope** in the late 1600s, Anton von Leeuwenhoek was perhaps the first to observe microscopic parasites. As Westerners began to travel and work more often in tropical parts of the world, medical researchers had to study and treat a variety of new infections, many of which were caused by parasites. By the early 1900s, parasitology had developed as a specialized field of study.

Typically, a parasitic infection does not directly kill a host, though the drain on the organism's resources can affect its growth, reproductive capability, and survival, leading to premature death. Parasites, and the diseases they cause and transmit, have been responsible for tremendous human suffering and loss of life throughout history. Although the majority of parasitic infections occur within tropical regions and among low-income populations, most all regions of the world sustain parasitic species, and all humans are susceptible to infection.

Although many species of **viruses**, bacteria, and **fungi** exhibit parasitic behavior and can be transmitted by parasites, scientists usually study them separately as infectious diseases. Types of organisms that are studied by parasitologists include species of **protozoa**, helminths or worms, and arthropods.

Protozoa are one-celled organisms that are capable of carrying out most of the same physiological functions as multicellular organisms by using highly developed organelles within their cell. Many of the over 45,000 species of known protozoa are parasitic. As parasites of humans, this group of organisms has historically been the cause of more suffering and death than any other category of disease causing organisms.

Intestinal protozoa are common throughout the world and particularly in areas where food and water sources are subject to **contamination** from animal and human waste. Typically, protozoa that infect their host through water or food do so while in an inactive state, called a cyst, where they have encased themselves in a protective outer membrane, and are released through the digestive tract of a previous host. Once inside the host, they develop into a mature form that feeds and reproduces.

Amebic dysentery is one of the more common diseases that often afflicts travelers who visit tropical and sub-tropical regions. This condition, characterized by diarrhea, vomiting and weakness, is caused by a protozoan known as *Entamoeba histolytica*. Another protozoan that causes severe diarrhea, but is also found in more temperate regions, is *Giardia lamblia*. Among Leeuwenhoek's discoveries was *G. lamblia*, which is a now well-publicized parasite that can infect hikers who drink untreated water in the back country.

Other types of parasitic protozoa infect the blood or tissues of their hosts. These protozoa are typically transmitted through another organism, called a vector, which carries the parasite before it enters the final host. Often the vector is an invertebrate, such as an insect, that itself feeds on the host and passes the protozoan on through the bite wound. Some of the most infamous of these protozoa are members of the genera *Plasmodium*, that cause **malaria**; *Trypanosoma*, that cause African **sleeping sickness**; and *Leishmania*, which leads to a number of debilitating and disfiguring diseases.

Helminths are worm-like organisms of which several classes of parasites are found including nematodes (roundworms), cestodes (tapeworms), and trematodes (flukes). Leeches, of the phylum Annelid, are also helminths and considered as ectoparasitic, attaching themselves to the outside skin of their hosts. Nematodes, or roundworms, have an estimated 80,000 species that are known to be parasitic. The general morphology of these worms is consistent with their name; they are usually long and cylindrical in shape. One of the most infamous nematodes is *Trichinella spiralis*, a parasite that lives its larval stage encysted in the muscle tissue of animals, including swine, and make their way into the intestinal tissue of humans who happen to digest infected, undercooked pork.

Arthropods are organisms characterized by exoskeletons and segmented bodies such as crustaceans, insects, and arachnids. They are the most diverse and widely distributed animals on the planet. Many arthropod species serve as carriers of bacterial and viral diseases, as intermediate hosts for protozoan and helminth parasites, and as parasites themselves.

Certain insect species are the carriers of some of humanity's most dreaded diseases, including malaria, **typhus**, and plague. As consumers of agricultural crops and parasites of our livestock, insects are also humankind's number one competitor for resources.

Mosquitoes, are the most notorious carriers, or vectors, of disease and parasites. Female mosquitoes rely on warm-blooded hosts to serve as a blood meal to nourish their eggs. During the process of penetrating a host's skin with their long, sucking mouth parts, saliva from the mosquito is transferred into the bite area. Any viral, protozoan, or helminth infections carried in the biting mosquito can be transferred directly into the blood stream of its host. Among these are malaria, **yellow fever**, *W. bancrofti* (filariasis and elephantiasis), and *D. immitis* (heartworm).

Flies also harbor diseases that can be transmitted to humans and other mammals when they bite to obtain a blood meal for themselves. For example, black flies can carry river blindness, sandflies can carry leishmaniasis and kala-azar, and tsetse flies, found mainly in Africa, carry the trypanosomes that cause sleeping sickness. Livestock, such as horses and cattle, can be infected with a variety of botflies and warbles that can infest and feed on the skin, throat, nasal passages, and stomachs of their hosts.

Fleas and lice are two of the most common and irritating parasitic insects of humans and livestock. Lice commonly live among the hairs of their hosts, feeding on blood. Some species are carriers of the epidemic inducing typhus fever. Fleas usually infest birds and mammals, and can feed on humans when they are transferred from pets or livestock. Fleas are known to carry a variety of devastating diseases, including the plague.

Another prominent class of arthropods that contains parasitic species is the arachnids. Though this group is more commonly known for spiders and scorpions, its parasitic members include ticks and mites. Mites are very small arachnids that infest both plants and animals. One common type is chiggers, which live in grasses and, as larva, grab onto passing animals and attach themselves to the skin, often leading to irritating rashes or bite wounds. Ticks also live their adult lives among grasses and short shrubs. They are typically larger than mites, and it is the adult female that attaches itself to an animal host for a blood meal. Tick bites themselves can be painful and irritating. More importantly, ticks can carry a number of diseases that affect humans. The most common of these include Rocky Mountain spotted fever, Colorado tick fever, and the latest occurrence of tick-borne infections, **Lyme disease**.

Most parasitic infections can be treated by use of medical and surgical procedures. The best manner of controlling infection, though, is prevention. Scientists have developed and continue to test a number of drugs that can be taken as a barrier, or prophylaxis, to certain parasites. Other measures of control include improving sanitary conditions of water and food sources, proper cooking techniques, education about personal **hygiene**, and control of intermediate and vector host organisms.

PARKMAN, PAUL DOUGLAS (1932-)
American physician

Paul Parkman isolated the rubella (German **measles**) virus and, with Harry Martin Meyer (1928–2001), co-discovered the first widely applicable test for rubella antibodies and the **vaccine** against rubella.

Born in Auburn, New York, on May 29, 1932, the son of Stuart Douglas Parkman, a postal clerk, and his wife Mary née Klumpp, a homemaker, Parkman graduated from Weedsport, New York, High School in 1950. His father also served on the Weedsport Central School Board of Education and raised turkeys and chickens to help finance his son's education. Parkman took advantage of a special three-year premedical program at St. Lawrence University, majored in biology, and received both his M.D. from the State University of New York Upstate Medical Center College of Medicine (now Upstate Medical University) and his B.S. from St. Lawrence together in 1957.

After his internship at Mary Imogene Bassett Hospital, Cooperstown, New York, from 1957 to 1958, and his residency in pediatrics at the Upstate Medical Center Hospitals from 1958 to 1960, Parkman joined the army and was assigned to Walter Reed Army Medical Center, Washington, D.C. In 1963, he began working for the Division of Biologics Standards, National Institutes of Health (NIH), as a virologist. From 1963 to 1972, he was chief of the Section of General **Virology** in the Laboratory for Viral **Immunology** at the Division of Biologics Standards. In 1973, the Division of Biologics Standards was transferred to the Food and Drug Administration (FDA), where Parkman remained until he retired from federal government service on July 31, 1990. He served the FDA as director of the Division of Virology and from 1973 to 1987 in a variety of roles within the Bureau of Biology and the Center for Drugs and Biologics. From 1987 to 1990, he was the founding director of the Center for Biologics Evaluation. After his retirement, he remained in Kensington, Maryland, to consult on biological products, especially vaccines.

At Walter Reed in 1960, Parkman and his associates Edward Louis Buescher (b. 1925) and Malcolm Stewart Artenstein (b. 1930) found and used an opportunity to study rubella, which they noticed was common among military recruits. Simultaneously working on the same problem were Thomas Huckle Weller (b. 1915) and Franklin Allen Neva (b. 1922) at Harvard Medical School. In 1962 the two teams independently succeeded in isolating the virus, a member of the Togaviridae family, and each published its results in the same volume of the *Proceedings of the Society of Experimental Biology and Medicine*.

Upon developing the first reliable test for rubella antibodies, thus making accurate diagnosis of the disease possible, Parkman immediately began to create a vaccine from the attenuated virus. Meyer, Parkman, and Theodore Constantine Panos (b. 1915) reported successful clinical trials of their vaccine in the *New England Journal of Medicine* in 1966. The last major rubella epidemic was in 1964. In the 1970s, the rubella vaccine became a component of the measles-mumps-rubella vaccine (MMR), now commonly administered to children at 15 months.

See also Immunization; Virology

PASSIVE DIFFUSION • *see* CELL MEMBRANE TRANSPORT

PASTEUR, LOUIS (1822-1895)
French chemist

Louis Pasteur left a legacy of scientific contributions that include an understanding of how **microorganisms** carry on the biochemical process of **fermentation**, the establishment of the causal relationship between microorganisms and disease, and the concept of destroying microorganisms to halt the transmission of communicable disease. These achievements led him to be called the founder of microbiology.

After his early education, Pasteur went to Paris to study at the Sorbonne, then began teaching chemistry while still a student. After being appointed chemistry professor at a new university in Lille, France, Pasteur began work on **yeast** cells and showed how they produce alcohol and carbon dioxide from sugar during the process of fermentation. Fermentation is a form of cellular **respiration** carried on by yeast cells, a way of getting energy for cells when there is no oxygen present. Pasteur found that fermentation would take place only when living yeast cells were present.

Establishing himself as a serious, hard-working chemist, Pasteur was called upon to tackle some of the problems plaguing the French beverage industry at the time. Of special concern was the spoiling of wine and beer, which caused great economic loss, and tarnished France's reputation for fine vintage wines. Vintners wanted to know the cause of l'amer, a condition that was destroying France's best burgundy wines. Pasteur looked at wine under the **microscope** and noticed that when aged properly, the liquid contained little spherical yeast cells. But when the wine turned sour, there was a proliferation of bacterial cells that produced lactic acid. Pasteur suggested that heating the wine gently at about 120°F (49°C) would kill the **bacteria** that produced lactic acid and let the wine age properly. Pasteur's book *Etudes sur le Vin*, published in 1866, was a testament to two of his great passions—the scientific method and his love of wine. It caused another

French revolution—one in winemaking, as Pasteur suggested that greater cleanliness was need to eliminate bacteria and that this could be accomplished using heat. Some wine-makers were initially reticent to heat their wines, but the practice eventually saved the wine industry in France.

The idea of heating to kill microorganisms was applied to other perishable fluids, including milk, and the idea of **pasteurization** was born. Several decades later in the United States, the pasteurization of milk was championed by American bacteriologist Alice Catherine Evans, who linked bacteria in milk with the disease **brucellosis**, a type of fever found in different variations in many countries.

In his work with yeast, Pasteur also found that air should be kept from fermenting wine, but was necessary for the production of vinegar. In the presence of oxygen, yeasts and bacteria break down alcohol into acetic acid, or vinegar. Pasteur also informed the vinegar industry that adding more microorganisms to the fermenting mixture could increase vinegar production. Pasteur carried on many experiments with yeast. He showed that fermentation can take place without oxygen (anaerobic conditions), but that the process still involved living things such as yeast. He did several experiments to show (as Lazzaro Spallanzani had a century earlier) that living things do not arise spontaneously but rather come from other living things. To disprove the idea of spontaneous generation, Pasteur boiled meat extract and left it exposed to air in a flask with a long S-shaped neck. There was no decay observed because microorganisms from the air did not reach the extract. On the way to performing his experiment Pasteur had also invented what has come to be known as sterile technique, boiling or heating of instruments and food to prevent the proliferation of microorganisms.

In 1862, Pasteur was called upon to help solve a crisis in another ailing French industry. The silkworms that produced silk fabric were dying of an unknown disease. Armed with his microscope, Pasteur traveled to the south of France in 1865. Here Pasteur found the tiny **parasites** that were killing the silkworms and affecting their food, mulberry leaves. His solution seemed drastic at the time. He suggested destroying all the unhealthy worms and starting with new cultures. The solution worked, and soon French silk scarves were back in the marketplace.

Pasteur then turned his attention to human and animal diseases. He supposed for some time that microscopic organisms cause disease and that these tiny microorganisms could travel from person to person spreading the disease. Other scientists had expressed this thought before, but Pasteur had more experience using the microscope and identifying different kinds of microorganisms such as bacteria and **fungi**.

In 1868, Pasteur suffered a stroke and much of his work thereafter was carried out by his wife Marie Laurent Pasteur. After seeing what military hospitals were like during the Franco-Prussian War, Pasteur impressed upon physicians that they should boil and sterilize their instruments. This was still not common practice in the nineteenth century.

Pasteur developed techniques for culturing and examining several disease-causing bacteria. He identified *Staphylococcus pyogenes* bacteria in boils and *Streptococcus*

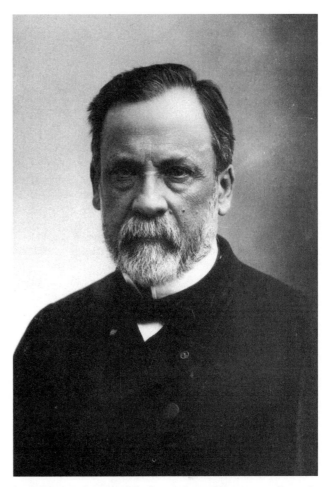

Louis Pasteur, who refuted the theory of spontaneous generation and developed the sterilization technique of pasteurization.

pyogenes in puerperal fever. He also cultured the bacteria that cause cholera. Once when injecting healthy chickens with cholera bacteria, he expected the chickens to become sick. Unknown to Pasteur, the bacteria were old and no longer virulent. The chickens failed to get the disease, but instead they received **immunity** against cholera. Thus, Pasteur discovered that weakened microbes make a good **vaccine** by imparting immunity without actually producing the disease.

Pasteur then began work on a vaccine for **anthrax**, a disease that killed many animals and infected people who contracted it from their sheep and thus was known as "wool sorters' disease." Anthrax causes sudden chills, high fever, pain, and can affect the brain. Pasteur experimented with weakening or attenuating the bacteria that cause anthrax, and in 1881 produced a vaccine that successfully prevented the deadly disease.

Pasteur's last great scientific achievement was developing a successful treatment for **rabies**, a deadly disease contracted from bites of an infected, rabid animal. Rabies, or hydrophobia, first causes pain in the throat that prevents swallowing, then brings on spasms, fever, and finally death. Pasteur knew that rabies took weeks or even months to become active. He hypothesized that if people were given an injection of a vaccine after being bitten, it could prevent the disease from manifesting. After methodically producing a rabies vaccine from the spinal fluid of infected rabbits, Pasteur sought to test it. In 1885, nine-year-old Joseph Meister, who had been bitten by a rabid dog, was brought to Pasteur, and after a series of shots of the new rabies vaccine, the boy did not develop any of the deadly symptoms of rabies.

To treat cases of rabies, the Pasteur Institute was established in 1888 with monetary donations from all over the world. It later became one of the most prestigious biological research institutions in the world. When Pasteur died in 1895, he was well recognized for his outstanding achievements in science.

See also Bacteria and bacterial infection; Colony and colony formation; Contamination, bacterial and viral; Epidemiology, tracking diseases with technology; Epidemiology; Food preservation; Germ theory of disease; History of microbiology; History of public health; Immunogenetics; Infection control; Winemaking

PASTEURELLA

Pasteurella is a genus, or subdivision, of **bacteria**. The genus is in turn a member of the family Pasteurellaceae, which includes the genus Hemophilus. Members of this genus *Pasteurella* are short rod-shaped bacteria that produce the negative reaction in the Gram stain procedure, are incapable of the active type of movement called motility, and can grow both in the presence and the absence of oxygen.

Pasteurella causes diseases in humans and many species of animals. One species in particular, *Pasteurella multocida* causes disease in both humans and animals. For example, almost all pet rabbits will at one time or another acquire infections of the nose, eyes, and lungs, or develop skin sores because of a *Pasteurella multocida* infection. The bacterium also causes a severe infection in poultry, including lameness and foul cholera, and illness in cattle and swine. Another species, *Pasteurella pneumotrophica*, infects mice, rats, guinea pigs, hamsters, and other animals that are often used in laboratory studies.

The annual economic cost of the losses due to these infections are several hundred million dollars in the United States alone.

In humans, *Pasteurella multocida* can be acquired from the bite of a cat or dog. From 20% to 50% of the one to two million Americans, mostly children, who are bitten by dogs and cats each year will develop the infection. Following some swelling at the site of the bite, the bacteria can migrate. An infection becomes established in nearby joints, where it produces swelling, arthritis, and pain.

Infections respond to common **antibiotics** including **penicillin**, tetracycline, and chloramphenicol. Despite the relative ease of treatment of the infection, little is still known of the genetic basis for the ability of the bacteria to establish an infection, and of the factors that allow the bacterium to evade the defense mechanisms of the host. In the controlled conditions of the laboratory, the adherent populations known as biofilms can be formed by *Pasteurella multocida*.

The recent completion of the genetic sequence of *Pasteurella multocida* will aid in determining the genes, and so their protein products, which are critical for infection.

See also Bacteria and bacterial infection; Proteomics

PASTEURIZATION

Pasteurization is a process whereby fluids such as wine and milk are heated for a predetermined time at a temperature that is below the boiling point of the liquid. The treatment kills any **microorganisms** that are in the fluid but does not alter the taste, appearance, or nutritive value of the fluid.

The process of pasteurization is named after the French chemist **Louis Pasteur** (1822–1895), who is regarded as the founder of the study of modern microbiology. Among Pasteur's many accomplishments was the observation that the heating of fluids destroys harmful **bacteria**.

The basis of pasteurization is the application of heat. Many bacteria cannot survive exposure to the range of temperatures used in pasteurization. The energy of the heating process is disruptive to the membrane(s) that enclose the bacteria. As well, the bacterial **enzymes** that are vital for the maintenance of the growth and survival of the bacteria are denatured, or lose their functional shape, when exposed to heat. The disruption of bacteria is usually so complete that recovery of the cells following the end of the heat treatment is impossible.

The pasteurization process is a combination of temperature, time, and the consistency of the product. Thus, the actual conditions of pasteurization can vary depending on the product being treated. For example heating at 145°F (63°C) for not less than 30 minutes or at 162°F (72°C) for not less than 16 seconds pasteurizes milk. A product with greater consistency, such ice cream or egg nog, is pasteurized by heating at a temperature of at least 156°F (69°C) for not less than 30 minutes or at a temperature of at least 176°F (80°C) for not less than 25 seconds.

Particularly in commercial settings, such as a milk processing plant, there are two long-standing methods of pasteurization. These are known as the batch method and the continuous method. In the batch method the fluid is held in one container throughout the process. This method of pasteurization tends to be used for products such as ice cream. Milk tends to be pasteurized using the continuous method.

In the continuous method the milk passes by a stack of steel plates that are heated to the desired temperature. The flow rate is such that the milk is maintained at the desired temperature for the specified period of time. The pasteurized milk then flows to another tank.

Several other more recent variations on the process of pasteurization have been developed. The first of these variations is known as flash pasteurization. This process uses a higher temperature than conventional pasteurization, but the temperature is maintained for a shorter time. The product is then rapidly cooled to below 50°F (10°C), a temperature at which it can then be stored. The intent of flash pasteurization is to eliminate harmful microorganisms while maintaining the product as close as possible to its natural state. Juices are candidates for this process. In milk, **lactic acid bacteria** can survive. While these bacteria are not a health threat, their subsequent metabolic activity can cause the milk to sour.

Another variation on pasteurization is known as ultra-pasteurization. This is similar to flash pasteurization, except that a higher than normal pressure is applied. The higher pressure greatly increases the temperature that can be achieved, and so decreases the length of time that a product, typically milk, needs to be exposed to the heat. The advantage of ultra-pasteurization is the extended shelf live of the milk that results. The milk, which is essentially sterile, can be stored unopened at room temperature for several weeks without compromising the quality.

In recent years the term cold pasteurization has been used to describe the **sterilization** of solids, such as food, using radiation. The applicability of using the term pasteurization to describe a process that does not employ heat remains a subject of debate among microbiologists.

Pasteurization is effective only until the product is exposed to the air. Then, microorganisms from the air can be carried into the product and growth of microorganisms will occur. The chance of this **contamination** is lessened by storage of milk and milk products at the appropriate storage temperatures after they have been opened. For example, even ultra-pasteurized milk needs to stored in the refrigerator once it is in use.

See also Bacteriocidal, bacteriostatic; Sterilization

PATHOGEN • *see* MICROBIOLOGY, CLINICAL

PENICILLIN

One of the major advances of twentieth-century medicine was the discovery of penicillin. Penicillin is a member of the class of drugs known as **antibiotics**. These drugs either kill (bactericidal) or arrest the growth of (bacteriostatic) **bacteria** and **fungi (yeast)**, as well as several other classes of infectious organisms. Antibiotics are ineffective against **viruses**. Prior to the advent of penicillin, bacterial infections such as **pneumonia** and sepsis (overwhelming infection of the blood) were usually fatal. Once the use of penicillin became widespread, fatality rates from pneumonia dropped precipitously.

The discovery of penicillin marked the beginning of a new era in the fight against disease. Scientists had known since the mid-nineteenth century that bacteria were responsible for some infectious diseases, but were virtually helpless to stop them. Then, in 1928, **Alexander Fleming** (1881–1955), a Scottish bacteriologist working at St. Mary's Hospital in London, stumbled onto a powerful new weapon.

Fleming's research centered on the bacteria *Staphylococcus*, a class of bacteria that caused infections such

as pneumonia, abscesses, post-operative wound infections, and sepsis. In order to study these bacteria, Fleming grew them in his laboratory in glass Petri dishes on a substance called **agar**. In August, 1928 he noticed that some of the Petri dishes in which the bacteria were growing had become contaminated with **mold**, which he later identified as belonging to the Penicillum family.

Fleming noted that bacteria in the vicinity of the mold had died. Exploring further, Fleming found that the mold killed several, but not all, types of bacteria. He also found that an extract from the mold did not damage healthy tissue in animals. However, growing the mold and collecting even tiny amounts of the active ingredient—penicillin—was extremely difficult. Fleming did, however, publish his results in the medical literature in 1928.

Ten years later, other researchers picked up where Fleming had left off. Working in Oxford, England, a team led by Howard Florey (1898–1968), an Australian, and Ernst Chain, a refugee from Nazi Germany, came across Fleming's study and confirmed his findings in their laboratory. They also had problems growing the mold and found it very difficult to isolate the active ingredient

Another researcher on their team, Norman Heatley, developed better production techniques, and the team was able to produce enough penicillin to conduct tests in humans. In 1941, the team announced that penicillin could combat disease in humans. Unfortunately, producing penicillin was still a cumbersome process and supplies of the new drug were extremely limited. Working in the United States, Heatley and other scientists improved production and began making large quantities of the drug. Owing to this success, penicillin was available to treat wounded soldiers by the latter part of World War II. Fleming, Florey, and Chain were awarded the Noble Prize in medicine. Heatley received an honorary M.D. from Oxford University in 1990.

Penicillin's mode of action is to block the construction of cell walls in certain bacteria. The bacteria must be reproducing for penicillin to work, thus there is always some lag time between dosage and response.

The mechanism of action of penicillin at the molecular level is still not completely understood. It is known that the initial step is the binding of penicillin to penicillin-binding proteins (PBPs), which are located in the cell wall. Some PBPs are inhibitors of cell autolytic **enzymes** that literally eat the cell wall and are most likely necessary during cell division. Other PBPs are enzymes that are involved in the final step of cell wall synthesis called transpeptidation. These latter enzymes are outside the cell membrane and link cell wall components together by joining glycopeptide polymers together to form **peptidoglycan**. The bacterial cell wall owes its strength to layers composed of peptidoglycan (also known as murein or mucopeptide). Peptidoglycan is a complex polymer composed of alternating N-acetylglucosamine and N-acetylmuramic acid as a backbone off of which a set of identical tetrapeptide side chains branch from the N-acetylmuramic acids, and a set of identical peptide cross-bridges also branch. The tetrapeptide side chains and the cross-bridges vary from species to species, but the backbone is the same in all bacterial species.

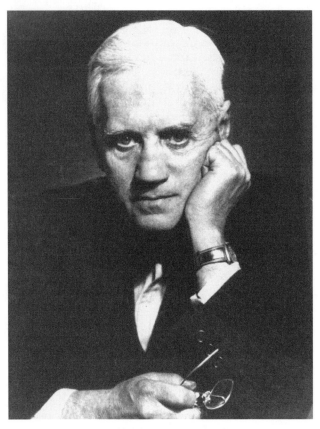

Sir Alexander Flemming, the discoverer of peniciliin.

Each peptidoglycan layer of the cell wall is actually a giant polymer molecule because all peptidoglycan chains are cross-linked. In gram-positive bacteria there may be as many as 40 sheets of peptidoglycan, making up to 50% of the cell wall material. In Gram-negative bacteria, there are only one or two sheets (about 5–10% of the cell wall material). In general, penicillin G, or the penicillin that Fleming discovered, has high activity against Gram-positive bacteria and low activity against Gram-negative bacteria (with some exceptions).

Penicillin acts by inhibiting peptidoglycan synthesis by blocking the final transpeptidation step in the synthesis of peptidoglycan. It also removes the inactivator of the inhibitor of autolytic enzymes, and the autolytic enzymes then lyses the cell wall, and the bacterium ruptures. This latter is the final bacteriocidal event.

Since the 1940s, many other antibiotics have been developed. Some of these are based on the molecular structure of penicillin; others are completely unrelated. At one time, scientists assumed that bacterial infections were conquered by the development of antibiotics. However, in the late twentieth century, bacterial resistance to antibiotics—including penicillin—was recognized as a potential threat to this success. A classic example is the *Staphylococcus* bacteria, the very species Fleming had found killed by penicillin on his Petri dishes. By 1999, a large percentage of *Staphylococcus* bacteria were resistant to penicillin G. Continuing research so far has been able to keep pace with emerging resistant strains of bacteria. Scientists and physicians must be judicious about the use of antibiotics, however, in order to minimize bacterial resistance and ensure that antibiotics such as penicillin remain effective agents for treatment of bacterial infections.

See also Antibiotic resistance, tests for; Bacteria and bacterial infection; Bacterial adaptation; Bacterial growth and division; Bacterial membranes and cell wall; History of the development of antibiotics

PENNINGER, JOSEF MARTIN (1964-   )
Austrian molecular immunologist

Josef Penninger is a medical doctor and molecular immunologist. In his short research career he has already made discoveries of fundamental significance to the understanding of bacterial infections and heart disease, osteoporosis, and the human **immune system**.

Penninger was born in Gurten, Austria. His education was in Austria, culminating with his receipt of a M.D. and Ph.D. from the University of Innsbruck in 1998. In 1990, he joined the Ontario Cancer Institute in Toronto. In 1994, he became principle investigator with the United States **biotechnology** company Amgen, joining the AMEN Research Institute that had just been established at the Department of Medical Biophysics at the University of Toronto.

In his decade at the AMEN Institute, Penninger has produced a steady stream of groundbreaking studies across the breath of **immunology**. He and his colleagues demonstrated that infection with the bacterial *Chlamydia trachomatis* caused heart damage in mice. The basis of the damage is an immune reaction to a bacterial protein that mimics the structure of the protein constituent of the heart valve.

As well, Penninger has shown that a protein called CD45 is responsible for regulating how a body's cells respond to developmental signals, coordinates the functioning of cells such as red and white blood cells, and regulates the response of the immune system to viral infection. The discovery of this key regulator and how it is co-opted in certain diseases is already viewed as a vital step to controlling diseases and preventing the immune system from attacking its own tissues (a response called an autoimmune reaction).

The research of Penninger and others, such as Barry Marshall and Stanley Pruisner, has caused a re-assessment of the nature of certain diseases. Evidence is consistent so far with a bacterial or biological origin for diseases such as schizophrenia, multiple sclerosis and Alzheimer's disease.

Penninger already has some 150 research papers published, many in the world's most prestigious scientific journals. Numerous prizes and distinctions have recognized the scope and importance of his work.

See also Chlamydial pneumonia; Immune system

PEPTIDOGLYCAN

Peptidoglycan is the skeleton of **bacteria**. Present in both Gram-positive and Gram-negative bacteria, the peptidoglycan is the rigid sac that enables the bacterium to maintain its shape.

This rigid layer is a network of two sugars that are cross-linked together by amino acid bridges. The sugars are N-acetyl glucosamine and N-acetyl muramic acid. The latter sugar is unique to the peptidoglycan, and is found no where else in nature.

The peptidoglycan in Gram-negative bacteria is only a single layer thick, and appears somewhat like the criss-cross network of strings on a tennis racket. The layer lies between the two membranes that are part of the cell wall of Gram-negative bacteria, and comprises only about twenty percent of the weight of the cell wall. In Gram-positive bacteria, the peptidoglycan is much thicker, some 40 sugars thick, comprising up to ninety percent of the weight of the cell wall. The cross bridging is three-dimensional in this network. The peptidoglycan layer is external to the single membrane, and together they comprise the cell wall of Gram-positive bacteria.

Research has demonstrated that the growth of the peptidoglycan occurs at sites all over a bacterium, rather than at a single site. Newly made peptidoglycan must be inserted into the existing network in such a way that the strength of the peptidoglycan sheet is maintained. Otherwise, the inner and outer pressures acting on the bacterium would burst the cell. This problem can be thought of as similar to trying to incorporate material into an inflated balloon without bursting the balloon. This delicate process is accomplished by the coordinate action of **enzymes** that snip open the peptidoglycan, insert new material, and bind the old and new regions together. This process is also coordinated with the rate of **bacterial growth**. The faster a bacterium is growing, the more quickly peptidoglycan is made and the faster the peptidoglycan sac is enlarged.

Certain **antibiotics** can inhibit the growth and proper linkage of peptidoglycan. An example is the beta-lactam class of antibiotics (such as **penicillin**). Also, the enzyme called lysozyme, which is found in the saliva and the tears of humans, attacks peptidoglycan by breaking the connection between the sugar molecules. This activity is one of the important bacterial defense mechanisms of the human body.

See also Bacterial ultrastructure

PERIPLASM

The periplasm is a region in the cell wall of Gram-negative **bacteria**. It is located between the outer membrane and the inner, or cytoplasmic, membrane. Once considered to be empty space, the periplasm is now recognized as a specialized region of great importance.

The existence of a region between the membranes of Gram-negative bacteria became evident when **electron microscopic** technology developed to the point where samples could be chemically preserved, mounted in a resin, and sliced very thinly. The so-called thin sections allowed electrons to pass through the sample when positioned in the electron **microscope**. Areas containing more material provided more contrast and so appeared darker in the electron image. The region between the outer and inner membranes presented a white appearance. For a time, this was interpreted as being indicative of a void. From this visual appearance came the notion that the space was functionless. Indeed, the region was first described as the periplasmic space.

Techniques were developed that allowed the outer membrane to be made extremely permeable or to be removed altogether while preserving the integrity of the underlying membrane and another stress-bearing structure called the **peptidoglycan**. This allowed the contents of the periplasmic space to be extracted and examined.

The periplasm, as it is now called, was shown to be a true cell compartment. It is not an empty space, but rather is filled with a periplasmic fluid that has a gel-like consistency. The periplasm contains a number of proteins that perform various functions. Some proteins bind molecules such as sugars, amino acids, vitamins, and ions. Via association with other cytoplasmic membrane-bound proteins these proteins can release the bound compounds, which then can be transported into the **cytoplasm** of the bacterium. The proteins, known as chaperons, are then free to diffuse around in the periplasm and bind another incoming molecule. Other proteins degrade large molecules such as nucleic acid and large proteins to a size that is more easily transportable. These periplasmic proteins include proteases, nucleases, and phosphatases. Additional periplasmic proteins, including beta lactamase, protect the bacterium by degrading incoming **antibiotics** before they can penetrate to the cytoplasm and their site of lethal action.

The periplasm thus represents a **buffer** between the external environment and the inside of the bacterium. Gram-positive bacteria, which do not have a periplasm, excrete degradative **enzymes** that act beyond the cell to digest compounds into forms that can be taken up by the cell.

See also Bacterial ultrastructure; Chaperones; Porins

PERTUSSIS

Pertussis, commonly known as whooping cough, is a highly contagious disease caused by the **bacteria** *Bordatella pertussis*. It is characterized by classic paroxysms (spasms) of uncontrollable coughing, followed by a sharp intake of air which creates the characteristic "whoop" from which the name of the illness derives.

B. pertussis is uniquely a human pathogen (a disease causing agent, such as a bacteria, virus, fungus, etc.) meaning that it neither causes disease in other animals, nor survives in humans without resulting in disease. It exists worldwide as a disease-causing agent, and causes **epidemics** cyclically in all locations.

B. pertussis causes its most severe symptoms by attacking specifically those cells in the respiratory tract which have cilia. Cilia are small, hair-like projections that beat constantly, and serve to constantly sweep the respiratory tract clean of such debris as mucus, bacteria, **viruses**, and dead cells. When *B. pertussis* interferes with this janitorial function, mucus and cellular debris accumulate and cause constant irritation to the respiratory tract, triggering the cough reflex and increasing further mucus production.

Although the disease can occur at any age, children under the age of two, particularly infants, are greatest risk. Once an individual has been exposed to *B. pertussis*, subsequent exposures result in a mild illness similar to the common **cold** and are thus usually not identifiable as resulting from *B. pertussis*.

Whooping cough has four somewhat overlapping stages: incubation, catarrhal stage, paroxysmal stage, and convalescent stage.

An individual usually acquires *B. pertussis* by inhaling droplets infected with the bacteria, coughed into the air by an individual already suffering from whooping cough symptoms. Incubation occurs during a week to two week period following exposure to *B. pertussis*. During the incubation period, the bacteria penetrate the lining tissues of the entire respiratory tract.

The catarrhal stage is often mistaken for an exceedingly heavy cold. The patient has teary eyes, sneezing, fatigue, poor appetite, and a very runny nose. This stage lasts about eight days to two weeks.

The paroxysmal stage, lasting two to four weeks, is heralded by the development of the characteristic whooping cough. Spasms of uncontrollable coughing, the "whooping" sound of the sharp inspiration of air, and vomiting are hallmarks of this stage. The whoop is believed to occur due to **inflammation** and mucous which narrow the breathing tubes, causing the patient to struggle to get air in, and resulting in intense exhaustion. The paroxysms can be caused by over activity, feeding, crying, or even overhearing someone else cough.

The mucus that is produced during the paroxysmal stage is thicker and more difficult to clear than the waterier mucus of the catarrhal stage, and the patient becomes increasingly exhausted while attempting to cough clear the respiratory tract. Severely ill children may have great difficulty maintaining the normal level of oxygen in their systems, and may appear somewhat blue after a paroxysm of coughing due to the low oxygen content of their blood. Such children may also suffer from encephalopathy, a swelling and degeneration of the brain which is believed to be caused both by lack of oxygen to the brain during paroxysms, and also by bleeding into the brain caused by increased pressure during coughing. Seizures may result from decreased oxygen to the brain. Some children have such greatly increased abdominal pressure during coughing, that hernias result (hernias are the abnormal protrusion of a loop of intestine through a weaker area of muscle). Another complicating factor during this phase is the development of **pneumonia** from infection with another bacterial agent, which takes hold due to the patient's weakened condition.

If the patient survives the paroxysmal stage, recovery occurs gradually during the convalescent stage, and takes about three to four weeks. Spasms of coughing may continue to occur over a period of months, especially when a patient contracts a cold or any other respiratory infection.

By itself, pertussis is rarely fatal. Children who die of pertussis infection usually have other conditions (e.g., pneumonia, metabolic abnormalities, other infections, etc.) that complicate their illness.

The presence of a pertussis-like cough along with an increase of certain specific white blood cells (lymphocytes) is suggestive of *B. pertussis* infection, although it could occur with other pertussis-like viruses. The most accurate method of diagnosis is to **culture** (grow on a laboratory plate) the organisms obtained from swabbing mucus out of the nasopharynx (the breathing tube continuous with the nose). *B. pertussis* can then be identified during microscopic examination of the culture.

In addition to the treatment of symptoms, Treatment with the antibiotic erythromycin is helpful against *B. pertussis* infection only at very early stages of whooping cough: during incubation and early in the catarrhal stage. After the cilia, and the cells bearing those cilia, are damaged, the process cannot be reversed. Such a patient will experience the full progression of whooping cough symptoms, which will only abate when the old, damaged lining cells of the respiratory tract are replaced over time with new, healthy, cilia-bearing cells. However, treatment with erythromycin is still recommended to decrease the likelihood of *B. pertussis* spreading. In fact, it is not uncommon that all members of the household in which a patient with whooping cough lives are treated with erythromycin to prevent spread of *B. pertussis* throughout the community.

The mainstay of prevention lies in the mass **immunization** program that begins, in the United States, when an infant is two months old. The pertussis **vaccine**, most often given as one immunization together with **diphtheria** and **tetanus**, has greatly reduced the incidence of whooping cough. Unfortunately, there has been some concern about serious neurologic side effects from the vaccine itself. This concern led huge numbers of parents in England, Japan, and Sweden to avoid immunizing their children, which in turn led to epidemics of disease in those countries. Multiple carefully constructed research studies, however, have provided evidence that pertussis vaccine was not the cause of neurologic damage.

See also Bacteria and bacterial infection; History of public health; Infection and resistance; Public health, current issues; Vaccination

PETRI DISH · *see* GROWTH AND GROWTH MEDIA

PETRI, RICHARD JULIUS (1852-1921)
German physician and bacteriologist

Richard Julius Petri's prominence in the microbiology community is due primarily to his invention of the growth container that bears his name. The Petri dish has allowed the growth of **bacteria** on solid surfaces under sterile conditions.

Petri was born in the German city of Barmen. Following his elementary and high school education he embarked on training as a physician. He was enrolled at the Kaiser

Wilhelm-Akademie for military physicians from 1871 to 1875. He then undertook doctoral training as a subordinate physician at the Berlin Charité. He received his doctorate in medicine in 1876.

From 1876 until 1882 Petri practiced as a military physician. Also, during this period, from 1877 to 1879, he was assigned to a research facility called the Kaiserliches Gesundheitsamt. There, he served as the laboratory assistant to **Robert Koch**. It was in Koch's laboratory that Petri acquired his interest in bacteriology. During his stay in Koch's laboratory, under Koch's direction, Petri devised the shallow, cylindrical, covered **culture** dish now known as the Petri dish or Petri plate.

Prior to this invention, bacteria were cultured in liquid broth. But Koch foresaw the benefits of a solid slab of medium as a means of obtaining isolated colonies on the surface. In an effort to devise a solid medium, Koch experimented with slabs of gelatin positioned on glass or inside bottles. Petri realized that Koch's idea could be realized by pouring molten **agar** into the bottom of a dish and then covering the agar with an easily removable lid.

While in Koch's laboratory, Petri also developed a technique for **cloning** (or producing exact copies) of bacterial strains on slants of agar formed in test tubes, followed by subculturing of the growth onto the Petri dish. This technique is still used to this day.

Petri's involvement in bacteriology continued after leaving Koch's laboratory. From 1882 until 1885 he ran the Göbersdorf sanatorium for **tuberculosis** patients. In 1886 he assumed the direction of the Museum of **Hygiene** in Berlin, and in 1889 he returned to the Kaiserliches Gesundheitsamt as a director.

In addition to his inventions and innovations, Petri published almost 150 papers on hygiene and bacteriology.

Petri died in the German city of Zeitz.

See also Bacterial growth and division; Growth and growth media; Laboratory techniques in microbiology

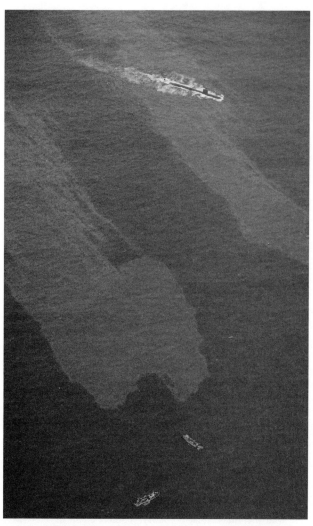

Oil spill from a damaged vessel (in this case, the Japanese training ship *Ehime Maru* after it was rammed by the American military submarine USS *Greeneville* near Hawaii).

PETROLEUM MICROBIOLOGY

Petroleum microbiology is a branch of microbiology that is concerned with the activity of **microorganisms** in the formation, recovery, and uses of petroleum. Petroleum is broadly considered to encompass both oil and natural gas. The microorganisms of concern are **bacteria** and **fungi**.

Much of the experimental underpinnings of petroleum microbiology are a result of the pioneering work of Claude ZoBell. Beginning in the 1930s and extending through the late 1970s, ZoBell's research established that bacteria are important in a number of petroleum related processes.

Bacterial degradation can consume organic compounds in the ground, which is a prerequisite to the formation of petroleum.

Some bacteria can be used to improve the recovery of petroleum. For example, experiments have shown that starved bacteria, which become very small, can be pumped down into an oil field, and then resuscitated. The resuscitated bacteria plug up the very porous areas of the oil field. When water is subsequently pumped down into the field, the water will be forced to penetrate into less porous areas, and can push oil from those regions out into spaces where the oil can be pumped to the surface.

Alternatively, the flow of oil can be promoted by the use of chemicals that are known as surfactants. A variety of bacteria produce surfactants, which act to reduce the surface tension of oil-water mixtures, leading to the easier movement of the more viscous oil portion.

In a reverse application, extra-bacterial polymers, such as **glycocalyx** and xanthan gum, have been used to make water more gel-like. When this gel is injected down into an oil formation, the gel pushes the oil ahead of it.

A third area of bacterial involvement involves the modification of petroleum hydrocarbons, either before or after collection of the petroleum. Finally, bacteria have proved very useful in the remediation of sites that are contaminated with petroleum or petroleum by-products.

The **bioremediation** aspect of petroleum microbiology has grown in importance in the latter decades of the twentieth century. In the 1980s, the massive spill of unprocessed (crude) oil off the coast of Alaska from the tanker *Exxon Valdez* demonstrated the usefulness of bacteria in the degradation of oil that was contaminating both seawater and land. Since then, researchers have identified many species of bacteria and fungi that are capable of utilizing the hydrocarbon compounds that comprise oil. The hydrocarbons can be broken down by bacteria to yield carbon dioxide and water. Furthermore, the bacteria often act as a consortium, with the degradation waste products generated by one microorganism being used as a food source by another bacterium, and so on.

A vibrant industry has been spawned around the use of bacteria as petroleum remediation agents and enhancers of oil recovery. The use of bacteria involves more than just applying an unspecified bacterial population to the spill or the oil field. Rather, the bacterial population that will be effective depends on factors, including the nature of the contaminant, **pH**, temperature, and even the size of the spaces between the rocks (i.e., permeability) in the oil field.

Not all petroleum microbiology is concerned with the beneficial aspects of microorganisms. Bacteria such as *Desulfovibrio hydrocarbonoclasticus* utilize sulfate in the generation of energy. While originally proposed as a means of improving the recovery of oil, the activity of such sulfate reducing bacteria (SRBs) actually causes the formation of acidic compounds that "sour" the petroleum formation. SRBs can also contribute to dissolution of pipeline linings that lead to the burst pipelines, and plug the spaces in the rock through which the oil normally would flow on its way to the surface. The growth of bacteria in oil pipelines is such as problem that the lines must regularly scoured clean in a process that is termed "pigging," in order to prevent pipeline blowouts. Indeed, the formation of acid-generating adherent populations of bacteria has been shown to be capable of dissolving through a steel pipeline up to 0.5 in (1.3 cm) thick within a year.

See also Biodegradable substances; Economic uses and benefits of microorganisms

PFEIFFER, RICHARD FRIEDRICH JOHANNES (1858-1945)

German physician

Richard Pfeiffer conducted fundamental research on many aspects of bacteriology, most notably bacteriolysis ("Pfeiffer's phenomenon"), which is the destruction of **bacteria** by dissolution, usually following the introduction of sera, specific antibodies, or hypotonic solutions into host animals.

Pfeiffer was born on March 27, 1858, to a German family in the Polish town of Zduny, Poznania, a province then governed by Prussia and later by Germany as Posen, but after World War II again by Poland as Ksiestwo Poznanskie. After studying medicine at the Kaiser Wilhelm Academy in Berlin from 1875 to 1879, he served Germany as an army physician and surgeon from 1879 to 1889. He received his M.D. at Berlin in 1880, taught bacteriology at Wiesbaden, Germany, from 1884 to 1887, then returned to Berlin to become the assistant of **Robert Koch** (1843–1910) at the Institute of **Hygiene** from 1887 to 1891. Upon earning his habilitation (roughly the equivalent of a Ph.D.) in bacteriology and hygiene at Berlin in 1891, he became head of the Scientific Department of the Institute for Infectious Diseases and three years later was promoted to full professor.

Pfeiffer accompanied Koch to India in 1897 to study **bubonic plague** and to Italy in 1898 to study cholera. He moved from Berlin to Königsberg, East Prussia (now Kaliningrad, Russia) in 1899 to become professor of hygiene at that city's university. He held the same position at the University of Breslau, Silesia, (now Wroclaw, Poland) from 1909 until his retirement in 1926, when he was succeeded by his friend Carl Prausnitz (1876–1963), a pioneer in the field of clinical allergy.

While serving the German army in World War I as a hygiene inspector on the Western front, Pfeiffer achieved the rank of general, won the Iron Cross, and personally intervened to save the lives of captured French microbiologists Lèon Charles Albert Calmette (1863–1933) and Camille Guèrin (1872–1961), co-inventors of the BCG (bacille biliè de Calmette-Guèrin) **vaccine** against **tuberculosis**.

Pfeiffer discovered many essential bacteriological facts, mostly in the 1890s. Several processes, phenomena, organisms, and items of equipment are named after him. A Petri dish of **agar** with a small quantity of blood smeared across the surface is called "Pfeiffer's agar." In 1891, he discovered a genus of bacteria, *Pfeifferella*, which has since been reclassified within the genus *Pseudomonas*. In 1892 he discovered and named *Haemophilus influenzae*, sometimes called "Pfeiffer's bacillus," which he incorrectly believed to be the cause of **influenza**. It does create some respiratory infections, as well as **meningitis** and conjunctivitis, but in the 1930s, other scientists learned that influenza is actually a caused by a virus.

Collaborating with Vasily Isayevich Isayev (1854–1911), he reported in 1894 and 1895 what became known as "Pfeiffer's phenomenon," **immunization** against cholera due to bacteriolysis, the dissolution of bacteria, by the injection of serum from an immune animal. In 1894, he noticed that a certain heat-resistant toxic substance was released into solution from the cell wall of *Vibrio cholerae* only after the cell had disintegrated. Following this observation he coined the term "endotoxin" to refer to potentially toxic polysaccharide or phospholipid macromolecules that form an integral part of the cell wall of Gram-negative bacteria. In 1895, he observed bactericidal substances in the blood and named them *Antikörper* ("antibodies").

Pfeiffer died on September 15, 1945 in the German-Silesian resort city of Bad Landeck, which, after the Potsdam Conference of July 17 to August 2, 1945, became Ladek Zdroj, Poland.

See also Antibody and antigen; Antibody formation and kinetics; Bacteria and bacterial infection; Bactericidal, bacteriostatic; Bubonic plague; Epidemics, bacterial; Infection and resistance; Meningitis, bacterial and viral; Pseudomonas; Serology; Typhoid fever; Typhus

PH

The term pH refers to the concentration of hydrogen ions (H+) in a solution. An acidic environment is enriched in hydrogen ions, whereas a basic environment is relatively depleted of hydrogen ions. The pH of biological systems is an important factor that determines which microorganism is able to survive and operate in the particular environment. While most **microorganisms** prefer pH's that approximate that of distilled water, some **bacteria** thrive in environments that are extremely acidic.

The hydrogen ion concentration can be determined empirically and expressed as the pH. The pH scale ranges from 0 to 14, with 1 being the most acidic and 14 being the most basic. The pH scale is a logarithmic scale. That is, each division is different from the adjacent divisions by a factor of ten. For example, a solution that has a pH of 5 is 10 times as acidic as a solution with a pH of 6.

The range of the 14-point pH scale is enormous. Distilled water has a pH of 7. A pH of 0 corresponds to 10 million more hydrogen ions per unit volume, and is the pH of battery acid. A pH of 14 corresponds to one ten-millionth as many hydrogen ions per unit volume, compared to distilled water, and is the pH of liquid drain cleaner.

Compounds that contribute hydrogen ions to a solution are called acids. For example, hydrochloric acid (HCl) is a strong acid. This means that the compounds dissociates easily in solution to produce the ions that comprise the compound (H+ and Cl−). The hydrogen ion is also a proton. The more protons there are in a solution, the greater the acidity of the solution, and the lower the pH.

Mathematically, pH is calculated as the negative logarithm of the hydrogen ion concentration. For example, the hydrogen ion concentration of distilled water is 10^{-7} and hence pure water has a pH of 7.

The pH of microbiological growth media is important in ensuring that growth of the target microbes occurs. As well, keeping the pH near the starting pH is also important, because if the pH varies too widely the growth of the microorganism can be halted. This growth inhibition is due to a numbers of reasons, such as the change in shape of proteins due to the presence of more hydrogen ions. If the altered protein ceases to perform a vital function, the survival of the microorganism can be threatened. The pH of growth media is kept relatively constant by the inclusion of compounds that can absorb excess hydrogen or hydroxyl ions. Another means of maintaining pH is by the periodic addition of acid or base in the amount needed to bring the pH back to the desired value. This is usually done in conjunction with the monitoring of the solution, and is a feature of large-scale microbial growth processes, such as used in a brewery.

Microorganisms can tolerate a spectrum of pHs. However, an individual microbe usually has an internal pH that is close to that of distilled water. The surrounding cell membranes and external layers such as the **glycocalyx** contribute to buffering the cell from the different pH of the surrounding environment.

Some microorganisms are capable of modifying the pH of their environment. For example, bacteria that utilize the sugar glucose can produce lactic acid, which can lower the pH of the environment by up to two pH units. Another example is that of **yeast**. These microorganisms can actively pump hydrogen ions out of the cell into the environment, creating more acidic conditions. Acidic conditions can also result from the microbial utilization of a basic compound such as ammonia. Conversely, some microorganisms can raise the pH by the release of ammonia.

The ability of microbes to acidify the environment has been long exploited in the pickling process. Foods commonly pickled include cucumbers, cabbage (i.e., sauerkraut), milk (i.e., buttermilk), and some meats. As well, the production of vinegar relies upon the pH decrease caused by the bacterial production of acetic acid.

See also Biochemistry; Buffer; Extremophiles

PHAGE GENETICS

Bacteriophages, **viruses** that infect **bacteria**, are useful in the study of how genes function. The attributes of bacteriophages include their small size and simplicity of genetic organization.

The most intensively studied **bacteriophage** is the phage called lambda. It is an important model system for the latent infection of mammalian cells by **retroviruses**, and it has been widely used for **cloning** purposes. Lambda is the prototype of a group of phages that are able to infect a cell and redirect the cell to become a factory for the production of new virus particles. This process ultimately results in the destruction of the host cell (lysis). This process is called the lytic cycle. On the other hand, lambda can infect a cell, direct the integration of its genome into the **DNA** of the host, and then reside there. Each time the host genome replicates, the viral genome undergoes replication, until such time as it activates and produces new virus particles and lysis occurs. This process is called the lysogenic cycle.

Lambda and other phages, which can establish lytic or lysogenic cycles, are called temperate phages. Other examples of temperate phages are bacteriophage mu and P1. Mu inserts randomly into the host chromosome causing insertional **mutations** where intergrations take place. The P1 genome exists in the host cell as an autonomous, self-replicating plasmid.

Phage **gene** expression during the lytic and lysogenic cycles uses the host **RNA** polymerase, as do other viruses. However, lambda is unique in using a type of regulation called antitermination.

As host RNA polymerase transcribes the lambda genome, two proteins are produced. They are called cro (for "control of repressor and other things") and N. If the lytic pathway is followed, **transcription** of the remainder of the viral genes occurs, and assembly of the virus particles will occur. The N protein functions in this process, ensuring that transcription does not terminate.

The path to **lysogeny** occurs differently, involving a protein called cI. The protein is a repressor and its function is to bind to operator sequences and prevent transcription. Expression of cI will induce the phage genome to integrate into the host genome. When integrated, only the cI will be produced, so as to maintain the lysogenic state.

The virus adopts the lytic or lysogenic path early following infection of the host bacterium. The fate of the viral genetic material is governed by a competition between the cro and cI proteins. Both can bind to the same operator region. The region has three binding zones—cro and cI occupy these zones in reverse order. The protein, which is able to occupy the preferred regions of the operator first, stimulates its further synthesis and blocks synthesis of the other protein.

Analysis of the genetics of phage activity is routinely accomplished using a **plaque** assay. When a phage infects a lawn or layer of bacterial cells growing on a flat surface, a clear zone of lysis can occur. The clear area is called a plaque.

Aside from their utility in the study of gene expression, phage genetics has been put to practical use as well. Cloning of the human insulin gene in bacteria was accomplished using a bacteriophage as a vector. The phage delivered to the bacterium a recombinant plasmid containing the insulin gene. M13, a single-stranded filamentous DNA bacteriophage, has long been used as a cloning vehicle for **molecular biology**. It is also valuable for use in DNA sequencing, because the viral particle contains single-stranded DNA, which is an ideal template for sequencing. T7 phage, which infects *Escherichia coli,* and some strains of *Shigella* and *Pasteurella,* is a popular vehicle for cloning of complimentary DNA. Also, the T7 promoter and RNA polymerase are in widespread use as a system for regulatable or high-level gene expression.

See also Bacteriophage and bacteriophage typing; Microbial genetics; Viral genetics

PHAGE THERAPY

Bacteriophage are well suited to deliver therapeutic payloads (i.e., deliver specific genes into a host organism). Characteristic of **viruses**, they require a host in which to make copies of their genetic material, and to assemble progeny virus particles. Bacteriophage are more specific in that they infect solely **bacteria**.

The use of phage to treat bacterial infections was popular early in the twentieth century, prior to the mainstream use of **antibiotics**. Doctors used phages as treatment for illnesses ranging from cholera to typhoid fevers. Sometimes, phage-containing liquid was poured into the wound. Oral, aerosol, and injection administrations were also used. With the advent of antibiotic therapy, the use of phage was abandoned. But now, the increasing resistance of bacteria to antibiotics has sparked a reassessment of phage therapy.

Lytic bacteriophage, which destroy the bacterial cell as part of their infectious process, are used in therapy. Much of the focus in the past 15 years has been on nosocomial, or hospital-acquired infections, where multi-drug-resistant organisms have become a particularly lethal problem.

Bacteriophage offer several advantages as therapeutic agents. Their target specificity causes less disruption to the normal host bacterial flora, some species of which are vital in maintaining the ecological balance in various areas of the body, than does the administration of a relatively less specific antibiotic. Few side effects are evident with phage therapy, particularly allergic reactions, such as can occur to some antibiotics. Large numbers of phage can be prepared easily and inexpensively. Finally, for localized uses, phage have the special advantage that they can continue multiplying and penetrating deeper as long as the infection is present, rather than decreasing rapidly in concentration below the surface like antibiotics.

In addition to their specific lethal activity against target bacteria, the relatively new field of **gene** therapy has also utilized phage. Recombinant phage, in which carry a bit of non-viral genetic material has been incorporated into their genome, can deliver the recombinant **DNA** or **RNA** to the recipient genome. The prime use of this strategy to date has been the replacement of a defective or deleterious host gene with the copy carried by the phage. Presently, however, technical safety issues and ethical considerations have limited the potential of phage genetic therapy.

See also Bacteriophage and bacteriophage typing; Microbial genetics; Viral genetics; Viral vectors in gene therapy

PHAGOCYTE AND PHAGOCYTOSIS

In the late 1800s and early 1900s, scientific researchers worked to uncover the mysteries of the body's immune system—the ways in which the body protects itself against harmful invading substances. One line of investigation showed that **immunity** is due to protective substances in the blood—antibodies—that act on disease organisms or toxins.

An additional discovery was made by the Russian-French microbiologist **Élie Metchnikoff** (1845–1916) in the 1880s. While studying transparent starfish larvae, Metchnikoff observed certain cells move to, surround, and engulf foreign particles introduced into the larvae. Metchnikoff then observed the same phenomenon in water fleas. Studying more complicated animals, Metchnikoff found similar cells moving freely in the blood and tissues. He was able to show that these mobile cells—the white blood corpuscles—in higher animals as well as humans also ingested **bacteria**.

The white blood cells responded to the site of an infection and engulfed and destroyed the invading bacteria. Metchnikoff called these bacteria-ingesting cells phagocytes, Greek for "eating cells," and published his findings in 1883.

The process of digestion by phagocytes is termed phagocytosis.

In 1905, English pathologist Almroth Wright (1861–1947) demonstrated that phagocytosis and **antibody** factors in the blood worked together in the immune response process.

See also Antibody and antigen; Antibody-antigen, biochemical and molecular reactions; Antibody formation and kinetics; Antibody, monoclonal; Antigenic mimicry; Immune system; Immunity, active, passive, and delayed; Immunity, cell mediated; Immunity, humoral regulation; Immunization; Immunogenetics; Immunology; Infection and resistance; Inflammation

PHAGOCYTE DEFECTS • *see* IMMUNODEFICIENCY DISEASE SYNDROMES

PHENOTYPE AND PHENOTYPIC VARIATION

The word **phenotype** refers to the observable characters or attributes of individual organisms, including their morphology, physiology, behavior, and other traits. The phenotype of an organism is limited by the boundaries of its specific genetic **complement (genotype)**, but is also influenced by environmental factors that impact the expression of genetic potential.

All organisms have unique genetic information, which is embodied in the particular nucleotide sequences of their **DNA (deoxyribonucleic acid)**, the genetic biochemical of almost all organisms, except for **viruses** and **bacteria** that utilize **RNA** as their genetic material. The genotype is fixed within an individual organism but is subject to change (**mutations**) from one generation to the next due to low rates of natural or spontaneous mutation. However, there is a certain degree of developmental flexibility in the phenotype, which is the actual or outward expression of the genetic information in terms of anatomy, behavior, and **biochemistry**. This flexibility can occur because the expression of genetic potential is affected by environmental conditions and other circumstances.

Consider, for example, genetically identical bacterial cells, with a fixed complement of genetic each plated on different gels. If one bacterium is colonized under ideal conditions, it can grow and colonize its full genetic potential. However, if a genetically identical bacterium is exposed to improper nutrients or is otherwise grown under adverse conditions, colony formation may be stunted. Such varying growth patterns of the same genotype are referred to as phenotypic plasticity. Some traits of organisms, however, are fixed genetically, and their expression is not affected by environmental conditions. Moreover, the ability of species to exhibit phenotypically plastic responses to environmental variations is itself, to a substantial degree, genetically determined. Therefore, phenotypic plasticity reflects both genetic capability and varying expression of that capability, depending on circumstances.

Phenotypic variation is essential for **evolution**. Without a discernable difference among individuals in a population there are no genetic **selection** pressures acting to alter the variety and types of alleles (forms of genes) present in a population. Accordingly, genetic mutations that do not result in phenotypic change are essentially masked from evolutionary mechanisms.

Phenetic similarity results when phenotypic differences among individuals are slight. In such cases, it may take a significant alteration in environmental conditions to produce significant selection pressure that results in more dramatic phenotypic differences. Phenotypic differences lead to differences in fitness and affect adaptation.

See also DNA (Deoxyribonucleic acid); Molecular biology and molecular genetics

PHENOTYPE • *see* GENOTYPE AND PHENOTYPE

PHOSPHOLIPIDS

Phospholipids are complex lipids made up of fatty acids, alcohols, and phosphate. They are extremely important components of living cells, with both structural and metabolic roles. They are the chief constituents of most biological membranes.

At one end of a phospholipid molecule is a phosphate group linked to an alcohol. This is a polar part of the molecule—it has an electric charge and is water-soluble (hydrophilic). At the other end of the molecule are fatty acids, which are non-polar, **hydrophobic**, fat soluble, and water insoluble.

Because of the dual nature of the phospholipid molecules, with a water-soluble group attached to a water-insoluble group in the same molecule, they are called amphipathic or polar lipids. The amphipathic nature of phospholipids make them ideal components of biological membranes, where they form a lipid bilayer with the polar region of each layer facing out to interact with water, and the non-polar fatty acid "tail" portions pointing inward toward each other in the interior of the bilayer. The lipid bilayer structure of cell membranes makes them nearly impermeable to polar molecules such as ions, but proteins embedded in the membrane are able to carry many substances through that they could not otherwise pass.

Phosphoglycerides, considered by some as synonymous for phospholipids, are structurally related to 3-phosphoglyceraldehyde (PGA), an intermediate in the catabolic **metabolism** of glucose. Phosphoglycerides differ from phospholipids because they contain an alcohol rather than an aldehyde group on the 1-carbon. Fatty acids are attached by an ester linkage to one or both of the free hydroxyl (-OH) groups of the glyceride on carbons 1 and 2. Except in phosphatidic acid, the simplest of all phosphoglycerides, the phosphate attached to the 3-carbon of the glyceride is also linked to another alcohol. The nature of this alcohol varies considerably.

See also Bacteremic; Bacterial growth and division; Bacterial membranes and cell wall; Bacterial surface layers; Bacterial ultrastructure; Biochemistry; Cell membrane transport; Membrane fluidity

Photosynthesis

PHOTOSYNTHESIS

Photosynthesis is the biological conversion of light energy into chemical energy. This occurs in green plants, algae, and photosynthetic **bacteria**.

Much of the early knowledge of bacterial photosynthesis came from the work of Dutch-born microbiologist **Cornelius van Neil** (1897–1985). During his career at the Marine Research Station in Monterey, California, van Neil studied photosynthesis in anaerobic bacteria. Like higher plants, these bacteria manufacture carbohydrates during photosynthesis. But, unlike plants, they do not produce oxygen during the photosynthetic process. Furthermore, the bacteria use a compound called bacteriochlorophyll rather than **chlorophyll** as a photosynthetic pigment. Van Neil found that all species of photosynthetic bacteria require a compound that the bacteria can oxidize (i.e., remove an electron from). For example, the purple sulfur bacteria use hydrogen sulfide.

Since van Neil's time, the structure of the photosynthetic apparatus has been deduced. The study of photosynthesis is currently an active area of research in biology. Crystals of the photosynthetic reaction center from the anaerobic photosynthetic bacterium *Rhodopseudomonas viridis* were created in the 1980s by Hartmut Michel and Johann Deisenhofer, who then used x-ray crystallography to determine the three-dimensional structure of the photosynthetic protein. In 1988, the two scientists shared the Nobel Prize in Chemistry with Robert Huber for this research.

Photosynthesis consists of two series of biochemical reactions, called the light reactions and the dark reactions. The light reactions use the light energy absorbed by chlorophyll to synthesize structurally unstable high-energy molecules. The dark reactions use these high-energy molecules to manufacture carbohydrates. The carbohydrates are stable structures that can be stored by plants and by bacteria. Although the dark reactions do not require light, they often occur in the light because they are dependent upon the light reactions. In higher plants and algae, the light and dark reactions of photosynthesis occur in chloroplasts, specialized chlorophyll-containing intracellular structures that are enclosed by double membranes.

In the light reactions of photosynthesis, light energy excites photosynthetic pigments to higher energy levels and this energy is used to make two high energy compounds, ATP (adenosine triphosphate) and NADPH (nicotinamide adenine dinucleotide phosphate). ATP and NADPH are consumed during the subsequent dark reactions in the synthesis of carbohydrates.

In algae, the light reactions occur on the so-called thylakoid membranes of the chloroplasts. The thylakoid membranes are inner membranes of the chloroplasts. These membranes are arranged like flattened sacs. The thylakoids are often stacked on top of one another, like a roll of coins. Such a stack is referred to as a granum. ATP can also be made by a special series of light reactions, referred to as cyclic photophosphorylation, which occurs in the thylakoid membranes of the **chloroplast**.

Algae are capable of photosynthetic generation of energy. There are many different groups of photosynthetic algae. Like higher plants, they all have chlorophyll-a as a photosynthetic pigment, two photosystems (PS-I and PS-II), and the same overall chemical reactions for photosynthesis. Algae differ from higher plants in having different complements of additional chlorophylls. *Chlorophyta* and *Euglenophyta* have chlorophyll-a and chlorophyll-b. *Chrysophyta*, *Pyrrophyta*, and *Phaeophyta* have chlorophyll-a and chlorophyll-c. *Rhodophyta* have chlorophyll-a and chlorophyll-d. The different chlorophylls and other photosynthetic pigments allow algae to utilize different regions of the solar spectrum to drive photosynthesis.

A number of photosynthetic bacteria are known. One example are the bacteria of the genus *Cyanobacteria*. These bacteria were formerly called the **blue-green algae** and were once considered members of the plant kingdom. However, unlike the true algae, cyanobacteria are prokaryotes, in that their **DNA** is not sequestered within a **nucleus**. Like higher plants, they have chlorophyll-a as a photosynthetic pigment, two photosystems (PS-I and PS-II), and the same overall equation for photosynthesis (equation 1). Cyanobacteria differ from higher plants in that they have additional photosynthetic pigments, referred to as phycobilins. Phycobilins absorb different wavelengths of light than chlorophyll and thus increase the wavelength range, which can drive photosynthesis. Phycobilins are also present in the Rhodophyte algae, suggesting a possible evolutionary relationship between these two groups.

Cyanobacteria are the predominant photosynthetic organism in anaerobic fresh and marine water.

Another photosynthetic bacterial group is called cloroxybacteria. This group is represented by a single genus called *Prochloron*. Like higher plants, *Prochloron* has chlorophyll-a, chlorophyll-b, and carotenoids as photosynthetic pigments, two photosystems (PS-I and PS-II), and the same overall equation for photosynthesis. *Prochloron* is rather like a free-living chloroplast from a higher plant.

Another group of photosynthetic bacteria are known as the purple non-sulfur bacteria (e.g., *Rhodospirillum rubrum*. The bacteria contain bacteriochlorophyll a or b positioned on specialized membranes that are extensions of the cytoplasmic membrane.

Anaerobic photosynthetic bacteria is a group of bacteria that do not produce oxygen during photosynthesis and only photosynthesize in environments that are devoid of oxygen. These bacteria use carbon dioxide and a substrate such as hydrogen sulfide to make carbohydrates. They have bacteriochlorophylls and other photosynthetic pigments that are similar to the chlorophylls used by higher plants. But, in contrast to higher plants, algae and cyanobacteria, the anaerobic photosynthetic bacteria have just one photosystem that is similar to PS-I. These bacteria likely represent a very ancient photosynthetic microbe.

The final photosynthetic bacteria are in the genus *Halobacterium*. Halobacteria thrive in very salty environments, such as the Dead Sea and the Great Salt Lake. Halobacteria are unique in that they perform photosynthesis without chlorophyll. Instead, their photosynthetic pigments are bacteriorhodopsin and halorhodopsin. These pigments are similar to sensory rhodopsin, the pigment used by humans and other animals for vision. Bacteriorhodopsin and halorhodopsin are embedded in the cell membranes of halobacteria and each pigment consists of retinal, a vitamin-A derivative, bound to a protein. Irradiation of these pigments causes a structural change in their retinal. This is referred to as photoisomerization. Retinal photoisomerization leads to the synthesis of ATP. Halobacteria have two additional rhodopsins, sensory rhodopsin-I and sensory rhodopsin-II. These compounds regulate phototaxis, the directional movement in response to light.

See also Evolutionary origin of bacteria and viruses

PHOTOSYNTHETIC MICROORGANISMS

Life first evolved in the primordial oceans of Earth approximately four billion years ago. The first life forms were prokaryotes, or non-nucleated unicellular organisms, which divided in two domains, the **Bacteria** and **Archaea**. They lived around hot sulfurous geological and volcanic vents on the ocean floor, forming distinct biofilms, organized in multilayered symbiotic communities, known as microbial mats. Fossil evidence suggests that these first communities were not photosynthetic, i.e., did not use the energy of light to convert carbon dioxide and water into glucose, releasing oxygen in the process. About 3.7 billions years ago, anoxygenic photosynthetic **microorganisms** probably appeared on top of pre-photosynthetic biofilms formed by bacterial and Archaean sulphate-processers. Anoxygenic photosynthesizers use electrons donated by sulphur, hydrogen sulfide, hydrogen, and a variety of organic chemicals released by other bacteria and Archaea. This ancestor species, known as protochlorophylls, did not synthesized **chlorophyll** and did not release oxygen during **photosynthesis**. Moreover, in that deep-water environment, they probably used infrared thermo taxis rather than sunlight as a source of energy.

Protochlorophylls are assumed to be the common ancestors of two evolutionary branches of oxygenic photosynthetic organisms that began evolving around 2.8 billion years ago: the bacteriochlorophyll and the chlorophylls. Bacteriochlorophyll gave origin to chloroflexus, sulfur green bacteria, sulfur purple bacteria, non-sulfur purple bacteria, and finally to oxygen-respiring bacteria. Chlorophylls originated Cyanobacteria, from which chloroplasts such as red algae, cryptomonads, **dinoflagellates**, crysophytes, brown algae, euglenoids, and finally green plants evolved. The first convincing paleontological evidence of eukaryotic microfossils (chloroplasts) was dated 1.5 at billion years old. In oxygenic photosynthesis, electrons are donated by water molecules and the energy source is the visible spectrum of visible light. However, the chemical elements utilized by oxygenic photosynthetic organisms to capture electrons divide them in two families, the Photosystem I Family and the Photosystem II Family. Photosystem II organisms, such as *Chloroflexus aurantiacus* (an ancient green bacterium) and sulfur purple bacteria, use pigments and quinones as electron acceptors, whereas member of the Photosystem I Family, such as green sulfur bacteria, Cyanobacteria, and chloroplasts use iron-sulphur centers as electron acceptors.

It is generally accepted that the **evolution** of oxygenic photosynthetic microorganisms was a crucial step for the increase of atmospheric oxygen levels and the subsequent burst of biological evolution of new aerobic species. About 3.5 billion years ago, the planet atmosphere was poor in oxygen and abundant in carbon dioxide and sulfuric gases, due to intense volcanic activity. This atmosphere favored the evolution of chemotrophic Bacteria and Archaea. As the populations of oxygenic photosynthetic microorganisms gradually expanded, they started increasing the atmospheric oxygen level two billion years ago, stabilizing it at its present level of 20% about 1.5 billion years ago, and additionally, reduced the carbon dioxide levels in the process. Microbial photosynthetic activity increased the planetary biological productivity by a factor of 100–1,000, opening new pathways of biological evolution and leading to biogeochemical changes that allowed life to evolve and colonize new environmental niches. The new atmospheric and biogeochemical conditions created by photosynthetic microorganisms allowed the subsequent appearance of plants about 1.2 billion years ago, and 600 million years later, the evolution of the first vertebrates, followed 70 million years later by the Cambrian burst of biological diversity.

See also Aerobes; Autotrophic bacteria; Biofilm formation and dynamic behavior; Biogeochemical cycles; Carbon cycle in microorganisms; Chemoautotrophic and chemolithotrophic bacteria; Electron transport system; Evolutionary origin of bacteria and viruses; Fossilization of bacteria; Hydrothermal vents; Plankton and planktonic bacteria; Sulfur cycle in microorganisms

PHYLOGENY

Phylogeny is the inferred evolutionary history of a group of organisms (including **microorganisms**). Paleontologists are interested in understanding life through time, not just at one time in the past or present, but over long periods of past time. Before they can attempt to reconstruct the forms, functions, and lives of once-living organisms, paleontologists have to place these organisms in context. The relationships of those organisms to each other are based on the ways they have branched out, or diverged, from a common ancestor. A phylogeny is usually represented as a phylogenetic tree or cladogram, which are like genealogies of species.

Phylogenetics, the science of phylogeny, is one part of the larger field of systematics, which also includes taxonomy. Taxonomy is the science of naming and classifying the diversity of organisms. Not only is phylogeny important for understanding paleontology (study of fossils), however, paleontology in turn contributes to phylogeny. Many groups of organisms are now extinct, and without their fossils we would not have as clear a picture of how modern life is interrelated.

There is an amazing diversity of life, both living and extinct. For scientists to communicate with each other about these many organisms, there must also be a classification of these organisms into groups. Ideally, the classification should be based on the evolutionary history of life, such that it predicts properties of newly discovered or poorly known organisms.

Phylogenetic systematics is an attempt to understand the evolutionary interrelationships of living things, trying to interpret the way in which life has diversified and changed over time. While classification is primarily the creation of names for groups, systematics goes beyond this to elucidate new theories of the mechanisms of **evolution**.

Cladistics is a particular method of hypothesizing relationships among organisms. Like other methods, it has its own set of assumptions, procedures, and limitations. Cladistics is now accepted as the best method available for phylogenetic analysis, for it provides an explicit and testable hypothesis of organismal relationships.

The basic idea behind cladistics is that members of a group share a common evolutionary history, and are "closely related," more so to members of the same group than to other organisms. These groups are recognized by sharing unique features that were not present in distant ancestors. These shared derived characteristics are called synapomorphies. Synapomorphies are the basis for cladistics.

In a cladistic analysis, one attempts to identify which organisms belong together in groups, or clades, by examining specific derived features or characters that those organisms share. For example, if a genus of **bacteria** forms a specific color or shaped **colony**, then those characters might be a useful character for determining the evolutionary relationships of other bacteria. Characters that define a clade are called synapomorphies. Characters that do not unite a clade because they are primitive are called plesiomorphies.

In a cladistic analysis, it is important to know which character states are primitive and which are derived (that is, evolved from the primitive state). A technique called outgroup comparison is commonly used to make this determination. In outgroup comparison, the individuals of interest (the ingroup) are compared with a close relative. If some of the individuals of the ingroup possess the same character state as the outgroup, then that character state is assumed to be primitive.

There are three basic assumptions in cladistics:

1. Any group of organisms are related by descent from a common ancestor.
2. There is a bifurcating pattern of cladogenesis.
3. Change in characteristics occurs in lineages over time.

The first assumption is a general assumption made for all evolutionary biology. It essentially means that life arose on Earth only once, and therefore all organisms are related in one way or another. Because of this, scientists can take any collection of organisms and determine a meaningful pattern of relationships, provided they have the right kind of information.

The second assumption is that new kinds of organisms may arise when existing species or populations divide into exactly two groups. The final assumption, that characteristics of organisms change over time, is the most important assumption in cladistics. It is only when characteristics change that different lineages or groups are recognized. The convention is to call the "original" state of the characteristic plesiomorphic and the "changed" state apomorphic. The terms *primitive* and *derived* have also been used for these

states, but they are often avoided by cladists, since those terms have been abused in the past.

Cladistics is useful for creating systems of classification. It is now the most commonly used method to classify organisms because it recognizes and employs evolutionary theory. Cladistics predicts the properties of organisms. It produces hypotheses about the relationships of organisms in a way that makes it possible to predict properties of the organisms. This can be especially important in cases when particular genes or biological compounds are being sought. Such genes and compounds are being sought all the time by companies interested in improving bacterial strains, disease resistance, and in the search for medicines. Only an hypothesis based on evolutionary theory, such as cladistic hypotheses, can be used for these endeavors.

As an example, consider the plant species *Taxus brevifolia*. This species produces a compound, taxol, which is useful for treating cancer. Unfortunately, large quantities of bark from this rare tree are required to produce enough taxol for a single patient. Through cladistic analysis, a phylogeny for the genus *Taxus* has been produced that shows *Taxus cuspidata*, a common ornamental shrub, to be a very close relative of *T. brevifolia*. *Taxus cuspidata*, then, may also produce large enough quantities of taxol to be useful. Having a classification based on evolutionary descent will allow scientists to select the species most likely to produce taxol.

Cladistics helps to elucidate mechanisms of evolution. Unlike previous systems of analyzing relationships, cladistics is explicitly evolutionary. Because of this, it is possible to examine the way characters change within groups over time, the direction in which characters change, and the relative frequency with which they change. It is also possible to compare the descendants of a single ancestor and observe patterns of origin and extinction in these groups, or to look at relative size and diversity of the groups. Perhaps the most important feature of cladistics is its use in testing long-standing hypotheses about adaptation.

See also Bacterial kingdoms; Evolution and evolutionary mechanisms; Evolutionary origin of bacteria and viruses; Microbial genetics; Viral genetics

PILI • *see* BACTERIAL APPENDAGES

PIPETTE

A pipette is a piece of volumetric glassware used to transfer quantitatively a desired volume of solution from one container to another. Pipettes are calibrated at a specified temperature (usually 68°F [20°C] or 77°F [25°C]) either to contain (TC) or to deliver (TD) the stated volume indicated by the etched/painted markings on the pipette side. Pipettes that are marked TD generally deliver the desired volume with free drainage; whereas in the case of pipettes marked TC the last drop must be blown out or washed out with an appropriate solvent.

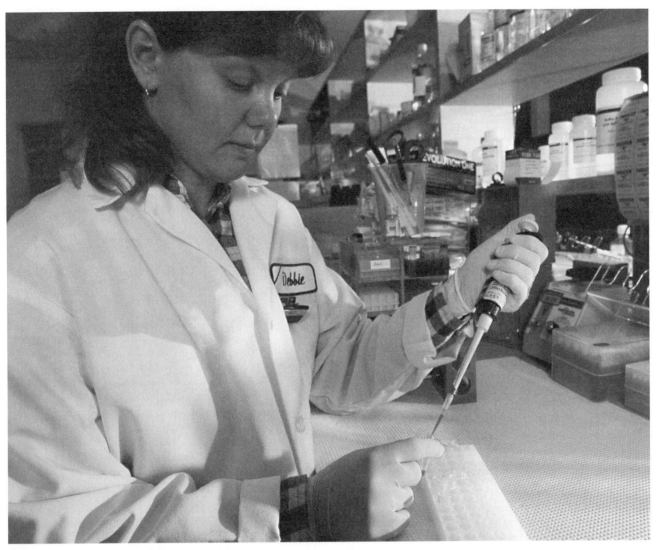

Researcher dispensing sample into an analysis tray.

For high-accuracy chemical analysis and research work, a volumetric transfer pipette is preferred. Volumetric transfer pipettes are calibrated to deliver a fixed liquid volume with free drainage, and are available in sizes ranging from 0.5–200 mL. Class A pipettes with volumes greater than 5 mL have a tolerance of +/-0.2% or better. The accuracy and precision of the smaller Class A pipettes and of the Class B pipettes are less. The Ostwald-Folin pipette is similar to the volumetric transfer pipette, except that the last drop should be blown out. Mohr and serological pipettes have graduated volumetric markings, and are designed to deliver various volumes with an accuracy of +/- 0.5-1.0%. The volume of liquid transferred is the difference between the volumes indicated before and after delivery. Serological pipettes are calibrated all the way to the tip, and the last drop should be blown out. The calibration markings on Mohr pipettes, on the other hand, begins well above the tip. Lambda pipettes are used to transfer very small liquid volumes down to 1 microliter. Dropping pipettes (i.e.,

medicine droppers) and Pasteur pipettes are usually uncalibrated, and are used to transfer liquids only when accurate quantification is not necessary.

Automatic dispensing pipettes and micropipettes are available commercially. Automatic dispensing pipettes, in sizes ranging from 1–2,000 mL, permit fast, repetitive delivery of a given volume of solution from a dispensing bottle. Micropipettes consist of a cylinder with a thumb-operated air-tight plunger. A disposable plastic tip attaches to the end of the cylinder, the plunger is depressed, and the plastic tip is immersed in the sample solution. The liquid enters the tip when the plunger is released. The solution never touches the plunger. Micropipettes generally have fixed volumes, however, some models have provisions for adjustable volume settings. Micropipettes are extremely useful in clinical and biochemical applications where errors of +/- 1% are acceptable, and where problems of **contamination** make disposable tips desirable.

See also Laboratory techniques in immunology; Laboratory techniques in microbiology

PITTMAN, MARGARET (1901-1995)
American bacteriologist

An expert in the development and standardization of bacterial vaccines, Margaret Pittman advanced the fight against such diseases as whooping cough (**pertussis**), **tetanus**, typhoid, cholera, **anthrax**, **meningitis**, and conjunctivitis.

Pittman was born on January 20, 1901 in Prairie Grove, Arkansas, the daughter of a physician, James ("Dr. Jim") Pittman, and the former Virginia Alice McCormick. The family moved to nearby Cincinnati, Arkansas, in 1909. Her father was the only doctor in that rural area, and she sometimes helped him on his rounds or with anesthesia. Her formal education was sporadic until three years of high school in Prairie Grove and two years of music seminary in Siloam Springs, Arkansas. As a member of the class of 1923 at Hendrix College, Conway, Arkansas, she double-majored in mathematics and biology, and won the Walter Edwin Hogan Mathematics Award in 1922. From 1923 until 1925 in Searcy, Arkansas, she taught and served as principal at Galloway Woman's College, which merged with Hendrix in 1933. She received her M.S. in 1926 and her Ph.D. in 1929, both in bacteriology from the University of Chicago.

Pittman's landmark article of 1931, "Variation and Type Specificity in the Bacterial Species *Haemophilus Influenzae*," showed that the pathogenicity (disease-causing quality) of this microbe is determined by minor differences in its physical nature, such as the presence or absence of a polysaccharide capsule. For all microbes, these differences can be classed as strains or types. Pittman identified six serotypes of *Haemophilus influenzae*, which she labeled "a" through "f." Serotype b (Hib) is the most pathogenic, causing meningitis and several other serious infections. Her work led to the development of polysaccharide vaccines that immunize against Hib.

Pittman conducted her bacteriological research at the Rockefeller Institute for Medical Research (later Rockefeller University) from 1928 to 1934, at the New York State Department of Health from 1934 to 1936, and from 1936 until the end of her career at the National Institutes of Health (NIH). Among the subjects of her research were tetanus, toxins and antitoxins, sera and antisera, the genus *Bordetella*, the Koch-Weeks bacillus, the standardization of vaccines, and cholera. Some of this work was done abroad under the auspices of the **World Health Organization** (**WHO**). In 1957, Pittman became the first woman director of an NIH laboratory when she was chosen chief of the Laboratory of Bacterial Products in the Division of Biologics Standards. She held that post until she retired in 1971. Thereafter she lived quietly but productively in Temple Hills, Maryland, serving occasionally as a guest researcher and consultant for NIH, the U.S. Food and Drug Administration (FDA), and WHO, and remaining active in the United Methodist Church, especially through Wesley

Theological Seminary in Washington, D.C. She died August 19, 1995.

In 1994, NIH inaugurated the Margaret Pittman Lect Series and the American Society for Microbiology presen its first Margaret Pittman Award. On October 19, 1995, Jc Bennett Robbins (b. 1932) and Ronald D. Sekura, both of National Institute of Child Health and Human Developm (NICHD) published an article in the *New England Journal Medicine*, announcing their new pertussis **vaccine**, based Pittman's research at the FDA.

See also Antiserum and antitoxin; Bacteria and bacter infection; Meningitis, bacterial and viral; Pneumonia, bact ial and viral; Serology; Tetanus and tetanus immunizati Typhoid fever

PLAGUE, BUBONIC • *see* BUBONIC PLAGUE

PLANKTON AND PLANKTONIC BACTERIA

Plankton and planktonic **bacteria** share two features. Fi they are both single-celled creatures. Second, they live floating organisms in the respective environments.

Plankton and planktonic bacteria are actually quite ferent from one another. Plankton is comprised of two m types, neither of which is bacterial. One type of plankton, one of most relevance to this volume, is phytoplankt Phytoplankton are plants. The second type of plankton is z **plankton**. These are microscopic animals. Phytoplankton fo the basis of the food chain in the ocean.

Phytoplankton are fundamentally important to life Earth for several reasons. In the oceans, they are the beginn of the food chain. Existing in the oceans in huge quantiti phytoplankton are eaten by small fish and animals that are turn consumed by larger species. Their numbers can be huge that they are detectable using specialized satellite im ing, which is exploited by the commercial fishing industry pinpoint likely areas in which to catch fish.

Phytoplankton, through their central role in the carl cycle, are also a critical part of the ocean chemistry. The carl dioxide content in the atmosphere is in balance with the cont in the oceans. The photosynthetic activity of phytoplank removes carbon dioxide from the water and releases oxyger a by-product to the atmosphere. This allows the oceans absorb more carbon dioxide from the air. Phytoplankton, the fore, act to keep the atmospheric level of carbon dioxide fr increasing, which causes the atmosphere to heat up, and a replenish the oxygen level of the atmosphere.

When phytoplankton die and sink to the ocean floor, carbon contained in them is lost from global circulation. T is beneficial because if the carbon from all dead matter recycled into the atmosphere as carbon dioxide, the balance carbon dioxide would be thrown off, and a massive atm pheric temperature increase would occur.

Phytoplankton are also being recognized as an indicator for the physical status of the oceans. They require a fairly limited range of water temperature for healthy growth. So, a downturn in phytoplankton survival can be an early indicator of changing conditions, both at a local level (such as the presence of pollutants) and at a global level (global warming).

Planktonic bacteria are free-living bacteria. They are the populations that grow in the familiar test tube and flask cultures in the microbiology laboratory. The opposite mode of growth is the adherent, or sessile, type of growth.

Planktonic bacteria have been recognized for centuries. They are some of the "animalcules" described by **Antoni van Leeuwenhoek** in 1673 using a **microscope** of his own design. Indeed, much of the knowledge of microbiology is based on work using these free-floating organisms. Research over the past two decades has shown that the planktonic mode of growth is secondary to the adherent type of growth. Additionally, the character of planktonic bacteria is very different from their adherent counterparts. Planktonic bacteria tend to have surfaces that are relatively hydrophilic (water loving), and the pattern of **gene** expression is markedly different from bacteria growing on a surface. Also, planktonic bacteria tend not to have a surrounding coat made of various sugars (this coat is also called a **glycocalyx**), and so the bacteria tend to be more susceptible to antibacterial agent such as **antibiotics**. Paradoxically, most of the knowledge of antibiotic activity has been based on experiments with planktonic bacteria.

When grown in a **culture** where no new nutrients are added, planktonic bacteria typically exhibit the four stages of population development that are known as lag phase, logarithmic (or exponential) phase, stationary phase, and death (or decline) phase. It is also possible to grow planktonic bacteria under conditions where fresh food is added at the same rate as culture is removed. Then, the bacteria will grow as fast as the rate of addition of the new food source and can remain in this state for as long as the conditions are maintained. Thus, planktonic bacteria display a great range in the speeds at which they can grow. These abilities, as well as other changes the bacteria are capable of, is possible because the bacteria are phenotypically "plastic;" that is, they are very adaptable. Their adherent counterparts tend to be less responsive to environmental change.

Planktonic bacteria are susceptible to eradication by the **immune system** of man and other animals. Examination of many infectious bacteria has demonstrated that once in a host, planktonic bacteria tend to adopt several strategies to evade the host reaction. These strategies include formation of the adherent, glycocalyx enclosed populations, the elaboration of the glycocalyx around individual bacteria, and entry into the cells of the host.

It is becoming increasingly evident that the planktonic bacteria first observed by Leeuwenhoek and which is the staple of lab studies even today is rather atypical of the state of the bacteria in nature and in infections. Thus, in a sense, the planktonic bacteria in the test tube culture is an artifact.

See also Carbon cycle in microorganisms

PLANT VIRUSES

Plant **viruses** are viruses that multiply by infecting plant cells and utilizing the plant cell's genetic replication machinery to manufacture new virus particles.

Plant viruses do not infect just a single species of plant. Rather, they will infect a group of closely related plant species. For example, the **tobacco mosaic virus** can infect plants of the genus *Nicotiana*. As the tobacco plant is one of the plants that can be infected, the virus has taken its name from that host. This name likely reflects the economic importance of the virus to the tobacco industry. Two other related viruses that were named for similar economic reasons are the potato-X and potato-Y viruses. The economic losses caused by these latter two viruses can be considerable. Some estimates have put the total worldwide damage as high as $60 billion a year.

The tobacco mosaic virus is also noteworthy as it was the first virus that was obtained in a pure form and in large quantity. This work was done by Wendall Meredith Stanley in 1935. For this and other work he received the 1946 Nobel Prize in Chemistry.

Plants infected with a virus can display lighter areas on leaves, which is called chlorosis. Chlorosis is caused by the degradation of the **chlorophyll** in the leaf. This reduces the degree of **photosynthesis** the plant can accomplish, which can have an adverse effect on the health of the entire plant. Infected plants may also display withered leaves, which is known as necrosis.

Sometimes plant viruses do not produce symptoms of infection. This occurs when the virus become latent. The viral nucleic acid becomes incorporated into the host material, just as happens with latent viruses that infect humans such as **herpes** viruses and **retroviruses**.

Most of the known plant viruses contain **ribonucleic acid (RNA)**. In a virus known as the wound tumor virus, the RNA is present as a double strand. The majority of the RNA plant viruses, however, possess a single strand of the nucleic acid. A group of viruses known as gemini viruses contain single stranded **deoxyribonucleic acid (DNA)** as their genetic material, and the cauliflower mosaic virus contains double stranded DNA.

As with viruses of other hosts, plant viruses display different shapes. Also as with other viruses, the shape of any particular virus is characteristic of that species. For example, a tobacco mosaic virus is rod-shaped and does not display variation in this shape. Other plant viruses are icosahedral in shape (an icosahedron is a 20-sided figure constructed of 20 faces, each of which is an equilateral triangle).

There are no plant viruses known that recognize specific receptors on the plant. Rather, plant viruses tend to enter plant cells either through a surface injury to a leaf or the woody stem or branch structures, or during the feeding of an insect or the microscopic worms known as nematodes. These methods of transmission allow the virus to overcome the barrier imposed by the plant cell wall and cuticle layer. Those viruses that are transmitted by insects or animals must be capable of multiplication in the hosts as well as in the plant.

Plant viruses may also be transmitted to a new plant host via infected seeds from another plant. In the laboratory, viral DNA can be introduced into the bacterium *Agrobacterium tumefaciens*. When the bacterium infects a plant, the viral DNA can be incorporated into the plant genome. Experimental infection of plants can be done by rubbing virus preparation into the leaves of the plant. The virus can enter the plant through the physical abrasion that is introduced.

As humans can mount an immune response against viral infection, so plants have defense strategies. One strategy is the presence of a tough cell wall on many plants that restricts the entry of viruses unless the surface barrier of the plant is compromised, as by injury. Many plants also display a response that is termed hypersensitivity. In this response the plant cells in the vicinity of the infected cell die. This acts to limit the spread of the virus, since the virus require living cells in which to replicate.

Some plants have been shown to be capable of warning each other of the presence of a viral infection. This communication is achieved by the airborne release of a specific compound. This behavior is similar to the cell to cell signaling found in bacterial populations, which is known as **quorum sensing**.

See also Viral genetics; Virology

PLAQUE

Plaque is the diverse community of **microorganisms**, mainly **bacteria**, which develops naturally on the surface of teeth. The microbes are cocooned in a network of sugary polymers produced by the bacteria, and by host products, such as saliva, epithelial and other host cells, and inorganic compounds such as calcium. The surface-adherent, enmeshed community of plaque represents a biofilm.

Plaque is important for two reasons, one beneficial and the other detrimental. The beneficial aspect of dental plaque is that the coverage of the tooth surface by microbes that are normally resident in the host can exclude the colonization of the tooth by extraneous bacteria that might be harmful. This phenomenon is known as competitive exclusion. However, despite this benefit, the plaque can position acid-producing bacteria near the tooth and protect those bacteria from attempts to kill or remove them. Plaque can become extremely hard, as the constituent inorganic components create a crystalline barrier. Protected inside the plaque, the acid-producing bacteria can dissolve the tooth enamel, which can lead to the production of a cavity.

A plaque is a complex community, consisting of hundreds of species of bacteria. Plaque formation generally begins with the adherence of certain bacteria, such as *Streptococcus sanguis*, *Streptococcus mutans*, and *Actinomyces viscosus*. Then, so-called secondary colonizers become established. Examples include *Fusobacterium nucleatum* and *Prevotella intermedia*. As the plaque matures, a varied variety of other bacteria can colonize the tooth surface.

Maturation of the plaque is associated with a shift in the type of bacteria that are predominant. Gram-positive bacteria that can exist in the presence or absence of oxygen give way to gram negative bacteria that require the absence of oxygen.

Depending on how the community evolves, the plaque can become problematic in terms of a cavity. Even within the plaque, there are variations in the structure and bacterial composition. Thus, even though one region of the plaque is relatively benign is no guarantee that another region will house detrimental bacteria.

The prevalence of acid-producing bacteria is related to the diet. A diet that is elevated in the types of sugar typically found in colas and candy bars will lower the **pH** in the plaque. The lowered pH is harsh on all organisms except the acid-producing bacteria. Most dentists assert that a diet that contains less of these sugars, combined with good oral **hygiene**, will greatly minimize the threat posed by plaque and will emphasize the benefit of the plaque's presence.

See also Bacteria and bacterial infection; Biofilm formation and dynamic behavior; Microbial flora of the oral cavity, dental caries

PLASMIDS

Plasmids are extra-chromosomal, covalently closed circular (CCC) molecules of double stranded (ds) **DNA** that are capable of autonomous replication. The prophages of certain bacterial phages and some dsRNA elements in **yeast** are also called plasmids, but most commonly plasmids refer to the extra-chromosomal CCC DNA in **bacteria**.

Plasmids are essential tools of genetic engineering. They are used as vectors in **molecular biology** studies.

Plasmids are widely distributed in nature. They are dispensable to their host cell. They may contain genes for a variety of phenotypic traits, such as **antibiotic resistance**, virulence, or metabolic activities. The products plasmids encode may be useful in particular conditions of **bacterial growth**. Replication of plasmid DNA is carried out by subsets of **enzymes** used to duplicate the bacterial chromosome and is under the control of plasmid's own replicon. Some plasmids reach copy numbers as high as 700 per cell, whereas others are maintained at the minimal level of 1 plasmid per cell. One particular type of plasmid has the ability to transfer copies of itself to other bacterial stains or species. These plasmids have a tra **operon**. Tra operon encodes the protein that is the component of sex pili on the surface of the host bacteria. Once the sex pili contact with the recipient cells, one strand of the plasmid is transferred to the recipient cells. This plasmid can integrate into the host chromosomal DNA and transfer part of the host DNA to the recipient cells during the next DNA transfer process.

Ideally, plasmids as vectors should have three characteristics. First, they should have a multiple **cloning** site (MSC) which consists of multiple unique restriction enzyme sites and allows the insertion of foreign DNA. Second, they should have a relaxed replication control that allows suffi-

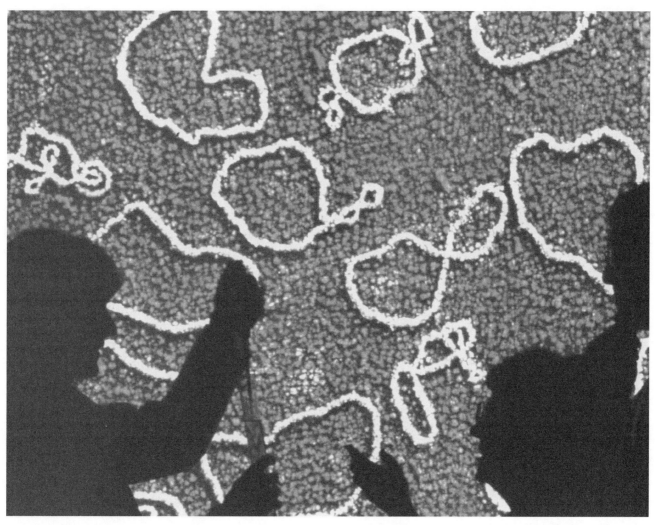

Transmission electron micrograph of plasmids.

cient plasmids to be produced. Last, plasmids should have selectable markers, such as **antibiotics** metabolite genes, which allow the identification of the transformed bacteria. Numerous plasmid vectors have been developed since the first plasmid vectors of the early 1970s. Some vectors have **bacteriophage** promoter sequences flanking the MSC that allows direct sequencing of the cloned DNA sequence. Some vectors have yeast or **virus replication** origin, which allows the plasmids to replicate in yeast and mammalian cells, hence enabling cloned cDNAs to express in these host cells. Many new features have and will be added into plasmids to make genetic engineering easier and faster.

See also Cloning, application of cloning to biological problems; DNA (Deoxyribonucleic acid); DNA hybridization; Molecular biology and molecular genetics

PLASMODIUM

Plasmodium is a genus of **protozoa** that has a life cycle that includes a human host and a mosquito. The genus consists predominantly of four species: *Plasmodium falciparum*, *Plasmodium vivax*, *Plasmodium ovale*, and *Plasmodium malariae*. With the exception of the latter species, *Plasmodium* are **parasites** of humans.

The main disease of concern with *Plasmodium* is **malaria**. This disease has been a problem for humans for millennia. There are still almost 20 million cases of malaria reported each year. The number of people who are actually infected is thought to be upwards of 500 million people annually. The death toll from malaria is one to two million people each year, mostly in underdeveloped countries. But even in developed countries, malaria can be a problem, especially if mosquito control programs are not vigilant.

The protozoan is spread to humans by the bite of a female Anopheline mosquito. A form of the parasite known as the sporozoite enters the bloodstream and makes its way to the liver. After multiplying in liver cells, the protozoan can penetrate red blood cells, which is a hallmark of the disease malaria. Multiplication occurs in a red blood cell, which ultimately bursts, releasing new forms of the protozoa that can infect neighbouring red blood cells. Such cycles lead to massive destruction of red blood cells.

Malaria can produce a myriad of symptoms, including high fever, generalized aches, tender spleen and liver, jaundice, and, in severe cases, convulsions, failure of the kidneys, shock, and collapse of the circulatory system. The fever tends to be cyclical, reflecting the cyclical pattern of protozoan release from red blood cells followed by a period of protozoan multiplication inside other red blood cells. These cycles can vary from 48 hours with *Plasmodium vivax* to about 72 hours with *Plasmodium malariae*.

Resistance of the protozoa, particularly *Plasmodium falciparum*, to the drugs such as chloroquinine and pyrimethamine that have previously been an effective control was first reported in 1961. Since that time, the occurrence of resistance has increased. A major factor in the development of the resistance is the adaptivity of the protozoan. The genome of the *Plasmodium* is very complex, and genetic alteration to new environmental pressures occurs quickly.

See also Parasites; Zoonoses

PLASTID · *see* PLASMIDS

PNEUMONIA, BACTERIAL AND VIRAL

Pneumonia is an infection of the lung, and can be caused by nearly any class of organism known to cause human infections, including **bacteria**, **viruses**, **fungi**, and **parasites**. In the United States, pneumonia is the sixth most common disease leading to death, and the most common fatal infection acquired by already hospitalized patients. In developing countries, pneumonia ties with diarrhea as the most common cause of death.

The main function of the respiratory system is to provide oxygen, the most important energy source for the body's cells. Inspired air travels down the respiratory tree to the alveoli, where the oxygen moves out of the alveoli and is sent into circulation throughout the body as part of the red blood cells. The oxygen in the inspired air is exchanged within the alveoli for the body's waste product, carbon dioxide, which leaves the alveoli during expiration.

The normal, healthy human lung is sterile, meaning that there are no normally resident bacteria or viruses (unlike the upper respiratory system and parts of the gastrointestinal system, where bacteria dwell even in a healthy state). There are multiple safeguards along the path of the respiratory system that are designed to keep invading organisms from leading to infection.

The first line of defense includes the hair in the nostrils, which serves as a filter for larger particles. The epiglottis is a

trap door of sorts, designed to prevent food and other swallowed substances from entering the larynx and then trachea. Sneezing and coughing, both provoked by the presence of irritants within the respiratory system, help to clear such irritants from the respiratory tract.

Mucous, produced throughout the respiratory system, also serves to trap dust and infectious organisms. Tiny hairlike projections (cilia) from cells lining the respiratory tract beat constantly, moving debris, trapped by mucus, upwards and out of the respiratory tract. This mechanism of protection is referred to as the mucociliary escalator.

Cells lining the respiratory tract produce several types of immune substances which protect against various organisms. Other cells (called macrophages) along the respiratory tract actually ingest and kill invading organisms.

The organisms that cause pneumonia, then, are usually carefully kept from entering the lungs by virtue of these host defenses. However, when an individual encounters a large number of organisms at once, either by inhaling contaminated air droplets, or by aspiration of organisms inhabiting the upper airways, the usual defenses may be overwhelmed and infection may occur.

In addition to exposure to sufficient quantities of causative organisms, certain conditions may predispose an individual to pneumonia. Certainly, the lack of normal anatomical structure could result in an increased risk of pneumonia. For example, there are certain inherited defects of cilia which result in less effective protection. Cigarette smoke, inhaled directly by a smoker or second-hand by an innocent bystander, interferes significantly with ciliary function, as well as inhibiting macrophage function.

Stroke, seizures, alcohol, and various drugs interfere with the function of the epiglottis, leading to a leaky seal on the trap door, with possible **contamination** by swallowed substances and/or regurgitated stomach contents. Alcohol and drugs also interfere with the normal cough reflex, further decreasing the chance of clearing unwanted debris from the respiratory tract.

Viruses may interfere with ciliary function, allowing themselves or other microorganism invaders, such as bacteria, access to the lower respiratory tract. One of the most important viruses which in recent years has resulted in a huge increase in the incidence of pneumonia is **HIV** (**Human Immunodeficiency Virus**), the causative virus in **AIDS** (Acquired Immunodeficiency Syndrome). Because AIDS results in a general decreased effectiveness of many aspects of the host's **immune system**, a patient with AIDS is susceptible to all types of pneumonia, including some previously rare parasitic types which would be unable to cause illness in an individual possessing a normal immune system.

The elderly have a less effective mucociliary escalator, as well as changes in their immune system, all of which cause them to be more at risk for the development of pneumonia.

Various chronic conditions predispose to pneumonia, including asthma, cystic fibrosis, neuromuscular diseases which may interfere with the seal of the epiglottis, and esophageal disorders which result in stomach contents passing upwards into the esophagus (increasing the risk of aspiration of those stomach contents with their resident bacteria), as well as diabetes, sickle cell anemia, lymphoma, leukemia, and emphysema.

Pneumonia is one of the most frequent infectious complications of all types of surgeries. Many drugs used during and after surgery may increase the risk of aspiration, impair the cough reflex, and cause a patient to underfill their lungs with air. Pain after surgery also discourages a patient from breathing deeply and coughing effectively.

The list of organisms which can cause pneumonia is very large, and includes nearly every class of infecting organism: viruses, bacteria, bacteria-like organisms, fungi, and parasites (including certain worms). Different organisms are more frequently encountered by different age groups. Furthermore, other characteristics of the host may place an individual at greater risk for infection by particular types of organisms.

Viruses, especially respiratory syncytial virus, parainfluenza and **influenza** viruses, and adenovirus, cause the majority of pneumonias in young children. Pneumonia in older children and young adults is often caused by the bacteria-like *Mycoplasma pneumoniae*. Adults are more frequently infected with bacteria (such as *Streptococcus* pneumoniae, *Hemophilus inflenzae*, and *Staphylococcus aureus*).

The parasite *Pneumocystis carinii* is an extremely important cause of pneumonia in patients with immune problems, such as patients being treated for cancer with **chemotherapy**, or patients with AIDS. People who have reason to come in contact with bird droppings, such as poultry workers, are at risk for pneumonia caused by the parasite *Chlamydia psittaci*. A very large, serious outbreak of pneumonia occurred in 1976, when many people attending an American Legion convention were infected by a previously unknown organism (subsequently named *Legionella pneumophila*) which was traced to air conditioning units in the convention hotel.

Pneumonia is suspected in any patient who presents with fever, cough, chest pain, shortness of breath, and increased respirations (number of breaths per minute). Fever with a shaking chill is even more suspicious, and many patients cough up clumps of mucus (sputum) that may appear streaked with pus or blood. Severe pneumonia results in the signs of oxygen deprivation, including blue appearance of the nail beds (cyanosis).

The invading organism causes symptoms, in part, by provoking an overly exuberant immune response in the lungs. The small blood vessels in the lungs (capillaries) become leaky, and protein-rich fluid seeps into the alveoli. This results in less functional area for oxygen-carbon dioxide exchange. The patient becomes relatively oxygen deprived, while retaining potentially damaging carbon dioxide. The patient breathes faster, in an effort to bring in more oxygen and blow off more carbon dioxide.

Mucus production is increased, and the leaky capillaries may tinge the mucus with blood. Mucus plugs actually further decrease the efficiency of gas exchange in the lung. The alveoli fill further with fluid and debris from the large number of white blood cells being produced to fight the infection.

Consolidation, a feature of bacterial pneumonias, occurs when the alveoli, which are normally hollow air spaces within the lung, instead become solid, due to quantities of fluid and debris.

Viral pneumonias and mycoplasma pneumonias do not result in consolidation. These types of pneumonia primarily infect the walls of the alveoli and the parenchyma of the lung.

Diagnosis is for the most part based on the patient's report of symptoms, combined with examination of the chest. Listening with a stethoscope will reveal abnormal sounds, and tapping on the patient's back (which should yield a resonant sound due to air filling the alveoli) may instead yield a dull thump if the alveoli are filled with fluid and debris.

Laboratory diagnosis can be made of some bacterial pneumonias by staining sputum with special chemicals and looking at it under a **microscope**. Identification of the specific type of bacteria may require culturing the sputum (using the sputum sample to grow greater numbers of the bacteria in a lab dish).

X-ray examination of the chest may reveal certain abnormal changes associated with pneumonia. Localized shadows obscuring areas of the lung may indicate a bacterial pneumonia, while streaky or patchy appearing changes in the x-ray picture may indicate viral or mycoplasma pneumonia. These changes on x-ray, however, are known to lag in time behind the patient's actual symptoms.

Antibiotics, especially given early in the course of the disease, are very effective against bacterial causes of pneumonia. Erythromycin and tetracycline improve recovery time for symptoms of mycoplasma pneumonia, but do not eradicate the organisms. Amantadine and acyclovir may be helpful against certain viral pneumonias.

Because many bacterial pneumonias occur in patients who are first infected with the influenza virus (the flu), yearly **vaccination** against influenza can decrease the risk of pneumonia for certain patients, particularly the elderly and people with chronic diseases (such as asthma, cystic fibrosis, other lung or heart diseases, sickle cell disease, diabetes, kidney disease, and forms of cancer). A specific **vaccine** against *Streptococcus* pneumoniae is very protective, and should be administered to patients with chronic illnesses. Patients who have decreased immune resistance (due to treatment with chemotherapy for various forms of cancer or due to infection with the AIDS virus), and therefore may be at risk for infection with *Pneumocystis carinii*, are frequently put on a regular drug regimen of Trimethoprim sulfa and/or inhaled pentamidine to avoid Pneumocystis pneumonia.

POLIOMYELITIS AND POLIO

Poliomyelitis is a contagious infectious disease that is caused by three types of poliovirus. The **viruses** cause damage and destruction of cells in the nervous system. Paralysis can result in about 2% of those who contract the disease, which is called polio. Most people who contract polio either have mild symptoms or no symptoms at all.

Poliomyelitis has been part of human history for millennia. An Egyptian stone engraving depicting the debilitating effects of poliomyelitis dates from over 3,000 years ago. In that time, the occurrence of polio was rare, as sanitation was poor. The close proximity between people and raw sewage bestowed protective **immunity** against the polioviruses, which reside in the feces. As sewage treatment became better and indoor plumbing became widespread in the twentieth century, exposure to the virus became less and the protective immunity was less likely to develop in children. By the time the disease was first described in Britain in 1789 by Michael Underwood, outbreaks in children were occurring. From the latter decades of the nineteenth century through to the 1950s, polio **epidemics** occurred frequently. Children were most at risk and could be crippled from polio, or suffer muscle damage severe enough to require the assistance of iron lungs, early mechanical ventilators, because their lungs had been damaged to the point of incapacity.

The word poliomyelitis derives from the Greek word *polio* (grey) and *myelon* (marrow, indicating the spinal cord). It is the poliomyelitis effect on the spinal cord that is associated with the devastating paralysis of the severe form of the disease.

Poliovirus is a member of the enterovirus group of the family Picornaviridae. Poliovirus serotypes (an antigenic means of categorizing viruses) P1, P2, and P3 are the agents of poliomyelitis. The viruses are very susceptible to heat, ultraviolet light and chemicals such as formaldehyde and chlorine.

Poliovirus is spread most commonly via contact with feces. Only humans are involved in the transmission, as only humans harbor the virus. Typically, feces-soiled hands are not washed properly and then are put into or round the mouth. Spread of the virus by coughing or sneezing can also occur. The virus multiplies in the pharynx or the gastrointestinal tract. From there the virus invades adjacent lymph tissue, enters the blood stream and can infect cells of the central nervous system. When neurons of the brain stem are infected, the paralytic symptoms of poliomyelitis result.

About 95% of those who are infected by the poliovirus may not exhibit symptoms. In those people who do exhibit symptoms, about 4–8% exhibit a fever and flu-like malaise and nausea. Recovery is complete within a short time. These people can continue to excrete the virus in their feces for a time after recovery, and so can infect others. About 2% of those with symptoms develop a more sever form of nonparalytic aseptic **meningitis**. The symptoms include muscular pain and stiffness. In the severe paralytic poliomyelitis, which occurs in less than 2% of all polio infections, breathing and swallowing become difficult and paralysis of the bladder and muscles occurs. Paralysis of the legs and the lung muscles is common. This condition is known as flaccid paralysis.

The paralytic form of polio can be of three types. Spinal polio is the most common, accounting for 79% of paralytic polio in the Unites States from 1969 to 1979. Bulbar polio, which accounts for 2% of cases, produces weakness in those muscles that receive impulses from the cranial nerves. Finally, bulbospinal polio, which is a combination of the two, accounts for about 20% of all cases.

At the time of the development of the vaccines to polio, in the early 1950s, there were nearly 58,000 cases of polio annually in the United States, with almost 20,000 of these people being rendered paralyzed. Earlier, President Franklin Roosevelt committed funds to a "war on polio." Roosevelt was himself a victim of polio.

Jonas Salk developed a **vaccine** to the three infectious forms of the poliovirus (out of the 125 known strains of the virus) in the early 1950s. His vaccine used virus that had been inactivated by the chemical formaldehyde. An immune response was still mounted to the virus particles when they were injected into humans. The vaccine was effective (except for one early faulty batch) and quickly became popular.

Soon after the Salk vaccine appeared, **Albert Sabin** developed a vaccine that was based on the use of still-live, but weakened, polio virus. The vaccine was administered as an oral solution. While effective as a vaccine, the weakened virus can sometimes mutate to a disease-causing form, and the vaccine itself, rarely, can cause poliomyelitis (vaccine-associated paralytic poliomyelitis). As of January 2000, the **Centers for Disease Control** has recommended that only the Salk version of the polio vaccine be used.

There is still no cure for poliomyelitis. In the post-vaccine era, however, poliomyelitis is virtually non-existent in developed countries. For example, in the United States there are now only approximately eight reported cases of polio each year, mostly due to the vaccine-associated paralytic phenomenon. The last cases of poliomyelitis in the Unites States caused by wild virus occurred in 1979. Elsewhere, there are still bout 250,00 cases every year, mainly in the India subcontinent, the Eastern Mediterranean, and Africa. However, an ongoing **vaccination** campaign by the **World Health Organization** aims to eradicate poliomyelitis by 2010.

See also History of public health

POLYMERASE CHAIN REACTION (PCR)

PCR (polymerase chain reaction) is a technique in which cycles of denaturation, annealing with primer, and extension with **DNA** polymerase, are used to amplify the number of copies of a target DNA sequence by more than 106 times in a few hours. American molecular biologist Kary Mullis developed the idea of PCR in the 1970s. For his ingenious invention, he was awarded the 1993 Nobel Prize in physiology or medicine.

The extraction of DNA polymerase from thermophilic **bacteria** allowed major advances in PCR technology.

PCR amplification of DNA is like any DNA replication by DNA polymerase *in vivo* (in living cells). The difference is that PCR produces DNA in a test tube. For a PCR to happen, four components are necessary: template, primer, deoxyribonecleotides (adenine, thymine, cytosine, guanine), and DNA polymerase. In addition, part of the sequence of the targeted DNA has to be known in order to design the according primers. In the first step, the targeted double stranded DNA is heated to over 194°F (90°C) for denaturation. During this process, two strands of the targeted DNA are separated from each other. Each strand is capable of being a template. The second step is carried out around 122°F (50°C). At this lowered temperature, the two primers anneal to their complementary sequence on each template. The DNA polymerase then extends the primer using the provided nucleotides. As a result, at the end of each cycle, the numbers of DNA molecules double.

PCR was carried out manually in incubators of different temperatures for each step until the discovery of DNA polymerase from thermophilic bacteria. The bacterium *Thermus aquaticus* was found in Yellow Stone National Park. This bacterium lives in the hot springs at 203°F (95°C). The DNA polymerase from *T. aquaticus* keeps its activity at above 203°F (95°C) for many hours. Several additional heat-resistant DNA polymerases have also now been identified.

Genetic engineered heat resistant DNA polymerases, that have proofreading functions and make fewer **mutations** in the amplified DNA products, are available commercially. PCR reactions are now carried out in different thermocyclers. Thermocyclers are designed to change temperatures automatically. Researchers set the temperatures and the time, and at the end of the procedure take the test tube out of the machine.

The invention of PCR was revolutionary to **molecular biology**. PCR is valuable to researchers because it allows them to multiply the quantity of a unique DNA sequence to a large and workable amount in a very short time. Researchers in the Human Genome Project are using PCR to look for markers in cloned DNA segments and to order DNA fragments in libraries. Molecular biologists use PCR to **cloning** DNA. PCR is also used to produce biotin or other chemical-labeled probes. These probes are used in nucleic acid hybridization, *in situ* hybridization and other molecular biology procedures.

PCR, coupled with fluorescence techniques and computer technology, allows the real time amplification of DNA. This enables quantitative detection of DNA molecules that exist in minute amounts. PCR is also used widely in clinical tests. Today, it has become routine to use PCR in the diagnosis of infectious diseases such **AIDS**.

See also Chromosomes, eukaryotic; Chromosomes, prokaryotic; DNA (Deoxyribonucleic acid); DNA chips and micro arrays; DNA hybridization; Immunogenetics; Laboratory techniques in immunology; Laboratory techniques in microbiology; Molecular biology and molecular genetics

PORINS

Porins are proteins that are located in the outer membrane of Gram-negative **bacteria**. They function to form a water-filled pore through the membrane, from the exterior to the **periplasm**, which is a region located between the outer and inner membranes. The porin channel allows the diffusion of small hydrophilic (water-loving) molecules through to the periplasm. The size of the diffusing molecule depends on the size of the channel.

A porin protein associates with two other porin proteins of the same type in the outer membrane. This may act to stabilize the three-dimensional structure of each porin molecule. Each porin contains a pore, so that there are three pores in the triad of porins.

The size of the water-filled channel that is created by a porin depends on the particular porin protein. For example, in the bacterium *Escherichia coli*, the so-called maltoporin and phosphoporin have different specificities (for the sugar maltose and phosphorus, respectively).

Since the discovery of porins in the 1970s in *Escherichia coli*, these proteins have been shown to be a general feature of the Gram-negative outer membrane. Much of the early work on porins came from the laboratories of Hiroshi Nikaido and Robert Hancock. Some examples of the bacteria known to possess porins are *Pseudomonas aeruginosa*, many other species of *Pseudomonas*, *Aeromonas salmonicida*, *Treponema pallidum*, and *Helicobacter pylori*.

A bacterium typically contains a variety of porins. Possession of porins of different sizes and chemistries is very advantageous for a bacterium. The various channels allow for the inward diffusion of a variety of nutrients required by the bacterium for survival and growth. Moreover, the diffusional nature of the molecule's entry means that a bacterium is able to acquire some needed nutrients without having to expend energy.

Another example of porin importance is found in *Escherichia coli*. In this bacterium, a duo of porins, which are designated OmpF and OmpC, function in response to changes in osmolarity. The production of these porins is under the control of a protein that senses the osmotic character of the environment. Depending on the ionic conditions, the amounts of OmpF and OmpC in the outer membrane can be altered so as to control the types of ions that enter the bacterium.

Porins share the same function in these bacteria from various habitats. This similar function is mirrored by the similarity in the three-dimensional structure of the proteins. Each porin is visually reminiscent of a barrel that is open to both ends. The slats of the barrel are arrangements of the constituent amino acids of the protein (beta sheets). The sequence of amino acids that makes up a beta sheet region allows the region to assume a zigzag configuration of the amino acids in one plane. The result is a narrow, flat strip of amino acids. When such strips are linked together, the barrel shape can be created. The outer surface of the porin barrel is more **hydrophobic** (water-hating) and so the partitioning of this surface into the hydrophobic interior of the membrane will be favored. The inner surface of the porin barrel contains side groups of the amino acids that prefer to interact with water.

The function of porin proteins was discovered by isolating the particular protein and then inserting the protein into model systems, that consisted either of lipid membranes floating in solution (liposomes) or floating as a sheet on the surface of a liquid (black lipid bilayer membranes). The passage of radioactive sugars of various sizes out of the liposomes or across the black lipid bilayer membranes could be measured, and the various so-called exclusion limits for each porin could be determined.

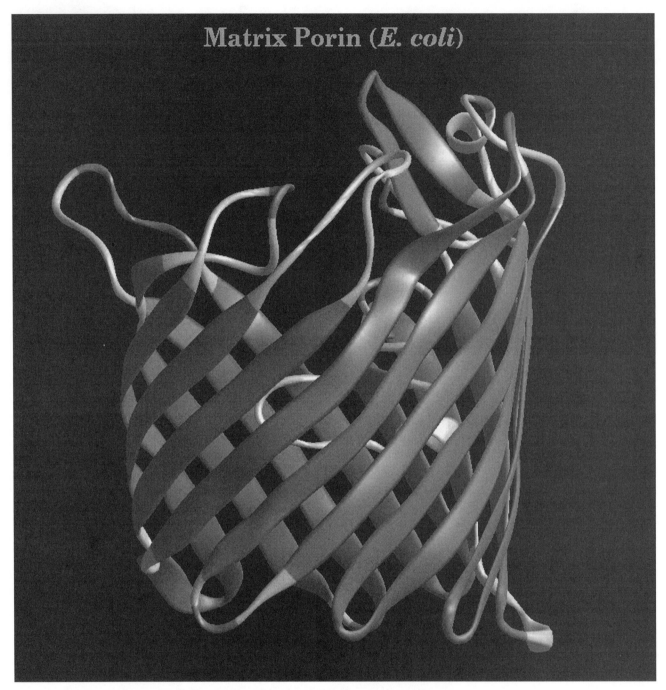

Matrix Porin (*E. coli*)

Three-dimensional computer model of a protein molecule of matrix porin found in *E. coli* bacteria.

Porins also have relevance in the **antibiotic resistance** of bacteria, particularly *Pseudomonas aerugionsa*, which is the cause of lung infections in those afflicted with cystic fibrosis, and can cause so-called "opportunistic infections" in those whose **immune system** is impaired. For example, the porin designated OprD is specifically utilized for the diffusion of the antibiotic imipenem into the bacterium. Imipenem resistance is associated with an alteration in the three-dimensional struc-

ture of OprD such that imipenem is excluded from entering the bacterium. The resistance of a number of clinical isolates of *Pseudomonas aeruginosa* is the result of porin alteration. Knowledge of the molecular nature of the alterations will help in the design of **antibiotics** that overcome the channel barrier.

See also Bacterial membranes and cell wall; Protein export

PRESUMPTIVE TESTS • *see* LABORATORY TECH-
NIQUES IN MICROBIOLOGY

PRIONS

Prions are proteins that are infectious. Indeed, the name prion is derived from "proteinaceous infectious particles." The discovery of prions and confirmation of their infectious nature overturned a central dogma that infections were caused by intact organisms, particularly **microorganisms** such as **bacteria**, **fungi**, **parasites**, or **viruses**. Since prions lack genetic material, the prevailing attitude was that a protein could not cause disease.

Prions were discovered and their role in brain degeneration was proposed by Stanley Pruisner. This work earned him the 1997 Nobel Prize in medicine or physiology.

In contrast to infectious agents that are not normal residents of a host, prion proteins are a normal constituent of brain tissue in humans and in all mammals studied thus far. The prion normally is a constituent of the membrane that surrounds the cells. The protein is also designated PrP (for proteinaceous infectious particle). PrP is a small protein, being only some 250 amino acids in length. The protein is arranged with regions that have a helical conformation and other regions that adopt a flatter, zigzag arrangement of the amino acids. The normal function of the prion is still not clear. Studies from mutant mice that are deficient in prion manufacture indicate that the protein may help protect the brain tissue from destruction that occurs with increasing frequency as someone ages. The normal prions may aid in the survival of brain cells known as Purkinje cells, which predominate in the cerebellum, a region of the brain responsible for movement and coordination.

The so-called prion theory states that PrP is the only cause of the prion-related diseases, and that these disease results when a normally stable PrP is "flipped" into a different shape that causes disease. Regions that are helical and zigzag are still present, but their locations in the protein are altered. This confers a different three-dimensional shape to the protein.

As of 2002, the mechanism by which normally functioning protein is first triggered to become infectious is not known. One hypothesis, known as the virino hypothesis, proposes that the infectious form of a prion is formed when the PrP associates with nucleic acid from some infectious organism. Efforts to find prions associated with nucleic acid have, as of 2001, been unsuccessful.

If the origin of the infectious prion is unclear, the nature of the infectious process following the creation of an infectious form of PrP is becoming clearer. The altered protein is able to stimulate a similar structural change in surrounding prions. The change in shape may result from the direct contact and binding of the altered and infectious prion with the unaltered and still-normally functioning prions. The altered proteins also become infective and encourage other proteins to

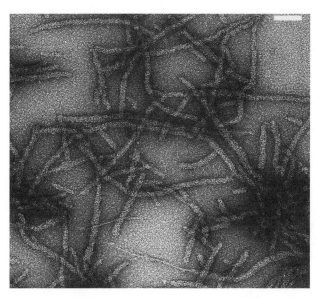

Negative stain electron micrograph of prions.

undergo the conformational change. The cascade produces proteins that adversely effect neural cells and the cells lose their ability to function and die.

The death of regions of the brain cells produces holes in the tissue. This appearance leads to the designation of the disease as spongiform encephalopathy.

The weight of evidence now supports the contention that prion diseases of animals, such as scrapie in sheep and bovine spongiform encephalopathy (BSE—popularly known as Mad cow disease) can cross the species barrier to humans. In humans, the progressive loss of brain function is clinically apparent as Creutzfeld-Jacob disease, kuru, and Gerstmann-Sträussler-Scheinker disease. Other human disease that are candidates (but as yet not definitively proven) for a prion origin are Alzheimer's disease and Parkinson's disease.

In the past several years, a phenomenon that bears much similarity to prion infection has been discovered in **yeast**. The prion-like protein is not involved in a neurological degeneration. Rather, the microorganism is able to transfer genetic information to the daughter cell by means of a shape-changing protein, rather than by the classical means of genetic transfer. The protein is able to stimulate the change of shape of other proteins in the interior of the daughter cell, which produces proteins having a new function.

The recent finding of a prion-related mechanism in yeast indicates that prions my be a ubiquitous feature of many organisms and that the protein may have other functions than promoting disease.

See also BSE and CJD disease; BSE and CJD disease, advances in research

PROBIOTICS

Probiotics is a term that refers to the consumption of certain **microorganisms** in an effort to improve overall health and the functioning of the body's microflora.

The use of microorganisms as a health aid is not new. People have asserted the health fortifying attributes of yogurt and fermented milk for thousands of years. However, the cause of the beneficial effect was unknown. A century ago, the Russian microbiologist **Élie Metchnikoff** (1845–1916) began the scientific assessment of the probiotic role of microorganisms.

Based on Metchnikoff's work and that of others, it appeared well established (but not clinically proven) by the 1920s that *Lactobacillus acidophilus* acted to relieve the conflicting conditions of constipation and diarrhea. Capsules containing living **bacteria** were popular items in drug stores of the day. However, with the advent of **antibiotics** as a cure for many ailments, the public interest in probiotics waned. The emphasis shifted to the treatment of infections, as opposed to the prevention of infections.

In the 1990s the interest in probiotics surged. A number of studies established the clinical significance of *Lactobacillus* and *Bifidobacterium* in improving the efficiency of lactose absorption, in the treatment of diarrhea in children, and in combating recurrent vaginal **yeast** infections.

Probiotic bacteria exert their effect by colonizing surfaces, such as found in the intestinal tract or the vagina. Compounds can also be produced by the adherent bacteria that are inhibitory to other types of bacteria. The net effect of these processes is the competitive exclusion of potentially harmful bacteria by the beneficial probiotic bacteria.

The exclusion process can extend to other infectious agents as well. For example, colonization of the intestinal tract with *Lactobacillus* GG has been shown to significantly reduce the length of diarrheal illness caused by rotavirus. The rotavirus had no place to adhere and were washed out of the intestinal tract.

Probiotics also have shown potential in relieving skin disorders that are the result of an allergic reaction to a food. The colonization of the intestinal wall appears to restore the ability of nutrients to cross from the intestinal canal to the bloodstream. This ability to absorb food nutrients is disrupted in those with some food **allergies**.

The molecular basis for the competitive exclusion behavior of bacteria such as *Lactobacillus* and *Bifidobacterium* is the subject of continuing study. The identification of the precise molecular agents that are responsible for surface blocking will expand the use of probiotics.

See also Lactobacillus; Microbial flora of the stomach and gastrointestinal tract

PROKARYOTAE

Prokaryote is a kingdom, or division, in the classification scheme devised for all life on Earth. This kingdom, which is also designated as Monera, includes all **bacteria** and **blue-green algae** (which are also called Cyanobacteria). There are four other kingdoms in the classification system. The classification is based on the structure of a subunit of the ribosome. This criterion was selected because the structure of the subunit seems to have been maintained with little change throughout the millions of years that life has existed on Earth.

Besides the kingdom Prokaryotae, there are the Protista (eukaryotic organisms' organisms that have a **nucleus** enclosed in a well-defined membrane), **Fungi**, Animalia (**eukaryotes** organized into complex organisms), and Plantae.

The use of kingdoms in the classification of organisms arose with the work of Carolus Linneus who, in the mid-1700s, devised the system that is still used today. The Linnean system of classification has kingdoms as the highest level, with six other subdivisions down to the species level. Bacteria are divided into various genera. A group of bacteria derived from a single cell is called a strain. Closely related strains constitute a bacterial species. For example, the complete classification of the bacterium *Escherichia coli* is as follows:

- Kingdom: Prokaryotae (Monera)
- Division (also called Phylum): Gracilicutes
- Class: Scotobacteria
- Order: Enterobacteriales
- Family: Enterobacteriaceae
- Genus: *Escherichia*
- Species: *Escherichia coli*

The Prokaryotae are further divided into two subkingdoms. These are called the Eubacteriobonta (which contains the so-called **Eubacteria**) and the Archaebacteriobonta (which contains the so-called Archaebacteria). This split arose from the research of Carl Woese. He showed that the so-called 16 S ribosomal subunit of bacteria divide bacteria into two groups; the Eubacteria and the Archaeobcteria.

Archaebacteria are a very diverse group of bacteria and have several features that set them apart from the other Prokaryotae. Their cell walls lack a structure called the **peptidoglycan**, which is a rigid and stress-bearing network necessary for the survival of other bacteria. Archaebacteria live in extreme environments such as deep-sea vents, hot springs, and very salty water. Finally, some metabolic processes of Archaebacteria are different from other bacteria.

The feature that most distinguishes the bacteria and blue-green algal members of the Prokaryote from the members of the other kingdoms is the lack of membrane-bound structure around the genetic material. The genetic material, **deoxyribonucleic acid** (**DNA**), is dispersed through the inside of the microorganism, a region that is typically referred to as the **cytoplasm**. In contrast, eukaryotic organisms have their genetic material compartmentalized inside a specialized membrane.

A second distinctive feature of the Prokaryotae concerns their method of reproduction. Most bacteria reproduce by growing and then splitting in two. This is called binary fission. Eukaryotic organisms have a more complex process that involves the replication of their differently organized genetic material and the subsequent migration of the material to specific regions of the cell.

Blue-green algae and some bacteria are able to manufacture their own food from sunlight through the process of **photosynthesis**. Green plants likewise have this capability. This type of bacteria are the photoautotrophs. Other bacteria are able to utilize elements like nitrogen, sulphur, hydrogen, or iron to make their food. This type of Prokaryote are the chemoautotrophs. But the bulk of the Prokaryotae exists by decomposing and using compounds made by other organisms. This decomposition is a vital process. Without this bacterial activity, the wastes of other organisms would blanket Earth.

The relative simplicity of the Prokaryotae, as compared to eukaryotes, extends to the genetic level. The prototypical bacterial species *Escherichia coli* contains approximately 5,000 genes. On average, about one in every 200 bacteria is likely to have a mutation in at least one of the genes. In a 100 ml **culture** containing one million bacteria per milliliter, this translates to 500,000 mutant bacteria. This ability of members of the Prokaryotae to mutant and so quickly adapt to a changing environment is the principle reason for their success through time.

The ecological distribution of the Prokaryotae is vast. Bacteria have adapted to live almost everywhere, in environments as diverse as the thermal deep-sea vents to the boiling hot springs of Yellowstone National Park, from the soil to the intestinal tract of man and animals. The diversity of bacteria led to the design of a classification system just for them. **David Hendricks Bergey** spearheaded this classification scheme in the first half of the twentieth century. His efforts culminated in the publication (and ongoing revisions) of the *Bergey's Manual of Systematic Bacteriology*.

See also Bacterial kingdoms; Evolutionary origin of bacteria and viruses

PROKARYOTIC CELLS, GENETIC REGULATION OF • *see* GENETIC REGULATION OF PROKARYOTIC CELLS

PROKARYOTIC MEMBRANE TRANSPORT

The ability of Prokaryotic **microorganisms** to move compounds into the cell, and to remove waste products of **metabolism** out of the cell, is crucial for the survival of the cell. Some of these functions are achieved by the presence of water-filled channels, particularly in the outer membrane of Gram-negative **bacteria**, which allow the diffusion of molecules through the channel. But this is a passive mechanism and does not involve the input of energy by the bacterium to accomplish the movement of the molecules across the membrane. Mechanisms that depend on the input of energy from the microorganism are active membrane transport mechanisms.

Prokaryotic membrane transport depends on the presence of specific proteins. These proteins are located within a membrane that surrounds the cell. Gram-positive bacteria have only a single membrane surrounding the contents of the

bacterium. So, it is within this membrane that the transport proteins reside. In Gram-negative bacteria, the transport proteins are important constituents of the inner of the two membranes that are part of the cell wall. The inner membrane is also referred to as the cytoplasmic membrane.

There are a number of proteins that can participate in transport of molecules across Prokaryotic membranes. Different proteins have different modes of operation. In general, there are three different functional types of protein. These are termed uniporters, antiporters, and symporters.

Uniporters can actually be considered analogous to the water-filed channels of the Gram-negative outer membrane, in that a uniporter is a single protein or a collection of several like proteins that produces a channel through which molecules can passively diffuse. No energy is required for this process. Some degree of selectivity as to the types of molecules that can pass down a channel is achieved, based on the diameter of the channel. Thus, a small channel excludes large molecules.

A uniporter can also function in a process known as facilitated diffusion. This process is governed by the concentrations of the molecule of interest on either side of the membrane. If the concentration on one side of the membrane barrier is higher than on the other side, the movement of molecules through the connecting channel will naturally occur, in order to balance the concentrations on both sides of the membrane.

An antiporter is a membrane protein that can transport two molecules across the membrane in which it is embedded at the same time. This is possible as one molecule is transported in one direction while the other molecule is simultaneously transported in the opposite direction. Energy is required for this process, and functions to allow a change in the shape of the protein or to permit all or part of the protein to swivel upon binding of the molecules to be transported. One model has the molecules binding to the protein that is exposed at either surface of the membrane, and then, by an internal rotation of the transport protein, both molecules are carried to the other membrane surface. Then, each molecule is somehow released from the transport protein.

The third type of transport protein is termed a symport. This type of protein can simultaneously transport two molecules across a membrane in the same direction. The most widely held model for this process has the molecules binding to the transport protein that is exposed on the external surface of the membrane. In an energy-dependent process, these molecules are driven through a central region of the protein to emerge on the opposite side of the membrane. The protein molecule remains stationary.

The energy for prokaryotic membrane transport can come from the breakdown, or hydrolysis, of an energy-containing molecule called adenosine triphosphate (ATP). The hydrolysis of ATP provides energy to move molecules from a region of lower concentration to a region of higher concentration (i.e., transport is against a concentration gradient).

Alternatively, energy for transport in the antiport and symport systems can be provided by the molecules themselves. The fact that the molecules prefer to be associated with the protein, rather than in solution, drives the transport process.

The outer membrane of Gram-negative bacteria does contain proteins that participate in the active transport of specific molecules to the periplasmic space, which separates the outer and inner membranes. Examples of such transport proteins include the FhuA of *Escherichia coli* and FepA of this and other bacteria. This type of active transport is important for disease processes, as iron can be crucial in the establishment of an infections, and because available iron is normally in very low concentration in the body.

See also Bacterial membranes and cell wall; Protein export

PROKARYOTIC REPLICATION • *see* CELL CYCLE (PROKARYOTIC), GENETIC REGULATION OF

PROMED • *see* EPIDEMIOLOGY, TRACKING DISEASES WITH TECHNOLOGY

PROPRIONIC ACID BACTERIA • *see* ACNE, MICROBIAL BASIS OF

PROSTHECATE AND NON-PROSTHECATE APPENDAGES • *see* BACTERIAL APPENDAGES

PROTEIN CRYSTALLOGRAPHY

Protein crystallography is a technique that utilizes x rays to deduce the three-dimensional structure of proteins. The proteins examined by this technique must first be crystallized.

When x rays are beamed at a crystal, the electrons associated with the atoms of the crystal are able to alter the path of the x rays. If the x rays encounter a film after passing through the crystal, a pattern can be produced following the development of the film. The pattern will consist of a limited series of dots or lines, because a crystal is composed of many repeats of the same molecule. Through a series of mathematical operations, the pattern of dots and lines on the film can be related to the structure of the molecule that makes up the crystal.

Crystallography is a powerful tool that has been used to obtain the structure of many molecules. Crystallography data was used, for example, in the determination of the structure of the double helix of **deoxyribonucleic acid** by American molecular biologist James Watson and British molecular biologist **Francis Crick** in the 1950s. **Bacteria** and virus are also amenable to x-ray crystallography study. For example, the structure of the toxin produced by *Vibrio cholerae* has been deduced by this technique. Knowledge of the shape of cholera toxin will help in the tailoring of molecules that will bind to the active site of the toxin. In this way, the toxin's activity can be neutralized. Another example is that of the tail region of the virus that specifically infects bacteria (**bacteriophage**). The tail is the portion of the bacteriophage that binds to the bacteria. Subsequently, the viral nucleic acid is injected into the bacterium via the tail. Details of the three-dimensional structure of the tail are crucial in designing ways to thwart the binding of the virus and the infection of the bacterium.

Proteins are also well suited to crystallography. The determination of the three-dimensional structure of proteins at a molecular level is necessary for the development of drugs that will be able to bind to the particular protein. Not surprisingly, the design of **antibiotics** relies heavily on protein crystallography.

The manufacture of a crystal of a protein species is not easy. Proteins tend to form three-dimensional structures that are quire irregular in shape because of the arrangement of the amino acid building blocks within the molecule. Some arrangements of the amino acids will produce flat sheets; other arrangements will result in a helix. Irregularly shaped molecules will not readily stack together with their counterparts. Moreover, once a crystal has formed, the structure is extremely fragile and can dissolve easily. This fragility does have an advantage, however, as it allows other molecules to be incorporated into the crystal during its formation. Thus, for example, an enzyme can become part of a crystal of its protein receptor, allowing the structure of the enzyme-receptor binding site to be studied.

A protein is crystallized by first making a very concentrated solution of the protein and then exposing the solution to chemicals that slowly increase the protein concentration. With the right combination of conditions the protein can spontaneously precipitate. The ideal situation is to have the precipitate begin at one site (the nucleation site). This site acts as the seed for more protein to come out of solution resulting in crystal formation.

Once a crystal has formed it must be delicately transferred to the machine where the x-ray diffraction will be performed. The crystal must be kept in an environment that maintains the crystal throughout the transfer of crystallographic procedures.

The entire process of protein crystallography is delicate and prone to error. Usually many failures occur before a successful experiment occurs. Yet, despite the effort and frustration, the information that can be obtained about protein structure is considerable.

See also Antibody-antigen, biochemical and molecular reactions; Biochemical analysis techniques; DNA (Deoxyribonucleic acid); Laboratory techniques in immunology; Laboratory techniques in microbiology; Molecular biology and molecular genetics; Proteins and enzymes; Vaccine

PROTEIN ELECTROPHORESIS • *see* ELECTROPHORESIS

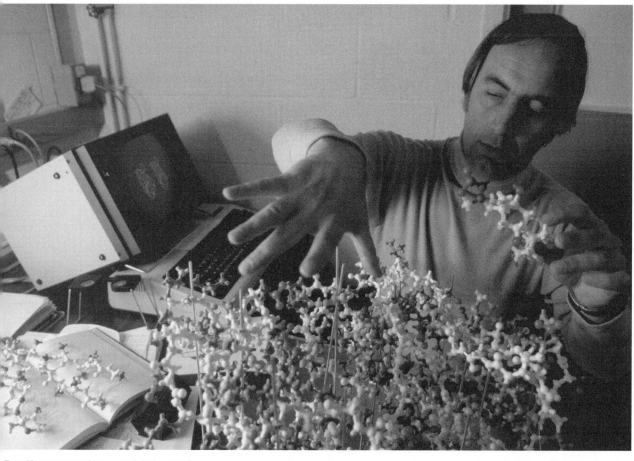

Ergo Novotny examines a model of a protein.

PROTEIN EXPORT

Protein export is a process whereby protein that has been manufactured in a cell is routed to the surface of the cell. Export
of proteins occurs in all **microorganisms**, but has been particularly well-studied in certain species of **bacteria** and **yeast**.

The ability of a cell to export protein is crucial to the
survival or pathogenicity of the cell. Bacteria that have protein
appendages for movement (e.g., flagella) and attachment (e.g.,
pili), and protective protein surface coatings (e.g., S layers)
depend on the efficient export of the proteins. Exotoxins that
are ultimately excreted by some bacteria need to get across the
cell wall before being released from the bacterium.

Defects in protein export can produce or contribute to a
number of maladies in eukaryotic cells including human cells
(e.g., cystic fibrosis, diabetes, osteopororsis).

A general feature of protein export is the manufacture of
the protein destined for secretion in a slightly longer form than
the exported form of the protein. The additional stretch is
known as the signal sequence, and its role in protein export
forms the so-called **signal hypothesis**. Gunter Blobel garnered
the 1999 Nobel Prize in Physiology or Medicine for his pioneering efforts in this area.

The "pre-protein" contains sequences of amino acids
that give the precursor stretch of protein blocks that are
hydrophilic (water-loving) and **hydrophobic** (water-hating).
This allows a portion of the precursor region to spontaneously
bury itself in the membrane layer that surrounds the interior of
a bacterium, or the membrane of the endoplasmic reticulum of
cells such as yeast. The hydrophilic sequences that flank the
hydrophobic region associate with either side of the membrane. Thus, the precursor region is a membrane anchor.

Anchoring of the protein to the membrane is assisted by
the action of two proteins. One of these proteins (designated
SecB) associates with the precursor sequence of the newly
made protein. The SecB protein then recognizes and binds to
a protein called SecA that is embedded in the membrane. The
SecB-SecA complex acts to guide the precursor region into
position at the membrane. As the remainder of the protein is
made, it is pushed out of the opposite side of the membrane.
An enzyme associated with the outer surface of the membrane
can snip off the precursor.

This process is sufficient for protein export in Gram-
negative bacteria that have the single membrane. However, in
Gram-negative bacteria the protein must be transported across
the **periplasm** and the outer membrane before being truly
exported. Furthermore, yeast cells require additional mecha-

nisms to route the protein from the Golgi apparatus to the exterior of the cell.

Proteins destined for export in Gram-negative bacteria are also synthesized as a precursor. The precursor functions at the outer membrane. Thus, the precursor must cross the inner membrane intact. This occurs because of an association that forms between a newly made precursor protein and a complex of several proteins. The protein complex is referred to as translocase. The translocase allows the precursor protein, with the hydrophobic region, to be completely transported across the inner membrane.

Studies using *Escherichia coli* and *Haemophilus influenzae* demonstrated the molecular nature of the translocase effect. The SecB protein is associated with the precursor region as a channel running alongside the precursor. The channel has a hydrophilic and a hydrophobic side. The latter is oriented outward so that it partitions into the hydrophobic interior of the bacterial inner membrane. The inner surface of SecB that is in intimate contact with the precursor region is hydrophilic. Thus, the precursor moves through the inner membrane in a watery channel.

As the precursor emerges into the periplasm, another protein present in the periplasm associates with the precursor region. This association also protects the precursor and allows the precursor to reach the inner surface of the outer membrane. Once there, the periplasmic protein is released, and the precursor sequence spontaneously inserts into the outer membrane.

Protein export has become an important target of strategies designed to thwart microorganism infections. By blocking the ability of certain proteins to be exported, the ability of bacteria to establish an infection can be hindered.

Conversely, the engineering of proteins to encourage their export can allow for the easier purification of commercially and clinically important proteins. For example, the engineering of human insulin in *Escherichia coli* relies on the export of the insulin protein. Once free of the bacteria, the insulin can be recovered in pure form much more easily and economically than if the protein needed to be extracted from the bacteria.

See also Bacteria and bacterial infection; Bacterial membranes and cell wall; Bacterial movement; Bacterial surface layers; Bacterial ultrastructure; Cell membrane transport; Enterotoxin and exotoxin; Molecular biology and molecular genetics; Prokaryotic membrane transport; Proteins and enzymes

PROTEIN SYNTHESIS

Protein synthesis represents the final stage in the **translation** of genetic information from **DNA**, via messenger **RNA** (mRNA), to protein. It can be viewed as a four-stage process, consisting of amino acid activation, translation initiation, chain elongation, and termination. The events are similar in both prokaryotes, such as **bacteria**, and higher eukaryotic

organisms, although in the latter there are more factors involved in the process.

To begin with, each of the 20 cellular amino acids are combined chemically with a transfer RNA (tRNA) molecule to create a specific aminoacyl-tRNA for each amino acid. The process is catalyzed by a group of **enzymes** called aminoacyl-tRNA synthetases, which are highly specific with respect to the amino acid that they activate. The initiation of translation starts with the binding of the small subunit of a ribosome, (30S in prokaryotes, 40S in **eukaryotes**) to the initiation codon with the nucleotide sequence AUG, on the mRNA transcript. In prokaryotes, a sequence to the left of the AUG codon is recognized. This is the Shine-Delgrano sequence and is complementary to part of the small ribosome subunit. Eukaryotic **ribosomes** start with the AUG nearest the 5'-end of the mRNA, and recognize it by means of a "cap" of 7-methylguanosine triphosphate. After locating the cap, the small ribosome subunit moves along the mRNA until it meets the first AUG codon, where it combines with the large ribosomal subunit.

In both prokaryotes and eukaryotes, the initiation complex is prepared for the addition of the large ribosomal subunit at the AUG site, by the release of initiation factor (IF) 3. In bacteria, the large 50S ribosomal subunit appears simply to replace IF–3, with IF–1 and IF–2. In eukaryotes, another factor eIF–5 (eukaryotic initiation factor 5), catalyses the departure of the previous initiation factors and the joining of the large 60S ribosomal subunit. In both cases, the release of initiation factor 2 involves the hydrolysis of the GTP bound to it. At this stage, the first aminoacyl-tRNA, Met-tRNA, is bound to the ribosome. The ribosome can accommodate two tRNA molecules at once. One of these carries the Met-tRNA at initiation, or the peptide-tRNA complex during elongation and is thus called the P (peptide) site, while the other accepts incoming aminoacyl-tRNA and is therefore called the A (acceptor) site. What binds to the A site is usually a complex of GTP, elongation factor EF-TU, and aminoacyl-tRNA. The tRNA is aligned with the next codon on the mRNA, which is to be read and the elongation factor guides it to the correct nucleotide triplet. The energy providing GTP is then hydrolysed to GDP and the complex of EF-TU:GDP leaves the ribosome. The GDP is released from the complex when the EF-TU complexes with EF-TS, which is then replaced by GTP. The recycled EF-TU: GTP is then ready to pick up another aminoacyl-tRNA for addition to the growing polypeptide chain. On the ribosome, a reaction is catalysed between the carboxyl of the P site occupant and the free amino group of the A site occupant, linking the two together and promoting the growth of the polypeptide chain. The peptidyl transferase activity which catalyses this transfer is intrinsic to the ribosome. The final step of elongation is the movement of the ribosome relative to the mRNA accompanied by the translocation of the peptidyl-tRNA from the A to the P. Elongation factor EF-G is involved in this step and a complex of EF-G and GTP binds to the ribosome, GTP being hydrolysed in the course of the reaction. The de-acylated tRNA is also released at this time.

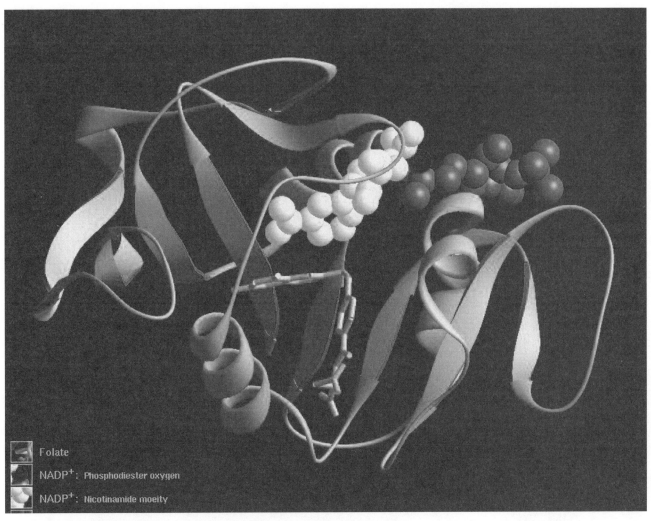

Folate

NADP$^+$: Phosphodiester oxygen

NADP$^+$: Nicotinamide moeity

Computer image of a protein moleucle, showing regions of different three-dimensional shape.

The end of polypeptide synthesis is signalled by a termination codon contacting the A site. Three prokaryotic release factors (RF) are known: RF–1 is specific for termination codons UAA and UAG, while RF–2 is specific for UAA and UGA. RF–3 stimulates RF–1 and RF–2, but does not in itself recognize the termination codons. RF–3 also has GTPase activity and appears to accelerate the termination at the expense of GTP. Only one eukaryotic release factor is known and it has GTPase activity.

At any one time, there can be several ribosomes positioned along the mRNA and thus initiation, elongation and termination proceed simultaneously on the same length of mRNA. The three dimensional structure of the final protein begins to appear during protein synthesis before translation is completed. In many cases, after the synthesis of the amino acid chain, proteins are subjected to further reactions which convert them to their biologically active forms, e.g., by the attachment of chemical groups or by removal of certain amino acids—a processes known as post-translational modification.

See also Deoxyribonucleic acid (DNA); Genetic code; Molecular biology and molecular genetics; Ribonucleic acid (RNA)

PROTEINS AND ENZYMES

The building blocks of proteins and **enzymes** are molecules formed by carboxyl acids attached to amino groups (–NH$_2$), known as amino acids. Most protein structures consist of combinations of only about twenty of the most commonly found amino acids.

Amino acids bind to each other to form peptides and proteins. Conventionally, the term protein is used to designate chains of several peptides, known as polypeptides, with a molecular weight higher than thousands of Daltons. Peptides with a biological function go in length from dipeptides and tripeptides, up to polymers with thousands of Daltons.

Most proteins have well-defined structures and their specific biological functions depend upon the correct conforma-

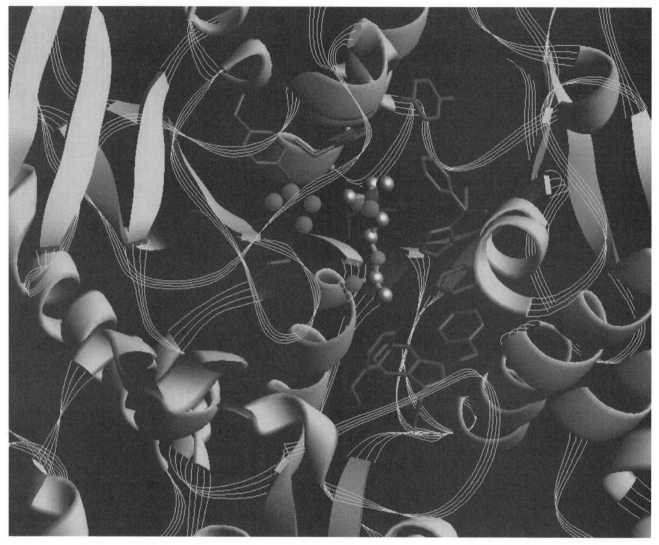

Computer representation of the three-dimensional structure of a protein.

tion of the molecular structure. For instance, the majority of soluble proteins of an organism, such as blood proteins, have globular structures, like small eggs. Some proteins are fiber-like and are associated in bundles, forming fibrils such as those of wool and hair. Myosin, the protein that makes muscles contract, has both globular and fibrous elements in its structure; whereas collagen, the protein of connective tissues, is constituted by three triple helices of fibrils that form super structures in the shape of a fibrous rope. Collagen represents one third of all proteins of the human body and together with elastin is responsible for both cohesion and elasticity of tissues.

Every enzyme is also a protein. Enzymes are proteins that function as catalysts of biochemical reactions. Most physiological activities in organisms are mediated by enzymes, from unicellular life forms to mammals. Enzymes speed up chemical reactions, allowing organic systems to reach equilibrium in a faster pace. For instance, every phase of the **cell cycle** is controlled by enzymes that alternately inhibit or stim-

ulate specific cellular activities as well as **gene** expression or repression, hence affecting the time of specific physiological activities within each phase of the cell cycle. Enzymes are highly selective in their activities, with each enzyme acting over a specific substrate or group of substrates. Substrate is a term designating any molecule that suffers enzymatic action, whether being activated or inhibited.

The main property of catalyst molecules is that they are not altered by the chemical reactions they induce, although some rare exceptions are known where some enzymes are inactivated by the reactions they catalyze. Enzymatic catalysis involves the formation of protein complexes between substrate and enzyme, where the amount of enzymes is generally much greater than the amount of substrate.

Some families of enzymes play an important role during the process of **DNA** replication. For example, when DNA synthesis activates, helicases break hydrogen bridges and some topoisomerases separate the two DNA strands. DNA-polymerases synthesize the fragments of the new DNA strand, while topoisomerase III does the proofreading of the transcribed sequences, eliminating those containing errors. Ribonuclease H removes **RNA** sequences from polymers containing complexed RNA/DNA, and DNA-ligase unites the newly transcribed fragments, thus forming the new DNA strand.

In the last decade, researchers discovered that many proteins involved in intracellular communication are structured in a modular way. In other words, they are constituted by relatively short amino acid sequences of about 100 amino acids, and have the basic role of connecting one protein to another. Some proteins of such signaling pathways are entirely comprised of connecting modules and deprived of enzymatic activity. These non-enzymatic modules are termed protein dominium or protein modules, and they help enzymes in the transmission of signals to the cell **nucleus** in an orderly and controlled way. Proteins containing only connecting (or binding) modules, such as SH2 and SH3, act as important molecular adaptors to other proteins. While one of its modules binds to a signaling complex, such as a transmembrane tyrosine-kinase receptor, other binding modules permit the docking of other proteins that, once complexed, amplifies the signal to the nucleus. Such adaptor proteins also allow the cell to utilize certain enzymes that otherwise would not be activated in a given signaling pathway. The structure of adaptor proteins also displays binding sites that connect to DNA, where they recognize specific nucleotide sequences of a given gene, thus inducing **transcription**. In this case, the only enzyme in the cascade of signals to the nucleus is the receptor in the surface of the cell, and all the events that follow occur through the recognition among proteins and through the protein recognition of a locus in DNA.

Proteins are encoded by genes. A gene usually encodes a nucleotide sequence that can be first transcribed in pre-messenger RNA, and then read and translated on the **ribosomes** into a group of similar proteins with different lengths and functions, known as protein isoforms. A single polypeptide may be translated and then cut by enzymes into different proteins of variable lengths and molecular weights.

During transcription, the non-coding DNA sequences (introns) are cut off, and the coding sequences (exons) are transcribed into pre-messenger RNA, which in turn is spliced to a continuous stretch of exons before protein **translation** begins. The spliced stretch subdivides in codons, where any of the four kinds of nucleotide may occupy one or more of the three positions, and each triplet codes for one specific amino acid. The sequence of codons is read on the ribosomes, three nucleotides at a time. The order of codons determine the sequence of amino acids in the protein molecule that is formed.

Introns may have a regulatory role of either the splicing or the translational process, and may even serve as exons to other genes. After translation, proteins may also undergo biochemical changes, a process known as post-translation processing. They may be either cut by enzymes or receive special bonds, such as disulfide bridges, in order to fold into a functional structure.

See also Biochemistry; Cell cycle (eukaryotic), genetic regu-

lation of; Cell cycle (prokaryotic), genetic regulation of; DNA (Deoxyribonucleic acid); Transcription; Translation

PROTEOMICS

Proteomics is a discipline of microbiology and **molecular biology** that has arisen from the **gene** sequencing efforts that culminated in the sequencing of the human genome in the last years of the twentieth century. In addition to the human genome, sequences of disease-causing **bacteria** are being deduced. Although fundamental, knowledge of the sequence of nucleotides that comprise **deoxyribonucleic acid** reveals only a portion of the protein structure encoded by the **DNA**. Because proteins are an essential element of bacterial structure and function (e.g., role in causing infection), the knowledge of the three-dimensional structure and associations of proteins is vital. Proteomics is an approach to unravel the structure and function of proteins.

The word proteomics is derived from PROTEin **complement** to a genOME. Essentially, this is the spectrum of proteins that are produced from the template of an organism's genetic material under a given set of conditions. Proteomics compares the protein profiles of proteomes under different conditions in order to unravel biological processes.

The origin of proteomics dates back to the identification of the double-stranded structure of DNA by Watson and Crick in 1953. More recently, the development of the techniques of protein sequencing and gel **electrophoresis** in the 1960s and 1970s provided the technical means to probe protein structure. In 1986, the first protein sequence database was created (SWISS-PROT, located at the University of Geneva). By the mid-1990s, the concept of the proteome and the discipline of proteomics were well established. The power of proteomics was manifest in March 2000, when the complete proteome of a whole organism was published, that of the bacterium *Mycoplasma genitalium*

Proteomics research often involves the comparison of the proteins produced by a bacterium (example, *Escherichia coli*) grown at different temperatures, or in the presence of different food sources, or a population grown in the lab versus a population recovered from an infection. *Escherichia coli* responds to changing environments by altering the proteins it produces. However, the full extent of the various alterations and their molecular bases are largely unknown. Proteomics research essentially attempts to provide a molecular explanation for bacterial behavior.

Proteomics can be widely applied to research of diverse microbes. For example, the **yeast *Saccharomyces cerevisiae*** is being studied to reveal the proteins produced and their functional associations with one another.

The task of sorting out all the proteins that can be produced by a bacterium or yeast cell is formidable. Targeting of the research effort is essential. For example, the comparison of the protein profile of a bacterium obtained directly from an infection (*in vivo*) with populations of the same microbe grown under defined conditions in the lab (*in vitro*) could identify proteins that are unique to the infection. Some of these could become targets for diagnosis, therapy, or for prevention of the infection.

The study of proteins is difficult. The amount of protein cannot be amplified as easily as can the amount of DNA, making the detection of minute amounts of protein challenging. The structure of proteins must be maintained, which can be difficult. For example, **enzymes**, heat, light, or the energy of mixing can break down some proteins.

With the advent of the so-called **DNA chips**, the expression of thousands of genes can be monitored simultaneously. But DNA is static. It exists and is either expressed or not. Moreover, the expression of a protein does not necessarily mean that the protein is active. Also, proteins can be modified after being produced. Proteins can adopt different shapes, which can determine different functions and levels of activity after they have been produced. These functions provide the structural and operational framework for the life of the bacterium. Proteomics represents the next step after gene expression analysis

Proteomics utilizes various techniques to probe protein expression and structure. The migration of proteins can depend on their net charge and on the size of the protein molecule. When these migrations are in two dimensions, as in 2-D polyacrylamide gel electrophoresis, thousands of proteins can be distinguished in a single experiment. A technique called mass spectrometry analyzes a trait of proteins known as the mass-to-charge ratio, which essentially enables the sequence of amino acids comprising the protein to be determined. Techniques exist that detect modifications after protein manufacture, such as the addition of phosphate groups. Analogous to DNA chips, so-called protein microarrays have been developed. In these, a solid support holds various molecules (antibodies and receptors, as two examples) that will specifically bind protein. The binding pattern of proteins to the support can help determine what proteins are being made and when they are synthesized.

Proteomics typically operates in tandem with **bioinformatics**, which is an integration of mathematical, statistical, and computational methods to unravel biological data. The vast amount of protein information emerging from a single experiment would be impossible to analyze by manual computation or analysis. Accordingly, comparison of the data with other databases and the use of computer modeling programs, such as those that calculate three-dimensional structures, are invaluable in proteomics.

The knowledge of protein expression and structure, and the potential changes in structure and function under different conditions, could allow the tailoring of treatment strategies. For example, in the lungs of those afflicted with cystic fibrosis, the bacterium *Pseudomonas aeuruginosa* forms adherent populations on the surface of the lung tissue. These populations, which are enclosed in a **glycocalyx** that the bacteri produce, are very resistant to treatments and directly and indirectly damage the lung tissue to a lethal extent. Presently, it is known that the bacteria change their genetic expression as they become more firmly associated with the surface. Through proteomics, more details of the proteins involved in the initial

approach to the surface and the subsequent, irreversible surface adhesion could be revealed. Once the targets are known, it is conceivable that they can be blocked. Thus, biofilms would not form and the bacteria could be more expeditiously eliminated from the lungs.

See also Biotechnology; Molecular biology and molecular genetics

PROTISTS

The kingdom Protista is the most diverse of all the five Eukaryotic kingdoms. There are more than 200,000 known species of protists with many more yet to be discovered. Protists can be found in countless colors, sizes, and shapes. They inhabit just about any area where water is found some or all of the time. They form the base of ecosystems by making food, as is the case with photosynthetic protists, or by themselves being eaten by larger organisms. They range in size from microscopic, unicellular organisms to huge seaweeds that can grow up to 300 ft (100 m) long.

The German zoologist Ernst Haeckel (1834–1919) first proposed the kingdom Protista in 1866. This early classification included any microorganism that was not a plant or an animal. Biologists did not readily accept this kingdom, and even after the American botanist Herbert F. Copeland again tried to establish its use 90 years later, there was not much support from the scientific community. Around 1960, R. Y. Stanier and **C. B. van Neil** (1897–1985) proposed the division of all organisms into two groups, the prokaryotes and the **eukaryotes**. Eukaryotes are organisms that have membrane-bound organelles in which metabolic processes take place, while prokaryotes lack these structures. In 1969, Robert Whittaker proposed the five-kingdom system of classification. The kingdom Protista was one of the five proposed kingdoms. At this time, only unicellular eukaryotic organisms were considered protists. Since then, the kingdom has expanded to include multicellular organisms, although biologists still disagree about what exactly makes an organism a protist.

Protists are difficult to characterize because of the great diversity of the kingdom. These organisms vary in body form, nutrition, and reproduction. They may be unicellular, colonial, or multicellular. As eukaryotes, protists can have many different organelles, including a **nucleus**, mitochondria, contractile vacuoles, food vacuoles, eyespots, plastids, pellicles, and flagella. The nuclei of protists contain **chromosomes**, with **DNA** associated with proteins. Protists are also capable of sexual, as well as asexual reproduction, meiosis, and mitosis. Protists can be free-living, or they may live symbiotically with another organism. This symbiosis can be mutalistic, where both partners benefit, or it can be parasitic, where the protist uses its host as a source of food or shelter while providing no advantage to the other organism. Many protists are economically important and beneficial to mankind, while others cause fatal diseases. Protists make up the majority of the **plankton** in aquatic systems, where they serve as the base of the food chain. Many protists are motile, using structures such as cilia, flagella, or pseudopodia (false feet) to move, while others are sessile. They may be autotrophs, producing their own food from sunlight, or heterotrophs, requiring an outside source of nutrition. It is unknown whether protists were the precursors to plants, animals, or **fungi**. It is possible that several evolutionary lines of protists developed separately. Biologists consider the protists as a polyphyletic group, meaning they probably do not share a common ancestor. The word protist comes from the Greek word for the very first, which indicates that researchers assume protists may have been the first eukaryotes to evolve on Earth.

Despite the great diversity evident in this kingdom, scientists have been able to classify the protists into several groups. The protists can be classified into one of three main categories, animal-like, plant-like, and fungus-like. Grouping into one of the three categories is based on an organism's mode of reproduction, method of nutrition, and motility. The animal-like protists are known as the **protozoa**, the plant-like protists are the algae, and the fungus-like protists are the **slime molds** and water molds.

The protozoa are all unicellular heterotrophs. They obtain their nutrition by ingesting other organisms or dead organic material. The word protozoa comes from the Latin word for first animals. The protozoans are grouped into various phyla based on their modes of locomotion. They may use cilia, flagella, or pseudopodia. Some protozoans are sessile, meaning they do not move. These organisms are parasitic because they cannot actively capture food. They must live in an area of the host organism that has a constant food supply, such as the intestines or bloodstream of an animal. The protozoans that use pseudopodia to move are known as amoebas, those that use flagella are called flagellates, those that use cilia are known as the ciliates, and those that do not move are called the sporozoans.

The amoebas belong to the phylum Rhizopoda. These protists have no wall outside of their cell membrane. This gives the cell flexibility and allows it to change shape. The word amoeba, in fact, comes from the Greek word for change. Amoebas use extensions of their cell membrane, called pseudopodia, to move as well as to engulf food. When the pseudopodium traps a bit of food, the cell membrane closes around the meal. This encasement forms a food vacuole. Digestive **enzymes** are secreted into the food vacuole, which break down the food. The cell then absorbs the nutrients. Because amoebas live in water, dissolved nutrients from the environment can diffuse directly through their cell membranes. Most amoebas live in marine environments, although some freshwater species exist. Freshwater amoebas live in a hypotonic environment, so water is constantly moving into the cell by osmosis. To remedy this problem, these amoebas use contractile vacuoles to pump excess water out of the cell. Most amoebas reproduce asexually by pinching off a part of the cell membrane to form a new organism. Amoebas may form cysts when environmental conditions become unfavorable. These cysts can survive conditions such as lack of water or nutrients. Two forms of amoebas have shells, the foraminiferans and the radiolarians.

The foraminiferans have a hard shell made of calcium carbonate. These shells are called tests. Foraminiferans live in marine environments and are very abundant. When they die, their shells fall to the ground where they become a part of the muddy ocean floor. Geologists use the fossilized shells to determine the ages of rocks and sediments. The shells at the ocean floor are gradually converted into chalky deposits, which can be uplifted to become a land formation, such as the white cliffs of Dover in England. Radiolarians have shells made of silica instead of calcium carbonate. Both organisms have many tiny holes in their shells, through which they extend their pseudopodia. The pseudopodia act as a sticky net, trapping bits of food.

The flagellates have one or more flagella and belong to the phylum Zoomastigina. These organisms whip their flagella from side to side in order to move through their aquatic surroundings. These organisms are also known as the zooflagellates. The flagellates are mostly unicellular with a spherical or oblong shape. A few are also amoeboid. Many ingest their food through a primitive mouth, called the oral groove. While most are motile, one class of flagellates, called the Choanoflagellates, is sessile. These organisms attach to a rock or other substrate by a stalk.

The ciliates are members of the phylum Ciliopa. There are approximately 8,000 species of ciliates. These organisms move by the synchronized beating of the cilia covering their bodies. They can be found almost anywhere, in freshwater or marine environments. Probably the best-known ciliate is the organism **Paramecium**. Paramecia have many well-developed organelles. Food enters the cell through the oral groove (lined with cilia, to "sweep" the food into the cell), where it moves to the gullet, which packages the meal into a food vacuole. Enzymes released into the food vacuole break down the food, and the nutrients are absorbed into the cell. Wastes are removed from the cell through an anal pore. Contractile vacuoles pump out excess water, since paramecia live in freshwater (hypotonic) surroundings. Paramecia have two nuclei, a macronucleus and a micronucleus. The larger macronucleus controls most of the metabolic functions of the cell. The smaller micronucleus controls much of the pathways involved in sexual reproduction. Thousands of cilia appear through the pellicle, a tough, protective covering surrounding the cell membrane. These cilia beat in a synchronized fashion to move the Paramecium in any direction. Underneath the pellicle are trichocysts, which discharge tiny spikes that help trap prey. Paramecia usually reproduce asexually, when the cell divides into two new organisms after all of the organelles have been duplicated. When conditions are unfavorable, however, the organism can reproduce sexually. This form of sexual reproduction is called **conjugation**. During conjugation, two paramecia join at the oral groove, where they exchange genetic material. They then separate and divide asexually, although this division does not necessarily occur immediately following the exchange of genetic material.

The sporozoans belong to the phylum **Sporozoa**. These organisms are sessile, so they cannot capture prey. Therefore, the sporozoans are all **parasites**. As their name suggests, many of these organisms produce spores, reproductive cells that can give rise to a new organism. Sporozoans typically have complex life cycles, as they usually live in more than one host in their lifetimes.

The plant-like protists, or algae, are all photosynthetic autotrophs. These organisms form the base of many food chains. Other creatures depend on these protists either directly for food or indirectly for the oxygen they produce. Algae are responsible for over half of the oxygen produced by photosynthesizing organisms. Many forms of algae look like plants, but they differ in many ways. Algae do not have roots, stems, or leaves. They do not have the waxy cuticle plants have to prevent water loss. As a result, algae must live in areas where water is readily available. Algae do not have multicellular gametangia as the plants do. They contain **chlorophyll**, but also contain other photosynthetic pigments. These pigments give the algae characteristic colors and are used to classify algae into various phyla. Other characteristics used to classify algae are energy reserve storage and cell wall composition.

Members of the phylum Euglenophyta are known as euglenoids. These organisms are both autotrophic as well as heterotrophic. There are hundreds of species of euglenoids. Euglenoids are unicellular and share properties of both plants and animals. They are plant-like in that they contain chlorophyll and are capable of **photosynthesis**. They do not have a cell wall of cellulose, as do plants; instead, they have a pellicle made of protein. Euglenoids are like animals in that they are motile and responsive to outside stimuli. One particular species, Euglena, has a structure called an eyespot. This area of red pigments is sensitive to light. An Euglena can respond to its environment by moving towards areas of bright light, where photosynthesis best occurs. In conditions where light is not available for photosynthesis, euglenoids can be heterotrophic and ingest their food. Euglenoids store their energy as paramylon, a type of polysaccharide.

Members of the phylum Bacillariophyta are called **diatoms**. Diatoms are unicellular organisms with silica shells. They are autotrophs and can live in marine or freshwater environments. They contain chlorophyll as well as pigments called carotenoids, which give them an orange-yellow color. Their shells resemble small boxes with lids. These shells are covered with grooves and pores, giving them a decorated appearance. Diatoms can be either radially or bilaterally symmetrical. Diatoms reproduce asexually in an unique manner. The two halves of the shell separate, each producing a new shell that fits inside the original half. Each new generation, therefore, produces offspring that are smaller than the parent. As each generation gets smaller and smaller, a lower limit is reached, approximately one quarter the original size. At this point, the diatom produces gametes that fuse with gametes from other diatoms to produce zygotes. The zygotes develop into full sized diatoms that can begin asexual reproduction once more. When diatoms die, their shells fall to the bottom of the ocean and form deposits called diatomaceous earth. These deposits can be collected and used as abrasives, or used as an additive to give certain paints their sparkle. Diatoms store their energy as oils or carbohydrates.

The **dinoflagellates** are members of the phylum Dinoflagellata. These organisms are unicellular autotrophs. Their cell walls contain cellulose, creating thick, protective plates. These plates contain two grooves at right angles to each other, each groove containing one flagellum. When the two flagella beat together, they cause the organism to spin through the water. Most dinoflagellates are marine organisms, although some have been found in freshwater environments. Dinoflagellates contain chlorophyll as well as carotenoids and red pigments. They can be free-living, or live in symbiotic relationships with jellyfish or corals. Some of the free-living dinoflagellates are bioluminescent. Many dinoflagellates produce strong toxins. One species in particular, Gonyaulax catanella, produces a lethal nerve toxin. These organisms sometimes reproduce in huge amounts in the summertime, causing a **red tide**. There are so many of these organisms present during a red tide that the ocean actually appears red. When this occurs, the toxins that are released reach such high concentrations in the ocean that many fish are killed. Dinoflagellates store their energy as oils or polysaccharides.

The phylum **Rhodophyta** consists of the red algae. All of the 4,000 species in this phylum are multicellular (with the exception of a few unicellular species) and live in marine environments. Red algae are typically found in tropical waters and sometimes along the coasts in cooler areas. They live attached to rocks by a structure called a holdfast. Their cell walls contain thick polysaccharides. Some species incorporate calcium carbonate from the ocean into their cell walls as well. Red algae contain chlorophyll as well as phycobilins, red and blue pigments involved in photosynthesis. The red pigment is called phycoerythrin and the blue pigment is called phycocyanin. Phycobilins absorb the green, violet, and blue light waves that can penetrate deep water. These pigments allow the red algae to photosynthesize in deep water with little light available. Reproduction in these organisms is a complex alternation between sexual and asexual phases. Red algae store their energy as floridean starch.

The 1,500 species of brown algae are the members of the phylum Phaeophyta. The majority of the brown algae live in marine environments, on rocks in cool waters. They contain chlorophyll as well as a yellow-brown carotenoid called fucoxanthin. The largest of the brown algae are the **kelp**. The kelp use holdfasts to attach to rocks. The body of a kelp is called a thallus, which can grow as long as 180 ft (60 m). The thallus is composed of three sections, the holdfast, the stipe, and the blade. Some species of brown algae have an air bladder to keep the thallus floating at the surface of the water, where more light is available for photosynthesis. Brown algae store their energy as laminarin, a carbohydrate.

The phylum **Chlorophyta** is known as the green algae. This phylum is the most diverse of all the algae, with greater than 7,000 species. The green algae contain chlorophyll as their main pigment. Most live in fresh water, although some marine species exist. Their cell walls are composed of cellulose, which indicates the green algae may be the ancestors of modern plants. Green algae can be unicellular, colonial, or multicellular. An example of a unicellular green alga is Chlamydomonas. An example of a colonial algae is Volvox. A Volvox **colony** is a hollow sphere of thousands of individual cells. Each cell has a single flagellum that faces the exterior of the sphere. The individual cells beat their flagella in a coordi-

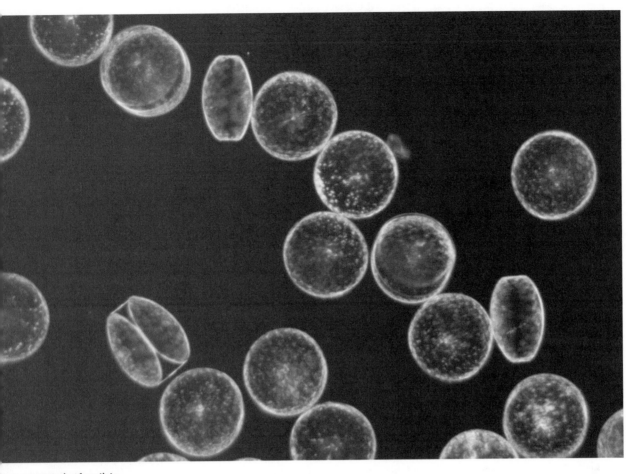

ms, an example of protists.

d fashion, allowing the colony to move. Daughter colonies
inside the sphere, growing until they reach a certain size
are released when the parent colony breaks open.
ogyra and Ulva are both examples of multicellular green
e. Reproduction in the green algae can be both sexual and
ual. Green algae store their energy as starch.

The fungus-like protists resemble the fungi during some
of their life cycle. These organisms exhibit properties of
fungi and protists. The slime molds and the water molds
members of this group. They all obtain energy by decom-
ng organic materials, and as a result, are important for
cling nutrients. They can be brightly colored and live in
, moist, dark habitats. The slime molds are classified as
er plasmodial or cellular by their modes of reproduction.

plasmodial slime molds belong to the phylum
omycota, and the cellular slime molds belong to the phy-
Acrasiomycota.

The plasmodial slime molds form a structure called a
modium, a mass of **cytoplasm** that contains many nuclei
has no cell walls or membranes to separate individual
s. The plasmodium is the feeding stage of the slime **mold**.
oves much like an amoeba, slowly sneaking along decay-
organic material. It moves at a rate of 1 in (2.5 cm) per
r, engulfing **microorganisms**. The reproductive structure of

plasmodial slime molds occurs when the plasmodium forms a
stalked structure during unfavorable conditions. This structure
produces spores that can be released and travel large distances.
The spores land and produce a zygote that grows into a new
plasmodium.

The cellular slime molds exist as individual cells during
the feeding stage. These cells can move like an amoeba as
well, engulfing food along the way. The feeding cells reproduce asexually through cell division. When conditions become
unfavorable, the cells come together to form a large mass of
cells resembling a plasmodium. This mass of cells can move
as one organism and looks much like a garden slug. The mass
eventually develops into a stalked structure capable of sexual
reproduction.

The water molds and downy mildews belong to the phylum Oomycota. They grow on the surface of dead organisms or
plants, decomposing the organic material and absorbing nutrients. Most live in water or in moist areas. Water molds grow as
a mass of fuzzy white threads on dead material. The difference
between these organisms and true fungi is the water molds
form flagellated reproductive cells during their life cycles.

Many protists can cause serious illness and disease.
Malaria, for example, is caused by the protist Plasmodium.
Plasmodia are sporozoans and are transferred from person to

person through female Anopheles mosquitoes. People who suffer from malaria experience symptoms such as shivering, sweating, high fevers, and delirium. African **sleeping sickness**, also known as African trypanosomiasis, is caused by another sporozoan, Trypanosoma. Trypanosoma is transmitted through the African tsetse fly. This organism causes high fever and swollen lymph nodes. Eventually the protist makes its way into the victim's brain, where it causes a feeling of uncontrollable fatigue. Giardiasis is another example of a disease caused by a protist. This illness is caused by **Giardia**, a sporozoan carried by muskrats and beavers. Giardiasis is characterized by fatigue, cramps, diarrhea, and weight loss. Amoebic **dysentery** occurs when a certain amoeba, *Entamoeba histolytica,* infects the large intestine of humans. It is spread through infected food and water. This organism causes bleeding, diarrhea, vomiting, and sometimes death.

Members of the kingdom Protista can also be very beneficial to life on Earth. Many species of red algae are edible and are popular foods in certain parts of the world. Red algae are rich in vitamins and minerals. Carageenan, a polysaccharide extracted from red algae, is used as a thickening agent in ice cream and other foods. Giant kelp forests are rich ecosystems, providing food and shelter for many organisms. Trichonymphs are flagellates that live in the intestines of termites. These protozoans break down cellulose in wood into carbohydrates the termites can digest.

The kingdom Protista is a diverse group of organisms. Some protists are harmful, but many more are beneficial. These organisms form the foundation for food chains, produce the oxygen we breathe, and play an important role in nutrient recycling. Many protists are economically useful as well. As many more of these unique organisms are discovered, humans will certainly enjoy the new uses and benefits protists provide.

See also Eukaryotes

PROTOPLASTS AND SPHEROPLASTS

Protoplasts and spheroplasts are altered forms of **bacteria** or **yeast**, in which the principal shape-maintaining structure of the bacteria is weakened. Each bacterium forms a sphere, which is the shape that allows the bacterium to withstand the rigors, particularly osmotic, of the fluid in which it resides.

The term protoplast refers to the spherical shape assumed by Gram-positive bacteria. Spheroplast refers to the spherical shape assumed by Gram-negative bacteria. The difference is essentially the presence of a single membrane, in the case of the protoplast, and the two membranes (inner and outer) of the Gram-negative spheroplasts. It is also possible to generate a gram-negative protoplast by the removal of the outer membrane. Thus, in essence, protoplast refers to a bacterial sphere that is bounded by a single membrane and spheroplast refers to a sphere that is bounded by two membranes.

Bacteria are induced to form protoplasts or spheroplasts typically by laboratory manipulation. However, formation of the structures can occur naturally. Such bacteria are referred to as L-forms. Examples of bacterial genera that can produce L-

forms include *Bacillus*, *Clostridium*, *Haemophilus*, *Pseudomonas*, *Staphylococcus*, and *Vibrio*.

The **peptidoglycan** is the main stress-bearing layer of the bacterial cell wall and the peptidoglycan also gives the bacterium its shape. In the laboratory, weakening the peptidoglycan network in the cell wall generates both protoplasts and spheroplasts.

By exposing bacteria to an enzyme called lysozyme, the interconnecting strands of the two particular sugars that form the peptidoglycan can be cut. When this is done, the peptidoglycan loses the ability to serve as a mechanical means of support.

The situation in yeast is slightly different, as other components of the yeast cell wall are degraded in order to form the protoplast.

The process of creating protoplasts and spheroplasts must be done in a solution in which the ionic composition and concentration of the fluid outside of the bacteria is the same as that inside the bacteria. Once the structural support of the peptidoglycan is lost, the bacteria are unable to control their response to differences in the ionic composition between the bacterial interior and exterior. If the inner concentration is greater than the outer ionic concentration, water will flow into the bacterium in an attempt to achieve an ionic balance. The increased volume can be so severe that the bacteria will burst. Conversely, if the inner ionic concentration is less than the exterior, water will exit the bacterium, in an attempt to dilute the surroundings. The bacteria can shrivel to the point of death.

Preservation of ionic balance is required to ensure that bacteria will not be killed during their **transformation** into either the protoplast or the spheroplast form. Living protoplasts and spheroplasts are valuable research tools. The membrane balls that are the protoplasts or spheroplasts can be induced to fuse more easily with similar structures as well as with eukaryotic cells. This facilitates the transfer of genetic material between the two cells. As well, the sequential manufacture of spheroplasts and protoplasts in Gram-negative bacteria allows for the selective release of the contents of the **periplasm**. This approach has been popular in the identification of the components of the periplasm, and in the localization of proteins to one or the other of the Gram-negative membranes. For example, if a certain protein is present in a spheroplast population—but is absent from a protoplast population—then the protein is located within the outer membrane.

See also Bacterial ultrastructure; Biotechnology; Transformation

PROTOZOA

Protozoa are a very diverse group of single-celled organisms, with more than 50,000 different types represented. The vast majority are microscopic, many measuring less than 1/200 mm, but some, such as the freshwater Spirostomun, may reach 0.17 in (3 mm) in length, large enough to enable it to be seen with the naked eye.

Scientists have discovered fossilized specimen of protozoa that measured 0.78 in (20 mm) in diameter. Whatever the size, however, protozoans are well-known for their diversity and the fact that they have evolved under so many different conditions.

One of the basic requirements of all protozoans is the presence of water, but within this limitation, they may live in the sea, in rivers, lakes, stagnant ponds of freshwater, soil, and in some decaying matters. Many are solitary organisms, but some live in colonies; some are free-living, others are sessile; and some species are even **parasites** of plants and animals (including humans). Many protozoans form complex, exquisite shapes and their beauty is often greatly overlooked on account of their diminutive size.

The protozoan cell body is often bounded by a thin pliable membrane, although some sessile forms may have a toughened outer layer formed of cellulose, or even distinct shells formed from a mixture of materials. All the processes of life take place within this cell wall. The inside of the membrane is filled with a fluid-like material called **cytoplasm**, in which a number of tiny organs float. The most important of these is the **nucleus**, which is essential for growth and reproduction. Also present are one or more contractile vacuoles, which resemble air bubbles, whose job it is to maintain the correct water balance of the cytoplasm and also to assist with food assimilation.

Protozoans living in salt water do not require contractile vacuoles as the concentration of salts in the cytoplasm is similar to that of seawater and there is therefore no net loss or gain of fluids. Food vacuoles develop whenever food is ingested and shrink as digestion progresses. If too much water enters the cell, these vacuoles swell, move towards the edge of the cell wall and release the water through a tiny pore in the membrane.

Some protozoans contain the green pigment **chlorophyll** more commonly associated with higher plants, and are able to manufacture their own foodstuffs in a similar manner to plants. Others feed by engulfing small particles of plant or animal matter. To assist with capturing prey, many protozoans have developed an ability to move. Some, such as Euglena and Trypanosoma are equipped with a single whip like flagella which, when quickly moved back and forth, pushes the body through the surrounding water body. Other protozoans (e.g., Paramecium) have developed large numbers of tiny cilia around the membrane; the rhythmic beat of these hairlike structures propel the cell along and also carry food, such as **bacteria**, towards the gullet. Still others are capable of changing the shape of their cell wall. The Amoeba, for example, is capable of detecting chemicals given off by potential food particles such as **diatoms**, algae, bacteria or other protozoa. As the cell wall has no definite shape, the cytoplasm can extrude to form pseudopodia (Greek *pseudes*, "false"; *pous*, "foot") in various sizes and at any point of the cell surface. As the Amoeba approaches its prey, two pseudopodia extend out from the main cell and encircle and engulf the food, which is then slowly digested.

Various forms of reproduction have evolved in this group, one of the simplest involves a splitting of the cell in a process known as binary fission. In species like amoeba, this process takes place over a period of about one hour: the nucleus divides and the two sections drift apart to opposite ends of the cell. The cytoplasm also begins to divide and the cell changes shape to a dumb-bell appearance. Eventually the cell splits giving rise to two identical "daughter" cells that then resume moving and feeding. They, in turn, can divide further in this process known as asexual reproduction, where only one individual is involved.

Some species that normally reproduce asexually, may occasionally reproduce through sexual means, which involves the joining, or fusion, of the nuclei from two different cells. In the case of **paramecium**, each individual has two nuclei: a larger macronucleus that is responsible for growth, and a much smaller micronucleus that controls reproduction. When paramecium reproduce by sexual means, two individuals join in the region of the oral groove—a shallow groove in the cell membrane that opens to the outside. When this has taken place, the macronuclei of each begins to disintegrate, while the micronucleus divides in four. Three of these then degenerate and the remaining nucleus divides once again to produce two micronuclei that are genetically identical. The two cells then exchange one of these nuclei that, upon reaching the other individual's micronucleus, fuse to form what is known as a zygote nucleus. Shortly afterwards, the two cells separate but within each cell a number of other cellular and cytoplasmic divisions will continue to take place, eventually resulting in the production of four daughter cells from each individual.

Protozoans have evolved to live under a great range of environmental conditions. When these conditions are unfavorable, such as when food is scarce, most species are able to enter an inactive phase, where cells become non-motile and secrete a surrounding cyst that prevents **desiccation** and protects the cell from extreme temperatures. The cysts may also serve as a useful means of dispersal, with cells being borne on the wind or on the feet of animals. Once the cyst reaches a more favorable situation, the outer wall breaks down and the cell resumes normal activity.

Many species are of considerable interest to scientists, not least because of the medical problems that many cause. The tiny **Plasmodium** protozoan, the cause of **malaria** in humans, is responsible for hundreds of millions of cases of illness each year, with many deaths occurring in poor countries. This parasite is transferred from a malarial patient to a healthy person by the bite of female mosquitoes of the genus Anopheles. As the mosquito feeds on a victim's blood the parasites pass from its salivary glands into the open wound. From there, they make their way to the liver where they multiply and later enter directly into red blood cells. Here they multiply even further, eventually causing the blood cell to burst and release from 6-36 infectious bodies into the blood plasma. A mosquito feeding on such a patient's blood may absorb some of these organisms, allowing the parasite to complete its life cycle and begin the process all over again. The shock of the release of so many parasites into the human blood stream results in a series of chills and fevers—typical symptoms of malaria. Acute cases of malaria may continue for some days or even weeks, and may subside if the body is able to develop **immunity** to the disease. Relapses, however, are common and malaria is still a major cause of death in the tropics. Although certain drugs have been developed to protect people from Plasmodium many forms of malaria have now developed, some of which are even immune to the strongest medicines.

While malaria is one of the best known diseases known to be caused by protozoans, a wide range of other equally devastating ailments are also caused by protozoan infections. Amoebic **dysentery**, for example, is caused by *Entamoeba histolytica.*; African **sleeping sickness**, which is spread by the bite of the tsetse fly, is caused by the flagellate protozoan Trypanosoma; a related species *T. cruzi* causes Chagas' disease in South and Central America; Eimeria causes coccidiosis in rabbits and poultry; and Babesia, spread by ticks, causes red water fever in cattle.

Not all protozoans are parasites however, although this is by far a more specialized life style than that adopted by free-living forms. Several protozoans form a unique, nondestructive, relationship with other species, such as those found in the intestine of wood-eating termites. Living in the termites' intestines the protozoans are provided with free board and lodgings as they ingest the wood fibers for their own nutrition. In the process of doing so, they also release proteins which can be absorbed by the termite's digestive system, which is otherwise unable to break down the tough cellulose walls of the wood fibers. Through this mutualistic relationship, the termites benefit from a nutritional source that they could otherwise not digest, while the protozoans receive a safe home and steady supply of food.

See also Amoebic dysentery; Entamoeba histolytica; Epidemiology, tracking diseases with technology; Waste water treatment; Water quality

PRUSINER, STANLEY (1942-   )

American physician

Stanley Prusiner performed seminal research in the field of neurogenetics, identifying the prion, a unique infectious protein agent containing no **DNA** or **RNA**.

Prusiner was born on in Des Moines, Iowa. His father, Lawrence, served in the United States Navy, moving the family briefly to Boston where Lawrence Prusiner enrolled in Naval officer training school before being sent to the South Pacific. During his father's absence, the young Stanley lived with his mother in Cincinnati, Ohio. Shortly after the end of World War II, the family returned to Des Moines where Stanley attended primary school and where his brother, Paul, was born. In 1952, the family returned to Ohio where Lawrence Prusiner worked as a successful architect.

In Ohio, Prusiner attended the Walnut Hills High School, before being accepted by the University of Pennsylvania where he majored in Chemistry. At the University, besides numerous science courses, he also had the opportunity to broaden his studies in subjects such as philosophy, the history of architecture, economics, and Russian history. During the summer of 1963, between his junior and senior years, he began a research project on hypothermia with

Sidnez Wolfson in the Department of Surgery. He worke the project throughout his senior year and then decided to on at the University to train for medical school. Durin second year of medicine, Prusiner decided to study the su fluorescence of brown adipose tissue (fatty tissue) in S golden hamsters as they arose from hibernation. This rese allowed him to spend much of his fourth study year a Wenner-Gren Institute in Stockholm working on the **me lism** of isolated brown adipocytes. At this he began to ously consider pursuing a career in biomedical research.

Early in 1968, Prusiner returned to the U.S. to com his medical studies. The previous spring, he had been giv position at the National Institutes of Health (NIH) on pleting an internship in medicine at the Universit California San Francisco (UCSF). During that year, he me wife, Sandy Turk, who was teaching mathematics to school students. At the NIH, he worked on the glutami family of **enzymes** in *Escherichia coli* and as the end o time at the NIH began to near, he examined the possibili taking up a postdoctoral fellowships in neurobio Eventually, however, he decided that a residency in neuro was a better route to developing a rewarding career in rese as it offered him direct contact with patients and therefo opportunity to learn about both the normal and abnormal n ous system. In July 1972, Prusiner began a residency at U in the Department of Neurology. Two months later, he ad ted a female patient who was exhibiting progressive los memory and difficulty performing some routine tasks. was his first encounter with a Creutzfeldt-Jakob disease (C patient and was the beginning of the work to which he dedicated most of his life.

In 1974, Prusiner accepted the offer of an assistant fessor position from Robert Fishman, the Chair of Neuro at UCSF, and began to set up a laboratory to study scrap parallel disease of human CJD found in sheep. Early on in endeavor, he collaborated with William Hadlow and Eklund at the Rocky Mountain Laboratory in Hami Montana, from whom he learnt much about the technique handling the scrapie agent. Although the agent was believed to be a virus, data from the very beginning sugge that this was a novel infectious agent, which containe nucleic acid. It confirmed the conclusions of Tikvah Alper J. S. Griffith who had originally proposed the idea of an in tious protein in the 1960s. The idea had been given little dence at that time. At the beginning of his research into p diseases, Prusiner's work was fraught with technical diffi ties and he had to stand up to the skepticism of his colleag Eventually he was informed by the Howard Hughes Med Institute (HHMI) that they would not renew their finan support and by UCSF that he would not be promoted to ter The tenure decision was eventually reversed, howe enabling Prusiner to continue his work with financial sup from other sources. As the data for the protein nature of scrapie agent accumulated, Prusiner grew more confident his findings were not artifacts and decided to summarize work in a paper, published in 1982. There he introduced term "prion," derived from "proteinaceous" and 'infectio particle and challenged the scientific community to attemp find an associated nucleic acid. Despite the strong convictions of many, none was ever found.

In 1983, the protein of the prion was found in Prusiner's laboratory and the following year, a portion of the amino acid sequence was determined by Leroy Hood. With that knowledge, molecular biological studies of **prions** ensued and an explosion of new information followed. Prusiner collaborated with Charles Weissmann on the molecular **cloning** of the **gene** encoding the prion protein (PrP). Work was also done on linking the PrP gene to the control of scrapie incubation times in mice and on the discovery that **mutations** within the protein itself caused different incubation times. Antibodies that provided an extremely valuable tool for prion research were first raised in Prusiner's lab and used in the discovery of the normal form of PrP protein. By the early 1990s, the existence of prions as causative agents of diseases like CJD in humans and bovine spongiform encephalopathy (BSE) in cows, came to be accepted in many quarters of the scientific community. As prions gained wider acceptance among scientists, Prusiner received many scientific prizes. In 1997, Prusiner was awarded the Nobel Prize for medicine.

See also BSE and CJD disease; Infection and resistance; Viral genetics

PSEUDOMEMBRANOUS COLITIS

Pseudomembranous colitis is severe **inflammation** of the colon in which raised, yellowish plaques, or pseudomembranes, develop on the mucosal lining. The plaques consist of clumps of dead epithelial cells from the colon, white blood cells, and fibrous protein.

Pseudomembranous colitis is usually associated with antibiotic use. When the normal balance of the flora in the colon is disturbed, pathogenic strains of the bacillus *Clostridium difficile* may proliferate out of control and produce damaging amounts of cytotoxins known as cytotoxins A and B.

C. difficile toxins often cause diarrhea and mild inflammation of the colon. Less frequently, the condition may progress further, causing ulceration and formation of the pseudomembranous plaques. Pseudomembranous colitis is most common in health care facilities such as hospitals and nursing homes, where an individual is most likely to be immune-compromised and to come into contact with persistent, heat-resistant *C. difficile* spores by the fecal-oral route. Thus, the best way to prevent it is meticulous cleanliness, coupled with avoiding the overuse of **antibiotics**.

Mild symptoms such as diarrhea often disappear spontaneously soon after the antibiotics are discontinued. Ironically, severe antibiotic-associated colitis must generally be treated with additional antibiotics to target the *C. difficile* pathogen. Benign intestinal flora such as **lactobacillus** or non-pathogenic **yeast** may be administered orally or rectally. Supportive therapies such as intravenous fluids are used as in other cases of ulcerative colitis. In rare cases, surgery to remove the damaged section of colon may be required.

While antibiotic use is the most common precipitating cause of pseudomembranous colitis, occasionally the condition may result from **chemotherapy**, bone marrow transplantation, or other causes.

See also Microbial flora of the stomach and gastrointestinal tract

PSEUDOMONAS

The genus *Pseudomonas* is made up of Gram-negative, rod-shaped **bacteria** that inhabit many niches. *Pseudomonas* species are common inhabitants of the soil, water, and vegetation. The genus is particularly noteworthy because of the tendency of several species to cause infections in people who are already ill, or whose immune systems are not operating properly. Such infections are termed opportunistic infections.

Pseudomonas rarely causes infections in those whose immune systems are fully functional. The disease-causing members of the genus are therefore prevalent where illness abounds. *Pseudomonas* are one of the major causes of nosocomial (hospital acquired) infections.

Bacteria in this genus not only cause infections in man, but also cause infections in plants and animals (e.g., horses). For example, *Pseudomonas mallei* causes ganders disease in horses.

The species that comprise the genus *Pseudomonas* are part of the wider family of bacteria that are classified as *Pseudomonadaceae*. There are more than 140 species in the genus. The species that are associated with opportunistic infections include *Pseudomonas aeruginosa*, *Pseudomonas maltophilia*, *Pseudomonas fluorescens*, *Pseudomonas putida*, *Pseudomonas cepacia*, *Pseudomonas stutzeri*, and *Pseudomonas putrefaciens*. *Pseudomonas aeruginosa* is probably the most well-known member of the genus.

Pseudomonas are hardy **microorganisms**, and can grow on almost any available surface where enough moisture and nutrients are present. Members of the genus are prone to form the adherent bacterial populations that are termed biofilms. Moreover, *Pseudomonas aeruginosa* specifically change their genetic behavior when on a surface, such that they produce much more of the **glycocalyx** material than they produce when floating in solution. The glycocalyx-enmeshed bacteria become extremely resistant to antibacterial agents and immune responses such as **phagocytosis**.

In the hospital setting *Pseudomonas aeruginosa* can cause very serious infections in people who have cancer, cystic fibrosis, and burns. Other infections in numerous sites in the body, can be caused by *Pseudomonas spp*. Infections can be site-specific, such as in the urinary tract or the respiratory system. More widely disseminated infections (termed systemic infections) can occur, particularly in burn victims and those whose immune systems are immunosuppressed.

For those afflicted with cystic fibrosis, the long-lasting lung infection caused by *Pseudomonas aeruginosa* can ultimately prove to be fatal. The bacteria have a surface that is altered from their counterparts growing in natural environments. One such alteration is the production of a glycocalyx around the bacteria. The bacteria become very hard for the **immune system** to eradicate. The immune response eventually damages the epithelial cells of the lung. So much so, sometimes, that lung function is severely compromised or ceases.

Another bacterium, *Pseudomonas cepacia*, is also an opportunistic cause of lung infections in those afflicted with cystic fibrosis. This species is problematic because it is resistant to more **antibiotics** than is *Pseudomonas aeruginosa*.

Glycocalyx production in some strains of *Pseudomonas aeruginosa* can be so prodigious that colonies growing on solid media appear slimy. Indeed, some species produce such mucoid colonies that the colonies will drip onto the lid of the **agar** plate when the plate is turned upside down. These slimy growths are described as mucoid colonies, and are often a hallmark of a sample that has been recovered from an infection.

Disease-causing species of *Pseudomonas* can possess a myriad of factors in addition to the glycocalyx that enable a bacterium to establish an infection. The appendages known as pili function in adherence to host cells. A component of the outer membrane possesses an endotoxin. Finally, a number of exotoxins and extracellular **enzymes** can cause damage at a distance from the bacterium. One such exotoxin, which is called toxin A, is extremely potent, and may be the prime cause of damage by the bacteria in infections.

Some species, especially *Pseudomonas aeruginosa* are a problem in hospitals. By virtue of their function, hospitals are a place where many immunocompromised people are found. This is an ideal environment for an opportunistic disease-causing bacterium. Moreover, *Pseudomonas aeruginosa* has acquired resistance to a number of commonly used antibiotics. As yet, a **vaccine** to the bacterium does not exist. Prevention of the spread of *Pseudomonas* involves the observance of proper **hygiene**, including handwashing.

See also Bacteria and bacterial infection; Infection and resistance; Lipopolysaccharide and its constituents

PSYCHROPHILIC BACTERIA

Psychrophilic ("cold loving") **microorganisms**, particularly **bacteria**, have a preferential temperature for growth at less than 59° Fahrenheit (15° Celsius). Bacteria that can grow at such cold temperatures, but which prefer a high growth temperature, are known as psychrotrophs.

The discovery of psychrophilic microorganisms and the increasing understanding of their functioning has increased the awareness of the diversity of microbial life on Earth. So far, more than 100 varieties of psychrophilic bacteria have been isolated from the deep sea. This environment is very cold and tends not to fluctuate in temperature. Psychrophilic bacteria are abundant in the near-freezing waters of the Arctic and the Antarctic. Indeed, in Antarctica, bacteria have been isolated from permanently ice-covered lakes. Other environments where psychrophilic bacteria have been include high altitude cloud droplets.

Psychrophilic bacteria are truly adapted for life at cold temperatures. The **enzymes** of the bacteria are structurally unstable and fail to operate properly even at room (or ambient) temperature. Furthermore, the membranes of psychrophilic bacteria contain much more of a certain kind of lipid than is found in other types of bacteria. The lipid tends to be more pliable at lower temperature, much like margarine is more pliable than butter at refrigeration temperatures. The increased fluidity of the membrane makes possible the chemical reactions that would otherwise stop if the membrane were semi-frozen. Some psychrophiles, particularly those from the Antarctic, have been found to contain polyunsaturated fatty acids, which generally do not occur in prokaryotes. At room temperature, the membrane of such bacteria would be so fluid that the bacterium would die.

Aside from their ecological curiosity, psychrophilic bacteria have practical value. Harnessing the enzymes of these organisms allows functions such as the cleaning of clothes in cold water to be performed. Furthermore, in the Arctic and Antarctic ecosystems, the bacteria form an important part of the food chain that supports the lives of more complex creatures. In addition, some species of psychrophiles, including *Listeria monocytogenes* are capable of growth at refrigeration temperatures. Thus, spoilage of contaminated food can occur, which can lead to disease if the food is eaten. Listeriosis, a form of **meningitis** that occurs in humans, is a serious health threat, especially to those whose **immune system** is either not mature or is defective due to disease or therapeutic efforts. Other examples of such disease-causing bacteria include *Aeromonas hydrophila*, *Clostridium botulinum*, and *Yersinia enterocolitica*.

See also Extremophiles

PUBLIC HEALTH, CURRENT ISSUES

Public health is the establishment and maintenance of healthful living conditions for the general population. This goal requires organized effort from all levels of government. Underlying the current concerns in public health are three principle aims of public health efforts. First is the assessment and monitoring of populations, from the community level to the national level, to identify populations who are at risk for whatever health problem is being considered. For example, public health efforts have shown that aboriginals in Canada are especially prone to developing diabetes. The second "plank" of public health is the formulation of policies to deal with the significant problems. Returning to the example, policies and strategies for action are now being formulated to reverse the trend. The third core public health function is to assure that everyone is able to receive adequate and affordable care and disease prevention services.

There are many microbiological threats to public health. In order to maintain the three cores of public health, priorities must be established. In organizations such as the **Centers for Disease Control** and the **World Health Organization**, different divisions have been created to address the different concerns. Within each division the particular area of concern, such as

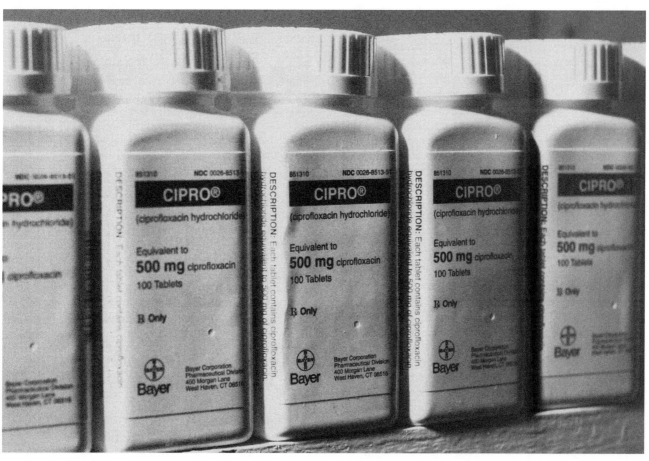

Ciprofloxacin used to treat anthrax.

food safety, can be simultaneously addressed at various levels, including basic research, policy development, and public awareness.

In the aftermath of the September 11, 2001, terrorist attacks on targets in the United States, public perception of the health risks of what is commonly known as **bioterrorism** has been heightened. The ability to transport harmful **microorganisms** or their products, such as **anthrax**, through the mail or via dispersal in the air has made clear how vulnerable populations are to attack. Public health agencies have realized that the ability to promptly respond to an incident is critical to any successful containment of the disease causing microbial threat. But the achievement of this response will require a huge effort from many public and private agencies, and will be extremely expensive. For example, it has been estimated that a response to each incident of bioterrorism, real or not, costs on the order of 50,000 dollars. Repeated mobilization of response teams would quickly sap the public health budget, at the cost of other programs. Thus, in the latter years of the twentieth century and the new century, the issue of bioterrorism and how to deal with it in a safe and economically prudent way has become a paramount public health issue.

Another public health issue that has become more important is the emergence of certain microbial diseases. In the emergence category, **hemorrhagic diseases** of viral origin, such as Ebola and Lassa fever are appearing more frequently. These diseases are terrifying due to their rapid devastation inflicted on the victim of infection, and because treatments are as yet rudimentary. The emergence of such diseases, which seems to be a consequence of man's encroachment on environments that have been largely untouched until now, is a harbinger of things to come. Public health agencies are moving swiftly to understand the nature of these diseases and how to combat them.

Diseases are also re-emerging. **Tuberculosis** is one example. Diseases such as tuberculosis were once thought to be a thing of the past, due to **antibiotics** and public health initiatives. Yet, the numbers of people afflicted with such diseases is on the rise. One factor in the re-emergence of certain diseases is the re-acquisition of **antibiotic resistance** by **bacteria**. Another factor in the re-emergence of tuberculosis is the sharp increase in the number of immunocompromised individuals that are highly susceptible to tuberculosis, such as those with acquired immune deficiency syndrome (**AIDS**). The overuse and incomplete use of antibiotics has also enabled bacteria to develop resistance that can be passed on to subsequent generations. Public health efforts and budgets are being re-directed to issues thought at one time to be dealt with and no longer a concern.

Certain infectious diseases represent another increasingly important public health issue. Just a few decades ago AIDS was more of a curiosity, given its seeming confinement to groups of people who were often marginalized and ostracized. In the past decade, however, it has become clear that AIDS is an all-inclusive disease. Aside from the suffering that the illness inflicts, the costs of care for the increasingly debilitated and dependent patients will constitute a huge drain on health care budgets in the decades to come. As a result, AIDS research to develop an effective **vaccine** or strategies that prolong the vitality of those infected with the AIDS virus is a major public health issue and priority.

Another public health issue of current importance is chronic bacterial and viral diseases. Conditions like fibromyalgia may have a bacterial or viral cause. The chronic and debilitating **Lyme disease** certainly has a bacterial cause. Moreover, the increasing use of surgical interventions to enhance the quality of life, with the installation of heart pacemakers, artificial joints, and the use of catheters to deliver and remove fluids from patients, has created conditions conducive for the explosion in the numbers of bacterial infections that result from the colonization of the artificial surfaces. Such bacterial biofilms have now been proven to be the source of infections that persist, sometimes without symptoms, in spite of the use of antibiotics. Such infections can be life threatening, and their numbers are growing. As with the other current public health issues, chronic infections represent both a public health threat and a budget drain.

A final area that has long been a public health concern is the safety of food and water. These have always been susceptible to **contamination** by bacteria, **protozoa** and **viruses**, in particular. With the popularity of prepared foods, the monitoring of foods and their preparation has become both more urgent and more difficult for the limited number of inspectors to do. Water can easily become contaminated. The threat to water has become greater in the past twenty years, because of the increasing encroachment of civilization on natural areas, where the protozoan pathogens *Giardia* and *Cryptosporidium* normally live, and because of the appearance of more dangerous bacterial pathogens, in particular *Escherichia coli* O157:H7. The latter organism is a problem in food as well.

See also Bacteria and bacterial infection; Epidemics and pandemics; Food safety; History of public health; Viruses and responses to viral infection

PUBLIC HEALTH SYSTEMS • *see* HISTORY OF PUBLIC HEALTH

PULSE-CHASE EXPERIMENT • *see* LABORATORY TECHNIQUES IN IMMUNOLOGY

PYREX: CONSTRUCTION, PROPERTY, AND USES IN MICROBIOLOGY

Pyrex is a brand name of a type of glass that is constructed of borosilicate. The Corning Glass Company of Corning, New York, developed Pyrex. Chemically, as borosilicate implies, this type of glass is composed of silica and at least five percent (of the total weight of the elements in the glass) of a chemical called boric oxide. The combination and concentrations of these constituents confers great resistance to temperature change and corrosion by harsh chemicals, such as strong acids and alkalis, to whatever vessel is made of the borosilicate glass. This durability has made Pyrex glassware extremely useful in the microbiology laboratory.

The development of Pyrex in 1924 by scientists at the Corning Company satisfied the demand for high quality scientific glassware that had began in the nineteenth century. Then, the glassware in existence was degraded by laboratory chemicals and became brittle when exposed to repeated cycles of heating and cooling. The formulation of Pyrex minimized the tendency of the material to expand and contract. This maintained the accuracy of measuring instruments such as graduated cylinders, and overcame the brittleness encountered upon repeated autoclave **sterilization** of the laboratory glassware.

Pyrex glassware immediately found acceptance in the microbiology research community. The popularity of the glassware continues today, despite the development of heat and chemical resistant plastic polymers. Glass is still the preferred container for growing **bacteria**. This is because the glass can be cleaned using harsh chemicals, which will completely remove any organic material that might otherwise adhere to the sides of the vessel. For applications where the chemical composition and concentrations of the medium components are crucial, such organic contaminants must be removed.

Pyrex glassware is also used to manufacture graduated cylinders that are extremely accurate. In some applications, the exact volume of a liquid is important to achieve. This type of glassware is known as volumetric glassware. Plastic still cannot match the accuracy or the unchanging efficiency of volume delivery that is achieved by Pyrex volumetric glassware.

Another application for borosilicate glass is in the measurement of optical density. For this application, typically specially designed vials are filled with the solution or suspension of interest and then placed in the path of a beam of light in a machine known as a **spectrophotometer**. The amount of light that passes through the sample can be recorded and, with the inclusion of appropriate controls, can be used, for example, to determine the number of bacteria in the sample. Plastic material does not lend itself to optical density measurements, as the plastic can be cloudy. Thus, the vial itself would absorb some of the incoming light. Pyrex, however, can be made so as to be optically transparent. Growth flasks have even been made in which a so-called "side arm," basically a test tube that is fused onto the flask, can be used to directly obtain optical density measurements without removing the **culture** from the flask.

In the same vein, the use of optically transparent slabs of Pyrex as **microscope** slides is a fundamental tool in the micro-

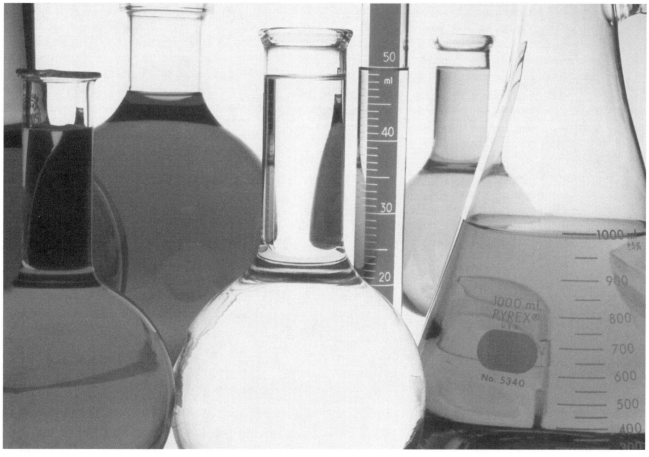

Pyrex labware filled with colored liquid.

biology laboratory. The heat resistance of the slide allows a specimen to be heated directly on the slide. This is important for stains such as the acid-fast stain for mycobacteria, in which heating of the samples is essential for the accurate staining of the bacteria. Also, as for the optical density measurements, the light microscopic examination of the bacterial sample depends upon the transparency of the support surface. Plastic is not an appropriate support material for slides.

Another area in which Pyrex glassware is essential in a microbiology laboratory is in the pipelines required for the delivery of distilled water. Distillation of water is a process that requires the boiling of the water. The pipelines must be heat resistant. Also, because physical scrubbing of the pipelines is not feasible, the pipes must withstand the application of caustic chemicals to scour organic material off the interior surface of the pipes.

Other applications of borosilicate glassware in the microbiology laboratory include nondisposable Petri plates for the use of solid media, centrifuge tubes, titration cylinders, and the stopcocks that control the flow rate.

Heat and chemically resistant plastics are widely used in the typical microbiology laboratory, particularly for routine, high-volume operations where cleaning and preparation of glassware for re-use is time-consuming and prone to error.

However, the accuracy and advantages of Pyrex glassware ensure its continued use in the most modern of microbiology laboratories.

See also Laboratory methods in microbiology; Microscopy

PYRROPHYTA

Approximately 2000 species of Pyrrophyta (from the Greek *pyrrhos,* meaning flames, and *phyton,* meaning plant) are known at present. Pyrrophyta have been identified in fossil deposits around the globe, from arctic to tropical seas, as well as in hypersaline waters, freshwater, and river deltas. Pyrrophyta are mostly unicellular microorganic **Protists** divided by botanists in two phyla, **dinoflagellates** and criptomonads.

The taxonomic classification of Pyrrophyta is disputed by some zoologists who consider them members of the **Protozoa** kingdom. Cryptomonads for instance, are considered red-brownish algae of Cryptomonadida Order by botanists, and protozoans of Cryptophycea Class by zoologists. This controversy is due to the unusual characteristics of these two phyla, sharing features with both plants and animals. For instance, most species swim freely because of the spiraling agitation of two flagella, and have multiple cell walls with two valves. Some Pyrrophyta are photosynthetic species, however, whereas others are not. They come in a variety of shapes and sizes and the photosynthetic species have golden-brown or yellowish-green chloroplasts. They can synthesize both types of **chlorophyll**, type a and type c, and contain high levels of carotenoids (yellow pigments). Some Pyrrophyta, such as *Gymnodium* and *Gonyaulax* are dinoflagellates responsible for red tides and secrete neurotoxins that cause massive fish death. If these toxins are airborne in a closed room, or if they get in contact with the skin, they may contaminate humans and cause temporary or more severe neurological disorders. Some species such as the *Ceratium* can deplete water from oxygen, also leading to massive fish death, a phenomenon known as black tide.

Photosynthetic Pyrrophyta are autotrophs, whereas the non-photosynthetic ones may be heterotrophs, existing as **parasites** in fish and aquatic invertebrates as well. Some autothrophic species also feed on other dinoflagellates and unicellular organisms, by engulfing them. Symbiotic species (zooxanthellae) are also known, which live in sponges, jelly-fish, anemones, growing coral reefs, etc, where they supply carbon to their hosts. Cryptomonads themselves are the evolutionary result of endosymbiosis, and are chimeric species that evolved from ancestral red algae and a non-photosynthetic host that retained the red alga **nucleus** under the form of a bead-like nucleomorph chromosome. The highly condensed chromosome of this Pyrrophyta consists of three different bead-like nucleomorphic units.

See also Chromosomes, eukaryotic; Photosynthesis

Q

Q FEVER

Q (or Query) fever is a disease that is caused by the bacterium *Coxiella burnetii*. The bacterium is passed to humans by contact with infected animals such as sheep, cattle, and goats, which are the main reservoirs of the microorganism. The disease, which was first described in Australia in 1935, can have a short-term (acute) stage and, in some people, a much longer, chronic stage.

The bacterium that causes Q fever is a **rickettsia**. Other rickettsia are responsible for Rocky Mountain Spotted Fever and trench fever, as examples. *Coxiella burnetti* and the other rickettsia are Gram-negative organisms, which need to infect host cells in order to grow and divide. Outside of the host the **bacteria** can survive, but do not replicate. Q fever differs from the other rickettsial diseases in that it is caused by the inhalation of the bacteria, not by the bite of a tick.

Groups most at risk to acquire Q fever are those who are around animals. These include veterinarians, sheep, cattle and dairy farmers, and workers in processing plants.

The bacteria are excreted into the environment in the milk, urine, and feces of the animals. Also, bacteria can be present in the amniotic fluid and the placenta in the birthing process. The latter is particularly relevant, as humans tend to be near the animals during birth, and so the chances of transfer of the bacterium from animal to human are great.

In addition, the **microorganisms** are hardy and can endure environmental stress. The chances for human infection are also increased because of the persistence of the bacteria in the environment outside of the animal host. *Coxiella burnetii* are very hardy bacteria, being resistant to antibacterial compounds, and to environmental stresses such as heat and lack of moisture. When present in a dry area, such as in hay or the dust of a barnyard, the organisms can be easily inhaled.

The entry of only a few live bacteria or even one living bacterium is required to cause an infection in humans. The environmental hardiness and low number of microbes required for an infection has made *Coxiella burnetii* a potential agent of **bioterrorism.**

Of those who become infected, only about half display symptoms. When symptoms of Q fever appear, they can include the sudden development of a high fever, severe headache, nausea, vomiting, abdominal pain, and an overall feeling of illness. **Pneumonia** and liver damage can develop in some people. Usually the symptoms pass in several months. However, the establishment of a chronic disease can occur, and is fatal in over 60 per cent of cases. The chronic form may not develop immediately after the transient disease. In fact, cases have been documented where the lapse between the initial disease and the chromic form was several decades. The chronic disease can lead to heart valve damage.

Why some people display symptoms of infection while others do not is still not resolved. Neither are the reasons why the disease is self-limiting within a short time in some people but develops into a lengthy, debilitating, and potentially lethal disease in other people.

Coxiella burnetii has two different forms, which have differing surface chemistries. These are called phase I and phase II. The phase I form is associated more with the chronic Q fever than is phase II.

Diagnosis of Q fever is most reliably obtained by the detection of antibodies to the infecting bacterium. Following diagnosis, treatment consists of antibiotic therapy. The **antibiotics** that have achieved the most success are fluoroquinolone, rifampin, and trimethoprim-sulfamethoxazole. In the chronic form of Q fever, the antibiotics may need to be administered for several years. If the disease has damaged body parts, such as heart valve, then treatment may also involve the replacement of the damaged tissues.

Vaccination against Q fever is not yet a standard option. A **vaccine** is available in Australia and parts of Europe, but has not yet been approved in North America.

Prevention of the transmission of the bacterium to humans involves the wearing of masks when around domestic

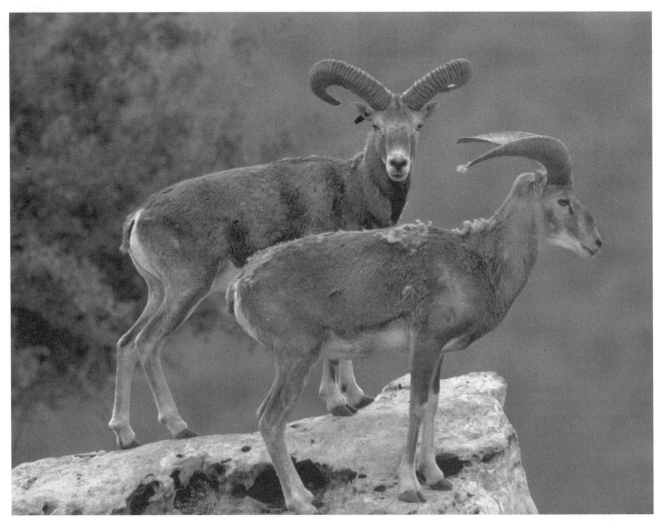

Mountain sheep, one of the natural hosts of the Q-fever bacterium *Coxiella burnetii*.

animals and the prompt disposal of placenta and other tissues resulting from the birth process.

See also Bacteria and bacterial diseases; Zoonoses

QUALITATIVE AND QUANTITATIVE ANALYSIS IN MICROBIOLOGY

Various techniques have been devised to permit the analysis of the structure and function of **microorganisms**. Some techniques are qualitative in their intent. That is, they provide a "yes or no" answer. Other techniques are quantitative in their intent. These techniques provide numerical information about a sample.

Assessing the growth of a bacterial sample provides examples of both types of analysis techniques. An example of a qualitative technique would be the growth of a bacterial sample on a solid growth medium, in order to solely assess whether the **bacteria** in the sample are living or dead. An

example of a quantitative technique is the use of that solid growth media to calculate the actual number of living bacteria in a sample.

Microscopic observation of microorganisms can reveal a wealth of qualitative information. The observation of a suspension of bacteria on a **microscope** slide (the wet mount) reveals whether the bacteria are capable of self-propelled motion. Microorganisms, particularly bacteria, can be applied to a slide as a so-called smear, which is then allowed to dry on the slide. The dried bacteria can be stained to reveal, for example, whether they retain the primary stain in the Gram stain protocol (Gram positive) or whether that stain is washed out of the bacteria and a secondary stain retained (Gram negative). Examination of such smears will also reveal the shape, size, and arrangement (singly, in pairs, in chains, in clusters) of the bacteria. These qualitative attributes are important in categorizing bacteria.

Microscopy can be extended to provide qualitative information. The incorporation of antibodies to specific components of the sample can be used to calculate the proportion

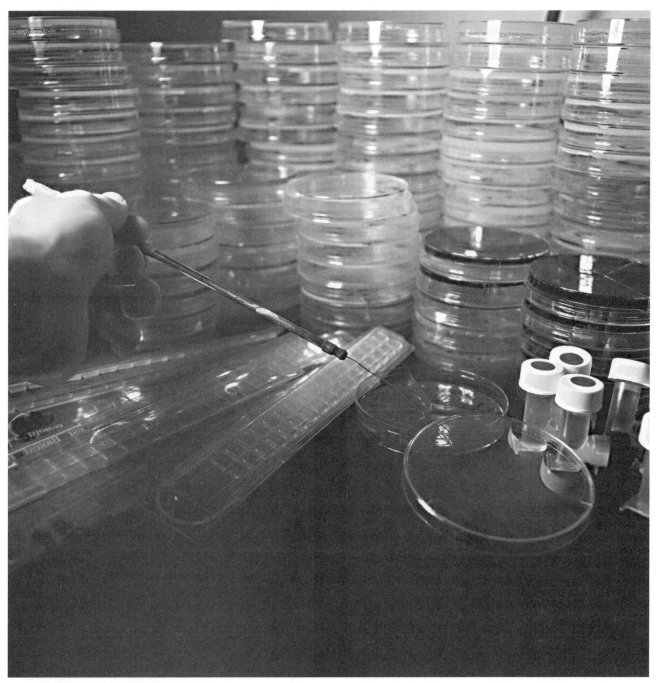

Growth of bacteria on agar is a qualitative result.

of the samples in a population that possess the target of interest. Fluorescent-labeled antibodies, or antibodies combined with a dark appearing molecule such as ferritin, are useful in such studies. The scanning confocal microscope is proving to be tremendously useful in this regard. The optics of the microscope allows visual data to be obtained at various depths through a sample (typically the sample is an adherent population of microorganisms). These optical thin sections can be reconstructed via computer imaging to produce a three-dimensional image of the specimen. The use of fluorescent-tagged antibodies allows the location of protein within the living biofilm to be assessed.

The self-propelled movement of living microorganisms, a behavior that is termed motility, can also provide quantitative information. For example, recording a moving picture image of the moving cells is used to determine their speed of movement, and whether the presence of a compound acts as an attractant or a repellant to the microbes.

Bacterial growth is another area that can yield qualitative or quantitative information. Water analysis for the bacterium *Escherichia coli* provides an example. A specialized growth medium allows the growth of only *Escherichia coli*. Another constituent of the growth medium is utilized by the growing bacteria to produce a by-product that fluoresces when exposed to ultraviolet light. If the medium is dispensed in bottles, the presence of growing *Escherichia coli* can be detected by the development of fluorescence. However, if the medium is dispensed in smaller volumes in a grid-like pattern, then the number of areas of the grid that are positive for growth can be related to a mathematical formula to produce a most probable number of living *Escherichia coli* in the water sample. Viable bacterial counts can be determined for many other bacteria by several other means.

The ability of bacteria to grow or not to grow on a media containing controlled amounts and types of compounds yields quantitative information about the nutritional requirements of the microbes.

The advent of molecular techniques has expanded the repertoire of quantitative information that can be obtained. For example, a technique involving reporter genes can show whether a particular **gene** is active and can indicate the number of copies of the gene product that is manufactured. Gene probes have also been tagged to fluorescent or radioactive labels to provide information as to where in a population a certain metabolic activity is occurring and the course of the activity over time.

Many other qualitative and quantitative techniques exist in microbiological analysis. A few examples include **immunoelectrophoresis**, immunoelectron microscopy, biochemical dissection of metabolic pathways, the molecular construction of cell walls and other components of microorganisms, and mutational analysis. The scope of the techniques is ever-expanding.

See also Laboratory techniques in immunology; Laboratory techniques in microbiology

QUORUM SENSING

Quorum sensing is a term that refers to the coordinated behavior exhibited by a population of **bacteria**. The phenomenon involves a communication between the bacterial members of the population and, via a triggering signal, the carrying out of a particular function.

Examples of quorum sensing are the coordinated feeding behavior and the formation of spores that occur in large populations of myxobacteria and actinomycetes. Quorum sensing also occurs in bacterial biofilms, where signals between bacteria can stimulate and repress the production of the extracellular polysaccharide in different regions of the biofilm, and the exodus of portions of the population from the biofilm, in order to establish a new biofilm elsewhere.

Historically, the first indication of quorum sensing was the discovery of the chemical trigger for luminescence in the bacterium *Photobacterium fischeri* in the 1990s. At high densities of bacteria, luminescence occurs. Light production, however, does not occur at lower numbers or densities of bacteria. The phenomenon was correlated with the production of a compound whose short name is homoserine lactone. The same molecule has since been shown to trigger responses in other quorum sensing systems in other bacteria. Examples of these responses include the production of disease-causing factors by *Pseudomonas aeruginosa* and cell division in *Escherichia coli*.

Quorum sensing enables a bacterial population to respond quickly to changing environmental conditions and, in the case of biofilms, to enable regions within the mature biofilm to perform the different functions necessary to sustain the entire community.

In *Photobacterium fischeri* the relatively **hydrophobic** ("water-hating") nature of the homoserine lactone molecule drives its diffusion into the cell wall surrounding a bacterium. Once inside the bacterium, the molecule interacts with a protein known as LuxR. The LuxR then induces the **transcription** of a region the genetic material that contains the genes that code for the luminescent proteins.

The molecular nature of the means by which quorum sensing triggers such homoserine lactone evoke a bacterial response in other bacteria is still unclear. Furthermore, the discovery of several quorum sensing systems in bacteria such as *Pseudomonas aeruginosa* indicate that multiple sensing pathways are operative, at different times or even simultaneously. For example, within a biofilm, bacteria may be actively manufacturing exopolysaccharide, repressed in the polymer's construction, growing slowly, or resuming the active growth that is the hallmark of free-floating bacteria. Resolving the molecular nature of the spectrum of quorum sensing activities could lead to strategies to disrupt the inter-cellular communication in disease processes.

See also Biofilm formation and dynamic behavior

R

RABIES

Rabies is a viral brain disease that is almost always fatal if it is not prevented with prompt treatment. The disease, which typically spreads to humans from animals through a scratch or a bite, causes **inflammation** of the brain. The disease is also called hydrophobia (meaning fear of water) because it causes painful muscle spasms in the throat that prevent swallowing. In fact, this is what leads to most fatalities in untreated cases: victims become dehydrated and die. Carriers of rabies include dogs, cats, bats, skunks, raccoons, and foxes; rodents are not likely to be infected. About 70% of rabies cases develop from wild animal bites that break the skin. Though a **vaccine** used first in 1885 is widely used, fatalities still occur due to rabies. Most fatalities take place in Africa and Asia, but some also occur in the United States. The cost of efforts to prevent rabies in the United States may be as high as $1 billion per year.

While many animal diseases cannot be passed from animal to man, rabies has long been known as an easy traveler from one species to the next. The disease was known among ancient people. The very name rabies, Latin for rage or madness, suggests the fear with which early men and women must have viewed the disease. For centuries there was no treatment, and the disease was left to run its rapid course leading to death.

Rabies is described in medical writings dating from 300 B.C., but the method of transmission or contagion was not recognized until 1804. In 1884, the French bacteriologist **Louis Pasteur** developed a preventive vaccine against rabies, and modifications of Pasteur's methods are still used in rabies therapy today. The Pasteur program, or variations of it, has greatly reduced the fatalities in humans from rabies. Modern treatment, following a bite by a rabid or presumed rabid animal, consists of immediate and thorough cleansing of the bite wound and injection into the wound and elsewhere of hyperimmune antirabies serum. Post exposure treatment consists of five injections of vaccine given over a one-month period, along with one dose of rabies immune globulin injected near the wound and intramuscularly.

The standard vaccine contains inactivated rabies virus grown in duck eggs. It is highly effective but causes neuroparalysis in about one in 30,000 persons receiving it. In the 1970s, a new vaccine was developed in France and the United States that contains virus prepared from human cells grown in the laboratory. This vaccine is safer and requires a shorter course of injections. With the widespread use of vaccine, rabies cases in the U.S. declined to fewer than five per year.

The transmission of rabies is almost invariably through the bite of an infected animal. The fact that the virus is eliminated in the saliva is of great significance, and unless saliva is introduced beneath the skin, the disease is seldom transmitted. The virus has been demonstrated in the saliva of dogs 3–8 days before the onset of symptoms. However, it has also been reported that only about 50–60% of the infected dogs shed the virus in the saliva. Rare cases of rabies have been reported where only clawing and scratching occurred, or where the skin was contaminated with saliva. The virus is most concentrated in the central nervous system and saliva, but it has also been demonstrated in various organs of the body and milk from infected animals.

In humans, the rabies virus, in addition to entering the body by the usual route through skin broken by a bite or scratch, can enter the body through intact mucous membranes, can be inhaled as an aerosol, and can be transplanted in an infected corneal graft. These four cases are the only virologically documented examples of transmission of rabies from one person to another. Vertical transmission from mother to fetus and from lactating mother to suckling young has been described in nonhuman mammals.

The incubation period in natural cases of rabies is variable. In general, the quantity of virus introduced into the wound is correlated with the length of incubation before symptoms occur. In dogs, the minimum period is ten days, the average 21–60 days, but may be as long as six months. In man, the incubation period is one to three months, with the minimum of ten days.

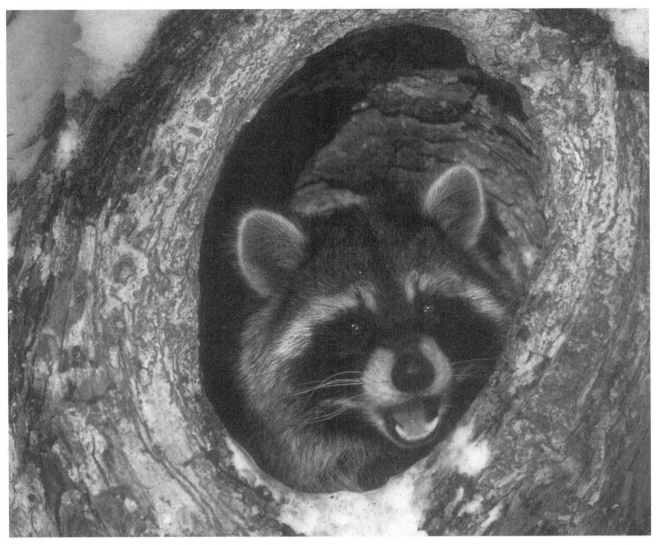

The raccoon is a common transmitter of the rabies virus to humans.

Rabies is caused by a number of different **viruses** that vary depending on geographic area and species. While the viruses are different, the disease they cause is singular in its course. The bullet-shaped virus is spread when it breaks through skin or has contact with a mucous membrane. The virus begins to reproduce itself initially in muscle cells near the place of first contact. At this point, within the first five days or so, treatment by **vaccination** has a high rate of success.

Once the rabies virus passes to the nervous system, **immunization** is no longer effective. The virus passes to the central nervous system, where it replicates itself in the system and moves to other tissues such as the heart, the lung, the liver, and the salivary glands. Symptoms appear when the virus reaches the spinal cord.

A bite from a rabid animal does not guarantee that one will get rabies; only about 50% of people who are bitten and do not receive treatment ever develop the disease. If one is bitten by or has had any exposure to an animal that may have rabies,

medical intervention should be sought immediately. Treatment virtually ensures that one will not come down with the disease. Any delay could diminish the treatment's effectiveness.

In humans and in animals, rabies may be manifest in one of two forms: the furious (agitated) type or the paralytic (dumb) type. Furious rabies in animals, especially in the dog, is characterized by altered behavior such as restlessness, hiding, depraved appetite, excitement, unprovoked biting, aimless wandering, excessive salivation, altered voice, pharyngeal paralysis, staggering, general paralysis, and finally death. Death usually occurs within three to four days after the onset of symptoms. The paralytic form of rabies is frequently observed in animals inoculated with fixed virus, and is occasionally observed in other animals with street virus contracted under natural conditions. Animals showing this type usually show a short period of excitement followed by uncoordination, ataxia, paralysis, dehydration, loss of weight, followed by death.

In humans, furious rabies patients typically show bizarre behavior, ranging from episodes of severe agitation to periods of depression. Confusion becomes extreme as the disease progresses, and the patient may become aggressive. Hydrophobia is always seen with this type of disease, until the patient becomes comatose while showing intermittently uncontrollable inspiratory spasms. This type of rabies is also characterized by hypersalivation, from 1–1.6 qt (1–1.5 L) of saliva in 24 hours, and excessive sweating.

The paralytic form of rabies in humans is often indistinguishable from that of most viral encephalitis, except for the fact that a patient suffering from rabies remains conscious during the course of the disease. Paralysis usually begins at the extremity exposed to the bite and gradually involves other extremities finally affecting the pharyngeal and respiratory muscles.

The dog is a most important animal as a disseminator of rabies virus, not only to man but also to other animals. Wild carnivora may be infected and transmit the disease. In the United States, foxes, raccoons and skunks are the most commonly involved. These animals are sometimes responsible for infecting domestic farm animals.

The disease in wildlife (especially skunks, foxes, raccoons, and bats) has become more prevalent in recent years, accounting for approximately 85% of all reported cases of animal rabies every year since 1976. Wildlife now constitutes the most important potential source of infection for both human and domestic animals in the United States. Rabies among animals is present throughout the United States with the exception of Hawaii, which has remained consistently rabies-free. The likelihood of different animals contracting rabies varies from one place to the next. Dogs are a good example. In areas where **public health** efforts to control rabies have been aggressive, dogs make up less than 5% of rabies cases in animals. These areas include the United States, most European countries, and Canada.

However, dogs are the most common source of rabies in many countries. They make up at least 90% of reported cases of rabies in most developing countries of Africa and Asia and many parts of Latin America. In these countries, public health efforts to control rabies have not been as aggressive. Other key carriers of rabies include the fox in Europe and Canada, the jackal in Africa, and the vampire bat in Latin America.

In the United States, 60% of all rabies cases were reported in raccoons. The high number of cases in raccoons reflects an animal epidemic, or, more properly, an epizootic. The epizootic began when diseased raccoons were carried from further south to Virginia and West Virginia. Since then, rabies in raccoons has spread up the eastern seaboard of the United States. Concentrations of animals with rabies include coyotes in southern Texas, skunks in California and in south and north central states, and gray foxes in southeastern Arizona. Bats throughout the United States also develop rabies. When rabies first enters a species, large numbers of animals die. When it has been around for a long time, the species adapts, and smaller numbers of animals die.

There are few deaths from rabies in the United States. Between 1980 and the middle of 1994, a total of 19 people in the United States died of rabies, far fewer than the 200 Americans killed by lightning, for example. Eight of these cases were acquired outside the United States. Eight of the 11 cases contracted in the United States stemmed from bat-transmitted strains of rabies.

Internationally, more than 33,000 people die annually from rabies, according to the World Health Association. A great majority of cases internationally stem from dog bites. Different countries employ different strategies in the fight against rabies. The United States depends primarily on vaccination of domestic animals and on immunization following exposure to possibly rabid animals. Great Britain, in which rabies has never been established, employs a strict quarantine for all domestic animals entering the country.

Continental Europe, which has a long history of rabies, developed an aggressive program in the 1990s of airdropping a new vaccine for wild animals. The vaccine is mixed with pellets of food for red foxes, the primary carrier there. Public health officials have announced that fox rabies may be eliminated from Western Europe by the end of the decade. The **World Health Organization** is also planning to use the vaccine in parts of Africa.

Though the United States have been largely successful in controlling rabies in humans, the disease remains present in the animal population, a constant reminder of the serious threat rabies could become without successful prevention efforts.

See also Viruses and responses to viral infection

RADIATION MUTAGENESIS

Mutations are caused by **DNA** damage and genetic alterations that may occur spontaneously at a very low rate. The frequency of these mutations can be increased by using special agents called mutagens. Ionizing radiation was the first mutagen that efficiently and reproducibly induced mutations in a multicellular organism. Direct damage to the cell **nucleus** is believed to be responsible for both mutations and other radiation mediated genotoxic effects like chromosomal aberrations and lethality. Free radicals generated by irradiation of the **cytoplasm** are also believed to induce **gene** mutations even in the non-irradiated nucleus.

There are many kinds of radiations that can increase mutations. Radiation is often classified as ionizing or non-ionizing depending on whether ions are emitted in the penetrated tissues or not. X rays, gamma rays (γ), beta particle radiation (β), and alpha particle (α) radiation (also known as alpha rays) are ionizing form of radiation. On the other hand, UV radiation, like that in sunlight, is non-ionizing. Biologically, the differences between types of radiation effects fundamentally involve the way energy is distributed in irradiated cell populations and tissues. With alpha radiation, ionizations lead to an intense but more superficial and localized deposition of energy. Primary ionization in x rays or gamma radiation traverses deeper into tissues. This penetration leads to a more even distribution of energy as opposed to the more concentrated or localized alpha rays.

This principle has been used experimentally to deliver radiation to specific cellular components. A cumulative effect of radiation has been observed in animal models. This means that if a population is repeatedly exposed to radiation, a higher frequency of mutations is observed that is due to additive effect. Intensive efforts to determine the mutagenic risk of low dose exposure to ionizing radiation have been an ongoing concern because of the use of nuclear energy and especially because of the exposure to radon gas in some indoor environments. Radon is estimated by the United States Environmental Protection Agency to be the cause of more than 20,000 cases of lung cancer annually.

The relative efficiencies of the different types of radiations in producing mutations is assessed as the mutagenic effect. The mutagenic effect of radiation is generally assumed to be due to direct damage to DNA, but the identity of the specific lesions remains uncertain.

Investigation of radiation's mutagenic effects on different tissues, cells, and subcellular compartments is becoming possible by the availability of techniques and tools that allow the precise delivery of small doses of radiation and that provide better monitoring of effects. Reactive oxygen species released in irradiated cells are believed to act directly on nuclear DNA and indirectly by modifying bases that will be incorporated in DNA, or deactivating DNA repair **enzymes**. Novel microbeam alpha irradiation techniques have allowed researchers to investigate radiation-induced mutations in non-irradiated DNA. There is evidence that radiation induces changes in the cytosol that—in eukaryotes—are transmitted to the nucleus and even to neighboring cells. Direct measurement of DNA damage caused by ionizing radiation is performed by examining micronucleus formation or analysis of DNA fragments on agarose gels following treatment with specific endonucleases such as those that only cleave at certain sites. The **polymerase chain reaction (PCR)** is also used to detect the loss of some marker genes by large deletions. The effect of ionizing radiation on cells can also be measured by evaluating the expression level of the stress inducible p21 protein.

Critical lesions leading to mutations or killing of a cell include induction of DNA strand breaks, damaged bases, and production of abasic sites (where a single base is deleted), and—in multichromosomal organisms—large chromosomal deletions. Except for large deletions, most of these lesions can be repaired to a certain extent, and the lethal and mutagenic effect of radiation is assumed to result principally from incompletely or incorrectly repaired DNA. This view is supported by experimental studies which showed that mice given a single radiation dose, called acute dose, develop a significantly higher level of mutations than mice given the same dose of radiation over a period of weeks or months. The rapid activation of the DNA-repair pathway through p53 protein and the stress-inducible p21 protein as well as the extreme sensitivity of cells with genetic defects in DNA repair machinery support the view that the ability of the cell to repair irradiation-induced DNA damage is a limiting factor in deciding the extent of the mutagenic effects.

See also Evolution and evolutionary mechanisms; Evolutionary origin of bacteria and viruses; Immunogenetics; Molecular biology and molecular genetics; Phage genetics; Radiation resistant bacteria; Radioisotopes and their uses; Viral genetics

RADIATION-RESISTANT BACTERIA

Radiation-resistant **bacteria** encompass eight species of bacteria in a genus known as *Deinococcus*. The prototype species is *Deinococcus radiodurans*. This and the other species are capable of not only survival but of growth in the presence of radiation that is lethal to all other known forms of life.

Radiation is measured in units called rads. An instantaneous dose of 500 to 1000 rads of gamma radiation is lethal to a human. However, *Deinococcus radiodurans* is unaffected by exposure to up to 3 million rads of gamma radiation. Indeed, the bacterium, whose name translates to "strange berry that withstands radiation," holds a place in The Guinness Book of World Records as "the world's toughest bacterium."

The bacterium was first isolated in the 1950s from tins of meat that had spoiled in spite of being irradiated with a dose that was thought to be sterilizing. The classification of the bacterium as *Deinococcus radiodurans*, and the isolation, characterization, and designation of the other species has been almost exclusively due to **Robert Murray** and his colleagues at the University of Western Ontario. The various species of *Deinococcus* have been isolated from a variety of locations as disperse as elephant feces, fish, fowl, and Antarctic rocks.

The reason for the development of such radiation resistance is still speculative. But, the current consensus is that it enabled the ancient form of the bacterium to survive in regions where available water was scarce. Other organisms developed different survival strategies, one example being the ability to form the metabolically dormant spore.

Deinococcus is an ancient bacteria, believed to be some two billion years old. They may have evolved at a time when Earth was bathed in more energetic forms of radiation than now, due to a different and less screening atmosphere. One theory even suggests that the bacteria originated on another world and were brought to Earth via a meteorite.

The extraterrestrial theory is likely fanciful, however, because the bacteria are not heat resistant. Exposure to temperatures as low as 113ºF (45ºC) can be lethal to the microorganism.

There are two known reasons for the radiation resistance of species of *Deinococcus*. Firstly, the structure of the two membranes that surround the Gram-negative bacterium contributes, albeit in a minor way. By far the major reason for the radiation resistance is the bacterium's ability to rapidly and correctly repair the extensive damage caused to its genetic material by radiation.

The high energy of radioactive waves literally cut apart the double stranded molecule of **deoxyribonucleic acid (DNA)**. These cuts occur in many places, effectively shattering the genome into many, very small fragments. *Deinococcus* is able to quickly reassemble the fragments in their correct order and then slice them back together. In contrast, bacteria such as

Escherichia coli can only tolerate one or several cuts to the DNA before the radiation damage is either lethal or causes the formation of drastic **mutations**.

The molecular nature of this repair ability is not yet clear. However, the completion of the sequencing of the genome of *Deinococcus radiodurans* in late 1999 should provide the raw material to pursue this question. The genome is unique among bacteria, being comprised of four to ten pieces of DNA and a large piece of extrachromosomal DNA that is part of a structure called a plasmid. The genome of other bacteria typically consists of a single circle of DNA (although plasmid DNA can also be present). Within the chromosome-like regions of *Deinococcus* there are many repeated stretches of DNA. In an analogy to a computer, the bacterium has designed many backup copies of its information. If some back up copies are impaired, the information can be recovered from the other DNA.

This DNA repair ability has made the genus the subject of intense scrutiny by molecular biologists interested in the process of DNA manufacture and repair. Furthermore, the radiation resistance of *Deinococcus* has made the bacteria an attractive microorganism for the remediation of radioactive waste. While this use is not currently feasible at the scale that would be required to clean up nuclear contamination, small-scale tests have proved encouraging. The bacteria still need to be engineered to cope with the myriad of organic contaminants and heavy metals that are also typically part of nuclear waste sites.

See also Bioremediation; Extremophiles

RADIOISOTOPES AND THEIR USES IN MICROBIOLOGY AND IMMUNOLOGY

Radioisotopes, containing unstable combinations of protons and neutrons, are created by neutron activation that involves the capture of a neutron by the **nucleus** of an atom. Such a capture results in an excess of neutrons (neutron rich). Proton rich radioisotopes are manufactured in cyclotrons. During radioactive decay, the nucleus of a radioisotope seeks energetic stability by emitting particles (alpha, beta or positron) and photons (including gamma rays).

The history of radioisotopes in microbiology and **immunology** dates back to their first use in medicine. Although nuclear medicine traces its clinical origins to the 1930s, the invention of the gamma scintillation camera by American engineer Hal Anger in the 1950s brought major advances in nuclear medical imaging and rapidly elevated the use of radioisotopes in medicine. For example, cancer and other rapidly dividing cells are usually sensitive to damage by radiation. Accordingly, some cancerous growths can be restricted or eliminated by radioisotope irradiation. The most common forms of external radiation therapy use gamma and x rays. During the last half of the 20th century the radioisotope cobalt-60 was a frequently used source of radiation used in such treatments. Iodine-131 and phosphorus-32 are also commonly used in radiotherapy. More radical uses of radioisotopes include the use of Boron-10 to specifically attack tumor cells. Boron-10 concentrates in tumor cells and is then subjected to neutron beams that result in highly energetic alpha particles that are lethal to the tumor tissue. More modern methods of irradiation include the production of x rays from linear accelerators.

Because they can be detected in low doses, radioisotopes can also be used in sophisticated and delicate biochemical assays or analysis. There are many common laboratory tests utilizing radioisotopes to analyze blood, urine and hormones. Radioisotopes are also finding increasing use in the labeling, identification and study of immunological cells.

The study of **microorganisms** also relies heavily on the use of radioisotopes. The identification of protein species, labeling of surface components of **bacteria**, and tracing the **transcription** and **translation** steps involved in nucleic acid and protein manufacture all utilize radioisotopes.

A radioisotope can emit three different types of radiation. The first of these is known as alpha radiation. This radiation is due to alpha particles, which have a positive charge. An example is the decay of an atom of a substance called Americium to an atom of Neptunium. The decay is possible because of the release of an alpha particle.

The second type of radiation is called beta radiation. This radiation results from the release of a beta particle. A beta particle has a negative charge. An example is the decay of a carbon atom to a nitrogen atom, with the release of a beta particle.

The final type of radiation is known as gamma radiation. This type of radiation is highly energetic.

The various types of radiations can be selected to provide information on a sample of interest. For example, to examine how quickly a protein is degraded, an isotope that decays very quickly is preferred. However, to study the adherence of bacteria to a surface, a radiolabel that persisted longer would be more advantageous.

Furthermore, various radioactive compounds are used in microbiological analyses to label different constituents of the bacterial cell. Radioactive hydrogen (i.e., tritium) can be used to produce radioactive **deoxyribonucleic acid**. The radioactive **DNA** can be detected by storing the DNA sample in contact with X-ray film. The radioactive particles that are emitted from the sample will expose the film. When the film is developed, the result is an image of the DNA. This process, which is known as autoradiography, has long been used to trace the elongation of DNA, and so determine the speed at which the DNA is replicating.

DNA can also be labeled, but in a different location within the molecule, by the use of radioactive phosphorus.

Bacterial and viral proteins can be labeled by the addition of radioactive methionine to the growth mixture. The methionine, which is an amino acid, will be incorporated into proteins that are made. Several paths can then be followed. For instance, in what is known as a pulse-chase experiment, the radioactive label is then followed by the addition of nonradioactive (or "cold") methionine. The rate at which the radioactivity disappears can be used to calculate the rate of turnover of the particular protein. In another experimental approach, the protein constituents of bacteria or **viruses** can be separated on an electrophoretic gel. The gel is then brought into contact with X-ray film. Wherever a radioactive protein band is present in the gel, the overlaying film will be exposed. Thus, the proteins that are radioactive can be determined.

The use of radiolabeled compounds that can be utilized as nutrients by bacteria allows various metabolic pathways to be determined. For example, glucose can be radiolabeled and its fate followed by various techniques, including chromatography, autoradiography, and gel **electrophoresis**. Furthermore, a molecule such as glucose can be radiolabeled at various chemical groups within the molecule. This allows an investigator to assess whether different regions of a molecule are used preferentially.

Radiolabeling has allowed for great advances in microbiological research. A well-known example is the 1952 experiment by Hershey and Chase, which established that DNA was the reservoir of genetic information. Bacterial viruses were exposed to either radioactive sulfur or phosphorus. The sulfur radiolabeled the surface of the virus, while the phosphorus labeled the DNA. Viruses were allowed to infect bacteria and then were mechanically sheared off of the bacteria. The sheared viruses were then collected separately from the bacteria. Radioactive sulfur was found in the virus suspension and radioactive phosphorus was found in the bacteria. Furthermore, the bacteria eventually produced new virus, some of which had radioactive DNA. Thus, radiolabeling demonstrated the relationship between DNA and genetic information.

See also Laboratory methods in microbiology

RARE GENOTYPE ADVANTAGE

Rare **genotype** advantage is the evolutionary theory that genotypes (e.g., the genes of a bacterium or parasite) that have been rare in the recent past should have particular advantages over common genotypes under certain conditions.

Rare genotype advantage can be best illustrated by a host-parasite interaction. Successful **parasites** are those carrying genotypes that allow them to infect the most common host genotype in a population. Thus, hosts with rare genotypes, those that do not allow for infection by the pathogen, have an advantage because they are less likely to become infected by the common-host pathogen genotypes. This advantage is transient, as the numbers of this genotype will increase along with the numbers of pathogens that infect this formerly rare host. The pattern then repeats. This idea is tightly linked to the so-called Red Queen Hypothesis first suggested in 1982 by evolutionary biologist Graham Bell (1949–) (so named after the Red Queen's famous remark to Alice in Lewis Carroll's *Through the Looking Glass:* "Now here, you see, you have to run as fast as you can to stay in the same place."). In other words, genetic variation represents an opportunity for hosts to produce offspring to which pathogens are not adapted. Then, sex, mutation, and genetic **recombination** provide a moving

target for the **evolution** of virulence by pathogens. Thus, hosts continually change to stay one step ahead of their pathogens, likened to the Red Queen's quote.

This reasoning also works in favor of pathogens. An example can be derived from the use of **antibiotics** on bacterial populations. Bacterial genomes harbor genes conferring resistance to particular antibiotics. Bacterial populations tend to maintain a high level of variation of these genes, even when they seem to offer no particular advantage. The variation becomes critical, however, when the **bacteria** are first exposed to an antibiotic. Under those conditions, the high amount of variation increases the likelihood that there will be one rare genotype that will confer resistance to the new antibiotic. That genotype then offers a great advantage to those individuals. As a result, the bacteria with the rare genotype will survive and reproduce, and their genotype will become more common in future generations. Thus, the rare genotype had an advantage over the most common bacterial genotype, which was susceptible to the drug.

See also Antibiotic resistance, tests for; Evolution and evolutionary mechanisms; Evolutionary origin of bacteria and viruses

RECOMBINANT DNA MOLECULES

Recombinant **deoxyribonucleic acid** (**DNA**) is genetic material from different organisms that has been chemically bonded together to form a single macromolecule. The **recombination** can involve the DNA from two eukaryotic organisms, two prokaryotic organisms, or between an eukaryote and a prokaryote. An example of the latter is the production of human insulin by the bacterium *Escherichia coli,* which has been achieved by splicing the **gene** for insulin into the *E. coli* genome such that the insulin gene is expressed and the protein product formed.

The splicing of DNA from one genome to another is done using two classes of **enzymes**. Isolation of the target DNA sequence is done using **restriction enzymes**. There are well over a hundred restriction enzymes, each cutting in a very precise way a specific base of the DNA molecule. Used singly or in combination, the enzymes allow target segments of DNA to be isolated. Insertion of the isolated DNA into the recipient genome is done using an enzyme called DNA ligase.

Typically, the recombinant DNA forms part of the DNA making up a plasmid. The mobility of the plasmid facilitates the easy transfer of the recombinant DNA from the host organism to the recipient organism.

Paul Berg of Stanford University first achieved the manufacture of recombinant DNA in 1972. Berg isolated a gene from a human cancer-causing monkey virus, and then ligated the **oncogene** into the genome of the bacterial virus lambda. For this and subsequent recombinant DNA studies (which followed a voluntary one-year moratorium from his research while safety issues were addressed) he was awarded the 1980 Nobel Prize in chemistry.

In 1973, Stanley Cohen and Herbert Boyer created the first recombinant DNA organism, by adding recombinant **plasmids** to *E. coli*. Since that time, advances in **molecular biology** techniques, in particular the development of the **polymerase chain reaction**, have made the construction of recombinant DNA swifter and easier.

Recombinant DNA has been of fundamental importance in furthering the understanding of genetic regulatory processes and shows great potential in the genetic design of therapeutic strategies.

See also Chromosomes, eukaryotic; Chromosomes, prokaryotic; DNA (Deoxyribonucleic acid); Genetic regulation of eukaryotic cells; Genetic regulation of prokaryotic cells; Laboratory techniques in immunology; Laboratory techniques in microbiology; PCR; Plasmid and plastid

RECOMBINATION

Recombination, is a process during which genetic material is shuffled during reproduction to form new combinations. This mixing is important from an evolutionary standpoint because it allows the expression of different traits between generations. The process involves a physical exchange of nucleotides between duplicate strands of **deoxyribonucleic acid (DNA)**.

There are three types of recombination; homologous recombination, specific recombination and **transposition**. Each type occurs under different circumstances. Homologous recombination occurs in **eukaryotes**, typically during the first phase of the meiotic cell division cycle. In most eukaryotic cells, genetic material is organized as **chromosomes** in the **nucleus**. A nick is made on the chromosomal DNA of corresponding strands and the broken strands cross over, or exchange, with each other. The recombinant region is extended until a whole **gene** is transferred. At this point, further recombination can occur or be stopped. Both processes require the creation of another break in the DNA strand and subsequent sealing of the nicks by special **enzymes**.

Site specific recombination typically occurs in prokaryotes. It is the mechanism by which viral genetic material is incorporated into bacterial chromosomes. The event is site-specific, as the incorporation (integration) of viral genetic material occurs at a specific location on the bacterial genome, called the attachment site, which is homologous with the phage genome. Under appropriate conditions alignment and merging of the viral and bacterial genomes occurs.

Transposition is a third type of recombination. It involves transposable elements called **transposons**. These are short segments of DNA found in both prokaryotes and eukaryotes, which contain the information enabling their movement from one genome to another, as well as genes encoding other functions. The movement of a transposon, a process of transposition, is initiated when an enzyme cuts DNA at a target site. This leaves a section that has unpaired nucleotides. Another enzyme called transposase facilitates insertion of the transposon at this site. Transposition is important in genetic engineer-

ing, as other genes can be relocated along with the transposon DNA. As well, transposition is of natural significance. For example, the rapid reshuffling of genetic information possible with transposition enables immunocytes to manufacture the millions of different antibodies required to protect eukaryotes from infection.

See also Cell cycle (eukaryotic), genetic regulation of; Cell cycle (prokaryotic), genetic regulation of; Microbial genetics

RED TIDE

Red tides are a marine phenomenon in which water is stained a red, brown, or yellowish color because of the temporary abundance of a particular species of pigmented **dinoflagellates** (these events are known as "blooms"). Also called phytoplankton, or planktonic algae, these single-celled organisms of the class Dinophyceae move using a tail-like structure called a flagellum. They also photosynthesize, and it is their photosynthetic pigments that can tint the water during blooms. Dinoflagellates are common and widespread. Under appropriate environmental conditions, various species can grow very rapidly, causing red tides. Red tides occur in all marine regions with a temperate or warmer climate.

The environmental conditions that cause red tides to develop are not yet understood. However, they are likely related to some combination of nutrient availability, nutrient ratios, and water temperature. Red tides are ancient phenomena. Scientists suspect that human activities that affect nutrient concentrations in seawater may be having an important influence on the increasingly more frequent occurrences of red tides in some areas. In particular, the levels of nitrogen, phosphorous, and other nutrients in coastal waters are increasing due to runoff from fertilizers and animal waste. Complex global changes in climate also may be affecting red tides. Water used as ballast in ocean-going ships may be introducing dinoflagellates to new waters.

Sometimes the dinoflagellates involved with red tides synthesize toxic chemicals. Genera that are commonly associated with poisonous red tides are *Alexandrium, Dinophysis,* and *Ptychodiscus*. The algal poisons can accumulate in marine organisms that feed by filtering large volumes of water, for example, shellfish such as clams, oysters, and mussels. If these shellfish are collected while they are significantly contaminated by red-tide toxins, they can poison the human beings who eat them. Marine toxins can also affect local ecosystems by poisoning animals. Some toxins, such as that from *Ptychodiscus brevis,* the organism that causes Florida red tides, are airborne and can cause throat and nose irritations.

Red tides can cause ecological damage when the algal bloom collapses. Under some conditions, so much oxygen is consumed to support the decomposition of dead algal biomass that anoxic (lack of oxygen) conditions develop. This can cause severe stress or mortality in a wide range of organisms that are intolerant of low-oxygen conditions. Some red-tide

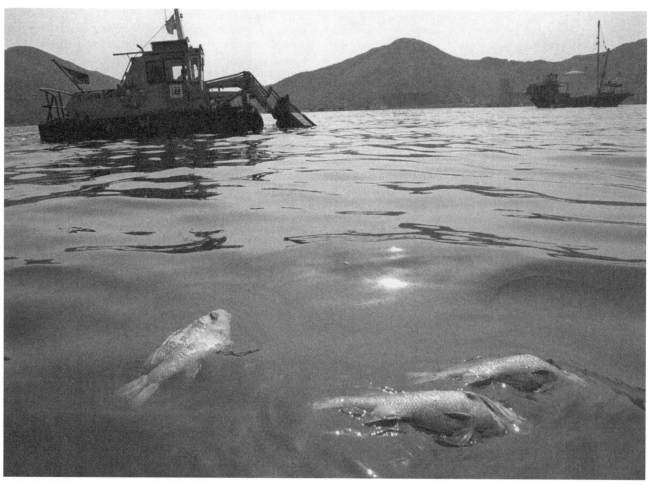

Red tide caused by the growth of algae in the sea.

algae can also clog or irritate the gills of fish and can cause stress or mortality by this physical effect.

Saxitoxin is a natural but potent neurotoxin that is synthesized by certain species of marine dinoflagellates. Saxitoxin causes paralytic shellfish poisoning, a toxic syndrome that affects humans who consume contaminated shellfish. Other biochemicals synthesized by dinoflagellates are responsible for diarrhetic shellfish poisoning, another toxic syndrome. Some red tide dinoflagellates produce reactive forms of oxygen—superoxide, hydrogen peroxide, and hydroxyl radical—which may be responsible for toxic effects. A few other types of marine algae also produce toxic chemicals. **Diatoms** in the genus *Nitzchia* synthesize domoic acid, a chemical responsible for amnesic shellfish poisoning in humans.

Marine animals can also be poisoned by toxic chemicals synthesized during blooms. For example, in 1991, a bloom in Monterey Bay, California, of the diatom *Nitzchia occidentalis* resulted in the accumulation of domoic acid in filter-feeding **zooplankton**. These small animals were eaten by small fish, which also accumulated the toxic chemical and then poisoned fish-eating cormorants and pelicans that died in large num-

bers. In addition, some humans who ate shellfish contaminated by domoic acid were made ill.

In another case, a 1988 bloom of the planktonic alga *Chrysochromulina polylepis* in the Baltic Sea caused extensive mortalities of various species of seaweeds, invertebrates, and fish. A bloom in 1991 of a closely related species of alga in Norwegian waters killed large numbers of salmon that were kept in aquaculture cages. In 1996, a red tide killed 149 endangered manatees in the coastal waters of Florida.

Even large whales can be poisoned by algal toxins. In 1985, 14 humpback whales died in Cape Cod Bay, Massachusetts, during a five-week period. This unusual mortality was caused by the whales eating mackerel that were contaminated by saxitoxin synthesized during a dinoflagellate bloom. In one observed death, a whale was seen to be behaving in an apparently normal fashion, but only 90 minutes later, it had died. The symptoms of the whale deaths were typical of the mammalian neurotoxicity that is associated with saxitoxin, and fish collected in the area had large concentrations of this poisonous chemical in their bodies.

See also Photosynthetic microorganisms; Plankton and planktonic bacteria

REPLICA PLATING • *see* LABORATORY TECHNIQUES IN
MICROBIOLOGY

REPRODUCTIVE IMMUNOLOGY

Pregnant women experience many physiological changes before implantation of the early embryo (blastocyst) takes place. Ovulation, copulation, and fertilization directly or indirectly induce dramatic changes in uterine physiology that resemble classical **inflammation** at the mucosal surfaces of the female reproductive tract, and it is quite likely that these changes impact the maternal **immune system** well before the blastocyst implants in the uterus. Consequently, the outcome of the immune response differs during pregnancy, when compared to outcomes in nonpregnant women. Thus, the uterus may be preconditioned to accept the blastocyst.

Blastocyst implantation is a crucial point in the process of reproduction because it is the moment of highest spontaneous embryo loss for humans. It is characterized by the invasion of trophoblastic cells in the maternal decidua, a mucosal tissue derived from the endometrium. Antigenically, the fetus and placenta have half of the **histocompatibility** genes because of the paternal origin of the conceptus. The reasons why the fetus and placenta are accepted by the maternal immune system are still largely unknown. It is, however, a harmonic equilibrium among maternal cells of the immune system. Originally, British immunologist Peter Medawar proposed three broad hypotheses to explain the paradox of maternal immunological tolerance to the fetus: (a) physical separation of mother and fetus; (b) antigenic immaturity of the fetus; and (c) immunologic inertness of the mother. At the present time, several factors have been included in the mechanisms of fetal protection: (1) general aspecific immunosuppression due to hormonal and proteic patterns of pregnancy, (2) reduced fetal immunogenicity by alteration of expression of fetal **MHC** antigens by placental trophoblast cells, (3) IgG production toward paternal lymphocyte antigens and toward maternal lymphocytes (blocking antibodies), also called trophoblast-lymphocyte cross-reactive antigens (TLX) for their cross reactivity with antigens of the trophoblast. These blocking antibodies could bind and protect fetal antigens from maternal lymphocytes, and (4) modification of the cellular mediated response driven by **cytokines**. Cytokines are produced in the feto-placental unit and have a positive activity on the development of pregnancy.

Spontaneous human fetal loss is a significant clinical problem. Studies on recurrent spontaneous abortion syndromes are dominated by suggestions of immunologic causation. This evidence includes genetic (epidemiological) analyses, anatomical, physiological, and evidence for cytokine dysregulation linked to inappropriate activation of the innate and adaptive immune systems during human pregnancy. However, it is difficult to discriminate whether abnormalities of pregnancies are causes or effects of immune dysfunction.

Autoimmunity is defined as the pathologic condition where humoral or cellular immune response is also directed against self-antigens, leading to severe and debilitating clinical conditions. Systemic autoimmune conditions such as systemic lupus erythematosus (SLE) are associated with higher risk for pregnancy loss. In the general population, about 15% of clinical pregnancies are spontaneously aborted, and about 50% of fertilized eggs fail implantation as a blastocyst. The higher rate of fetal loss in women with SLE occurs in association with antiphospholipid antibodies (aPL), which are also associated with miscarriage in otherwise healthy women. Clinical relevance is also given to lupus anticoagulant (LAC), anticardiolipin antibodies (aCL), and antinuclear antibodies (ANA). These are associated with several medical conditions the description of which is beyond the aim of this article.

Association of LAC with recurrent miscarriage has been described in the past twenty years. The lupus anticoagulant test (LAC) is a clotting time test used to detect women's antibodies against components of the blood clotting system, such as negatively charged **phospholipids** or prothrombin. These antibodies cause a prolongation in the clotting time.The aCL test measures 3 different species of antibodies to the phospholipid cardiolipin. This test is essentially an antiphospholipid **antibody** test, with all features similar to those of the aPL. ANA are antibodies against one or more elements within a biological cell, involved in the machinery of translating genomic message into proteins. These antibodies can destroy cells, and their effect usually leads to SLE.

When the immune system is the cause of miscarriage, the mother has a 30% chance of having a successful pregnancy without intervention after three miscarriages, a 25% chance after four miscarriages, and a 5% chance after five miscarriages. More epidemiological studies report a 90% chance of failure in untreated patients, whereas, in the presence of aPL, a 70% chance of reproductive failure was reported. Prevalence of LA in women with recurrent miscarriage has been quoted in a range between five and fifteen percent of fetal loss. Pathogenesis of fetal loss in the presence of aPL includes the presence of extensive infarction and necrosis in the placenta due the recurrent thrombosis of the placental vascular bed. In particular, intraluminal thromboses of the uterine spiral arteries and necrotizing decidual vasculopathy, histologically characterized by fibrinoid necrosis, atherosis, and intimal thickening have been observed.

Among immune system causes of miscarriage are the inability to properly detect fetal antigens and the lack of producing blocking antibodies. Another cause is maternal production of anti-sperm antibodies (IgG and IgA).

Endometriosis is a disease in which abnormal endometrial tissue grows in the abdomen and other places in the body. It causes internal bleeding, inflammation, scarring, severe pain, fatigue, and sometimes infertility. Endometriosis is related to the functional deficit of NK cells and cytoplasmic granules of cytotoxic lymphocytes (CTL) that allow the development of autoantibodies. In premature ovarian failure, autoantibodies against ovarian tissue and against gonadotropin receptors have been found. Oocyte reduction has been detected in women affected with premature ovarian failure.

Several male factors can influence the ability of successful fertilization, including the presence of male anti-sperm antibodies (IgG and IgM) that bind to the surface of the spermatozoa and may mask receptors or other functionally important proteins, thus interfering with the sperm-egg interaction, and reducing the probability for successful fertilization. Male anti-sperm antibody production is more likely to occur after vasectomy, or with undescended testicles, or epididymitis.

See also Autoimmunity and autoimmune diseases; Immunochemistry; Immunologic therapies; Immunological analysis techniques

RESPIRATION

Respiration is the physiological process that produces high-energy molecules such as adenosine triphosphate (ATP). The high-energy compounds become the fuel for the various manufacturing and growth processes of the cell. Respiration involves the transfer of electrons in a chemically linked series of reactions. The final electron acceptor in the respiration process is oxygen.

Respiration occurs in all types of organisms, including **bacteria**, **protists**, **fungi**, plants, and animals. In **eukaryotes**, respiration is often separated into three separate components. The first is known as external respiration, and is the exchange of oxygen and carbon dioxide between the environment and the organism (i.e., breathing). The second component of respiration is internal respiration. This is the exchange of oxygen and carbon dioxide between the internal body fluids, such as blood, and individual cells. Thirdly, there is cellular respiration, which is the biochemical oxidation of glucose and consequent synthesis of ATP.

Cellular respiration in prokaryotes and eukaryotes is similar. Cellular respiration is an intracellular process in which glucose is oxidized and the energy is used to make the high-energy ATP compound. ATP in turn drives energy-requiring processes such as biosynthesis, transport, growth, and movement.

In prokaryotes and eukaryotes, cellular respiration occurs in three sequential series of reactions; glycolysis, the citric acid cycle, and the electron transport chain. In prokaryotes such as bacteria, respiration involves components that are located in the **cytoplasm** of the cell as well as being membrane-bound.

Glycolysis is the controlled breakdown of sugar (predominantly, glucose, a 6-carbon carbohydrate) into pyruvate, a 3-carbon carbohydrate. Organisms frequently store complex carbohydrates, such as glycogen or starch, and break these down into glucose that can then enter into glycolysis. The process involves the controlled breakdown of the 6-carbon glucose into two molecules of the 3-carbon pyruvate. At least 10 **enzymes** are involved in glucose degradation. The oxidation of glucose is controlled so that the energy in this molecule can be used to manufacture other high-energy compounds. Each round of glycolysis generates only a small amount of ATP, in a process known as substrate-level phosphorylation.

For each glucose molecule that is broken down by glycolysis, there is a net gain of two molecules of ATP. Glycolysis produces reduced nicotinamide adenine dinucleotide (NADH), a high-energy molecule that can subsequently used to make ATP in the electron transfer chain. For each glucose molecule that is broken down by glycolysis, there is a net gain of two molecules of NADH. Finally, glycolysis produces compounds that can be used to manufacture compounds that are called fatty acids. Fatty acids are the major constituents of lipids, and are important energy storage molecules.

Each pyruvate molecule is oxidized to form carbon dioxide (a 1-carbon molecule) and acetyl CoA (a two carbon molecule). Cells can also make acetyl CoA from fats and amino acids. Indeed, this is how cells often derive energy, in the form of ATP, from molecules other than glucose or complex carbohydrates. Acetyl CoA enters into a series of nine sequential enzyme-catalyzed reactions, known as the citric acid cycle. These reactions are so named because the first reaction makes one molecule of citric acid (a 6-carbon molecule) from one molecule of acetyl CoA (a 2-carbon molecule) and one molecule of oxaloacetic acid (a 4-carbon molecule). A complete round of the citric acid cycle expels two molecules of carbon dioxide and regenerates one molecule of oxaloacetic acid.

The citric acid cycle produces two high-energy compounds, NADH and reduced flavin adenine dinucleotide ($FADH_2$), that are used to make ATP in the electron transfer chain. One glucose molecule produces 6 molecules of NADH and 2 molecules of $FADH_2$. The citric acid cycle also produces guanosine triphosphate (GTP; a high-energy molecule that can be easily used by cells to make ATP) by a process known as substrate-level phosphorylation. Finally, some of the intermediates of the citric acid cycle reactions are used to make other important compounds, in particular amino acids (the building blocks of proteins), and nucleotides (the building blocks of **DNA**).

The electron transfer chain is the final series of biochemical reactions in respiration. The series of organic electron carriers are localized inside the mitochondrial membrane of eukaryotes and the single membrane of Gram-positive bacteria or the inner membrane of Gram-negative bacteria. Cytochromes are among the most important of these electron carriers. Like hemoglobin, cytochromes are colored proteins, which contain iron in a nitrogen-containing heme group. The final electron acceptor of the electron transfer chain is oxygen, which produces water as a final product of cellular respiration.

The main function of the electron transfer chain is the synthesis of 32 molecules of ATP from the controlled oxidation of the eight molecules of NADH and two molecules of $FADH_2$, made by the oxidation of one molecule of glucose in glycolysis and the citric acid cycle. The electron transfer chain slowly extracts the energy from NADH and $FADH_2$ by passing electrons from these high-energy molecules from one electron carrier to another, as if along a chain. As this occurs, protons (H+) are pumped across the membrane, creating a proton gradient that is subsequently used to make ATP by a process known as chemiosmosis.

Respiration is often referred to as aerobic respiration, because the electron transfer chain utilizes oxygen as the final electron acceptor. When oxygen is absent or in short supply, cells may rely upon glycolysis alone for their supply of ATP. Glycolysis presumably originated in primitive cells early in the Earth's history when very little oxygen was present in the atmosphere. The glycolysis process has been referred to as anaerobic respiration, although this term is little used today to avoid confusion.

See also Bacterial growth and division; Biochemistry

RESTRICTION ENZYMES

Restriction **enzymes** are proteins that are produced by **bacteria** as a defense mechanism against **viruses** that infect the bacteria (bacterial phages). Most bacteria have restriction modification systems that consist of methylases and restriction enzymes. In such systems a bacteria's own **DNA** is modified by methylation (the addition of a methyl group, CH_3) at a specific location determined by a specific pattern of nucleotide residue and protected from degradation by specialized enzymes termed endonucleases.

The names of restriction enzymes are created from the first letter of the bacterial genus followed by the first two letters of the species plus a Roman numeral if more than one restriction enzyme has been identified in a particular species. Thus, the fifth restriction enzyme from *E. coli* is called EcoRV (pronounced e, ko, r five). Besides **cloning**, restriction enzymes are used in **genetic mapping** techniques, linking the genome directly to a conventional genetic marker.

Any DNA molecule, from viruses to humans, contains restriction-enzyme target sites purely by chance and, therefore, may be cut into defined fragments of size suitable for cloning. Restriction sites are not relevant to the function of the organism, nor would they be cut *in vivo,* because most organisms do not have restriction enzymes.

There are three types of restriction endonucleases in bacteria. Type I cuts unmodified DNA at a non-specific site 1000 base pairs beyond the recognition site. Type III recognizes a short asymmetric sequence and cuts at a site 24-26 base pairs from the recognition site. Type II recognizes short DNA of four to eight nucleotides. Type II restriction enzymes are widely used in **molecular biology**. Type II restriction enzymes have two properties useful in recombinant DNA technology. First, they cut DNA into fragments of a size suitable for cloning. Second, many restriction enzymes make staggered cuts generating single-stranded ends conducive to the formation of recombinant DNA. Hamilton Smith identified the first type II restriction enzyme, HindII, in 1970 at Johns Hopkins University.

Most type II restriction endonucleases cut DNA into staggered ends. For example, restriction enzyme EcoRI (from the bacterium *Escherichia coli*) recognizes the following six-nucleotide-pair sequence in the DNA of any organism: 5'–GAATTC–3', 3'–CTTAAG–5'. This type of segment is called a DNA palindrome, which means that both strands have the same nucleotide sequence but in antiparallel orientation. EcoRI cuts in the six-base-pair DNA between the G and the A nucleotides. This staggered cut leaves a pair of identical single

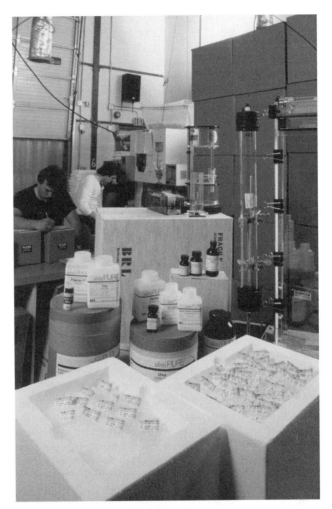

Restriction enzymes ready for use.

stranded ends. Some enzymes cut DNA at the same position of both strands, leaving both ends blunt.

See also Cell cycle (prokaryotic), genetic regulation of; DNA (Deoxyribonucleic acid); Gene amplification; Gene; Genetic code; Genetic identification of microorganisms; Genetic mapping; Genetic regulation of eukaryotic cells; Molecular biology and molecular genetics

RETROPOSONS AND TRANSPOSABLE ELEMENTS

Transposable elements are relatively long **DNA** sequences in prokaryotic and eukaryotic genomes that act as mobile genetic elements. These elements, which represent a large part of the genomes of many species transpose by a mechanism that involves DNA synthesis followed by random integration at a new target site in the genome.

All transposable elements encode for transposase, the special enzyme activity that helps in the insertion of **trans-**

posons at a new site, and most of them contain inverted repeats at their ends. The major difference between bacterial transposable elements and their eukaryotic counterparts is the mechanism of **transposition**. Only eukaryotic genomes contain a special type of transposable elements, called retroposons, which use reverse transcriptase to transpose through an **RNA** intermediate.

Transposition may result in splicing of DNA fragments into or out of the genome. During replicative transposition, the transposon is first replicated giving a new copy that is transferred to a new site, with the old copy being left at the original site. Nonreplicative transposition however describes the movement of a transposon that is excised from a donor site, usually generating a double, and is integrated in a new site.

The most basic transposable elements in **bacteria** are **insertion sequences**, which encode only for one enzyme, the transposase. Longer bacterial transposons contain at least one more protein-coding **gene**, which most frequently is an **antibiotic resistance** gene. In **eukaryotes**, retroposons are more common than transposons. They are either retroviral or nonviral. Viral retroposons encode for the **enzymes** reverse transcriptase and integrase and are flanked by long terminal repeats (LTRs) in the same way as **retroviruses**. The typical and most abundant nonviral retroposons are the short interspersed elements (SINEs) and the long interspersed elements (LINEs), which are usually repeated, many times in the mammalian genome. Both SINEs and LINEs lack LTRs and are thought to transpose through a special retrotransposition mechanism that involves **transcription** of one strand of the retroposon into RNA. This RNA undergoes conformation change (looping) and provides a primer for the synthesis of single stranded cDNA. The cDNA later serve as template for the synthesis of a double stranded DNA that is inserted in the genome by yet unknown mechanisms.

Transposons and retroposons seem to play a role in **evolution** and biology by promoting rearrangement and restructuring of genomes. Transposition may directly cause both deletion and inversion mutagenesis. Furthermore, transposable elements mediate the movement of host DNA sequences to new locations, enrich the genome with identical sequences positioned at different locations, and promote homologous **recombination**. Such recombination may eventually result in deletions, inversions, and translocations.

Transposons usually influence the expression of the genes in proximity of their insertion sites. They have therefore been extensively used as tools to create random insertion **mutants** in bacteria, **yeast** and higher eukaryotes. They are also used in large-scale functional genomic studies. They are valuable both during the **cloning** of genes and the generation of transgenic animals.

See also Microbial genetics; Transposition

RETROVIRUSES

Retroviruses are **viruses** in which the genetic material consists of **ribonucleic acid** (**RNA**) instead of the usual **deoxyribonu-**

cleic acid (**DNA**). Retroviruses produce an enzyme known as reverse transcriptase that can transform RNA into DNA, which can then be permanently integrated into the DNA of the infected host cells.

Many **gene** therapy treatments and experiments use disabled mouse retroviruses as a carrier (vector) to inject new genes into the host DNA. Retroviruses are rendered safe by adding, mutating, or deleting viral genes so that the virus cannot reproduce after acting as a vector for the intended delivery of new genes. Although viruses are not normally affected by **antibiotics**, genes can be added to retroviruses that make them susceptible to specific antibiotics.

As of 2002, researchers have discovered only a handful of retroviruses that infect humans. **Human immunodeficiency virus** (**HIV**), the virus that causes acquired immune deficiency syndrome (**AIDS**), is a retrovirus. Another human retrovirus, **human T-cell leukemia virus** (**HTLV**), was discovered three years prior to the discovery of HIV. Both HTLV and HIV attack human immune cells called **T cells**. T cells are the linchpin of the human immune response. When T cells are infected by these retroviruses, the **immune system** is disabled and several serious illnesses result. HTLV causes a fatal form of cancer called adult T cell leukemia. HTLV infection of T cells changes the way the T cells work in the body, causing cancer. HIV infection of T cells, however, eventually kills T cells, rendering the immune system powerless to stave off infections from **microorganisms**.

Retroviruses are sphere-shaped viruses that contain a single strand or a couple of strands of RNA. The sphere-shaped capsule of the virus consists of various proteins. The capsule is studded on the outside with proteins called receptor proteins. In HIV, these receptor proteins bind to special proteins on T cells called CD4 receptors. CD4 stands for cluster of differentiation, and CD type 4 is found on specific T cells called helper cells. The human retroviruses discovered so far bind only to CD4 receptors, which makes their affinity for T helper cells highly specific.

The retrovirus receptor docks with a CD4 receptor on a T cell, and enters the T cell through the T cell membrane. Once inside, the retrovirus begins to replicate. But because the retrovirus's genetic material consists of RNA, not DNA, replication is more complicated in a retrovirus than it is for a virus that contains DNA.

In all living things, DNA is the template by which RNA is transcribed. DNA is a double-stranded molecule that is located within the **nucleus** of cells. Within the nucleus, DNA transcribes RNA, a single-stranded nucleic acid. The RNA leaves the nucleus through tiny pores and enters the **cytoplasm**, where it directs the synthesis of proteins. This process has been called the "central dogma" of genetic **transcription**. No life form has been found that violates this central dogma—except retroviruses. In retroviruses, the RNA is used to transcribe DNA, which is exactly opposite to the way genetic material is transcribed in all other living things. This reversal is why they are named retrograde, or backwards, viruses.

In addition to RNA, retroviruses contain an enzyme called reverse transcriptase. This is the enzyme that allows the retrovirus to make a DNA copy from RNA. Once this DNA copy is made, the DNA inserts itself into the T cell's DNA. The inserted DNA then begins to produce large numbers of viral RNA that are identical to the infecting virus's RNA. This new RNA is then transcribed into the proteins that make up the infecting retrovirus. In effect, the T cell is transformed into a factory that produces more retroviruses. Because reverse transcriptase enzyme is unique to retroviruses, drugs that inhibit the action of this enzyme are used to treat retroviral infection, such as HIV. Reverse transcriptase is vital for retrovirus replication, but not for human cell replication. Therefore, modern reverse transcriptase inhibitor drugs are specific for retroviruses. Often, reverse transcriptase inhibitors are used in combination with other drugs to treat HIV infection.

Retroviruses are especially lethal to humans because they cause a permanent change in the T cell's DNA. Other viruses merely commandeer their host cell's cytoplasm and chemical resources to make more viruses; unlike retroviruses, they do not insert their DNA into the host cell's DNA. Nor do most viruses attack the body's T cells. Most people's cells, therefore, can recover from an attack from a virus. Eventually, the body's immune system discovers the infection and neutralizes the viruses that have been produced. Any cells that contain viruses are not permanently changed by the viral infection. Because retroviruses affect a permanent change within important cells of the immune system, cellular recovery from a retrovirus infection does not occur.

In 1980, researchers headed by Robert Gallo at the National Cancer Institute discovered the first human retrovirus. They found the virus within leukemic T cells of patients with an aggressive form of T cell cancer. These patients were from the southern United States, Japan, and the Caribbean. Almost all patients with this form of cancer were found to have antibodies (immune system proteins made in response to an infection) to HTLV.

HIV is perhaps the most famous retrovirus. Discovered independently by several researchers in 1983, HIV is now known to be the causative agent of AIDS. People with AIDS test positive for HIV antibodies, and the virus itself has been isolated from people with the disease.

HIV attacks T cells by docking with the CD4 receptor on its surface. Once inside the cell, HIV begins to transcribe its RNA into DNA, and the DNA is inserted into the T cell's DNA. However, new HIV is not released from the T cell right away. Instead, the virus stays latent within the cell, sometimes for 10 years or more. For reasons that are not yet clear, at some point the virus again becomes active within the T cell, and HIV particles are made within the cell. The new HIV particles bud out from the cell membrane and attack other T cells. Soon, all of the T cells of the body are infected and die. This infection cycle explains why very few virus particles are found in people with the HIV infection (those who do not yet have AIDS); many particles are found in people who have fulminate AIDS.

No cure has yet been found for AIDS. Researchers are still unsure about many aspects of HIV infection, and research into the immune system is still a relatively new science. Several anti-retroviral drugs, such as AZT, ddI, and ddC, have been administered to people with AIDS. These drugs do not cure HIV infection; but they usually postpone the development of AIDS. AIDS is almost invariably fatal.

Simian **immunodeficiency** virus (SIV) is the primate version of HIV. In fact, monkeys infected with SIV are used to test AIDS drugs for humans. Rous sarcoma virus (RSV) causes cancer in chickens and was the first retrovirus identified. Feline leukemia virus (FELV) causes feline leukemia in cats and is characterized by symptoms similar to AIDS. Feline leukemia is a serious disease that, like AIDS, is fatal. Unlike AIDS, a **vaccine** has been developed to prevent this disease.

See also AIDS, recent advances in research and treatment; Immunogenetics; T cells or T lymphocytes; Viral genetics; Viral vectors in gene therapy; Virus replication; Viruses and responses to viral infection

REVERSE TRANSCRIPTION • *see* TRANSCRIPTION

RH AND RH INCOMPATIBILITY

Human red blood cells contain protein molecules (antigens) in their cell membranes that determine the blood type of an individual. There are several kinds of antigens present on human red blood cells, as well as the Rh **antigen**. People with the Rh antigen are distinguished with a blood type ending in a plus (+); those without the Rh antigen have a minus (–) in their blood type.

Rh disease occurs when an Rh-negative mother is exposed to Rh-positive fetal blood and develops antibodies. During pregnancy, and especially during labor and delivery, some of the fetus's Rh-positive red blood cells get into the mother's (Rh -) bloodstream. Higher passage of fetal cells is observed in women who have undergone amniocentesis and other invasive diagnostic procedures, and in women with placental anomalies. This triggering of the mother's immune response is referred to as sensitization, or isoimmunization. In pregnancies occurring after exposure (usually not in the first pregnancy), maternal antibodies may lyse (disintegrate) the red blood cells of an Rh-positive fetus, leading to red blood cell destruction and fetal anemia. In the case of Rh, the predominant maternal **antibody** belongs to the G type (igG) which can freely cross the placenta and enter the fetal circulation. The consequent anemia may be so profound that the fetus may die in the uterus. Reacting to the anemia, the fetal bone marrow may release immature red blood cells (erythroblasts) into the fetal peripheral circulation, causing erythroblastosis fetalis. After birth, affected newborns may develop kernicterus. At any further pregnancy, the Rh incompatibility mechanism tends to be accelerated.

Since 1968, there has been a treatment that can prevent Rh disease. Without prophylaxis (preventative treatment), about one in six Rh negative women who deliver a Rh positive infant will develop anti-Rh antibodies from fetomaternal hemorrhage occurring either during pregnancy or at delivery. No universal policy exists for postnatal prophylaxis. The standard dose of anti-D immunoglobulin varies in different countries. In the USA, it is standard practice for Rh– patients who deliver Rh+ infants to receive an intramuscular dose of Rh immune globulin within 72 hours after delivery. With this treatment, the risk of subsequent sensitization deceases from about 15% to 2%. However, in spite of the routine use of gammaglobulin for both antepartum and postpartum immunoprophylaxis, severe fetal Rh alloimmunization continues to be a serious medical problem. In the presence of severe fetal anemia, early intervention appears to offer substantial improvement in clinical outcome.

Prenatal antibody screening is recommended for all pregnant women at their first prenatal visit. Repeat antibody screening at 24–28 weeks gestation is recommended for unsensitized Rh-negative mothers. The goals of antepartum care are to accurately screen the pregnant woman for Rh incompatibility and sensitization, to start appropriate therapeutic interventions as quickly as possible, and to deliver a mature fetus who has not yet developed severe hemolysis.

Frequent blood tests (indirect Coombs' tests) are obtained from the mother, starting at 16 to 20 weeks' gestation. These tests identify the presence of Rh-positive antibodies in maternal blood. When the antibody titer rises to 1:16 or greater, the fetus should be monitored by amniocentesis, cordocentesis, or the delta optical density 450 test. Administration of a dose of Rh immune globulin to Rh– patients at 28 weeks was found to reduce the risk of sensitization to about 0.2%.

The early diagnosis of fetal Rh status represents the best approach for the management of the disease, and a promising non-invasive detection of incompatibility seems now possible by means of the **polymerase chain reaction** (**PCR**) analysis of cell-free fetal **DNA** circulating in the mother's blood.

See also Antibody and antigen; Antibody formation and kinetics

RHIZOBIUM-AGROBACTERIUM GROUP •

see ECONOMIC USES AND BENEFITS OF MICROORGANISMS

RHODOPHYTA

The red algae phylum Rhodophyta synthesizes a class of water-soluble pigments termed phycobilins, known to be produced only by another algae, the Cryptomonads. There are approximately 6,000 species of Rhodophyta. Some of them are unicellular species that grow as filaments or membrane-like sheet cells, and some multicellular coralline species deposit calcium carbonate inside and around their cell walls, which are very similar in appearance to pink and red corals. Some Rhodophyta have an important role in coral-reef formation in tropical seas due to the deposits of calcium carbonate crystals they release in the environment, and are therefore termed coralline algae.

Rhodophyta are ancient algae whose fossil remains are found under the form of coralline algal skeletons in limestone deposits of coral reef origin dating back to the Precambrian Era. They use the blue spectrum of visible light to accomplish **photosynthesis** that allows them to live in deep waters, storing energy under the form of Floridean starch. They make mostly chlorophyll-a, and the pigments alpha and beta-carotene, phycoerythrin, as well as others similar to those made by Cyanobacteria, such as allophycocyanin and r-phycocyanin. The cell walls are made mainly of cellulose (but some species use xylan), and colloidal substances, such as agars and carageenan; and the cells may be multinucleated. The Floridean starch, a carbohydrate molecule consisting of 15 units of glucose, is kept free in the **cytoplasm**, whereas in other algae it is attached to the **chloroplast**. Some species are consumed by humans such as the Japanese nori (*Porphyra*) and others are utilized as components in processed food and by the pharmaceutical industries, such as *Chondrus,* and *Gelidium.*

See also Blue-green algae; Petroleum microbiology; Protists; Xanthophylls

RIBONUCLEIC ACID (RNA)

Nucleic acids are complex molecules that contain a cell's genetic information and the instructions for carrying out cellular processes. In eukaryotic cells, the two nucleic acids, ribonucleic acid (RNA) and **deoxyribonucleic acid** (**DNA**), work together to direct **protein synthesis**. Although it is DNA that contains the instructions for directing the synthesis of specific structural and enzymatic proteins, several types of RNA actually carry out the processes required to produce these proteins. These include messenger RNA (mRNA), ribosomal RNA (rRNA), and transfer RNA (tRNA). Further processing of the various RNA's is carried out by another type of RNA called small nuclear RNA (snRNA). The structure of RNA is very similar to that of DNA, however, instead of the base thymine, RNA contains the base uracil. In addition, the pentose sugar ribose is missing an oxygen atom at position two in DNA, hence the name deoxy-.

Nucleic acids are long chain molecules that link together individual nucleotides that are composed of a pentose sugar, a nitrogenous base, and one or more phosphate groups.

The nucleotides, the building blocks of nucleic acids, in ribonucleic acid are adenylic acid, cytidylic acid, guanylic acid, and uridylic acid. Each of the RNA subunit nucleotides carries a nitrogenous base: adenylic acid contains adenine (A), cytidylic acid contains cytosine (C), guanylic acid contains guanine (G), and uridylic acid contains uracil.

In humans, the DNA molecule is made of phosphate-base-sugar nucleotide chains, and its three-dimensional shape affects its genetic function. In humans and other higher organisms, DNA is shaped in a two-stranded spiral helix organized into structures called **chromosomes**. In contrast, most RNA molecules are single-stranded and take various shapes.

Nucleic acids were first identified by the Swiss biochemist Johann Miescher (1844–1895). Miescher isolated a cellular substance containing nitrogen and phosphorus.

Thinking it was a phosphorus-rich nuclear protein, Miescher named it nuclein.

The substance identified by Miescher was actually a protein plus nucleic acid, as the German biochemist Albrecht Kossel discovered in the 1880s. Kossel also isolated nucleic acids' two purines (adenine and guanine) and three pyrimidines (thymine, cytosine, and uracil), as well as carbohydrates.

The American biochemist Phoebus Levene, who had once studied with Kossel, identified two nucleic acid sugars. Levene identified ribose in 1909 and deoxyribose (a molecule with less oxygen than ribose) in 1929. Levene also defined a nucleic acid's main unit as a phosphate-base-sugar nucleotide. The nucleotides' exact connection into a linear polymer chain was discovered in the 1940s by the British organic chemist Alexander Todd.

In 1951, American molecular biologist James Watson and the British molecular biologists **Francis Crick** and Maurice Wilkins developed a model of DNA that proposed its now accepted two-stranded helical shape in which adenine is always paired with thymine and guanine is always paired with the cytosine. In RNA, uracil replaces thymine.

During the 1960s, scientists discovered that three consecutive DNA or RNA bases (a codon) comprise the **genetic code** or instruction for production of a protein. A **gene** is transcribed into messenger RNA (mRNA), which moves from the **nucleus** to structures in the **cytoplasm** called **ribosomes**. Codons on the mRNA order the insertion of a specific amino acid into the chain of amino acids that are part of every protein. Codons can also order the **translation** process to stop. Transfer RNA (tRNA) molecules already in the cytoplasm read the codon instructions and bring the required amino acids to a ribosome for assembly.

Some proteins carry out cell functions while others control the operation of other genes. Until the 1970s cellular RNA was thought to be only a passive carrier of DNA instructions. It is now known to perform several enzymatic functions within cells, including transcribing DNA into messenger RNA and making protein. In certain **viruses** called **retroviruses**, RNA itself is the genetic information. This, and the increasing knowledge of RNA's dynamic role in DNA cells, has led some scientists to argue that RNA was the basis for Earth's earliest life forms, an environment termed the RNA World.

The first step in protein synthesis is the **transcription** of DNA into mRNA. The mRNA exits the nuclear membrane through special pores and enters the cytoplasm. It then delivers its coded message to tiny protein factories called ribosomes that consist of two unequal sized subunits. Some of these ribosomes are found floating free in the cytosol, but most of them are located on a structure called rough endoplasmic reticulum (rER). It is thought that the free-floating ribosomes manufacture proteins for use within the cell (cell proliferation), while those found on the rER produce proteins for export out of the cell or those that are associated with the cell membrane.

Genes transcribe their encoded sequences as a RNA template that plays the role of precursor for messenger RNA (mRNA), being thus termed pre-mRNA. Messenger RNA is formed through the splicing of exons from pre-mRNA into a sequence of codons, ready for protein translation. Therefore, mRNA is also termed mature mRNA, because it can be transported to the cytoplasm, where protein translation will take place in the ribosomal complex.

Transcription occurs in the nucleus, through the following sequence of the events. The process of gene transcription into mRNA in the nucleus begins with the original DNA nitrogenous base sequence represented in the direction of transcription (e.g. from the 5' [five prime] end to the 3' [three prime] end) as DNA 5'...AGG TCC TAG TAA...3' to the formation of pre-mRNA (for the exemplar DNA cited) with a sequence of 3'...TCC AGG ATC ATT...5' (exons transcribed to pre-mRNA template) then into a mRNA sequence of 5'...AGG UCC UAG UAA...3' (codons spliced into mature mRNA).

Messenger RNA is first synthesized by genes as nuclear heterogeneous RNA (hnRNA), being so called because hnRNAs varies enormously in their molecular weight as well as in their nucleotide sequences and lengths, which reflects the different proteins they are destined to code for translation. Most hnRNAs of eukaryotic cells are very big, up to 50,000 nucleotides, and display a poly-A tail that confers stability to the molecule. These molecules have a brief existance, being processed during transcription into pre-mRNA and then in mRNA through splicing.

The molecular weight of mRNAs also varies in accordance with the protein size they encode for during translation. Because three nucleotides are needed for the translation of each amino acid that will constitute the polypeptide chain during protein synthesis, they necessarily are much bigger than the protein itself. Prokaryotic mRNA molecules usually have a short existence of about 2–3 minutes, but the fast bacterial mRNA turnover allows for a quick response to environmental changes by these unicellular organisms. In mammals, the average life span of mRNA goes from 10 minutes up to two days. Therefore, eukaryotic cells in mammals have different molecules of mRNA that show a wide range of different degradation rates. For instance, mRNA of regulatory proteins, involved either in cell **metabolism** or in the **cell cycle** control, generally has a short life of a few minutes, whereas mRNA for globin has a half-life of 10 hours.

The enzyme RNA-polymerase II is the transcriptional element in human eukaryotic cells that synthesizes messenger RNA. The general chemical structure of most eukaryotic mRNA molecules contain a 7-methylguanosine group linked through a triphosphate to the 5' extremity, forming a cap. At the other end (i.e., 3' end), there is usually a tail of up to 150 adenylils or poly-A. One exception is the histone mRNA that does not have a poly-A tail. It was also observed the existence of a correlation between the length of the poly-A tail and the half-life of a given mRNA molecule.

At the biochemical level, RNA molecules are linear polymers that share a common basic structure comprised of a backbone formed by an alternating polymer of phosphate groups and ribose (a sugar containing five carbon atoms). Organic nitrogenous bases i.e., the purines adenine and guanine, and the pyrimidines cytosine and uracil are linked together through phosphodiester bridges. These four nitrogenous bases are also termed heterocyclic bases and each of

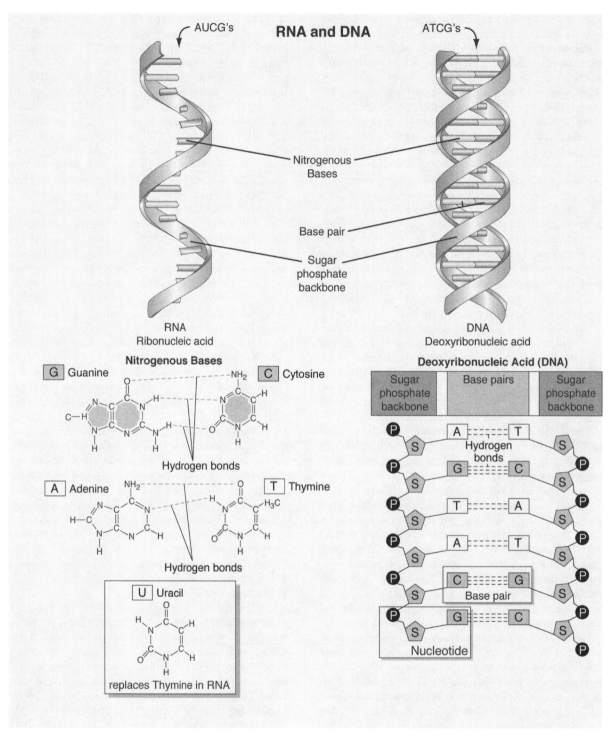

Diagram showing specific base pairing found in DNA and RNA.

them combines with one of the riboses of the backbone to form a nucleoside, such as adenosine, guanosine, cytidine, and uridine. The combination of a ribose, a phosphate, and a given nitrogenous base by its turn results in a nucleotide, such as adenylate, guanylate, cytidylate, uridylate. Each phosphodiester bridge links the 3' carbon at the ribose of one nucleotide to the 5' carbon at the ribose of the subsequent nucleotide, and so on. RNA molecules fold on themselves and form structures termed hairpin loops, because they have extensive regions of complementary guanine-cytosine (G-C) or adenine-uracil (A-U) pairs. Nevertheless, they are single polynucleotide chains.

The mRNA molecules contain at the 5' end a leader sequence that is not translated, known as UTR (untranslated region) and an initiation codon (AUG), that precedes the coding region formed by the spliced exons, which are termed codons in the mature mRNA. At the end of the coding region, three termination codons (UAG, UAA, UGA) are present, being followed by a trailer sequence that constitutes another UTR, which is by its turn followed by the poly-A tail. The stability of the mRNA molecule is crucial to the proper translation of the transcript into protein. The poly-A tail is responsible by such stability because it prevents the precocious degradation of mRNA by a 3' to 5' exonuclease (a cytoplasmatic enzyme that digests mRNA starting from the extremity 3' when the molecule leaves the cell nucleus). The mRNA of histones, the nuclear proteins that form the nucleosomes, do not have poly-A tails, thus constituting an exception to this rule. The poly-A tail also protects the other extremity of the mRNA molecule by looping around and touching the 7-methylguanosine cap attached to the 5' extremity. This prevents the decapping of the mRNA molecule by another exonuclease. The removal of the 7-methylguanosine exposes the 5' end of the mRNA to digestion by the 5' to 3' exonuclease (a cytoplasmatic enzyme that digests mRNA starting from the 5' end). When the translation of the protein is completed, the enzymatic process of deadenylation (i.e., enzymatic digestion of the poly-A tail) is activated, thus allowing the subsequent mRNA degradation by the two above mentioned exonucleases, each working at one of the ends of the molecule.

Transfer RNA (tRNA) is often referred to as the "Rosetta Stone" of genetics, as it translates the instructions encoded by DNA, by way of messenger RNA (mRNA), into specific sequences of amino acids that form proteins and polypeptides. This class of small globular RNA is only 75 to 90 nucleotides long, and there is at least one tRNA for every amino acid. The job of tRNA is to transport free amino acids within the cell and attach them to the growing polypeptide chain. First, an amino acid molecule is attached to its particular tRNA. This process is catalyzed by an enzyme called aminoacyl—tRNA synthetase that binds to the inside of the tRNA molecule. The molecule is now charged. The next step, joining the amino acid to the polypeptide chain, is carried out inside the ribosome. Each amino acid is specified by a particular sequence of three nucleotide bases called codons. There are four different kinds of nucleotides in mRNA. This makes possible 64 different codons (4^3). Two of these codons are called STOP codons; one of these is the START codon (AUG). With only 20 different amino acids, it is clear that some amino acids have more then one codon. This is referred to as the degeneracy of the genetic code. On the other end of the tRNA molecule are three special nucleotide bases called the anticodon. These interact with three complimentary codon bases in the mRNA by way of hydrogen bonds. These weak directional bonds are also the force that holds together the double strands of DNA.

In order to understand how this happens, it was necessary to first understand the three dimensional structure (conformation) of the tRNA molecule. This was first attempted in 1965, where the two-dimensional folding pattern was deduced from the sequence of nucleotides found in **yeast** alanine tRNA. Later work (1974), using x-ray diffraction analysis, was able to reveal the conformation of yeast phenylalanine tRNA. The molecule is shaped like an upside-down L. The vertical portion is made up of the D stem and the anti-codon stem, and the horizontal arm of the L is made up of the acceptor stem and the T stem. Thus, the translation depends entirely upon the physical structure. At one end of each tRNA is a structure that recognizes the genetic code, and at the other end is the particular amino acid for that code. Amazingly, this unusual shape is conserved between **bacteria**, plants, and animals.

Another unusual thing about tRNA is that it contains some unusual bases. The other classes of nucleic acids can undergo the simple modification of adding a methyl ($CH3^-$) group. However, tRNA is unique in that it undergoes a range of modifications from methylation to total restructuring of the purine ring. These modifications occur in all parts of the tRNA molecule, and increase its structural integrity and versatility.

Ribosomes are composed of ribosomal RNA (as much as 50%) and special proteins called ribonucleoproteins. In **eukaryotes** (an organism whose cells have chromosomes with nucleosomal structure and are separated from the cytoplasm by a two membrane nuclear envelope and whose functions are compartmentalized into distinct cytoplasmic organelles), there are actually four different types of rRNA. One of these molecules is called 18SrRNA; along with some 30–plus different proteins, it makes up the small subunit of the ribosome. The other three types of rRNA are called 28S, 5.8S, and 5S rRNA. One of each of these molecules, along with some 45 different proteins, is used to make the large subunit of the ribosome. There are also two rRNAs exclusive to the mitochondrial (a circular molecule of some 16,569 base pairs in the human) genome. These are called 12S and 16S. A mutation in the 12SrRNA has been implicated in non-syndromic hearing loss. Ribosomal RNA's have these names because of their molecular weight. When rRNA is spun down by ultracentrifuge, these molecules sediment out at different rates because they have different weights. The larger the number, the larger the molecule.

The larger subunit appears to be mainly involved in such biochemical processes as catalyzing the reactions of polypeptide chain elongation and has two major binding sites. Binding sites are those parts of large molecule that actively participate in its specific combination with another molecule. One is called the aminoacyl site and the other is called the peptidyl site. Ribosomes attach their peptidyl sites to the membrane surface of the rER. The aminoacyl site has been associated with binding transfer RNA. The smaller subunit appears to be concerned with ribosomal recognition processes such as mRNA. It is involved with the binding of tRNA also. The smaller subunit combines with mRNA and the first "charged " tRNA to form the initiation complex for translation of the RNA sequence into the final polypeptide.

The precursor of the 28S, 18S and the 5.83S molecules are transcribed by RNA polymerase I (Pol I) and the 5S rRNA is transcribed by RNA polymerase III (PoIII). Pol I is the most active of all the RNA polynmerases, and is one indication of how important these structures are to cellular function.

Ribosomal RNAs fold in very complex ways. Their structure is an important clue to the evolutionary relationships found between different kinds of organisms. Sequence comparisons of the various rRNAs across various species show that even though their base sequences vary widely, **evolution** has conserved their secondary structures, therefore, organization must be important for their function.

Since the 1970s, nucleic acids' cellular processes have become the basis for genetic engineering, in which scientists add or remove genes in order to alter the characteristics or behavior of cells. Such techniques are used in agriculture, pharmaceutical and other chemical manufacturing, and medical treatments for cancer and other diseases.

See also Biochemistry; Genetic regulation of eukaryotic cells

RIBOSOMES

Ribosomes are organelles that play a key role in the manufacture of proteins. Found throughout the cell, ribosomes are composed of ribosomal **ribonucleic acid** (rRNA) and proteins. They are the sites of **protein synthesis**.

Although **Robert Hooke** first used a light **microscope** to look at cells in 1665, it was only during the last few decades that the cell's organelles were discovered. This is primarily because light microscopes do not have the magnifying power required to see these tiny structures. Using an **electron microscope**, scientists have been able to see most of the cells substructures, including the ribosomes.

Ribosomes are composed of a variety of proteins and rRNA. They are organized in two functional subunits that are constructed in the cell's nucleolus. One is a small subunit that has a squashed shape, while another is a large subunit that is spherical in shape. The large subunit is about twice as big as the small unit. The subunits usually exist separately, but join when they are attached to a messenger **RNA** (mRNA). This initiates protein synthesis.

Production of a protein begins with initiation. In this step, the ribosomal small subunit binds to the mRNA along with the first transfer RNA (tRNA). The next step is elongation, where the ribosome moves along the mRNA and strings together the amino acids one by one. Finally, the ribosome encounters a stop sequence and the two subunits release the mRNA, the polypeptide chain, and the tRNA.

Protein synthesis occurs at specific sites within the ribosome. The P site of a ribosome contains the growing protein chain. The A site holds the tRNA that has the next amino acid. The two sites are held close together and a chemical reaction occurs. When the stop signal is present on the mRNA, protein synthesis halts. The polypeptide chain is released and the ribosome subunits are returned to the pool of ribosome units in the **cytoplasm**.

Ribosomes are found in two locations in the cell. Free ribosomes are dispersed throughout the cytoplasm. Bound ribosomes are attached to a membranous structure called the endoplasmic reticulum. Most cell proteins are made by the free ribosomes. Bound ribosomes are instrumental in producing proteins that function within or across the cell membrane. Depending on the cell type, there can be as many as a few million ribosomes in a single cell.

Because most cells contain a large number of ribosomes, rRNA is the most abundant type of RNA. rRNA plays an active role in ribosome function. It interacts with both the mRNA and tRNA and helps maintain the necessary structure. Transfer RNA is the molecule that interacts with the mRNA during protein synthesis and is able to read a three amino acid sequence. On the opposite end of the tRNAs, amino acids are bonded on a growing polypeptide chain. Generally, it takes about a minute for a single ribosome to make an average sized protein. However, several ribosomes can work on a single mRNA at the same time. This allows the cell to make many copies of a single protein rapidly. Sometimes these multiple ribosomes, or polysomes, can become so large that they can be seen with a light microscope.

The ribosomes in **eukaryotes** and prokaryotes are slightly different. Eukaryotic ribosomes are generally larger and are made up of more proteins. Since many diseases are caused by prokaryotes, these slight differences have important medical implications. Drugs have been developed that can inhibit the function of a prokaryotic ribosome, but leave the eukaryotic ribosome unaffected. One example is the antibiotic tetracycline.

See also Protein synthesis

RICKETTSIA AND RICKETTSIAL POX

Rickettsia are a group of **bacteria** that cause a number of serious human diseases, including the spotted fevers and **typhus**. Rod- or sphere-shaped, rickettsia lack both flagella (whip-like organs that allow bacteria to move) and pili (short, flagella-like projections that help bacteria adhere to host cells). Specific species of rickettsia include *Rickettsia rickettsii*, which causes the dangerous Rocky Mountain spotted fever; *R. akari*, which causes the relatively mild rickettsial pox; *R. prowazekii*, which causes the serious disease epidemic typhus; *R. typhi*, the cause of the more benign endemic or rat typhus; and *R. tsutsugamushi*, the cause of scrub typhus.

Rickettsia are transmitted to humans by insects such as ticks, mites, and chiggers. Usually the insect has acquired the bacteria from larger animals which they parasitize, such as rats, mice, and even humans. When an insect infected with rickettsia bites a human, the bacteria enter the bloodstream. From there, unlike most other bacteria that cause infection by adhering to cells, rickettsia enter specific human cells, where they reproduce. Eventually these host cells lyse (burst open), releasing more rickettsia into the bloodstream. Most rickettsial diseases are characterized by fever and a rash. Although all can be effectively cured with **antibiotics**, some of the rickettsial diseases, such as epidemic typhus and Rocky Mountain spotted fever, can be fatal if not treated promptly.

Rocky Mountain spotted fever is one of the most severe rickettsial diseases. First recognized in the Rocky Mountains, it has since been found to occur throughout the United States.

The **Centers for Disease Control** report about 600–1,000 cases occurring annually, but this number may be underestimated due to underreporting. *Rickettsia rickettsii* are carried and transmitted by four species of the hard-shelled tick, all of which feed on humans, wild and domestic animals, and small rodents. When a tick feeds on an infected animal, the bacteria are transmitted to the tick, which can in turn infect other animals with its bite. Human-to-human transmission of *R. rickettsii* does not occur. Once inside the human bloodstream, the bacteria invade cells that line the small blood vessels.

The symptoms of Rocky Mountain spotted fever reflect the presence of bacteria inside blood vessel cells. Within two to 12 days of being bitten by an infected tick, the infected person experiences a severe headache, fever, and malaise. After about two to four days, a rash develops, first on the extremities, then the trunk. A characteristic sign of this disease is that the rash involves the soles of the feet and palms of the hands. If the disease is not treated with antibiotics, the infected blood vessel cells lyse, causing internal hemorrhage, blockage of the blood vessels, and eventual death of the cells. Shock, kidney failure, heart failure, and stroke may then occur. Rocky Mountain spotted fever is often fatal if not treated.

A similar but milder disease is rickettsial pox, caused by *R. akari.* These bacteria are transmitted by mites which live preferentially on the common house mouse, only occasionally biting humans. Rickettsial pox is characterized by a rash that does not affect the palms or soles of the feet. The rash includes a lesion called an eschar-a sore that marks the spot of the infected mite bite. The mild course of this disease and the presence of the rash sometimes leads to its misdiagnosis as chicken pox, but the eschar clearly distinguishes rickettsial pox from chicken pox.

Outside of the United States, spotted fevers such as North Asian tick typhus, Queensland tick typhus, and boutonneuse fever are caused by other rickettsia species. As their names suggest, these diseases are found in Asia, Mongolia, and the Siberian region of Russia; in Australia; and in the Mediterranean region, Africa, and India, respectively. Symptoms of these spotted fevers resemble those of rickettsial pox. Although these spotted fevers share some of the symptoms of Rocky Mountain spotted fever, they are milder diseases and are usually not fatal.

Three forms of typhus are also caused by rickettsia. Epidemic typhus is caused by *R. prowazekii,* a bacterium that is transmitted by the human body louse. Consequently, episodes of this disease occur when humans are brought into close contact with each other under unsanitary conditions. Endemic typhus and scrub typhus are caused by *R. typhi* and *R. tsutsugamushi,* respectively. Transmitted by rat fleas, endemic typhus is a mild disease of fever, headache, and rash. Scrub typhus, named for its predilection for scrub habitats (although it has since been found to occur in rain forests, savannas, beaches, and deserts as well) is transmitted by chiggers. Unlike endemic typhus, scrub typhus is a serious disease that is fatal if not treated.

Not all rickettsia cause disease. Some species, such as *R. parkeri* and *R. montana,* normally live inside certain species of ticks and are harmless to the insect. These rickettsia are non-pathogenic (they do not cause disease) to humans as well.

With the exception of epidemic typhus, no **vaccine** exists to prevent rickettsial infection. Prevention of these diseases should focus on the elimination of insect carriers with insecticides and wearing heavy clothing when going into areas in which rickettsial carriers dwell. For instance, appropriate clothing for a forest expedition should include boots, long-sleeved shirts, and long pants. Treating the skin with insect **repellents** is also recommended to prevent insect bites.

RNA TUMOR VIRUSES

RNA tumor viruses contain **ribonucleic acid** as their genetic material. The **viruses** derive their designation from their association with tumors.

RNA tumor viruses are **retroviruses** that possess the reverse transcriptase enzyme that manufactures **deoxyribonucleic acid** (**DNA**) from the RNA template. Indeed, *retro* is the Latin word for backwards.

The history of RNA tumor viruses extends back to the first decade of the twentieth century. In 1908, it was demonstrated that fluid from a chicken that has leukemia could cause cells to be cancerous, even after the fluid had been filtered to remove all bacteria-sized organisms. Three years later, **Peyton Rous** identified one such factor, now named the Rous Sarcoma Virus. By the 1950s, many oncogenic viruses had been discovered and the RNA nature of these viruses had been established. In the 1960s, the reverse transcriptase enzyme was discovered. Finally, in 1981, the first human retrovirus was discovered, this being the **Human T-cell Leukemia Virus** (HTLV-1). The latter virus is a well-known tumor viruses.

There are two groups of RNA tumor viruses, the Oncovirinae and the Lentivirinae. Examples of the first group include the Rous Sarcoma Virus, HTLV-1, and HTLV-2 (which is also known as hairy cell leukemia virus). A prominent example of the second group is the **Human Immunodeficiency Virus** (**HIV**). A characteristic of HIV and other members of the second group is the long period of latency before symptoms of infection appear.

As for many viruses, the investigation of RNA tumor viruses involves growing the virus in a **culture** of whatever eukaryotic cell the virus is able to replicate inside. Then, the virus is purified. Subsequently, the virus can be studied using a variety of molecular and genetic techniques, and the **electron microscope** to assess the shape of the virus particles.

Some RNA tumor viruses never exist outside of the host cell, and lack an envelope around their genetic material. Viruses such as the mouse mammary tumor virus have an envelope that has spikes protruding from the surface. Other RNA tumor viruses contain spikes that are less prominent. Lentiviruses are an example of the latter shape.

The envelope of RNA tumor viruses comes from the membrane surrounding the host cell. The virus acquires this envelope as it emerges from the host cell. Within this envelope are distinctive proteins, which are coded for by the envelope, or env **gene**. Another characteristic component of RNA tumor viruses is the presence of a protein that coats the viral RNA. The gag gene codes for this latter protein. The protein encoded by the gag gene is also found in the envelope. The presence of these two protein species in RNA tumor viruses is being explored as a target for therapy to prevent RNA virus-induced cancer.

Another hallmark of RNA tumor viruses is the presence of a gene that is designated pol. The products of the pol gene include reverse transcriptase, another enzyme that helps integrate the viral genetic material into the host genome, and other **enzymes** that help process the genetic material and viral proteins so as to permit assembly of new virus. These essential functions have made the pol gene the target of antiviral strategies.

The infection process begins with the binding of the virus particles to a specific molecule on the surface of the host cell. Generically, such molecules are termed receptors. Once the virus is bound, it can be taken into the host by the process of endocytosis. Blocking the viral recognition of the host receptor and binding of the virus is yet another strategy to prevent tumor development.

The molecular basis for the **transformation** of cells by RNA tumor viruses was revealed by a number of scientists, including the Nobel laureate Harold Varmus. He and the others demonstrated that the cancer genes (oncogenes) of the viruses were similar or the same as certain genes with the nucleic acid of the host cell. When a virus infects the host, the host gene may become part of a new virus particle following viral replication. Over time, the host gene may become altered in subsequent rounds of viral replication. Eventually, this altered host gene may end up replacing a normal gene in a new host cell. The altered gene produces a protein that is involved in over-riding the controls on the division process of the host cell. The result is the uncontrolled cell division that is the hallmark of a cancer cell.

See also AIDS, recent advances in research and treatment; Immunodeficiency; Viral genetics

ROUS, PEYTON (1879-1970)
American physician

Francis Peyton Rous was a physician-scientist at the Rockefeller Institute for Medical Research (later the Rockefeller University) for over sixty years. In 1966, Rous won the Nobel Prize for his 1910 discovery that a virus can cause cancer tumors. His other contributions to scientific medicine include creating the first blood bank, determining major functions of the liver and gall bladder, and identifying factors that initiate and promote malignancy in normal cells.

Rous was born in Baltimore, Maryland, to Charles Rous, a grain exporter, and Frances Wood, the daughter of a Texas judge. His father died when Rous was eleven, and his mother chose to stay in Baltimore. His sisters were professionally successful, one a musician, the other a painter.

Rous, whose interest in natural science was apparent at an early age, wrote a "flower of the month" column for the *Baltimore Sun*. He pursued his biological interests at Johns Hopkins University, receiving a B.A. in 1900 and an M.D. in 1905. After a medical internship at Johns Hopkins, however, he decided (as recorded in *Les Prix Nobel en 1966*) that he was "unfit to be a real doctor" and chose instead to concentrate on research and the natural history of disease. This led to a full year of studying lymphocytes with Aldred Warthin at the University of Michigan and a summer in Germany learning morbid anatomy (pathology) at a Dresden hospital.

After Rous returned to the United States, he developed pulmonary **tuberculosis** and spent a year recovering in an Adirondacks sanatorium. In 1909, Simon Flexner, director of the newly founded Rockefeller Institute in New York City, asked Rous to take over cancer research in his laboratory. A few months later, a poultry breeder brought a Plymouth Rock chicken with a large breast tumor to the Institute and Rous, after conducting numerous experiments, determined that the tumor was a spindle-cell sarcoma. When Rous transferred a cell-free filtrate from the tumor into healthy chickens of the same flock, they developed identical tumors. Moreover, after injecting a filtrate from the new tumors into other chickens, a malignancy exactly like the original formed. Further studies revealed that this filterable agent was a virus, although Rous carefully avoided this word. Now called the Rous sarcoma virus RSV) and classed as an **RNA** retrovirus, it remains a prototype of animal **tumor viruses** and a favorite laboratory model for studying the role of genes in cancer.

Rous's discovery was received with considerable disbelief, both in the United States and in the rest of the world. His viral theory of cancer challenged all assumptions, going back to Hippocrates, that cancer was not infectious but rather a spontaneous, uncontrolled growth of cells and many scientists dismissed his finding as a disease peculiar to chickens. Discouraged by his failed attempts to cultivate **viruses** from mammal cancers, Rous abandoned work on the sarcoma in 1915. Nearly two decades passed before he returned to cancer research.

After the onset of World War I, Rous, J. R. Turner, and O. H. Robertson began a search for emergency blood transfusion fluids. Nothing could be found that worked without red blood corpuscles so they developed a citrate-sugar solution that preserved blood for weeks as well as a method to transfuse the suspended cells. Later, behind the front lines in Belgium and France, they created the world's first blood bank from donations by army personnel. This solution was used again in World War II, when half a million Rous-Turner blood units were shipped by air to London during the Blitz.

During the 1920s, Rous made several contributions to physiology. With P. D. McMaster, Rous demonstrated the concentrating activity of bile in the gall bladder, the acid-alkaline balance in living tissues, the increasing permeability along capillaries in muscle and skin, and the nature of gallstone formation. In conducting these studies, Rous devised **culture** techniques that have become standard for studying living tissues in the laboratory. He originated the method for growing viruses on chicken embryos, now used on a mass scale for producing viral vaccines, and found a way to isolate single cells from solid tissues by using the enzyme trypsin.

Moreover, Rous developed an ingenious method for obtaining pure cultures of Kupffer cells by taking advantage of their phagocytic ability; he injected iron particles in animals and then used a magnet to separate these iron-laden liver cells from suspensions.

In 1933, a Rockefeller colleague's report stimulated Rous to renew his work on cancer. Richard Shope discovered a virus that caused warts on the skin of wild rabbits. Within a year, Rous established that this papilloma had characteristics of a true tumor. His work on mammalian cancer kept his viral theory of cancer alive. However, another twenty years passed before scientists identified viruses that cause human cancers and learned that viruses act by invading genes of normal cells. These findings finally advanced Rous's 1910 discovery to a dominant place in cancer research.

Meanwhile, Rous and his colleagues spent three decades studying the Shope papilloma in an effort to understand the role of viruses in causing cancer in mammals. Careful observations, over long periods of time, of the changing shapes, colors, and sizes of cells revealed that normal cells become malignant in progressive steps. Cell changes in tumors were observed as always evolving in a single direction toward malignancy.

The researchers demonstrated how viruses collaborate with carcinogens such as tar, radiation, or chemicals to elicit and enhance tumors. In a report co-authored by W. F. Friedewald, Rous proposed a two-stage mechanism of carcinogenesis. He further explained that a virus can be induced by carcinogens or it can hasten the growth and transform benign tumors into cancerous ones. For tumors having no apparent trace of virus, Rous cautiously postulated that these spontaneous growths might contain a virus that persists in a masked or latent state, causing no harm until its cellular environment is disturbed.

Rous eventually ceased his research on this project due to the technical complexities involved with pursuing the interaction of viral and environmental factors. He then analyzed different types of cells and their nature in an attempt to understand why tumors go from bad to worse.

Rous maintained a rigorous workday schedule at Rockefeller. His meticulous editing and writing, both scientific and literary, took place during several hours of solitude at the beginning and end of each day. At midday, he spent two intense hours discussing science with colleagues in the Institute's dining room. Rous then returned to work in his laboratory on experiments that often lasted into the early evening.

Rous was appointed a full member of the Rockefeller Institute in 1920 and member emeritus in 1945. Though officially retired, he remained active at his lab bench until the age of ninety, adding sixty papers to the nearly three hundred he published. He was elected to the National Academy of Sciences in 1927, the American Philosophical Society in 1939, and the Royal Society in 1940. In addition to the 1966 Nobel Prize for Medicine, Rous received many honorary degrees and awards for his work in viral oncology, including the 1956 Kovalenko Medal of the National Academy of Sciences, the 1958 Lasker Award of the American Public Health Association, and the 1966 National Medal of Science.

As editor of the *Journal of Experimental Medicine,* a periodical renowned for its precise language and scientific excellence, Rous dominated the recording of forty-eight years of American medical research. He died of abdominal cancer in New York City, just six weeks after he retired as editor.

See also Viral genetics; Viral vectors in gene therapy; Virology; Virus replication; Viruses and responses to viral infection

ROUX, PIERRE-PAUL-ÉMILE (1853-1933)
French physician and bacteriologist

Soon after becoming a doctor, Émile Roux began doing research on bacterial diseases for **Louis Pasteur**. It has taken a century, however, for Roux's contribution to Pasteur's work—specifically his experiments utilizing dead **bacteria** to vaccinate against rabies—to be acknowledged. Roux is also credited, along with Alexandre Yersin, with the discovery of the **diphtheria** toxin secreted by *Corynebacterium diphtheriae* and **immunization** against the disease in humans. Both colleague and close friend to Pasteur, Roux eventually became the director of the Pasteur Institute in Paris.

Roux began his study of medicine at the Clermont-Ferrand Medical School in 1872. In 1874 Roux moved to Paris where he continued his studies at a private clinic. In 1878 he helped create lectures on **fermentation** for Emile Duclaux at the Sorbonne, Paris. Duclaux introduced Roux to Louis Pasteur, who was then in need of a doctor to assist with his research on bacterial diseases.

In 1879 Roux first began assisting Pasteur on his experiments with chicken cholera. The cholera bacillus was grown in pure **culture** and then injected into chickens, which would invariably die within 48 hours. However, one batch of culture was left on the shelf too long and when injected into chickens, failed to kill them. Later, these same chickens—in addition to a new group of chickens—were injected with new cultures of the cholera bacillus. The new group of chickens died while the first group of chickens remained healthy. Thus began the studies of the attenuation of chicken cholera.

In the 1880's Pasteur and Roux began research on rabid animals in hopes of finding a **vaccine** for **rabies**. Pasteur proceeded by inoculating dogs with an attenuated (weakened) strain of the bacteria from the brain tissue of rabid animals. Roux worked on a similar experiment utilizing dead rather than weakened bacteria from the dried spinal cords of infected rabbits.

On July 4, 1885, a 9-year-old boy named Joseph Meister was attacked on his way to school and repeatedly bitten by a rabid dog. A witness to the incident rescued Meister by beating the dog away with an iron bar; the dog's owner, Theodore Vone, then shot the animal. Meister's wounds were cauterized with carbolic acid and he was taken to a local doctor. This physician realized that Meister's chance of survival was minimal and suggested to Meister's mother that she take her son to Paris to see Louis Pasteur, who had successfully vaccinated dogs against rabies. The vaccine had never been tried on humans, and Pasteur was reluctant to give it to the boy; but when two physicians stated that Meister would die without it, Pasteur relented and administered the vaccine.

Pasteur stated that he utilized the attenuated strain of the vaccine; his lab notes, however, confirm that he treated Meister with the dead strain that Roux had been working on. (Why Pasteur maintained that he used his attenuated strain is not clear.) In any case, Meister received 13 shots of the rabies vaccine in the stomach in 10 days and was kept under close observation for an additional 10 days. The boy survived and became the first person to be immunized against rabies.

In 1883 Roux became the assistant director of Pasteur's laboratory. He undertook administrative responsibilities to help establish the Pasteur Institute, which opened in 1888 with Roux serving as director (from 1904) and teaching a class in microbiology.

Also in 1883 Roux and Yersin discovered the diphtheria toxin secreted by *Corynebacterium diphtheriae*. The two scientists filtered the toxin from cultures of the diphtheria bacterium and injected it into healthy laboratory animals. The animals exhibited the same symptoms (and eventual death) as those infected with the bacterium. Other data to support their discovery of the diphtheria toxin included urine obtained from children infected with the microorganism. Toxin excreted in the urine was sufficient to produce the same symptoms of the disease in laboratory animals. In 1894 Roux and Louis Martin began to study the immunization of horses against diphtheria in order to create a serum to be used in humans. The outcome of their research led them to successfully treat 300 children with the serum.

Beginning in 1896 Roux researched different aspects of diseases such as **tetanus**, **tuberculosis**, bovine **pneumonia**, and **syphilis** until he became the director of the Pasteur Institute in 1904. At that time Roux ceased all personal research and focused solely on running the Pasteur Institute until his death from tuberculosis in 1933.

See also Bacteria and bacterial infection; History of microbiology; History of public health

RUSKA, ERNST (1906-1988)

German physicist

The inventor of the **electron microscope**, Ernst Ruska, combined an academic career in physics and electrical engineering with work in private industry at several of Germany's top electrical corporations. He was associated with the Siemens Company from 1937 to 1955, where he helped mass produce the electron **microscope**, the invention for which he was awarded the 1986 Nobel Prize in physics. The Nobel Prize Committee called Ruska's electron microscope one of the most important inventions of the twentieth century. The benefits of electron microscopy to the field of microbiology and medicine allow scientists to study such structures as **viruses** and protein molecules. Technical fields such as electronics have also found new uses for Ruska's invention: improved

versions of the electron microscope became instrumental in the fabrication of computer chips.

Ruska was born in Heidelberg, Germany, on December 25, 1906. He was the fifth child of Julius Ferdinand Ruska, an Asian studies professor, and Elisabeth (Merx) Ruska. After receiving his undergraduate education in the physical sciences from the Technical University of Munich and the Technical University of Berlin, he was certified as an electrical engineer in 1931. He then went on to study under Max Knoll at Berlin, and received his doctorate in electrical engineering in 1933. During this period, Ruska and Knoll created an early version of the electron microscope, and Ruska concurrently was employed by the Fernseh Corporation in Berlin, where he worked to develop television tube technology. He left Fernseh to join Siemens as an electrical engineer, and at the same time accepted a position as a lecturer at the Technical University of Berlin. His ability to work in both academic and corporate milieus continued through his time at Siemens, and expanded when in 1954, he became a member of the Max Planck Society. In 1957, he was appointed director of the Society's Institute of Electron Microscopy, and in 1959, he accepted the Technical University of Berlin's invitation to become professor of electron optics and electron microscopy. Ruska remained an active contributor to his field until his retirement in 1972.

Prior to Ruska's invention of the electron microscope in 1931, the field of microscopy was limited by the inability of existing microscopes to see features smaller than the wavelength of visible light. Because the wavelength of light is about two thousand times larger than an atom, the mysteries of the atomic world were virtually closed to scientists until Ruska's breakthrough using electron wavelengths as the resolution medium. When the electron microscope was perfected, microscope magnification increased from approximately two thousand to one million times.

The French physicist, **Louis Victor de Broglie**, was the first to propose that subatomic particles, such as electrons, had wavelike characteristics, and that the greater the energy exhibited by the particle, the shorter its wavelength would be. De Broglie's theory was confirmed in 1927 by Bell Laboratory researchers. The conception that it was possible to construct a microscope that used electrons instead of light was realized in the late 1920s when Ruska was able to build a short-focus magnetic lens using a magnetic coil. A prototype of the electron microscope was then developed in 1931 by Ruska and Max Knoll at the Technical University in Berlin. Although it was less powerful than contemporary optical microscopes, the prototype laid the groundwork for a more powerful version, which Ruska developed in 1933. That version was ten times stronger than existing light microscopes. Ruska subsequently worked with the Siemens Company to produce for the commercial market an electron microscope with a resolution to one hundred angstroms (by contrast, modern electron microscopes have a resolution to one angstrom, or one ten-billionth of a meter).

Ruska's microscope—called a transmission microscope—captures on a fluorescent screen an image made by a focused beam of electrons passing through a thin slice of metalized material. The image can be photographed. In 1981,

Gerd Binnig and Heinrich Rohrer took Ruska's concept further by using a beam of electrons to scan the surface of a specimen (rather than to penetrate it). A recording of the current generated by the intermingling of electrons emitted from both the beam and specimen is used to build a contour map of the surface. The function of this scanning electron microscope complements, rather than competes against, the transmission microscope, and its inventors shared the 1986 Nobel Prize in physics with Ruska.

In 1937, Ruska married Irmela Ruth Geigis, and the couple had two sons and a daughter. In addition to the Nobel Prize, Ruska's work was honored with the Senckenberg Prize of the University of Frankfurt am Main in 1939, the Lasker Award in 1960, and the Duddell Medal and Prize of the Institute of Physics in London in 1975, among other awards. He also held honorary doctorates from the University of Kiev, the University of Modena, the Free University of Berlin, and the University of Toronto. Ruska died in West Berlin on May 30, 1988.

See also Microscope and microscopy

S

S LAYER • *see* SHEATHED BACTERIA

SABIN, ALBERT (1906-1993)
Russian American virologist

Albert Sabin developed an oral **vaccine** for polio that led to the once-dreaded disease's virtual extinction in the Western Hemisphere. Sabin's long and distinguished research career included many major contributions to **virology**, including work that led to the development of attenuated live-virus vaccines. During World War II, he developed effective vaccines against **dengue fever** and Japanese B encephalitis. The development of a live polio vaccine, however, was Sabin's crowning achievement.

Although Sabin's polio vaccine was not the first, it eventually proved to be the most effective and became the predominant mode of protection against polio throughout the Western world. In South America, "Sabin Sundays" were held twice a year to eradicate the disease. The race to produce the first effective vaccine against polio was marked by intense and often acrimonious competition between scientists and their supporters; in addition to the primary goal of saving children, fame and fortune were at stake. Sabin, however, allowed his vaccine to be used free of charge by any reputable organizations as long as they met his strict standards in developing the appropriate strains.

Albert Bruce Sabin was born in Bialystok, Russia (now Poland), on August 26, 1906. His parents, Jacob and Tillie Sabin, immigrated to the United States in 1921 to escape the extreme poverty suffered under the czarist regime. They settled in Paterson, New Jersey, and Sabin's father became involved in the silk and textile business. After Albert Sabin graduated from Paterson High School in 1923, one of his uncles offered to finance his college education if Sabin would agree to study dentistry. Later, during his dental education, Sabin read the *Microbe Hunters* by Paul deKruif and was

drawn to the science of virology, as well as to the romantic and heroic vision of conquering epidemic diseases.

After two years in the New York University (NYU) dental school, Sabin switched to medicine and promptly lost his uncle's financial support. He paid for school by working at odd jobs, primarily as a lab technician and through scholarships. He received his B.S. degree in 1928 and enrolled in NYU's College of Medicine. In medical school, Sabin showed early promise as a researcher by developing a rapid and accurate system for typing (identifying) *Pneumococci,* or the **pneumonia viruses**. After receiving his M.D. degree in 1931, he went on to complete his residency at Bellevue Hospital in New York City, where he gained training in pathology, surgery, and internal medicine. In 1932, during his internship, Sabin isolated the B virus from a colleague who had died after being bitten by a monkey. Within two years, Sabin showed that the B virus's natural habitat is the monkey and that it is related to the human **Herpes** Simplex virus. In 1934, Sabin completed his internship and then conducted research at the Lister Institute of Preventive Medicine in London.

In 1935, Sabin returned to the United States and accepted a fellowship at the Rockefeller Institute for Medical Research. There, he resumed in earnest his research of **poliomyelitis** (or polio), a paralytic disease that had reached epidemic proportions in the United States at the time of Sabin's graduation from medical school. By the early 1950s, polio afflicted 13,500 out of every 100 million Americans. In 1950 alone, more than 33,000 people contracted polio. The majority of them were children.

Ironically, polio was once an endemic disease (or one usually confined to a community, group, or region) propagated by poor sanitation. As a result, most children who lived in households without indoor plumbing were exposed early to the virus; the vast majority of them did not develop symptoms and eventually became immune to later exposures. After the **public health** movement at the turn of the century began to improve sanitation and more and more families had indoor toilets, children were not exposed at an early age to the virus and thus did not develop a natural **immunity**. As a result, polio became an epidemic disease and spread quickly through communities to other children without immunity, regardless of race, creed, or social status. Often victims of polio would lose complete control of their muscles and had to be kept on a respirator, or in a low-pressure iron lung, to help them breathe.

In 1936, Sabin and Peter K. Olitsky used a test tube to grow some poliovirus in the central nervous tissue of human embryos. Not a practical approach for developing the huge amounts of virus needed to produce a vaccine, this research nonetheless opened new avenues of investigation for other scientists. However, their discovery did reinforce the mistaken assumption that polio only affected nerve cells.

Although primarily interested in polio, Sabin was "never able to be a one-virus virologist," as he told Donald Robinson in an interview for Robinson's book *The Miracle Finders*. Sabin also studied how the **immune system** battled viruses and conducted basic research on how viruses affect the central nervous system. Other interests included investigations of **toxoplasmosis**, a usually benign viral disease that sometimes caused death or severe brain and eye damage in prenatal infections. These studies resulted in the development of rapid and sensitive serologic diagnostic tests for the virus.

During World War II, Sabin served in the United States Army Medical Corps. He was stationed in the Pacific theater where he began his investigations into insect-borne encephalitis, sandfly fever, and dengue. He successfully developed a vaccine for dengue fever and conducted an intensive **vaccination** program on Okinawa using a vaccine he had developed at Children's Hospital of Cincinnati that protected more than 65,000 military personnel against Japanese encephalitis. Sabin eventually identified a number of antigenic (or immune response-promoting) types of sandfly fever and dengue viruses that led to the development of several attenuated (avirulent) live-virus vaccines.

After the war, Sabin returned to the University of Cincinnati College of Medicine, where he had previously accepted an appointment in 1937. With his new appointments as professor of research pediatrics and fellow of the Children's Hospital Research Foundation, Sabin plunged back into polio research. Sabin and his colleagues began performing autopsies on everyone who had died from polio within a four-hundred-mile radius of Cincinnati, Ohio. At the same time, Sabin performed autopsies on monkeys. From these observations, he found that the poliovirus was present in humans in both the intestinal tract and the central nervous system. Sabin disproved the widely held assumption that polio entered humans through the nose to the respiratory tract, showing that it first invaded the digestive tract before attacking nerve tissue. Sabin was also among the investigators who identified the three different strains of polio.

Sabin's discovery of polio in the digestive tract indicated that perhaps the polio virus could be grown in a test tube in tissue other than nerve tissue, as opposed to costly and difficult-to-work-with nerve tissue. In 1949, John Franklin Enders, Frederick Chapman Robbins, and Thomas Huckle

Sweller grew the first polio virus in human and monkey non-nervous tissue cultures, a feat that would earn them a Nobel Prize. With the newfound ability to produce enough virus to conduct large-scale research efforts, the race to develop an effective vaccine accelerated.

At the same time that Sabin began his work to develop a polio vaccine, a young scientist at the University of Pittsburgh, **Jonas Salk**, entered the race. Both men were enormously ambitious and committed to their own theory about which type of vaccine would work best against polio. While Salk committed his efforts to a killed polio virus, Sabin openly expressed his doubts about the safety of such a vaccine as well as its effectiveness in providing lasting protection. Sabin was convinced that an attenuated live-virus vaccine would provide the safe, long-term protection needed. Such a vaccine is made of living virus that is diluted, or weakened, so that it spurs the immune system to fight off the disease without actually causing the disease itself.

In 1953, Salk seemed to have won the battle when he announced the development of a dead virus vaccine made from cultured polio virus inactivated, or killed, with formaldehyde. While many clamored for immediate mass field trials, Sabin, Enders, and others cautioned against mass inoculation until further efficacy and safety studies were conducted. Salk, however, had won the entire moral and financial support of the National Foundation for Infantile Paralysis, and in 1954, a massive field trial of the vaccine was held. In 1955, to worldwide fanfare, the vaccine was pronounced effective and safe.

Church and town hall bells rang throughout the country, hailing the new vaccine and Salk. However, on April 26, just fourteen days after the announcement, five children in California contracted polio after taking the Salk vaccine. More cases began to occur, with eleven out of 204 people stricken eventually dying. The United States Public Health Service (PHS) ordered a halt to the vaccinations, and a virulent live virus was found to be in certain batches of the manufactured vaccine. After the installation of better safeguards in manufacturing, the Salk vaccine was again given to the public and greatly reduced the incidence of polio in the United States. But Sabin and Enders had been right about the dangers associated with a dead-virus vaccine; and Sabin continued to work toward a vaccine that he believed would be safe, long lasting, and orally administered without the need for injection like Salk's vaccine.

By orally administering the vaccine, Sabin wanted it to multiply in the intestinal tract. Sabin used Enders's technique to obtain the virus and tested individual virus particles on the central nervous system of monkeys to see whether the virus did any damage. According to various estimates, Sabin's meticulous experiments were performed on anywhere from nine to fifteen thousand monkeys and hundreds of chimpanzees. Eventually, he diluted three mutant strains of polio that seemed to stimulate **antibody** production in chimpanzees. Sabin immediately tested the three strains on himself and his family, as well as research associates and volunteer prisoners from Chillicothe Penitentiary in Ohio. Results of these tests showed that the viruses produced immunity to polio with no harmful side effects. By this time, however, the public and much of the scientific community were committed to the Salk vaccine. Two scientists working for Lederle Laboratories had also developed a live-virus vaccine. However, the Lederle vaccine was tested in Northern Ireland in 1956 and proved dangerous, as it sometimes reverted to a virulent state.

Although Sabin lacked backing for a large-scale clinical trial in the United States, he remained undaunted. He was able to convince the Health Ministry in the Soviet Union to try his vaccine in massive trials. At the time, the Soviets were mired in a polio epidemic that was claiming eighteen to twenty thousand victims a year. By this time, Sabin was receiving the political backing of the **World Health Organization** in Geneva, Switzerland, which had previously been using Salk's vaccine to control the outbreak of polio around the world; they now believed that Sabin's approach would one day eradicate the disease.

Sabin began giving his vaccine to Russian children in 1957, inoculating millions over the next several years. Not to be outdone by Salk's public relations expertise, Sabin began to travel extensively, promoting his vaccine through newspaper articles, issued statements, and scientific meetings. In 1960, the U.S. Public Health Service, finally convinced of Sabin's approach, approved his vaccine for manufacture in the United States. Still, the PHS would not order its use and the Salk vaccine remained the vaccine of choice until a pediatrician in Phoenix, Arizona, Richard Johns, organized a Sabin vaccine drive. The vaccine was supplied free of charge, and many physicians provided their services without a fee on a chosen Sunday. The success of this effort spread, and Sabin's vaccine soon became "the vaccine" to ward off polio.

The battle between Sabin and Salk persisted well into the 1970s, with Salk writing an op-ed piece for the New York Times in 1973 denouncing Sabin's vaccine as unsafe and urging people to use his vaccine once more. For the most part, Salk was ignored, and by 1993, health organizations began to report that polio was close to extinction in the Western Hemisphere.

Sabin continued to work vigorously and tirelessly into his seventies, traveling to Brazil in 1980 to help with a new outbreak of polio. He antagonized Brazilian officials, however, by accusing the government bureaucracy of falsifying data concerning the serious threat that polio still presented in that country. He officially retired from the National Institute of Health in 1986. Despite his retirement, Sabin continued to be outspoken, saying in 1992 that he doubted whether a vaccine against the **human immunodeficiency virus**, or **HIV**, was feasible. Sabin died from congestive heart failure at the Georgetown University Medical Center on March 3, 1993. In an obituary in the *Lancet,* Sabin was noted as the "architect" behind the eradication of polio from North and South America. Salk issued a statement praising Sabin's work to vanquish polio.

See also Antibody and antigen; Antibody formation and kinetics; History of immunology; History of public health; Poliomyelitis and polio

SACCHAROMYCES CEREVISIAE

Unicellular **Fungi** (**Yeast** Phylum) are one of the most studied single-cell **Eukaryotes**. Among them, *Saccharomyces cerevisiae* is perhaps the biological model most utilized for decades in order for scientists to understand the molecular anatomy and physiology of eukaryotic cells, such as membrane and trans-membrane receptors, **cell cycle** controls, and **enzymes** and proteins involved in signal **transduction** to the **nucleus**.

Many strands of *S. cerevisiae* are used by the wine and beer industry for **fermentation**. *S. cerevisiae* is a member of the group of budding yeasts that replicate (reproduce) through the formation of an outgrowth in the parental cell known as a bud. After nuclear division into two daughter nuclei, one nucleus migrates to the bud, which continues to grow until it breaks off to form an independent daughter cell. Most eukaryotic cells undergo symmetric cell division, resulting in two daughter cells with the same size. In budding yeast, however, cell division is asymmetric and produces at cell separation a large parental cell and a small daughter cell. Moreover, after separation, the parental cell starts the production of a new bud, whereas the daughter cell continues to grow into its mature size before producing its own bud. Cell cycle times are also different between parental and young daughter cells. Parental (or mother cells) have a cell cycle of 100 minutes, whereas daughter cells in the growing process have a cycle time of 146 minutes from birth to first budding division.

The study of cell cycle controls, enzymatic systems of **DNA** repair, programmed cell death, and DNA **mutations** in *S. cerevisiae* and *S. pombe* greatly contributed to the understanding of pre-malignant cell transformations and the identification of genes involved in carcinogenesis. They constitute ideal biological models for these studies because they change the cellular shape in each phase of the cell cycle and in case of genetic mutation, the position defect is easily identified and related to the specific phase of the cell cycle. Such mutations are known as cdc mutations (cell division cycle mutations).

See also Cell cycle (eukaryotic), genetic regulation of; Yeast genetics

SALK, JONAS (1914-1995)

American physician

Jonas Salk was one of the United States's best-known microbiologists, chiefly celebrated for his discovery of his polio **vaccine**. Salk's greatest contribution to **immunology** was the insight that a "killed virus" is capable of serving as an **antigen**, prompting the body's **immune system** to produce antibodies that will attack invading organisms. This realization enabled Salk to develop a polio vaccine composed of killed polio **viruses**, producing the necessary antibodies to help the body to ward off the disease without itself inducing polio.

The eldest son of Orthodox Jewish-Polish immigrants, Jonas Edward Salk was born in East Harlem, New York, on October 28, 1914. His father, Daniel B. Salk, was a garment worker, who designed lace collars and cuffs and enjoyed sketching in his spare time. He and his wife, Dora Press, encouraged their son's academic talents, sending him to Townsend Harris High School for the gifted. There, young Salk was both highly motivated and high achieving, graduating at the age of fifteen and enrolling in the legal faculty of the City College of New York. Ever curious, he attended some science courses and quickly decided to switch fields. Salk graduated with a bachelor's degree in science in 1933, at the age of nineteen, and went on to New York University's School of Medicine. Initially he scraped by on money his parents had borrowed for him; after the first year, however, scholarships and fellowships paid his way. In his senior year, Salk met the man with whom he would collaborate on some of the most important work of his career, Dr. Thomas Francis, Jr.

On June 7, 1939, Salk was awarded his M.D. The next day, he married Donna Lindsay, a psychology major who was employed as a social worker. The couple eventually had three sons. After graduation, Salk continued working with Francis, and concurrently began a two-year internship at Mount Sinai Hospital in New York. Upon completing his internship, Salk accepted a National Research Council fellowship and moved to The University of Michigan to join Dr. Francis, who had been heading up Michigan's department of **epidemiology** since the previous year. Working on behalf of the U.S. Army, the team strove to develop a flu vaccine. Their goal was a "killed-virus" vaccine—able to kill the live flu viruses in the body, while simultaneously producing antibodies that could fight off future invaders of the same type, thus producing **immunity**. By 1943, Salk and Francis had developed a formalin-killed-virus vaccine, effective against both type A and B **influenza** viruses, and were in a position to begin clinical trials.

In 1946, Salk was appointed assistant professor of epidemiology at Michigan. Around this time he extended his research to cover not only viruses and the body's reaction to them, but also their epidemic effects in populations. The following year he accepted an invitation to move to the University of Pittsburgh School of Medicine's Virus Research Laboratory as an associate research professor of bacteriology. When Salk arrived at the Pittsburgh laboratory, what he encountered was not encouraging. The laboratory had no experience with the kind of basic research he was accustomed to, and it took considerable effort on his part to bring the lab up to par. However, Salk was not shy about seeking financial support for the laboratory from outside benefactors, and soon his laboratory represented the cutting edge of viral research.

In addition to building a respectable laboratory, Salk also devoted a considerable amount of his energies to writing scientific papers on a number of topics, including the polio virus. Some of these came to the attention of Daniel Basil O'Connor, the director of the National Foundation for Infantile Paralysis—an organization that had long been involved with the treatment and rehabilitation of polio victims. O'Connor eyed Salk as a possible recruit for the polio vaccine research his organization sponsored. When the two finally met, O'Connor was much taken by Salk—so much so, in fact, that he put almost all of the National Foundation's money behind Salk's vaccine research efforts.

Poliomyelitis, traceable back to ancient Egypt, causes permanent paralysis in those it strikes, or chronic shortness of breath often leading to death. Children, in particular, are especially vulnerable to the polio virus. The University of Pittsburgh was one of four universities engaged in trying to sort and classify the more than one hundred known varieties of polio virus. By 1951, Salk was able to assert with certainty that all polio viruses fell into one of three types, each having various strains; some of these were highly infectious, others barely so. Once he had established this, Salk was in a position to start work on developing a vaccine.

Salk's first challenge was to obtain enough of the virus to be able to develop a vaccine in doses large enough to have an impact; this was particularly difficult since viruses, unlike culture-grown **bacteria**, need living cells to grow. The breakthrough came when the team of **John F. Enders**, **Thomas Weller**, and Frederick Robbins found that the polio virus could be grown in embryonic tissue—a discovery that earned them a Nobel Prize in 1954.

Salk subsequently grew samples of all three varieties of polio virus in cultures of monkey kidney tissue, then killed the virus with formaldehyde. Salk believed that it was essential to use a killed polio virus (rather than a live virus) in the vaccine, as the live-virus vaccine would have a much higher chance of accidentally inducing polio in inoculated children. He therefore, exposed the viruses to formaldehyde for nearly 13 days. Though after only three days he could detect no virulence in the sample, Salk wanted to establish a wide safety margin; after an additional ten days of exposure to the formaldehyde, he reasoned that there was only a one-in-a-trillion chance of there being a live virus particle in a single dose of his vaccine. Salk tested it on monkeys with positive results before proceeding to human clinical trials.

Despite Salk's confidence, many of his colleagues were skeptical, believing that a killed-virus vaccine could not possibly be effective. His dubious standing was further compounded by the fact that he was relatively new to polio vaccine research; some of his chief competitors in the race to develop the vaccine—most notably **Albert Sabin**, the chief proponent for a live-virus vaccine—had been at it for years.

As the field narrowed, the division between the killed-virus and the live-virus camps widened, and what had once been a polite difference of opinion became a serious ideological conflict. Salk and his chief backer, the National Foundation for Infantile Paralysis, were lonely in their corner. Salk failed to let his position in the scientific wilderness dissuade him and he continued, undeterred, with his research. To test his vaccine's strength, in early 1952, Salk administered a type I vaccine to children who had already been infected with the polio virus. Afterwards, he measured their **antibody** levels. His results clearly indicated that the vaccine produced large amounts of antibodies. Buoyed by this success, the clinical trial was then extended to include children who had never had polio.

In May 1952, Salk initiated preparations for a massive field trial in which over four hundred thousand children would be vaccinated. The largest medical experiment that had ever been carried out in the United States, the test finally got underway in April 1954, under the direction of Dr. Francis and sponsored by the National Foundation for Infantile Paralysis. More than one million children between the ages of six and nine took part in the trial, each receiving a button that proclaimed them a "Polio Pioneer." A third of the children were given doses of the vaccine consisting of three injections—one for each of the types of polio virus—plus a booster shot. A control group of the same number of children was given a placebo, and a third group was given nothing.

At the beginning of 1953, while the trial was still at an early stage, Salk's encouraging results were made public in the *Journal of the American Medical Association.* Predictably, media and public interest were intense. Anxious to avoid sensationalized versions of his work, Salk agreed to comment on the results thus far during a scheduled radio and press appearance.

Despite the doomsayers, on April 12, 1955, the vaccine was officially pronounced effective, potent, and safe in almost 90% of cases. The meeting at which the announcement was made was attended by five hundred of the world's top scientists and doctors, 150 journalists, and sixteen television and movie crews. The success of the trial catapulted Salk to instant stardom.

Wishing to escape from the glare of the limelight, Salk turned down the countless offers and tried to retreat into his laboratory. Unfortunately, a tragic mishap served to keep the attention of the world's media focused on him. Just two weeks after the announcement of the vaccine's discovery, eleven of the children who had received it developed polio; more cases soon followed. Altogether, about 200 children developed paralytic polio, eleven fatally. For a while, it appeared that the **vaccination** campaign would be railroaded. However, it was soon discovered that all of the rogue vaccines had originated from the same source, Cutter Laboratories in California. On May 7, the vaccination campaign was called to a halt by the Surgeon General. Following a thorough investigation, it was found that Cutter had used faulty batches of virus **culture**, which were resistant to the formaldehyde. After furious debate and the adoption of standards that would prevent such a reoccurrence, the inoculation resumed. By the end of 1955, seven million children had received their shots, and over the course of the next two years more than 200 million doses of Salk's polio vaccine were administered, without a single instance of vaccine-induced paralysis. By the summer of 1961, there had been a 96% reduction in the number of cases of polio in the United States, compared to the five-year period prior to the vaccination campaign.

After the initial inoculation period ended in 1958, Salk's killed-virus vaccine was replaced by a live-virus vaccine developed by Sabin; use of this new vaccine was advantageous because it could be administered orally rather than intravenously, and because it required fewer "booster" inoculations. To this day, though, Salk remains known as the man who defeated polio.

In 1954, Salk took up a new position as professor of preventative medicine at Pittsburgh, and in 1957 he became professor of experimental medicine. The following year he began work on a vaccine to immunize against all viral diseases of the central nervous system. As part of this research, Salk per-

formed studies of normal and malignant cells, studies that had some bearing on the problems encountered in cancer research. In 1960, he founded the Salk Institute for Biological Studies in La Jolla, California; heavily funded by the National Foundation for Infantile Paralysis (by then known as the March of Dimes), the institute attracted some of the brightest scientists in the world, all drawn by Salk's promise of full-time, uninterrupted biological research.

Salk died on 23 June 1995, at a San Diego area hospital. His death, at the age of 80, was caused by heart failure.

See also Antibody and antigen; Antibody formation and kinetics; Immunity, active, passive and delayed; Immunization; Poliomyelitis and polio

SALMONELLA

Salmonella is the common name given to a type of food poisoning caused by the **bacteria** *Salmonella enteritidis* (other types of illnesses are caused by other species of *Salmonella* bacteria, including **typhoid fever**. When people eat food contaminated by *S. enteritidis,* they suffer **gastroenteritis (inflammation** of the stomach and intestines, with diarrhea and vomiting).

Salmonella food poisoning is most often caused by improperly handled or cooked poultry or eggs. Because chickens carrying the bacteria do not appear ill, infected chickens can lay eggs or be used as meat.

Early in the study of *Salmonella* food poisoning, it was thought that *Salmonella* bacteria were only found in eggs which had cracks in them, and that the infecting bacteria existed on the outside of the eggshell. Stringent guidelines were put into place to ensure that cracked eggs do not make it to the marketplace, and to make sure that the outside of eggshells were all carefully disinfected. However, outbreaks of *Salmonella* poisoning continued. Research then ultimately revealed that, because the egg shell has tiny pores, even uncracked eggs which have been left for a time on a surface (such as a chicken's roost) contaminated with *Salmonella* could become contaminated. Subsequently, further research has demonstrated that the bacteria can also be passed from the infected female chicken directly into the substance of the egg prior to the shell forming around it.

Currently, the majority of *Salmonella* food poisoning occurs due to unbroken, disinfected grade A eggs, which have become infected through bacteria which reside in the hen's ovaries. In the United States, he highest number of cases of *Salmonella* food poisoning occur in the Northeast, where it is believed that about one out of 10,000 eggs is infected with *Salmonella.*

The most effective way to avoid *Salmonella* poisoning is to properly cook all food which could potentially harbor the bacteria. Neither drying nor freezing are reliable ways to kill *Salmonella.* While the most common source for human infection with *Salmonella* bacteria is poultry products, other carriers include pets such as turtles, chicks, ducklings, and iguanas.

Products containing animal tissues may also be contaminated with *Salmonella*.

While anyone may contract *Salmonella* food poisoning from contaminated foods, the disease proves most threatening in infants, the elderly, and individuals with weakened immune systems. People who have had part or all of their stomach or spleen removed, as well as individuals with sickle cell anemia, cirrhosis of the liver, leukemia, lymphoma, **malaria**, louse-borne relapsing fever, or acquired **immunodeficiency** syndrome (**AIDS**) are particularly susceptible to *Salmonella* food poisoning. In the United States, about 15% of all cases of food poisoning are caused by *Salmonella*.

Salmonella food poisoning occurs most commonly when people eat undercooked chicken or eggs, sauces, salad dressings, or desserts containing raw eggs. The bacteria can also be spread if raw chicken, for example, contaminates a cutting board or a cook's hands, and is then spread to some other uncooked food. Cases of *Salmonella* infections in children have been traced to the children handling a pet (such as a turtle or an iguana) and then eating without first washing their hands. An individual who has had *Salmonella* food poisoning will continue to pass the bacteria into their feces for several weeks after the initial illness. Poor handwashing can allow others to become infected.

Symptoms of *Salmonella* food poisoning generally occur about 12–72 hours after ingestion of the bacteria. Half of all patients experience fever; other symptoms include nausea, vomiting, diarrhea, and abdominal cramping and pain. The stools are usually liquid, but rarely contain mucus or blood. Diarrhea usually lasts about four days. The entire illness usually resolves itself within about a week.

While serious complications of *Salmonella* food poisoning are rare, individuals with other medical illnesses are at higher risk. Complications occur when the *Salmonella* bacteria make their way into the bloodstream. Once in the bloodstream, the bacteria can invade any organ system, causing disease. Infections which can be caused by *Salmonella* include: bone infections (osteomyelitis), infections of the sac containing the heart (pericarditis), infections of the tissues which cover the brain and spinal cord (**meningitis**), and liver and lung infections.

Salmonella food poisoning is diagnosed by examining a stool sample. Under appropriate laboratory conditions, the bacteria in the stool can be encouraged to grow, and then processed and viewed under a **microscope** for identification.

Simple cases of *Salmonella* food poisoning are usually treated by encouraging good fluid intake, to avoid dehydration. Although the illness is caused by a bacteria, studies have shown that using **antibiotics** may not shorten the course of the illness. Instead, antibiotics may have the adverse effect of lengthening the amount of time the bacteria appear in the feces, thus potentially increasing others' risk of exposure to *Salmonella*. Additionally, some strains of *Salmonella* are developing resistance to several antibiotics.

Efforts to prevent *Salmonella* food poisoning have been greatly improved now that it is understood that eggs can be contaminated during their development inside the hen. Flocks are carefully tested, and eggs from infected chickens can be pasteurized to kill the bacteria. Efforts have been made to carefully educate the public about safe handling and cooking practices for both poultry and eggs. People who own pets that can carry *Salmonella* are also being more educated about more careful handwashing practices. It is unlikely that a human **immunization** will be developed, because there are so many different types of *Salmonella* enteritidis. However, researchers in 1997 produced an oral **vaccine** for poultry from genetically altered live *Salmonella* bacteria, currently undergoing testing, that may show the prevention of *Salmonella* bacteria from infecting meat or eggs. In 2001, two teams of researchers in England sequenced the genomes of both *Salmonella Typhimurium* (a common cause of food poisoning) and *Salmonella Typhi* the cause of typhoid fever). Data gathered from the project will improve diagnosis of *Salmonella* infections, and may eventually lead to a method of blocking its transmission in humans.

See also Antibiotic resistance, tests for; Bacteria and bacterial infection; Bacterial adaptation; Food safety

SALMONELLA FOOD POISONING

Salmonella food poisoning, consistent with all food poisoning, results from the growth of the bacterium in food. This is in contrast to food intoxication, were illness results from the presence of toxin in the food. While food intoxication does not require the growth of the contaminating **bacteria** to reasonably high numbers, food poisoning does.

Salmonella is a Gram negative, rod-shaped bacterium. The gastrointestinal tracts of man and animals are common sources of the bacterium. Often the bacterium is spread to food by handling the food with improperly washed hands. Thus, proper **hygiene** is one of the keys to preventing *Salmonella* food poisoning.

The food poisoning caused by *Salmonella* is one of about ten bacterial causes of food poisoning. Other involved bacteria are *Staphylococcus aureus*, *Clostridium perfringens*, *Vibrio parahaemolyticus*, and certain types of ***Escherichia coli***. Between 24 and 81 million cases of food borne diarrhea due to *Salmonella* and other bacteria occur in the United States each year. The economic cost of the illnesses is between 5 and 17 billion dollars.

Poultry, eggs, red meat, diary products, processed meats, cream-based desserts, and salad-type sandwich filling (such as tuna salad or chicken salad) are prime targets for colonization by species of *Salmonella*. The high protein content of the foodstuffs seems to be one of the reasons for their susceptibility. **Contamination** is especially facilitated if improperly cooked or raw food is held at an improper storage temperature, for example at room temperature. Proper cooking and storage temperatures will prevent contamination, as **Salmonella** is destroyed at cooking temperatures above 150° F (65.5 °C) and will not grow at refrigeration temperatures (less than 40°F, or 4.4°C). Also, contamination can result if the food is brought into contact with contaminated surfaces or utensils.

The vulnerable foods offer *Salmonella* a ready source of nutrients and moisture. If the temperature conditions are right for growth, the increase in numbers of *Salmonella* can be explosive. For example, from a starting population of a single live bacterium with a division time of 30 minutes, a population of over 500 million bacteria can be generated in just 15 hours.

The ingestion of contaminated foods leads, within hours, to the development of one or all of the following ailments: stomach cramps, vomiting, fever, headache, chills, sweating, fatigue, loss of appetite, and watery or bloody diarrhea. Prolonged diarrhea is dangerous, as the body can be depleted of fluids and salts that are vital for the proper functioning of organs and tissues. The resulting shock to the body can be intolerably lethal to infants and the elderly. As well, there is a possibility that the bacteria can spread from the intestinal tract to the bloodstream, leading to infections in other parts of the body.

There are hundreds are different forms, or strains, of *Salmonella*, varying in the antigenic composition of their outer surface and in the maladies caused. Concerning food poisoning, *Salmonella enteriditis* is of particular concern. This strain causes **gastroenteritis** and other maladies because of several so-called virulence factors the organism is armed with.

One virulence factor is called adhesin. An adhesin is a molecule that functions in the recognition and adhesion of the bacterium to a receptor on the surface of a host cell. In the case of *Salmonella,* the tube-like structures called fimbriae can perform this function. Other molecules on the surface of the bacterium can be involved also.

Another virulence factor is a compound called lipopolysaccharide (LPS for short). Depending on the structure, LPS can help shield the *Salmonella* surface from host antibacterial compounds. As well, part of the LPS, can lipid A, can be toxic to the host. The lipid A toxic component is also referred to as endotoxin. Salmonella also produces another toxin called **enterotoxin**. Other bacteria produce enterotoxin as well. The *Salmonella* enterotoxin is readily degraded by heat, so proper cooking of food will destroy the activity of the toxin. The enterotoxin remains inside the bacteria, so the toxin concentration increases with the increase in bacterial numbers.

Salmonella is not particularly difficult to identify, as it produces distinctive visual reactions on standard laboratory growth media. For example, on bismuth sulfide media the bacteria produce hydrogen sulfide, which produces jet-black colonies. Unfortunately for the individual who experiences a food poisoning event, the diagnosis is always "after the fact." Knowledge of the cause often comes after the miseries of the poisoning have come and gone. But, in those instances where the spread of the bacteria beyond the gastrointestinal tract has occurred, diagnosis is helpful to treat the infection.

The prospects of eliminating of *Salmonella* food poisoning using **vaccination** are being explored. The most promising route is to block the adhesion of the bacteria to host epithelial cells of the intestinal tract. Such a strategy would require the development of a **vaccine** with long lasting **immunity**. However, vaccine development efforts will likely be devoted to other illnesses. For the foreseeable future, the best strategy in preventing *Salmonella* food poisoning will remain the proper cooking of foods and the observance of good hygiene practices when handling food.

See also Food preservation

SCANNING ELECTRON MICROSCOPE · *see*

ELECTRON MICROSCOPE, TRANSMISSION AND SCANNING

SCHICK, BELA (1877-1967)

Hungarian-born American physician

Bela Schick was a pioneer in the field of child care; not only did he invent the **diphtheria** test, which helped wipe out this disease in children, but he also formulated and publicized child care theories that were advanced for his day. Schick also defined the allergic reaction, was considered the leading pediatrician of his time, and made contributions to knowledge about scarlet fever, **tuberculosis**, and infant nutrition. Schick received many honors for his work, including the Medal of the New York Academy of Medicine and the Addingham Gold Medal, a British award. Schick was also the founder of the American Academy of Pediatrics.

Schick was born on July 16, 1877 in Boglar, Hungary, the child of Jacob Schick, a grain merchant, and Johanna Pichler Schick. He attended the Staats Gymnasium in Graz, Austria, graduating in 1894. He then received his M.D. degree at Karl Franz University, also in Graz. After a stint with the medical corps in the Austro-Hungarian army, Schick started his own medical practice in Vienna in 1902. From then on he devoted his ample energies to teaching, research, and medical practice at the University of Vienna, where he served from 1902 to 1923—first as an intern, then as an assistant in the pediatrics clinic, and finally as lecturer and professor of pediatrics.

It was in 1905 that Schick made one of his most significant contributions. While working with collaborator Clemens von Pirquet, Schick wrote his first research study describing the phenomenon of allergy, which was then called serum sickness. The study not only described the concept of allergy, but also recommended methods of treatment.

At age 36, Schick moved on to make one of the most important discoveries of the twentieth century—the test for diphtheria. The test, announced in 1913, was a remarkably simple one that could tell whether a person was vulnerable to the disease. It showed whether a patient had already been exposed to the diphtheria toxin, which would make him immune from getting it again. A tiny amount of the diluted toxin was injected into the patient's arm. If the spot turned red and swollen, the doctors would know whether or not the patient been exposed to the disease. The treatment was then injection with an antitoxin.

Diphtheria was a common disease in the early twentieth century and afflicted thousands of children in every city throughout the world. It was especially common in Europe, where the close quarters of many cities made infection more likely. At the time Schick embarked on his research, scientists had already isolated the microbe or toxin that caused diphtheria. A horse serum had also been developed that could prevent or even cure the disease. But the serum had so many side effects that doctors were unwilling to prescribe it unless they knew a patient was seriously in danger of catching diphtheria. Thus, Schick's discovery made it easier for them to treat those who were the most vulnerable.

In 1923, an antitoxin without side effects was developed and was then given to babies during their first year of life. Later on, the Schick test would show whether **immunity** persisted. Schick's test technique was also used years later to treat people with **allergies**, using the same technique of injecting small doses of an antitoxin.

Schick left Vienna in 1923 to become pediatrician-in-chief at Mt. Sinai Hospital in New York City. Schick became an American citizen that same year and two years later married his wife, Catherine C. Fries. He held his post at Mt. Sinai Hospital until his retirement in May 1943, when he became a consulting pediatrician. During his career, he also worked simultaneously at other hospitals, acting as director of pediatrics at Sea View Hospital in Staten Island, New York and consulting pediatrician at the Willard Parker Hospital, the New York Infirmary for Women and Children, and Beth Israel Hospital. He also taught as a professor of the diseases of children at Columbia University College of Physicians and Surgeons, starting in 1936.

Schick directed a private practice in New York City as well. His office held a collection of dolls and animals that he had acquired in travels throughout the world. He would often play the piano in his office, or take out one of his doll or animal figures to calm a child. He never displayed a stethoscope until he made sure a child was relaxed. At one time, he estimated that he had treated over a million children.

Childless himself, he had a great fondness for children and in 1932 authored a popular book titled *Child Care Today* that contained his firm beliefs about how children should be raised. Many of his ideas were advanced for his time. He advocated little punishment for children and no corporal punishment. He also said that trauma in a child's early life often had a lasting effect.

Schick and his wife lived in a large apartment in New York City and were frequent travelers around the world. On a cruise to South America with his wife during his later years, Schick fell ill with pleurisy. Eventually brought back to the United States to Mt. Sinai Hospital, he died on Dec. 6, 1967.

See also Allergies; History of immunology; History of microbiology; History of public health; Immune system; Immunology; Medical training and careers in microbiology

SCID · *see* SEVERE COMBINED IMMUNODEFICIENCY (SCID)

SECONDARY IMMUNE RESPONSE · *see*
IMMUNITY, ACTIVE, PASSIVE, AND DELAYED

SELECTION

Evolutionary selection pressures act on all living organisms, regardless whether they are prokaryotic or higher **eukaryotes**. Selection refers to an evolutionary pressure that is the result of a combination of environmental and genetic pressures that affect the ability of an organism to live and, equally importantly, to produce reproductively successful offspring (including prokaryotic strains of cells).

As implied, natural selection involves the natural (but often complex) pressures present in an organism's environment. Artificial selection is the conscious manipulation of mating, manipulation, and fusion of genetic material to produce a desired result.

Evolution requires genetic variation, and these variations or changes (**mutations**) are usually deleterious because environmental factors already support the extent genetic distribution within a population.

Natural selection is based upon expressed differences in the ability of organisms to thrive and produce biologically successful offspring. Importantly, selection can only act to exert influence (drive) on those differences in **genotype** that appear as phenotypic differences. In a very real sense, evolutionary pressures act blindly.

There are three basic types of natural selection: directional selection favoring an extreme **phenotype**; stabilizing selection favoring a **phenotype** with characteristics intermediate to an extreme phenotype (i.e., normalizing selection); and disruptive selection that favors extreme phenotypes over intermediate genotypes.

The evolution of pesticide resistance provides a vivid example of directional selection, wherein the selective agent (in this case DDT) creates an apparent force in one direction, producing a corresponding change (improved resistance) in the affected organisms. Directional selection is also evident in the efforts of human beings to produce desired traits in many organisms ranging from **bacteria** to plants and animals.

Not all selective effects are directional, however. Selection can also produce results that are stabilizing or disruptive. Stabilizing selection occurs when significant changes in the traits of organisms are selected against. An example of this is birth weight in humans. Babies that are much heavier or lighter than average do not survive as well as those that are nearer the mean (average) weight.

On the other hand, selection is said to be disruptive if the extremes of some trait become favored over the intermediate values. Although not a factor for **microorganisms**, sexual selection and sexual dimorphism can influence the immunologic traits and capacity of a population.

Sometimes the fitness of a phenotype in some environment depends on how common (or rare) it is; this is known as frequency-dependent selection. Perhaps an animal enjoys an increased advantage if it conforms to the majority phenotype in the population. Conversely, a phenotype could be favored if it is rare, and its alternatives are in the majority. Frequency-dependent selection provides an interesting case in which the **gene** frequency itself alters the selective environment in which the genotype exists.

Many people attribute the phrase "survival of the fittest" to Darwin, but in fact, it originated from another naturalist/philosopher, Herbert Spencer (1820–1903). Recently, many recent evolutionary biologists have asked: Survival of the fittest what? At what organismal level is selection most powerful? What is the biological unit of natural selection-the species, the individual, or even the gene?

Selection can provide interesting consequences for bacteria and **viruses**. For example, reduced virulence in **parasites**, who depend on the survival of their hosts for their own survival may increase the reproductive success of the invading parasite. The *myxoma* virus, introduced in Australia to control imported European rabbits (*Oryctolagus cuniculus*), at first caused the deaths of many individuals. However, within a few years, the mortality rate was much lower, partly because the rabbits became resistant to the pathogen, but also partly because the virus had evolved a lower virulence. The reduction in the virulence is thought to have been aided because the virus is transmitted by a mosquito, from one living rabbit to another. The less deadly viral strain is maintained in the rabbit host population because rabbits afflicted with the more virulent strain would die before passing on the virus. Thus, the viral genes for reduced virulence could spread by group selection. Of course, reduced virulence is also in the interest of every individual virus, if it is to persist in its host. Scientists argue that one would not expect to observe evolution by group selection when individual selection is acting strongly in an opposing direction.

Some biologists, most notably Richard Dawkins (1941–), have argued that the gene itself is the true unit of selection. If one genetic alternative, or allele, provides its bearer with an adaptive advantage over some other individual who carries a different allele then the more beneficial allele will be replicated more times, as its bearer enjoys greater fitness. In his book *The Selfish Gene*, Dawkins argues that genes help to build the bodies that aid in their transmission; individual organisms are merely the "survival machines" that genes require to make more copies of themselves.

This argument has been criticized because natural selection cannot "see" the individual genes that reside in an organism's genome, but rather selects among phenotypes, the outward manifestation of all the genes that organisms possess. Some genetic combinations may confer very high fitness, but they may reside with genes having negative effects in the same individual. When an individual reproduces, its "bad" genes are replicated along with its "good" genes; if it fails to do so, even its most advantageous genes will not be transmitted into the next generation. Although the focus among most evolutionary biologists has been on selection at the level of the individual, this example raises the possibility that individual genes in genomes are under a kind of group selection. The success of single genes in being transmitted to subsequent generations will depend on their functioning well together, collectively building the best possible organism in a given environment.

When selective change is brought about by human effort, it is known as artificial selection. By allowing only a selected minority of individuals or specimen to reproduce, breeders can produce new generations of organisms (e.g. a particular virus or bacterium) that feature desired traits.

See also Epidemiology; Evolution and evolutionary mechanisms; Evolutionary origin of bacteria and viruses; Rare genotype advantage

SELECTIVE MEDIA · *see* GROWTH AND GROWTH MEDIA

SEM · *see* ELECTRON MICROSCOPE, TRANSMISSION AND SCANNING

SEMMELWEIS, IGNAZ PHILIPP (1818-1865)
Hungarian physician

Along with American physician Oliver Wendell Holmes (1809–1894), Ignaz Semmelweis was one of the first two doctors worldwide to recognize the contagious nature of puerperal fever and promote steps to eliminate it, thereby dramatically reducing maternal deaths.

Semmelweis was born in Ofen, or Tabàn, then near Buda, now part of Budapest, Hungary, on July 1, 1818, the son of a Roman Catholic shopkeeper of German descent. After graduating from the Catholic Gymnasium of Buda in 1835 and the University of Pest in 1837, he went to the University of Vienna to study law, but immediately switched to medicine. He studied at Vienna until 1839, then again at Pest until 1841, then again at Vienna, earning his M.D. in 1844. Among his teachers were Karl von Rokitansky (1804–1878), Josef Skoda (1805–1881), and Ferdinand von Hebra (1816–1880). He did postgraduate work in Vienna hospitals in obstetrics, surgery, and, under Skoda, diagnostic methods. In 1846, he became assistant physician, tantamount to senior resident, at the obstetrical clinic of the Vienna General Hospital.

In the mid-nineteenth century, the maternal death rate for hospital births attended by physicians was much higher than for either home births or births attended by midwives. The principal killer was puerperal fever, or childbed fever, whose etiology was then unknown, but which **Louis Pasteur** (1822–1895) learned in 1879 was caused by a streptococcal infection of the open wound at the site of the placenta in women who had recently given birth. The infection could remain topical or it could pass through the uterus into the bloodstream and quickly become fatal. Before Semmelweis and Holmes, physicians generally assumed that puerperal fever was an unpreventable and natural consequence of some childbirths, and accepted the terrifying mortality statistics.

Witnessing so many healthy young mothers sicken and die greatly affected Semmelweis, and he grew determined to discover the cause and prevention of puerperal fever. Using Rokitanksy's pathological methods, he began a comparative study of autopsies of puerperal fever victims. The breakthrough came when his fellow physician, Jakob Kolletschka (1803–1847), died of blood poisoning after cutting his finger while performing an autopsy. Semmelweis noticed that the pathological features of the autopsy on Kolletschka's body matched those of the autopsies of the puerperal fever victims. Semmelweis then only suspected, and did not prove, that the fever was a septicemia, an intrusion of **microorganisms** from a local infection into the bloodstream, but he instantly took action. In May 1847, he ordered all personnel under his authority to wash their hands between patients. This was a novel, radical, and unpopular rule, but in just a month the maternal death rate at the Vienna General Hospital dropped from twelve to two percent.

Even though Semmelweis had solid results and statistics on his side, many physicians simply refused to believe that washing their hands, which they considered undignified, could save lives. Resistance to his rule stiffened. Semmelweis made many powerful enemies, and in March 1849, he was demoted from his supervisory role. He served at St. Rochus Hospital in Pest from 1851 to 1857, but never achieved his former professional status.

Holmes was facing a similar crisis in America. In 1843, Holmes first claimed in print that puerperal fever was contagious. Semmelweis first published his findings in 1848. Now having heard of Semmelweis, Holmes in 1855, expanded his original article into a small book that explicitly praised Semmelweis. Likewise, having now heard of Holmes, Semmelweis published *Die Aetiologie, der Begriff, und die Prophylaxis des Kindbettfiebers* [The Etiology, Concept, and Prophylaxis of Childbed Fever] in 1861. The book was not well received. Semmelweis was a poor prose stylist, and his lack of writing skill adversely affected his campaign. Holmes, on the other hand, an accomplished essayist and poet as well as a first-rate physician, proved more persuasive, although it would still be thirty years before sanitary and hygienic methods became standard in American and European hospitals.

While no one ridiculed Holmes, who had enough charm and grace to forestall such attacks, Semmelweis became subject of mockery in the central European medical community. In 1863, the frustration he had long felt finally took its toll on his spirit. He became chronically depressed, unpredictably angry, socially withdrawn, and increasingly bitter. In July 1865, a coalition of colleagues, friends, and relatives committed him to the Niederösterreichische Heil-und Pflegeanstalt, an insane asylum in Döbling, near Vienna. He died there a month later, on August 13, 1865, from bacteremia due to an infected cut on his finger, with symptoms markedly akin to those of puerperal fever.

See also Bacteria and bacterial infection; Contamination, bacterial and viral; Germ theory of disease; Hygiene; Infection control; Streptococci and streptococcal infections; Transmission of pathogens; Viruses and responses to viral infection

SERILITY • *see* REPRODUCTIVE IMMUNOLOGY

SEROCONVERSION

Seroconversion is a term that refers to the development in the blood of antibodies to an infectious organism or agent. Typically, seroconversion is associated with infections caused by **bacteria**, **viruses**, and protozoans. But seroconversion also occurs after the deliberate inoculation with an **antigen** in the process of **vaccination**. In the case of infections, the development of detectable levels of antibodies can occur quickly, in the case of an active infection, or can be prolonged, in the case of a latent infection. Seroconversion typically heralds the development of the symptoms of the particular infection.

The phenomenon of seroconversion can be important in diagnosing infections that are caused by latent viruses. Examples of viruses include **hepatitis** B and C viruses, the Epstein Barr virus, and the **Human Immunodeficiency Virus** (**HIV**). When these viruses first infect people, the viral nucleic acid can become incorporated into the genome of the host. As a result, there will not be an immune response mounted against the virus. However, once viral replication has commenced antibodies to viral proteins can accumulate to detectable levels in the serum.

Seroconversion is am important aspect of Acquired **Immunodeficiency** Syndrome (**AIDS**). Antibodies to HIV can sometimes be detected shortly after infection with the virus, and before the virus becomes latent. Symptoms of infection at this stage are similar to the flu, and disappear quickly, so treatment is often not sought. If, however, diagnosis is made at this stage, based on presence of HIV antibodies, then treatment can begin immediately. This can be important to the future outlook of the patient, because often at this stage of the infection the **immune system** is relatively undamaged. If seroconversion occurs following activation of the latent virus, then immune destruction may already be advanced.

The presence of antibodies in the serum occurs much earlier in the case of infections that occur very soon after the introduction of the infectious microorganism. The type of **antibody** present can be used in the diagnosis of the infection. Additionally, seroconversion in the presence of symptoms but in the absence of detectable **microorganisms** (particularly bacteria) can be a hallmark of a chronic infection caused by the adherent bacterial populations known as biofilms. Again, the nature of the antibodies can help alert a physician to the presence of a hitherto undetected **bacterial infection**, and treatment can be started.

See also Antibiotic resistance, tests for; Antibody and antigen; Antibody-antigen, biochemical and molecular reactions; Antibody formation and kinetics; Immunity, active, passive and delayed; Immunochemistry; Immunodeficiency disease syndromes; Serology

SEROLOGY

Serology is the study of antigen-antibody reactions outside of a living organism (i.e., *in vitro*, in a laboratory setting). The basis of serology is the recognition of an **antigen** by immune mechanisms, with the subsequent production of an **antibody**.

In medical terminology, serology refers to a blood test to detect the presence of antibodies against a microorganism. The detection of antibodies can be qualitative (i.e., determining whether the antibodies are present) or quantitative (i.e., determining the quantity of an antibody produced). Some **microorganisms** can stimulate the production of antibodies that persist in a person's blood for a long time. Thus, in a qualitative assay the detection of a particular antibody does not mean that the person has a current infection. However, it does mean that it is likely that at some time that person was infected with the particular microbial pathogen. Serology assays can be performed at various times and the level of antibody determined. If the antibody level rises, it usually is indicative of a response to an infection. The body produces elevated amounts of the antibody to help fight the challenging antigen.

Serology as a science began in 1901. Austrian American immunologist **Karl Landsteiner** (1868–1943) identified groups of red blood cells as A, B, and O. From that discovery came the recognition that cells of all types, including blood cells, cells of the body, and microorganisms carry proteins and other molecules on their surface that are recognized by cells of the **immune system**. There can be many different antigens on the surface of a microorganism, with many different antibodies being produced.

When the antigen and the antibody are in suspension together, they react together. The reaction can be a visible one, such as the formation of a precipitate made up of a complex of the antigen and the antibody. Other serology techniques are agglutination, complement-fixation and the detection of an antigen by the use of antibodies that have been complexed with a fluorescent compound.

Serological techniques are used in basic research, for example, to decipher the response of immune systems and to detect the presence of a specific target molecule. In the clinical setting, serology is used to confirm infections and to type the blood from a patient. Serology has also proven to be very useful in the area of forensics, where blood typing can be vital to establishing the guilt or innocence of a suspect, or the identity of a victim.

See also Antibody and antigen; Antibody formation and kinetics; Antibody-antigen, biochemical and molecular reactions; Bacteria and bacterial infection; Immune system; Laboratory techniques in immunology

SESSILE BACTERIA • *see* BIOFILM FORMATION AND DYNAMIC BEHAVIOR

SEVERE COMBINED IMMUNODEFICIENCY (SCID)

Severe combined **immunodeficiency** (SCID) is a rare genetic disease that is actually a group of inherited disorders charac-

terized by a lack of immune response, usually occurring in infants less than six months old. SCID is the result of a combination of defects of both **T-lymphocytes** and B-lymphocytes. Lymphocytes are white blood cells that are made in bone marrow, and many move to the thymus gland where they become specialized immune T and **B cells**. In healthy individuals, **T cells** attack antigens while B cells make plasma cells that produce antibodies (**immunoglobulins**). However, this immune response in SCID patients is absent making them very susceptible to invading diseases, and thus children with untreated SCID rarely live to the age of two years.

SCID is characterized by three main features. The helper T-lymphocytes are functioning poorly or are absent, the thymus gland may be small and functioning poorly or is absent, and the stem cells in bone marrow, from which mature T- and B-lymphocytes arise, are absent or defective in their function. In all of these situations, little or no antibodies are produced. If, for example, T-lymphocytes are never fully developed, then the **immune system** can never function normally. Moreover, the results of these defects include the following: impairment of normal functioning T- and B-lymphocytes, negative effects on the maturation process for T-helper and T-suppressor cells, and elimination and damage of the original source of the lymphocytes.

The immune disorders characterized in SCID arise because of the inheritance of abnormal genes from one or both parents. The most common form of SCID is linked to the X chromosome inherited from the mother; this makes SCID more common among males. The second most common defect is caused by the inheritance of both parents' abnormally inactive genes governing the production of a particular enzyme that is needed for the development of **immunity**, called adenosine deaminase (ADA). Although many defective genes for other forms of SCID have been identified in the last few years, scientists do not fully understand all of the forms of the disease.

There are many specific clinical signs that are associated with SCID. After birth, an infant with SCID is initially protected by the temporarily active maternal immune cells; however, as the child ages, his or her immune system fails to take over as the maternal cells become inactive. Pulmonary problems such as **pneumonia**, non-productive coughs, **inflammation** around the bronchial tubes, and low alveolar oxygen levels can affect the diseased infant repetitively. Chronic diarrhea is not uncommon, and can lead to severe weight loss, malnutrition, and other gastrointestinal problem. Infants with the disease have an unusual number of bacterial, fungal, viral, or protozoal infections that are much more resistant to treatment than in healthy children. Mouth **thrush** and **yeast** infections, both fungal, appear in SCID patients and are very resistant to treatment. Additionally, chronic bacterial and fungal **skin infections** and several abnormalities of the blood cells can persist.

Severe combined immunodeficiency is a disease that can be successfully treated if it is identified early. The most effective treatment has been hematopoietic stem cell transplants that are best done with the bone marrow of a sister or brother; however, the parent's marrow is acceptable if the infant is less than three months old. Early treatment can also help to avoid pre-transplant **chemotherapy** often necessary to prevent rejection of the marrow in older children. This is especially advantageous because chemotherapy can leave the patient even more susceptible to invading bodies. When successful, treatment for SCID corrects the patient's immune system defect, and as of 2002 success rates have been shown to be nearly 80% for the bone marrow transplant.

Gene therapy is the subject of ongoing research, and shows promise as a treatment for SCID. Researchers remove T cells of SCID patients and expose those cells to the ADA gene for ten days, and then return the cells intravenously. Although it was successful in one case, this treatment of SCID is still very much in the experimental stage. Nevertheless, these and other treatments hold potential for the development of a cure for SCID.

See also Immune system; Immunochemistry; Immunodeficiency disease syndromes; Immunodeficiency diseases; Immunogenetics; Immunoglobulins and immunoglobulin deficiency syndromes; Immunological analysis techniques; Immunology

SEXUALLY TRANSMITTED DISEASES (STDS)

Sexually transmitted diseases (STDs) vary in their susceptibility to treatment, their signs and symptoms, and the consequences if they are left untreated. Some are caused by **bacteria**. These usually can be treated and cured. Others are caused by **viruses** and can typically be treated but not cured. As of June 2002, recent advancements in diagnosis now allow the identification of more than 15 million new cases of STD in the United States each year.

Long known as venereal disease, after Venus, the Roman goddess of love, sexually transmitted diseases are increasingly common. The more than 20 known sexually transmitted diseases range from the life-threatening to painful and unsightly. The life-threatening sexually transmitted diseases include **syphilis**, which has been known for centuries, some forms of **hepatitis**, and Acquired Immune Deficiency Syndrome (**AIDS**), which was first identified in 1981.

Most sexually transmitted diseases can be treated successfully, although untreated sexually transmitted diseases remain a huge **public health** problem. Untreated sexually transmitted diseases can cause everything from blindness to infertility. While AIDS is the most widely publicized sexually transmitted disease, others are more common. More than 13 million Americans of all backgrounds and economic levels develop sexually transmitted diseases every year. Prevention efforts focus on teaching the physical signs of sexually transmitted diseases, instructing individuals on how to avoid exposure, and emphasizing the need for regular check-ups.

The history of sexually transmitted disease is controversial. Some historians argue that syphilis emerged as a new disease in the fifteenth century. Others cite Biblical and other ancient texts as proof that syphilis and perhaps **gonorrhea** were ancient as well as contemporary burdens. The dispute can best be understood with some knowledge of the elusive nature of gonorrhea and syphilis, called "the great imitator" by the eminent physician William Osler (1849–1919).

No laboratory tests existed to diagnose gonorrhea and syphilis until the late nineteenth and early twentieth centuries. This means that early clinicians based their diagnosis exclusively on symptoms, all of which could be present in other illnesses. Symptoms of syphilis during the first two of its three stages include chancre sores, skin rash, fever, fatigue, headache, sore throat, and swollen glands. Likewise, many other diseases have the potential to cause the dire consequences of late-stage syphilis. These range from blindness to mental illness to heart disease to death. Diagnosis of syphilis before laboratory tests were developed was complicated by the fact that most symptoms disappear during the third stage of the disease.

Symptoms of gonorrhea may also be elusive, particularly in women. Men have the most obvious symptoms, with **inflammation** and discharge from the penis from two to ten days after infection. Symptoms in women include a painful sensation while urinating or abdominal pain. However, women may be infected for months without showing any symptoms. Untreated gonorrhea can cause infertility in women and blindness in infants born to women with the disease.

The nonspecific nature of many symptoms linked to syphilis and gonorrhea means that historical references to sexually transmitted disease are open to different interpretations. There is also evidence that sexually transmitted disease was present in ancient China.

During the Renaissance, syphilis became a common and deadly disease in Europe. It is unclear whether new, more dangerous strains of syphilis were introduced or whether the syphilis which emerged at that time was, indeed, a new illness. Historians have proposed many arguments to explain the dramatic increase in syphilis during the era. One argument suggests that Columbus and other explorers of the New World carried syphilis back to Europe. In 1539, the Spanish physician Rodrigo Ruiz Diaz de Isla treated members of the crew of Columbus for a peculiar disease marked by eruptions on the skin. Other contemporary accounts tell of **epidemics** of syphilis across Europe in 1495.

The abundance of syphilis during the Renaissance made the disease a central element of the dynamic **culture** of the period. The poet John Donne (1572-1631) was one of many thinkers of that era who saw sexually transmitted disease as a consequence of man's weakness. Shakespeare (1564-1616) also wrote about syphilis, using it as a curse in some plays and referring to the "tub of infamy," a nickname for a common medical treatment for syphilis. The treatment involved placing syphilitic individuals in a tub where they received mercury rubs. Mercury, which is now known to be a toxic chemical, did not cure syphilis, but is thought to have helped relieve some symptoms. Other treatments for syphilis included the induction of fever and the use of purgatives to flush the system.

The sculptor Benvenuto Cellini (1500–1571) is one of many individuals who wrote about their own syphilis during the era: "The French disease, for it was that, remained in me more than four months dormant before it showed itself." Cellini's reference to syphilis as the "French disease" was typical of Italians at the time and reflects a worldwide eagerness to place the origin of syphilis far away from one's own home. The French, for their part, called it the "Neapolitan disease," and the Japanese called it the "Portuguese disease." The name syphilis was bestowed on the disease by the Italian Girolamo Fracastoro (1478–1553), a poet, physician, and scientist. Fracastoro created an allegorical story about syphilis in 1530 entitled "Syphilis, or the French Disease." The story proposed that syphilis developed on Earth after a shepherd named Syphilis foolishly cursed at the Sun. The angry Sun retaliated with a disease that took its name from the foolish shepherd, who was the first individual to get sick.

For years, medical experts used syphilis as a catch-all diagnosis for sexually transmitted disease. Physicians assumed that syphilis and gonorrhea were the same thing until 1837, when Philippe Ricord (1800–1889) reported that syphilis and gonorrhea were separate illnesses. The late nineteenth and early twentieth centuries saw major breakthroughs in the understanding of syphilis and gonorrhea. In 1879, Albert Neisser (1855–1916) discovered that gonorrhea was caused by a bacillus, which has since been named *Neisseria gonorrhoeae*. Fritz Richard Schaudinn (1871–1906) and Paul Erich Hoffmann (1868–1959) identified a special type of spirochete bacteria, now known as Treponema pallidum, as the cause of syphilis in 1905.

Further advances occurred quickly. August von Wassermann (1866–1925) developed a blood test for syphilis in 1906, making testing for syphilis a simple procedure for the first time. Just four years later in 1910, the first effective therapy for syphilis was introduced in the form of Salvarsan, an organic arsenical compound. The compound was one of many effective compounds introduced by the German physician **Paul Ehrlich** (1854–1915), whose argument that specific drugs could be effective against **microorganisms** has proven correct. The drug is effective against syphilis, but it is toxic and even fatal to some patients.

The development of Salvarsan offered hope for individuals with syphilis, but there was little public understanding about how syphilis was transmitted in the early twentieth century. In the United States, this stemmed in part from government enforcement of laws prohibiting public discussion of certain types of sexual information. One popular account of syphilis from 1915 erroneously warned that one could develop syphilis after contact with whistles, pens, pencils, toilets, and toothbrushes.

In a tragic chapter in American history, some members of the U.S. Public Health Service exploited the ignorance of the disease among the general public as late as the mid-twentieth century in order to study the ravages of untreated syphilis. The Tuskegee Syphilis Study was launched in 1932 by the U.S. Public Health Service. The almost 400 black men who participated in the study were promised free medical care and burial money. Although effective treatments had been available for decades, researchers withheld treatment, even when **penicillin** became available in 1943, and carefully observed the unchecked progress of symptoms. Many of the

participants fathered children with congenital syphilis, and many died. The study was finally exposed in the media in the early 1970s. When the activities of the study were revealed, a series of new regulations governing human experimentation were passed by the government.

A more public discussion of sexually transmitted disease was conducted by the military during World Wars I and II. During both wars, the military conducted aggressive public information campaigns to limit sexually transmitted disease among the armed forces. One poster from World War II showed a grinning skull on a woman dressed in an evening gown striding along with German Chancellor Führer Adolf Hitler and Japanese Emperor Hirohito. The poster's caption reads "V.D. Worst of the Three," suggesting that venereal disease could destroy American troops faster than either of America's declared enemies.

Concern about the human cost of sexually transmitted disease helped make the production of the new drug penicillin a wartime priority. Arthur Fleming (1881–1955), who is credited with the discovery of penicillin, first observed in 1928 that the penicillium **mold** was capable of killing bacteria in the laboratory; however, the mold was unstable and difficult to produce. Penicillin was not ready for general use or general clinical testing until after Howard Florey (1898–1968) and **Ernst Boris Chain** (1906–1979) developed ways to purify and produce a consistent substance.

The introduction of penicillin for widespread use in 1943 completed the **transformation** of syphilis from a life–threatening disease to one that could be treated relatively easily and quickly. United States rates of cure were 90–97% for syphilis by 1944, one year after penicillin was first distributed in the country. Death rates dropped dramatically. In 1940, 10.7 out of every 100,000 people died of syphilis. By 1970, it was 0.2 per 100,000.

Such progress infused the medical community with optimism. A 1951 article in the American Journal of Syphilis asked, "Are Venereal Diseases Disappearing?" By 1958, the number of cases of syphilis had dropped to 113,884 from 575,593 in 1943, the year penicillin was introduced.

Venereal disease was not eliminated, and sexually transmitted diseases continue to ravage Americans and others in the 1990s. Though penicillin has lived up to its early promise as an effective treatment for syphilis, the number of cases of syphilis has increased since 1956. In addition, millions of Americans suffer from other sexually transmitted diseases, many of which were not known a century or more ago, such as Acquired Immune Deficiency Syndrome (AIDS) caused by the **HIV** virus. By the 1990s, sexually transmitted diseases were among the most common infectious diseases in the United States.

Some sexually transmitted diseases are seen as growing at epidemic rates. For example, syphilis, gonorrhea, and chancroid, which are uncommon in Europe, Japan and Australia, have increased at epidemic rates among certain urban minority populations. A 1990 study found the rate of syphilis was more than four times higher among blacks than among whites. The Public Health Service reports that as many as 30 million Americans have been affected by genital **herpes**. Experts have also noted that sexually transmitted disease appears to increase in areas where AIDS is common.

Shifting sexual and marital habits are two factors behind the growth in sexually transmitted disease. Americans are more likely to have sex at an earlier age than they did in years past. They also marry later in life than Americans did two to three decades ago, and their marriages are more likely to end in divorce. These factors make Americans more likely to have many sexual partners over the course of their lives, placing them at greater risk of sexually transmitted disease.

Public health officials report that fear and embarrassment continue to limit the number of people willing to report signs of sexually transmitted disease.

All sexually transmitted diseases have certain elements in common. They are most prevalent among teenagers and young adults, with nearly 66% occurring in people under 25. In addition, most can be transmitted in ways other than through sexual relations. For example, AIDS and Hepatitis B can be transmitted through contact with tainted blood, but they are primarily transmitted sexually. In general, sexual contact should be avoided if there are visible sores, warts, or other signs of disease in the genital area. The risk of developing most sexually transmitted diseases is reduced by using condoms and limiting sexual contact—but can only be reduced to zero by having monogamous (one partner) sexual relations between partners who are free of disease or vectors of disease (e.g., the HIV virus).

Bacterial sexually transmitted diseases include syphilis, gonorrhea, chlamydia, and chancroid. Syphilis is less common than many other sexually transmitted diseases in the Unites States, with 134,000 cases in 1990. The disease is thought to be more difficult to transmit than many other sexually transmitted diseases. Sexual partners of an individual with syphilis have about a 10% chance of developing syphilis after one sexual contact, but the disease has come under increasing scrutiny as researchers have realized how easily the HIV virus which causes AIDS can be spread through open syphilitic chancre sores.

Gonorrhea is far more common than syphilis, with approximately 750,000 cases of gonorrhea reported annually in the United States. The gonococcus bacterium is considered highly contagious. Public health officials suggest that all individuals with more than one sexual partner should be tested regularly for gonorrhea. Penicillin is no longer the treatment of choice for gonorrhea, because of the numerous strains of gonorrhea that are resistant to penicillin. Newer strains of **antibiotics** have proven to be more effective. Gonorrhea infection overall has diminished in the United States, but the incidence of gonorrhea among certain populations (e.g., African-Americans) has increased.

Chlamydia infection is considered the most common sexually transmitted disease in the United States. About four million new cases of chlamydia infection are reported every year. The infection is caused by the bacterium Chlamydia trachomatis. Symptoms of chlamydia are similar to symptoms of gonorrhea, and the disease often occurs at the same time as gonorrhea. Men and women may have pain during urination or notice an unusual genital discharge one to three weeks after

exposure. However, many individuals, particularly women, have no symptoms until complications develop.

Complications resulting from untreated chlamydia occur when the bacteria has a chance to travel in the body. Chlamydia can result in pelvic inflammatory disease in women, a condition which occurs when the infection travels up the uterus and fallopian tubes. This condition can lead to infertility. In men, the infection can lead to epididymitis, inflammation of the epididymis, a structure on the testes where spermatozoa are stored. This too can lead to infertility. Untreated chlamydia infection can cause eye infection or **pneumonia** in babies of mothers with the infection. Antibiotics are successful against chlamydia.

The progression of chancroid in the United States is a modern-day indicator of the migration of sexually transmitted disease. Chancroid, a **bacterial infection** caused by *Haemophilus ducreyi*, was common in Africa and rare in the United States until the 1980s. Beginning in the mid-1980s, there were outbreaks of chancroid in a number of large cities and migrant-labor communities in the United States. The number of chancroid cases increased dramatically during the last two decades of the twentieth century.

In men, who are most likely to develop chancroid, the disease is characterized by painful open sores and swollen lymph nodes in the groin. The sores are generally softer than the harder chancre seen in syphilis. Women may also develop painful sores. They may feel pain urinating and may have bleeding or discharge in the rectal and vaginal areas. Chancroid can be treated effectively with antibiotics.

As of June 2002, there are no cures for the sexually transmitted diseases caused by viruses: AIDS, genital herpes, viral hepatitis, and genital warts. Treatment to reduce adverse symptoms is available for most of these diseases, but the virus cannot be eliminated from the body.

AIDS is the most life-threatening sexually transmitted disease, a disease which is usually fatal and for which there is no cure. The disease is caused by the **human immunodeficiency virus** (HIV), a virus which disables the **immune system**, making the body susceptible to injury or death from infection and certain cancers. HIV is a retrovirus which translates the **RNA** contained in the virus into **DNA**, the genetic information code contained in the human body. This DNA becomes a part of the human host cell. The fact that viruses become part of the human body makes them difficult to treat or eliminate without harming the patient.

HIV can remain dormant for years within the human body. More than 800,000 cases of AIDS have been reported in the United States **Centers for Disease Control** since the disease was first identified in 1981, and at least one million other Americans are believed to be infected with the HIV virus. Initial symptoms of AIDS include fever, headache, or enlarged lymph nodes. Later symptoms include energy loss, frequent fever, weight loss, or frequent **yeast** infections. HIV is transmitted most commonly through sexual contact or through use of contaminated needles or blood products. The disease is not spread through casual contact, such as the sharing of towels, bedding, swimming pools, or toilet seats.

Genital herpes is a widespread, recurrent, and incurable viral infection. Almost a million new cases are reported in the United States annually. The prevalence of herpes infection reflects the highly contagious nature of the virus. About 75% of the sexual partners of individuals with the infection develop genital herpes.

The herpes virus is common. Most individuals who are exposed to one of the two types of herpes simplex virus never develop any symptoms. In these cases, the herpes virus remains in certain nerve cells of the body, but does not cause any problems. Herpes simplex virus type 1 most frequently causes cold sores on the lips or mouth, but can also cause genital infections. Herpes simplex virus type 2 most commonly causes genital sores, though mouth sores can also occur due to this type of virus.

In genital herpes, the virus enters the skin or mucous membrane, travels to a group of nerves at the end of the spinal cord, and initiates a host of painful symptoms within about one week of exposure. These symptoms may include vaginal discharge, pain in the legs, and an itching or burning feeling. A few days later, sores appear at the infected area. Beginning as small red bumps, they can become open sores which eventually become crusted. These sores are typically painful and last an average of two weeks.

Following the initial outbreak, the virus waits in the nerve cells in an inactive state. A recurrence is created when the virus moves through the nervous system to the skin. There may be new sores or simply a shedding of virus which can infect a sexual partner. The number of times herpes recurs varies from individual to individual, ranging from several times a year to only once or twice in a lifetime. Occurrences of genital herpes may be shortened through use of an antiviral drug which limits the herpes virus's ability to reproduce itself.

Genital herpes is most dangerous to newborns born to pregnant women experiencing their first episode of the disease. Direct newborn contact with the virus increases the risk of neurological damage or death. To avoid exposure, physicians usually deliver babies using cesarean section if herpes lesions are present.

Hepatitis, an inflammation of the liver, is a complicated illness with many types. Millions of Americans develop hepatitis annually. The hepatitis A virus, one of four types of viral hepatitis, is most often spread by **contamination** of food or water. The hepatitis B virus is most often spread through sexual contact, through the sharing of intravenous drug needles, and from mother to child. Hospital workers who are exposed to blood and blood products are also at risk. Hepatitis C and Hepatitis D (less commonly) may also be spread through sexual contact.

A yellowing of the skin, or jaundice, is the best known symptom of hepatitis. Other symptoms include dark and foamy urine and abdominal pain. There is no cure for hepatitis, although prolonged rest usually enables individuals with the disease to recover completely.

Many people who develop hepatitis B become carriers of the virus for life. This means they can infect others and face a high risk of developing liver disease. There are as many as 350 million carriers worldwide, and about 1.5 million in the United States. A **vaccination** is available against hepatitis B.

The link between human papillomavirus, genital warts, and certain types of cancer has drawn attention to the potential risk of genital warts. There are more than 60 types of human papillomavirus. Many of these types can cause genital warts. In the United States, about 1 million new cases of genital warts are diagnosed every year.

Genital warts are very contagious, and about two-thirds of the individuals who have sexual contact with someone with genital warts develop the disease. There is also an association between human papillomavirus and cancer of the cervix, anus, penis, and vulva. This means that people who develop genital warts appear to be at a higher risk for these cancers and should have their health carefully watched. Contact with genital warts can also damage infants born to mothers with the problem.

Genital warts usually appear within three months of sexual contact. The warts can be removed in various ways, but the virus remains in the body. Once the warts are removed the chances of transmitting the disease are reduced.

Many questions persist concerning the control of sexually transmitted diseases. Experts have struggled for years with efforts to inform people about transmission and treatment of sexually transmitted disease. Frustration over the continuing increase in sexually transmitted disease is one factor which has fueled interest in potential vaccines against certain sexually transmitted diseases.

A worldwide research effort to develop a **vaccine** against AIDS has resulted in a series of vaccinations now in clinical trials. Efforts have focused in two areas, finding a vaccine to protect individuals against the HIV virus and finding a vaccine to prevent the progression of HIV to AIDS in individuals who already have been exposed to the virus. One of many challenges facing researchers has been the ability of the HIV virus to change, making efforts to develop a single vaccine against the virus futile.

Researchers also are searching for vaccines against syphilis and gonorrhea. Experiments conducted on prisoners more than 40 years ago proved that some individuals could develop **immunity** to syphilis after inoculation with live *Treponema pallidum*, but researchers have still not been able to develop a vaccine against syphilis which is safe and effective. In part this stems from the unusual nature of the syphilis bacteria, which remain potentially infectious even when its cells are killed. An effective gonorrhea vaccine has also eluded researchers.

Immunizations are available against Hepatitis A and Hepatitis B (Hepatitis D is prevented by the Hepatitis B vaccine). The virus that causes Hepatitis C, however, is able to change its form (mutate) quite rapidly, thereby hampering efforts to develop a vaccine against it.

Without vaccinations for most of the sexually transmitted diseases, health officials depend on public information campaigns to limit the growth of the diseases. Some critics have claimed that the increasing incidence of sexually transmitted diseases suggest that current techniques are failing. In other countries, however, the incidence of sexually transmitted disease has fallen during the same period it has risen in the

United States. For example, in Sweden the gonorrhea rate fell by more than 95% from 1970 to 1989 after vigorous government efforts to control sexually transmitted disease in Sweden.

Yet the role of government funding for community health clinics, birth control, and public information campaigns on sexually transmitted disease has long been controversial. Public officials continue to debate the wisdom of funding public distribution of condoms and other services that could affect the transmission of sexually transmitted disease. Although science has made great strides in understanding the causes and cures of many sexually transmitted diseases, society has yet to reach agreement on how best to attack them.

See also Bacteria and bacterial infection; Immunization; Immunogenetics; Public health, current issues; Virus replication; Viruses and responses to viral infection

SHEATHED BACTERIA

Sheathed **bacteria** are bacteria that grow as long filaments whose exterior is covered by a layer known as a sheath. Within the sheath, the bacteria can be capable of growth and division. Examples of sheathed bacteria include *Leptothrix discophora* (also known as "iron bacteria"), and *Sphaerotilus natans*.

Sheathed bacteria are common of the bacterial communities in water and in soil. In these environments, the sheath is often coated with precipitates of elements in the water or soil environments, such as oxides of iron and manganese. The elements are unstable in solution, and thus will readily come out of solution when presented with an appropriate site.

The sheath that covers the bacteria can be of varied construction. Much of the structural information has been gleaned from the observation of thin slices of sample using the transmission **electron microscope**. The sheath surrounding *Leptothrix* species is glycocalyx-like in appearance. Often the deposition of metals within the sheath network produces areas where the material has crystallized. In contrast, the sheath of *Sphaerotilus natans* presents the "railroad track" appearance, which is typical of a biological membrane consisting of two layers of lipid molecules.

Electron microscopic studies of *Leptothrix* species have shown that the bacterium is intimately connected with the overlying sheath. The connections consist of protuberances that are found all over the surface of the bacterium. In contrast, *Sphaerotilus natans* is not connected with the overlying sheath.

Both *Leptothrix* and *Sphaerotilus natans* can exist independently of the sheath. Bacteria in both genera have a life cycle that includes a free-swimming form (called a swarmer cell) that is not sheathed. The free-swimming forms have flagella at one end of the bacteria that propels the cells along. When encased in the sheath, the bacteria are referred to as sheathed or resting bacteria.

Bacterial sheaths tend to be manufactured when the bacteria are in an aquatic or soil environment that contains high amounts of organic matter. The sheath may serve to provide protection to the bacteria in these environments, Also, the ability of metallic compounds to precipitate on the sheath may pro-

vide the bacteria with a ready supply of such inorganic nutrients. For example, *Leptothrix* is able to utilize the manganese contained in the manganese oxide precipitate on the sheath.

Sheaths may also help the bacteria survive over a wide range of temperature and **pH**, by providing a relatively inert barrier to the external environment.

See also Bacterial appendages; Soil formation, involvement of microorganisms

SHIGELLA

Shigella is a genus of Gram-negative **bacteria** that is similar in behavior and habitat to **Escherichia coli**. The bacterium is named after its discoverer, Japanese scientist Kiyoshi Shiga. The bacteria were discovered over 100 years ago.

Some strains of the bacteria can produce toxins, including the so-called Shiga toxin, which is very similar to the destructive verotoxin of *Escherichia coli* O157:H7. Indeed, strain O157:H7 is now presumed to have arisen by virtue of a genetic **recombination** between strains of *Shigella* and *Escherichia coli* in the intestinal tract, which resulted in the acquisition of the verotoxin by *Escherichia coli*.

The similarity between *Shigella* and *Escherichia coli* extends to the structure of the bacteria and their utilization of certain compounds as nutrients. The similarity is so pronounced that *Shigella* has been regarded as a strain of *Escherichia coli*. However, this is now known not to be the case. *Shigella* does not produce gas from the utilization of carbohydrates, while *Escherichia coli* does.

Shigella is one of a group of bacteria, which includes *Escherichia coli*, that inhabits the intestinal tract of humans and other warm blooded animals. Most strains of the bacterium are innocuous. However, the strains that possess the destructive toxins can do much damage to the intestinal wall and other areas of the body.

There are a number of *Shigella* species that are noteworthy to humans. *Shigella sonnei*, which is also known as group D *Shigella*, is the cause of almost 70 percent of the reported cases of food-borne *Shigella* illness in the United States each year. *Shigella flexneri*, which is also called group B *Shigella*, is responsible for virtually all the remaining cases of food-borne illness. In underdeveloped countries of the world, the bacterium *Shigella dysenteriae* type 1 is epidemic in its scope.

The illness that is caused by *Shigella* species is called shigellosis. The illness is classified as a bacillary **dysentery**. An estimated 300,000 cases of shigellosis occurs in the United States each year. Production of the toxins following the ingested of *Shigella*-contaminated food produces the illness. The illness is characterized by pain in the abdomen, cramps, diarrhea that can become bloody as intestinal cells are damaged, vomiting, and fever. These symptoms typically begin from 12 hours to three days after consuming food that is contaminated with the microorganism. **Contamination** usually results from the exposure of the food to feces-contaminated water or from improper **hygiene** prior to the handling of the food. Both are routes of transfer of fecal material to the food. The amount of fecal material need not be great, as studies have proven that only 10 living *Shigella* are required to establish an infection in humans.

The infection tends to be fairly short in duration and clears without any therapeutic intervention. In some people, however, the primary infection can be the prelude to very damaging infections of the kidney and the joins. The latter infection, which is caused by *Shigella flexneri*, is known as Reiter's syndrome. This can persist for years. During this time, infections by other strains of *Shigella* are possible.

Shigellosis results from the attachment of the bacteria to epithelial cells that line the intestinal tract, and the entry of the bacteria into the cells. Within the host cells, the bacteria divide and can then spread laterally to infect other host cells. The interior location of the bacteria protects them from any host immune response or from **antibiotics**. Additionally, some strains of *Shigella* produce the toxins that can damage the epithelial cells.

The establishment of an infection is easier in people whose immune systems are compromised. For example, shigellosis is a significant problem in those afflicted with acquired **immunodeficiency** syndrome.

Treatment for *Shigella* infections is not always clinically prudent. Many infections, while very inconvenient and painful, pass relatively quickly. Management of the symptoms, particularly ensuring proper hydration, is preferred in immunocompetent people, as opposed to antibiotic therapy. The reason is that the bacteria can rather readily acquire resistance to antibiotics, which can make eradication of the bacteria even harder. Also, the antibiotic resistant bacteria can be excreted in the feces of the infected individual, and may then spread the resistant strain to other people.

Prevention of the spread of infection involves proper hygiene and thorough cooking of foods.

See also Enterobacteriaceae; Enterotoxin and exotoxin; Food safety

SHOTGUN CLONING

The shotgun method (also known as shotgun cloning) is a method in cloning genomic **DNA**. It involves taking the DNA to be cloned and cutting it either using a restriction enzyme or randomly using a physical method to smash the DNA into small pieces. These fragments are then taken together and cloned into a vector. The original DNA can be either genomic DNA (whole genome shotgun cloning) or a clone such as a **YAC (yeast artificial chromosome)** that contains a large piece of genomic DNA needing to be split into fragments.

If the DNA needs to be in a certain cloning vector, but the vector can only carry small amounts of DNA, then the shotgun method can be used. More commonly, the method is used to generate small fragments of DNA for sequencing. A DNA sequence can be generated at about 600 bases at a time, so if a DNA fragment of about 1100kb is cloned, then it can be sequenced in two steps, with 600 bases from each end, and a

hundred base overlap. The sequencing can always be primed with a known sequence from the vector and so any prior knowledge of the sequence that has been cloned is not necessary. This approach of shotgun cloning followed by DNA sequencing from both ends of the vector is called shotgun sequencing.

Shotgun sequencing was initially used to sequence small genomes such as that of the cauliflower mosaic virus (CMV), which is 8kb long. More recently, it has been applied to more complex genomes. Usually this involves creating a physical map and a contig (line of overlapping clones) of clones containing a large amount of DNA in a vector such as a YAC, which are then shotgun cloned into smaller vectors and sequenced. However, a whole genome shotgun approach has been used to sequence the mouse, fly and human genomes by the private company Celera. This involves shotgun cloning the whole genome and sequencing the clones without creating a physical map. It is faster and cheaper than creating a physical **gene** map and sequencing clones one by one, but the reliability of reassembling all the sequences of the small fragments into one genomic sequence has been doubted. For example, a part of the fly genome was sequenced by the one-by-one approach and the whole genome shotgun method. The two sequences were compared, and showed differences. 60% of the genes were identical, 31% showed minor differences and 9% showed major differences. The whole genome shotgun method generated the sequence much more quickly, but the one-by-one approach is probably more accurate because the genes were studied in more detail.

See also Cloning, application of cloning to biological problems; Yeast artificial chromosome (YAC); Yeast genetics

SIGNAL HYPOTHESIS

The signal hypothesis was proposed to explain how proteins that were destined for export from **bacteria** or for targeting to certain regions within eucaryotic **microorganisms** (e.g., **yeast**) achieved their target. The hypothesis was proposed in the 1970s by Günter Blobel, who was then as now a molecular biologist at the Rockefeller University in New York. Blobel's work received the 1999 Nobel Prize in medicine or physiology.

The signal hypothesis proposes that proteins destined for secretion, which involves the movement of the protein across a biological membrane, are originally manufactured with an initial sequence of amino acids that may or may not present in the mature protein.

Work by Blobel and others over two decades established the validity of the proposal. The so-called signal sequence is now known to be only some 20 amino acids in length. The arrangement of amino acids in the signal sequence is not random. Rather, the beginning of the sequence, along with a few amino acid residues in the center of the sequence, is comprised of amino acids that are hydrophilic ("water-loving"). Sandwiched between these regions is a central portion that is made up of amino acids that are **hydrophobic** ("water-hating").

The hydrophilic beginning of the signal sequence, which emerges first as the protein is made, associates with the inner hydrophilic surface of the membrane. As the hydrophilic region of the protein merges, it burrows into the core of the membrane bilayer. The short hydrophilic stretch within the signal sequence anchors in the hydrophilic region on the opposite side of the membrane. Thus, the sequence provides an anchor for the continued extrusion of the emerging protein. In some proteins, the signal sequence can be enzymatically clipped off the remainder of the protein. Proteins of Gram-negative bacteria that are exported from the inside of the cell to the periplasmic space between the inner and outer membranes are examples of such processed proteins. Alternatively, the protein may remain anchored to the membrane via the embedded signal sequence.

The signal hypothesis has been demonstrated in plant cells, animal cells, single-celled **eukaryotes** (e.g., yeast), and in bacteria. The malfunction of the signal mechanism can be detrimental in all these systems. In contrast, the use of signal sequences has proven beneficial for the export of bio-engineered drugs from bacteria.

See also Bacterial membranes and cell wall; Prokaryotic membrane transport

SINSHEIMER, ROBERT LOUIS (1920-)

American molecular biologist and biophysicist

Born in Washington, D.C., Robert Sinsheimer attended secondary school in Chicago before studying at the Massachusetts Institute of Technology (MIT). At MIT Sinsheimer took his undergraduate degree in quantitative biology before moving on to complete his Ph.D. in biophysics. Sinsheimer initially accepted a faculty position at MIT but moved to Iowa State College in 1949 to take up the post of professor of biophysics.

Sinsheimer became a professor of biophysics at the California Institute of Technology (Caltech) in 1957 and was Chairman of the Caltech Division of Biology from 1968 to 1977. During this period he conducted a series of investigations into the physical and genetic characteristics of a **bacteriophage** called Phi X 174. These breakthrough studies illuminated the viral genetic processes. Sinsheimer and his colleagues also succeeded for the first time in isolating, purifying, and synthetically replicating viral **DNA**.

The bacteriophage Phi X 174 was an ideal candidate for study because it contained only a single strand of DNA comprised of about 5,500 nucleotides forming approximately 11 genes. In addition it was easier to obtain samples of the bacteriophage DNA.

In 1977 Sinsheimer left Caltech to become a chancellor of the University of California, Santa Cruz. One reason the position of chancellor appealed to him was that it provided a forum to address his concerns that had developed concerning the social implications and potential hazards of recombinant DNA technology and **cloning** methods. Sinsheimer was one of the first scientists to question the potential hazardous uses of

molecular biology and the ethical implications of the developing technologies. In addition Sinsheimer became committed to promoting scientific literacy among non-scientists.

His early years at Santa Cruz were challenging. During his tenure the university re-established itself as a seat of research and academic excellence. Some of Sinsheimer's accomplishments included the establishment of the Keck telescope, the establishment of programs in agroecology, applied economics, seismological studies, and a major in computer engineering.

Sinsheimer also participated fundamentally in the genesis of the Human Genome Project. In May 1985 Sinsheimer organized a conference at Santa Cruz to consider the benefits of sequencing the human genome. From these and other such deliberations arose the Human Genome Project.

Author of more than 200 scientific papers, Sinsheimer's autobiography, *The Strands of a Life: The Science of DNA and the Art of Education,* was published in 1994.

See also Bacteriophage and bacteriophage typing; Containment and release prevention protocol; Molecular biology and molecular genetics; Phage genetics

SKIN INFECTIONS

The skin is the largest organ in the human body. It is the front line of defense against many types of pathogens, and remains disease-free over most of its area most of the time. However, breaks in the skin are particularly prone to invasion by **microorganisms**, and skin infections are a relatively common complaint. Skin infections may be bacterial, viral or fungal in nature.

Among the more common bacterial skin infections is impetigo, a usually mild condition caused by staphylococcal or streptococcal **bacteria**. It causes small skin lesions and typically spreads among schoolchildren. Folliculitis results in pustules at the base of hairs or, in more serious cases, in painful boils. Often it is caused by *Staphylococcus* species. A relatively recent manifestation called "hot tub folliculitis" results from *Pseudomonas* bacteria in poorly maintained hot tubs. Those bacterial skin infections that do not resolve spontaneously are treated with topical or oral **antibiotics**.

Among the more serious bacterial infections of the skin is cellulitis, a deep infection involving subcutaneous areas and the lymphatic circulation in the region as well as the skin itself. The affected area is painful, red, and warm to the touch, and the patient may be feverish. Cellulitis is usually caused by bacterial invasion of an injury to the skin. Treatment includes oral and/or intravenous antibiotics, and immobilization and elevation of the affected area.

Viral skin infections typically show up as warts caused by the Human Papillomavirus (HPV). Common warts usually appear on the extremities, especially in children and adolescents. Plantar warts often grow on the heel or sole of the foot, surrounded by overgrown, calloused skin. When they develop on weight-bearing surfaces such as the heel, plantar warts may become painful. HPV also causes genital warts, or condylo-

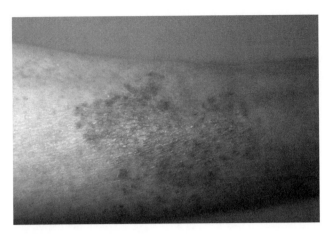
Skin infection caused by tinea.

mata, which may increase the risk for cervical or penile cancer. Many methods are used in attempts to remove warts, with varying degrees of success. These include cryotherapy, antiviral agents, application of salicylic acid, surgical removal, and laser treatment.

Skin infections caused by **fungi**, including **yeast**, are called dermatomycoses. A common subcategory consists of the dermatophytoses, caused by *Trichophyton* species. These infections include tinea capitis ("cradle cap"), tinea corporis ("ringworm"), tinea cruris ("jock itch"), and tinea pedis ("athlete's foot"). *Candida,* which often affects the mucous membranes, may also be responsible for skin infections. Obese patients are prone to fungal infections in skin folds, as are uncircumcised men. Candida is also involved in some cases of diaper rash. Fungal infections are typically treated with topical imidazole creams or sprays.

See also Bacteria and bacterial infection; Candidiasis; Infection and resistance; Viruses and responses to viral infection; Yeast, infectious

SLEEPING SICKNESS

Sleeping sickness (trypanosomiasis) is a protozoan infection passed to humans through the bite of the tsetse fly. It progresses to death within months or years if left untreated. Near-control of trypanosomiasis was achieved in the 1960s, but the disease has since re-emerged in Sub-Saharan Africa, where political instability and war have hampered **public health** efforts. As of 2002, the **World Health Organization**, in conjunction with Médicines Sans Frontièrs (Doctors Without Borders) and major pharmaceutical companies were in the midst of a five-year major effort to halt the spread of trypanosomiasis and treat its victims.

Protozoa are single-celled organisms considered to be the simplest animal life form. The protozoa responsible for sleeping sickness are a flagellated variety (flagella are hair-like projections from the cell which aid in mobility) which exist only in Africa. The type of protozoa causing sleeping sickness in humans is referred to as the *Trypanosoma brucei* complex. It is divided further into Rhodesian (Central and East Africa) and Gambian (Central and West Africa) subspecies.

The Rhodesian variety live within antelopes in savanna and woodland areas, causing no disruption to the antelope's health. (While the protozoa cause no illness in antelopes, they are lethal to cattle who may become infected.) The protozoa are acquired by tsetse flies who bite and suck the blood of an infected antelope or cow. Within the tsetse fly, the protozoa cycle through several different life forms, ultimately migrating to the salivary glands of the tsetse fly. Once the protozoa are harbored in the salivary glands, they can be deposited into the bloodstream of the fly's next blood meal.

Humans most likely to become infected by Rhodesian trypanosomes are game wardens or visitors to game parks in East Africa. The Rhodesian variety of sleeping sickness causes a much more severe illness with a greater likelihood of eventual death. The Gambian variety of Trypanosoma thrives in tropical rain forests throughout Central and West Africa, does not infect game or cattle, and is primarily a threat to people dwelling in such areas. It rarely infects visitors.

The first sign of sleeping sickness may be a sore appearing at the tsetse fly bite spot about two to three days after having been bitten. Redness, pain, and swelling occur. Two to three weeks later, Stage I disease develops as a result of the protozoa being carried through the blood and lymphatic circulations. This systemic (meaning that symptoms affect the whole body) phase of the illness is characterized by a high fever that falls to normal then re-spikes. A rash with intense itching may be present, and headache and mental confusion may occur. The Gambian form includes extreme swelling of lymph tissue, enlargement of the spleen and liver, and swollen lymph nodes. Winterbottom's sign is classic of Gambian sleeping sickness; it consists of a visibly swollen area of lymph nodes located behind the ear and just above the base of the neck. During this stage, the heart may be affected by a severe inflammatory reaction, particularly when the infection is caused by the Rhodesian form.

Many of the symptoms of sleeping sickness are actually the result of attempts by the patient's **immune system** to get rid of the invading organism. The overly exuberant cells of the immune system damage the patient's organs, causing anemia and leaky blood vessels. These leaky blood vessels help to spread the protozoa throughout the patient's body.

One reason for the immune system's intense reaction to the Trypanosomes is also the reason why the Trypanosomes survive so effectively. The protozoa are able to change rapidly specific markers on their outer coats. These kinds of markers usually stimulate the host's immune system to produce immune cells specifically to target the markers and allow quick destruction of these invading cells. Trypanosomes are able to express new markers at such a high rate of change that the host's immune system cannot catch up.

Stage II sleeping sickness involves the nervous system. The Gambian strain has a clearly delineated phase in which the predominant symptomatology involves the brain. The patient's speech becomes slurred, mental processes slow, and he or she sits and stares or sleeps for long periods of time.

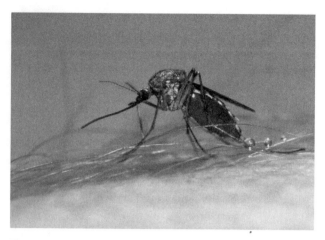

The trypanosome that causes sleeping sickness is commonly transferred to humans by mosquitoes.

Other symptoms resemble Parkinson's disease: imbalance when walking, slow and shuffling gait, trembling of the limbs, involuntary movement, muscle tightness, and increasing mental confusion. These symptoms culminate in coma, then death.

Diagnosis of sleeping sickness can be made by microscopic examination of fluid from the site of the tsetse fly bite or swollen lymph nodes for examination. A method to diagnose Rhodesian trypanosome involves culturing blood, bone marrow, or spinal fluid. These cultures are injected into rats to promote the development of blood-borne protozoan infection. This infection can be detected in blood smears within one to two weeks.

Medications effective against the *Trypanosoma brucei* complex protozoa have significant potential for side effects. Suramin, eflornithine, pentamidine, and several drugs which contain arsenic (a chemical which is potentially poisonous) are effective anti-trypanosomal agents. Each of these drugs requires careful monitoring to ensure that they do not cause serious complications such as a fatal hypersensitivity reaction, kidney or liver damage, or **inflammation** of the brain. Trials are underway to monitor the effectiveness of new medications for treatment of trypanosomiasis.

Prevention of sleeping sickness requires avoiding contact with the tsetse fly; insect **repellents**, mosquito netting, and clothing that covers the limbs to the wrists and ankles are mainstays. There are currently no immunizations available to prevent sleeping sickness.

See also Protists

SLIME LAYER · *see* GLYCOCALYX

SLIME MOLDS

Slime molds are organisms in two taxonomic groups, the cellular slime molds (Phylum Acrasiomycota) and the plasmodial slime molds (Phylum Myxomycota). Organisms in both groups are eukaryotic (meaning that their cells have nuclei) and are fungus-like in appearance during part of their life cycle. For this reason, they were traditionally included in **mycology** textbooks. However, modern biologists consider both groups to be only distantly related to the **fungi**. The two groups of slime molds are considered separately below.

Species in the cellular slime **mold** group are microscopic during most stages of their life cycle, when they exist as haploid (having one copy of each chromosome in the **nucleus**), single-celled amoebas. The amoebas typically feed on **bacteria** by engulfing them, in a process known as **phagocytosis**, and they reproduce by mitosis and fission. Sexual reproduction occurs but is uncommon. Most of what we know about this group is from study of the species *Dictyostelium discoideum*. When there is a shortage of food, the individual haploid amoebas of a cellular slime mold aggregate into a mass of cells called a pseudoplasmodium. A pseudoplasmodium typically contains many thousands of individual cells. In contrast to the plasmodial slime molds, the individual cells in a pseudoplasmodium maintain their own plasma membranes during aggregation. The migrating amoebas often form beautiful aggregation patterns, which change form over time.

After a pseudoplasmodium has formed, the amoebas continue to aggregate until they form a mound on the ground surface. Then, the mound elongates into a "slug." The slug is typically less than 0.04 in (1 mm) in length and migrates in response to heat, light, and other environmental stimuli.

The slug then develops into a sporocarp, a fruiting body with cells specialized for different functions. A sporocarp typically contains about 100,000 cells. The sporocarp of *Dictyostelium* is about 0.08 in (2 mm) tall and has cells in a base, stalk, and ball-like cap. The cells in the cap develop into asexual reproductive spores, which germinate to form new amoebas. The different species of cellular slime molds are distinguished by sporocarp morphology.

Dictyostelium discoideum has been favored by many biologists as a model organism for studies of development, **biochemistry**, and genetics. Aspects of its development are analogous to that of higher organisms, in that a mass of undifferentiated cells develops into a multicellular organism, with different cells specialized for different functions. The development of *Dictyostelium* is much easier to study in the laboratory than is the development of higher organisms.

A food shortage induces aggregation in *Dictyostelium*. In aggregation, individual amoebas near the center of a group of amoebas secrete pulses of cAMP (cyclic adenosine-3'5'-monophosphate). The cAMP binds to special receptors on the plasma membranes of nearby amoebas, causing the cells to move toward the cAMP source for about a minute. Then, these amoebas stop moving and in turn secrete cAMP, to induce other more distant amoebas to move toward the developing aggregation. This process continues until a large, undifferentiated mass of cells, the pseudoplasmodium, is formed.

Interestingly, cAMP is also found in higher organisms, including humans. In *Dictyostelium* and these higher organisms, cAMP activates various biochemical pathways and is synthesized in response to hormones, neurotransmitters, and other stimuli.

The plasmodial slime molds are relatively common in temperate regions and can be found living on decaying plant matter. There are about 400 different species. Depending on the species, the color of the amorphous cell mass, the **plasmodium**, can be red, yellow, brown, orange, green, or other colors. The color of the plasmodium and the morphology of the reproductive body, the sporocarp, are used to identify the different species.

The plasmodial slime molds are superficially similar to the cellular slime molds. Both have a haploid amoeba phase in when cells feed by phagocytosis, followed by a phase with a large amorphous cell mass, and then a reproductive phase with a stalked fruiting body.

However, the plasmodial slime molds are distinguished from the cellular slime molds by several unique features of their life cycle. First, the germinating spores produce flagellated as well as unflagellated cells. Second, two separate haploid cells fuse to produce a zygote with a diploid nucleus. Third, the zygote develops into a plasmodium, which typically contains many thousands of diploid nuclei, all surrounded by a continuous plasma membrane.

The **cytoplasm** of the plasmodium moves about within the cell, a process known as cytoplasmic streaming. This is readily visible with a **microscope**. The function of cytoplasmic streaming is presumably to move nutrients about within the giant cell.

In nature, plasmodial slime molds grow well in wet and humid environments, and under such conditions the plasmodium of some species can be quite large. After a particularly wet spring in Texas in 1973, several residents of a Dallas suburb reported a large, moving, slimy mass, which they termed "the Blob." One reporter in the local press speculated that the Blob was a mutant bacterium, able to take over the earth. Fortunately, a local mycologist soberly identified the Blob as *Fuligo septica,* a species of plasmodial slime mold.

Another plasmodial slime mold, *Physarum polycephalum,* is easily grown in the laboratory and is often used by biologists as a model organism for studies of cytoplasmic streaming, biochemistry, and cytology. The plasmodium of this species moves in response to various stimuli, including ultraviolet and blue light. The proteins actin and myosin are involved in this movement. Interestingly, actin and myosin also control the movement of muscles in higher organisms, including humans.

See also Mycology

SLOW VIRUSES

Historically, the term "slow virus infections" was coined for a poorly defined group of seemingly viral diseases which were later found to be caused by several quite different conventional **viruses**, also unconventional infectious agents. They nevertheless shared the properties of causing diseases with long incubation periods and a protracted course of illness, affecting largely the central nervous and/or the lymph system and usually culminating in death. The slow virus concept was first introduced by the Icelandic physician Bjorn Sigurdsson (1913–1959) in 1954. He and his co-workers had made pioneering studies on slow diseases in sheep including maedivisna and scrapie. Maedi is a slowly progressive interstitial **pneumonia** of adult sheep while visna is a slow, progressive encephalomyelitis and the same virus, belonging, to the lentivirus subgroup of **retroviruses**, was found to be responsible for both conditions.

Since the original isolation of the maedi-visna virus, concern with slow viral infections, both in animals and in humans, has grown. Research on sheep lentiviruses and their pathogenesis has continued to this day and received an important impetus in the 1980s with the recognition of the devastating condition in humans known as acquired **immunodeficiency** syndrome (**AIDS**). AIDS shared many of the attributes of slow virus infections in animals and led virologists to suspect, then to identify, the lentivirus causing AIDS: the **human immunodeficiency virus** or **HIV**. Questions posed by Bjorn Sigurdsson's work on maedi-visna also became the central pathogenic questions of HIV disease. For example: how and where does HIV persist despite an initially robust and long-sustained immune response? How does HIV actually destroy the tissues it infects? Why do these events unfold so slowly? Final answers to all these questions have still not been found and there is much research still to be done on the lentiviruses but Sigurdsson's contribution to HIV research through the study of maedi-visna is now recognized.

Other slow virus infections of humans due by conventional viruses include progressive multifocal leukoencephalopathy (PML) caused by the JC papovavirus. This is an opportunistic infection in hosts that have defective cell-mediated **immunity** and the majority of human cases now occur in HIV 1 infected individuals. Patients present with progressive multifocal signs including visual loss, aphasia (difficulty speaking), seizures, dementia, personality changes, gait problems, and less commonly, cerebellar, brain stem, and spinal cord features. Death occurs within weeks to months of clinical onset. Subacute sclerosing panencephalitis (SSPE), another slow infection, has been identified as a rare consequence of chronic persistant infection by the **measles** (rubella) virus, causing an insidious syndrome of behavioral changes in young children. Patients develop motor abnormalities, in particular myoclonic jerks, and ultimately become mute, quadriplegic, and in rigid stupor. SSPE is found worldwide with a frequency of one case per million per year. Progressive rubella panencephalitis is another very rare slow virus infection of children and young people caused by the same virus. Most patients have a history of congenital or acquired rubella and the clinical course is more protracted than in SSPE with progressive neurologic deficit occurring over several years. A third slow virus of humans that has had some publicity in recent years is the **human T-cell leukemia virus** (**HTLV**) types 1 and 2 which are associated with adult T-cell leukemia. It was initially thought that the causative agent of AIDS was related to HTLV though it later became clear that whereas HTLV 1 and 2 are both oncogenic ("cancer producing") retroviruses, HIV belongs to the lentivirus sub-group.

An unconventional agent causing slow infections has now been identified as a non-viral "proteinaceous, infectious" agent, or prion. **Prions** give rise to the group of diseases now called transmissible spongiform encephalopathies. In animals these include scrapie in sheep and bovine spongiform encephalopathy (BSE) in cows. Human prion infections include rare dementing diseases like kuru, Creutzfeldt-Jakob disease (CJD), Gerstmann-Straussler-Scheinker (GSS) syndrome, and fatal familial insomnia (FFI). The prion agent is replicated without provoking any **antibody** response, appears not to have any recognizable nucleic acid component, and is resistant to conventional inactivation techniques for infectious agents. Current evidence suggests that the prion protein is an abnormal isoform of a normal host encoded protein known as PrP, which is coded on the short arm of chromosome 20. Prions appear to "replicate" by a novel form of protein-protein information transfer, the abnormal PrP seemingly inducing the normal protein to undergo a structural change into the abnormal form. Most pathological changes observed with transmissible spongiform encephalopathies are confined to the brain; however, scrapie-induced disorders of the pancreas have also been described. The neuropathology sometimes shows a dramatic spongiform disruption of brain tissue but may also be subtle and non-characteristic, even at the terminal stages of the disease. In the latter cases, diagnosis has to rely on features like clinical signs, transmissibility, detection of abnormal PrP or identification of **mutations** in the PrP **gene**.

In humans, prion diseases may be sporadic, acquired or inherited. Iatrogenic transmissions of the prion have occurred following medical procedures such as pituitary growth hormone injections, where the hormone source was contaminated with prion tissue, or corneal transplants, where a patient accidentally received an infected cornea. The first recognized human prion disease was kuru, which emerged among the South Fore people of New Guinea and is now generally thought to have been transmitted by the practice of ritual cannibalism. CJD is today the most common human prion disease occurring worldwide with a frequency of about one per million per year. The peak incidence occurs in older people between the ages 55 and 65 although recently a "new variant" has emerged in the U.K., which affects individuals at a much earlier age. It is widely believed that the new variant CJD is closely related to the variety causing BSE in cattle and may be contracted by the ingestion of infected beef.

Inherited prion disease can arise from specific point mutations in the PrP gene. Perhaps 10–15% of CJD cases are familial with an autosomal dominant pattern of inheritance. Gerstmann-Straussler-Scheinker syndrome is another rare familial condition that is vertically transmitted in an apparently autosomal dominant way. As with other prion diseases it can be horizontally transmitted to non-human primates and rodents through intracerebral inoculation of brain homogenates from patients with the disease. The exact incidence of the syndrome is unknown but is estimated to be between one and ten per hundred million per year and the condition appears to be an allelic variant of familial Creutzfeldt-Jakob disease. Fatal familial insomnia is the third most common inherited human prion disease. The region of the brain most affected in this condition is the thalamus which monitors sleep patterns. The symptoms of the disease are characterized by progressive insomnia and, as with other prion diseases, eventual motor signs.

See also Viral genetics

SMALLPOX

Smallpox is an infection caused by the **variola virus**, a member of the poxvirus family. Throughout history, smallpox has caused huge **epidemics** resulting in great suffering and enormous death tolls worldwide. In 1980, the **World Health Organization** (**WHO**) announced that a massive program of **vaccination** against the disease had resulted in the complete eradication of the virus (with the exception of stored virus stocks in two laboratories).

Smallpox is an extraordinarily contagious disease. The virus can spread by contact with victims, as well as in contaminated air droplets and even on the surfaces of objects used by other smallpox victims (books, blankets, etc.). After acquisition of the virus, there is a 12–14 day incubation period, during which the virus multiplies, but no symptoms appear. The onset of symptoms occurs suddenly and includes fever and chills, muscle aches, and a flat, reddish-purple rash on the chest, abdomen, and back. These symptoms last about three days, after which the rash fades and the fever drops. A day or two later, the fever returns, along with a bumpy rash starting on the feet, hands, and face. This rash progresses from the feet along the legs, from the hands along the arms, and from the face down the neck, ultimately reaching and including the chest, abdomen, and back. The individual bumps, or papules, fill with clear fluid, and, over the course of 10–12 days, became pus-filled. The pox eventually scabs over, and when the scab falls off it leaves behind a pock-mark or pit, which remains as a permanent scar on the skin of the victim.

Death from smallpox usually follows complications such as **bacterial infection** of the open skin lesions, **pneumonia**, or bone infections. A very severe and quickly fatal form of smallpox was "sledgehammer smallpox," and resulted in hemorrhage from the skin lesions, as well as from the mouth, nose, and other areas of the body. No treatment was ever discovered for smallpox nor could anything shorten the course of the disease. Up until its eradication, smallpox was diagnosed most clearly from the patients' symptoms. **Electron microscopic** studies could identify the variola virus in fluid isolated from disease papules, from infected urine, or from the blood prior to the appearance of the papular rash.

Smallpox is an ancient disease. There is evidence that a major epidemic occurred towards the end of the eighteenth Egyptian dynasty. Studies of the mummy of Pharaoh Ramses V (d. 1157 B.C.) indicate that he may have died of smallpox. Several historical accounts, some dating to the sixth century, describe how different peoples attempted to vaccinate against smallpox. In China, India, and the Americas, from about the tenth century, it was noted that individuals who had even a mild case of smallpox could not be infected again. Material from people ill with smallpox (e.g., fluid or pus from the papules) was scratched into the skin of those who had never had the illness, in an attempt to produce a mild reaction and its accompanying protective effect. These efforts often resulted in full-fledged smallpox, and sometimes served only to effectively spread the infection throughout the community. In Colonial America, such crude vaccinations against smallpox were outlawed because of the dangers.

In 1798, **Edward Jenner** (1749–1823) published a paper in which he discussed an important observation that milkmaids who contracted a mild infection of the hands (caused by vaccinia virus, a relative of variola) appeared to be immune to smallpox. He created an **immunization** against smallpox that used the pus material found in the lesions of **cowpox** infection. Jenner's paper, although severely criticized at first, later led to much work in the area of vaccinations. Vaccination using Jenner's method proved instrumental in decreasing the number of smallpox deaths.

Smallpox is dangerous only to human beings. Animals and insects can neither be infected by smallpox, nor carry the virus in any form. Humans also cannot carry the virus unless they are symptomatic. These important facts entered into the decision by the WHO to attempt worldwide eradication of the smallpox virus. The methods used in the WHO eradication program were simple and included the careful surveillance of all smallpox infections worldwide to allow for quick diagnosis and immediate quarantine of patients. It also included the immediate vaccination of all contacts of any patient diagnosed with smallpox infection. The WHO program was extremely successful, and the virus was declared eradicated worldwide in May of 1980. Two laboratories (in Atlanta, Georgia and in Koltsovo, Russia) retain samples of the smallpox virus, because some level of concern exists that another poxvirus could mutate (undergo genetic changes) and cause human infection. Other areas of concern include the possibility of smallpox virus being utilized in a situation of **biological warfare**, or the remote chance that the smallpox virus could somehow escape from the laboratories where it is being stored. For these reasons, large quantities of **vaccine** are stored in different countries around the world, so that response to any future threat by the smallpox virus can be prompt.

See also Smallpox, eradication, storage, and potential use as a bacteriological weapon; Vaccine

SMALLPOX: ERADICATION, STORAGE, AND POTENTIAL USE AS A BACTERIO-LOGICAL WEAPON

Historically, **smallpox** was one of the most feared diseases in the ancient world. After an extensive and successful eradication program, the **World Health Organization** (**WHO**) certified the global eradication of smallpox infection in 1980. There has not been a single reported case of smallpox infection in over 20 years. However, smallpox was once a deadly disease with the power to decimate populations. Successful efforts to prevent

the spread of smallpox through **vaccination** changed the course of Western medicine and indeed, the history of smallpox is a fascinating testament to the effect of health and disease on the development of modern civilization. Today it is difficult to imagine the devastating effects of the disease on the human population. In 1981, smallpox was removed from the WHO list of diseases covered under the International Health Regulations, which detail notification requirements and measures that should be taken to contain an outbreak. The last reported case of smallpox occurred in Somalia in 1977, and on May 8, 1980, the WHO declared the global eradication of smallpox. This meant that smallpox vaccination was no longer required and the WHO indicated that only "investigators at special risk" should have the **vaccine**. It was also decided that seed lots of vaccinia virus would be maintained as well as stocks of 200 million doses of prepared vaccine in case of an accidental outbreak. There is a 30% case-fatality rate associated with smallpox infections among unvaccinated individuals and routine vaccinations have now not been performed in the United States in over 25 years. The fact that stocks of smallpox still exist means that an accidental or deliberate release of the virus could occur. Smallpox, if used as a biological weapon, clearly presents a threat to both civilian and military populations. Thus, although there is little risk of naturally occurring smallpox infections at this time, there is a significant potential for a smallpox epidemic of manmade origin.

The concept of using the variola (smallpox) virus in warfare is an old one. During the French and Indian Wars (1754–1767), British colonial commanders distributed blankets that were used by smallpox victims in order to initiate an epidemic among Native Americans. The mortality rate associated with these outbreaks was as high as 50% in certain tribes. More recently, in the years leading up to World War II, the Japanese military explored smallpox weaponization during operations of Unit 731 in Mongolia and China.

There are a number of characteristics that make the **variola virus** an excellent candidate for use as a biological weapon. An aerosol suspension of variola can spread widely and have a very low infectious dosage. In general, the dissemination of a pathogen by aerosol droplets is the preferred deployment method for biological weapons. Smallpox is highly contagious and is spread through droplet inhalation or ingestion. As there are no civilian or military smallpox vaccination requirements at this time, a large susceptible population is at risk from the infection. The incubation period in naturally occurring cases averages seven to 14 days. However, the period could be shortened to three to seven days, especially in the cases of aerosol application. People who have contracted the disease are contagious during the late stages of the incubation period, even though they remain asymptomatic. Thus, transmission of the disease can occur as early as two days after exposure to the virus. Depending on the climate, corpses of smallpox victims remain infectious for days to months. The duration of the disease is long and coupled with the complex isolation and protection requirements of smallpox treatment, each infected person would require the efforts of several medical support personnel.

In general, the worldwide practice of smallpox **immunization** greatly diminished the fear of an epidemic caused by a deliberate release of the virus. Although the disease was declared eradicated in 1980, stores of smallpox officially exist at the two WHO-approved repositories. The first is at the **Centers for Disease Control** and Prevention in Atlanta, USA. The second is the State Research Center for **Virology** and **Biotechnology** (also known as Vector) at Koltsovo, in the Novosibirsk region of Siberian Russia. In June 1995, WHO inspected the Koltsovo facility and determined that it was an acceptable storage facility after the virus stocks were moved there from the original storage site at the Institute of Viral Preparations in Moscow. All other laboratories around the world were required to destroy their remaining stores of smallpox virus. Concomitantly, WHO recommended that all countries discontinue vaccination against the disease.

Despite the provisions of the WHO and the 1972 **Biological Weapons Convention**, the former Soviet Union maintained a sophisticated and large-scale research and development program for biological weapons implementation. This research was carried out at both military and civilian level. It is now known that the Soviet Union successfully developed and adapted smallpox virus for use in strategic weapons.

Considerable debate has ensued regarding the officially remaining stores of smallpox virus. The WHO Ad hoc Committee on Orthopoxvirus Infections has, since 1986, consistently recommended destruction of the remaining reserves of the smallpox virus. The initial proposal was to destroy the remaining stocks in December 1990. However, the possibility that smallpox has been, and might be, incorporated into biological weapons has encouraged the scientific community to continue research on the pathogen. Although the tentative date set for the destruction of all remaining smallpox stores is late 2002, a consensus among scientists and military strategists has not yet been reached and in view of current political unrest in areas such as the Middle East, total destruction of all stores is not likely to happen.

Since many laboratories involved in biological weapons research and development in the former Soviet Union are now working with decreased funding, staff, and support, there is concern that bioweapons resources and expertise may spread to other countries. A report from the Washington Center for Strategic and International Studies states that at least 10 countries are involved in biological weapon research programs. The ability of a group to acquire variola and develop it as a biological weapon is limited by several factors. Specialized skills are required to grow smallpox in effectively large quantities and to adapt it for use as an aerosol-based weapon. It is unlikely that small, technically limited facilities or dissident groups would use smallpox as a weapon. Also, the open use of a biological weapon by any nation or political state would undoubtedly elicit severe retaliation. Lastly, the smallpox virus is not as readily available as other agents of biological terrorism, such as **anthrax** (*Bacillus anthraci*) or plague (*Yersinia pestis)*. Therefore, analysis of these and other factors have led bioweapons experts to conclude that well-financed and highly organized private groups

or politically/state financed terrorist groups would be the most likely to use smallpox as a bio-weapon.

See also Bioterrorism; Bioterrorism, protective measures; Epidemics, viral; Viruses and responses to viral infection

SNOW BLOOMS

Snow bloom refers to the rapid growth and increase in numbers of so-called snow algae on the surface and interior of snow fields. Typically occurring as the surface of the snow warms in the springtime sun, the algal growth confers various colors to the snow. Colors of different algal species include yellow, red, green, and orange.

Blooms occur when nutrients are abundant and conditions such as temperature are conducive to rapid growth. "Red tide," due to the growth of a **diatoms** in salt water, is another example of a bloom.

There are some 350 species of snow algae. A common species is *Chlamydomonas nivalis*.

Snow algae have been known for millennia. The Greek philosopher Aristotle described red snow over 2,000 years ago. The algal basis for the blooms was determined in the early nineteenth century, when some red-colored snow obtained by a British expedition near Greenland was analyzed.

Snow blooms occur most frequently in high altitude areas where snow persists over a long time and accumulates to great depths. Examples include the Sierra Nevada range in California and the Rocky Mountains of North America.

The various colors of snow blooms reflect the presence of various pigmented compounds in the algae. These compounds, which are called carotenoids, confer protection against the sunlight, particularly against the ultraviolet portion of the spectrum. Red algae are more sunlight tolerant than are green, orange, and yellow-pigmented algae. Non-red algae tend to shield themselves from the sunlight by growing beneath the snow's surface.

In another adaptation, the algal membrane is adapted for cold, in much the same way that cold-loving **bacteria** are, via the presence of lipids that remain pliable at low temperatures.

Another feature of snow algae that contributes to their tolerance is their ability to form cysts. These are analogous to bacterial spores, in that they provide the algae with a means of becoming metabolically dormant during inhospitable periods. During the winter, the cysts remain encased in snow. Indeed, experiments have determined that cysts are not inactivated even after a prolonged storage at -94° F (-70° C). As the snow melts in the springtime, resuscitation of the cysts occurs. The algal cells migrate to the surface of the snow in order to reproduce. After reproducing the cells drift down into the nutritionally poor subsurface, where their **transformation** into cyst form is again stimulated. The following spring the cycle is repeated.

See also Psychrophilic bacteria

SOIL FORMATION, INVOLVEMENT OF MICROORGANISMS

Microorganisms are essential to soil formation and soil ecology because they control the flux of nutrients to plants (i.e., control of carbon, nitrogen, and sulfur cycles,), promote nitrogen fixation, and promote soil detoxification of inorganic and naturally occurring organic pollutants. Soil microorganisms are also part of several food chains, thus serving as source nutrients to one another, and frequently serve as the primary members of food chains in soil biota.

The roots of plants are also part of soil biota and some **fungi**. Many **bacteria** live in symbiotic relation to plant roots, around which there is an area of elevated microbial activity, known as rhizosphere. The Animalia kingdom is also represented in soil biota by Nematodes, Earthworms, Mollusks, Acarina, Collembola, as well as several insects and larvae that feed mostly on decaying organic matter. They all take part in the soil food chain and help to promote the conversion of organic matter into bacterial and fungal biomass. Soil microbiology is a relatively recent discipline and it is estimated that about only one percent of soil microorganisms are so far identified.

The soil ecosystem is composed of inorganic matter (calcium, iron oxide, nitrates, sulfur, phosphates, ash, and stone particles), substrates (fallen leaves, dead organisms, rotten wood, dead roots), organisms (microbes, animals, and plants), air, and water. Bacteria and fungi are mostly heterotrophic organisms that feed on the existing organic matter by decomposing them in order to absorb the resultant micronutrients and minerals. Therefore, they are essential to the recycling process of nutrients that keeps soils in good condition for plant growth. The community of microorganisms in a given type of soil differs from that belonging to another soil type. They are highly dependent on environmental factors such as levels of carbon dioxide, oxygen, hydrogen, soil **pH** (whether acid, alkaline, or neutral), types of substrates, amounts of available substrates, levels of moisture, and temperature. Each community is highly complex, and so far, little is known about the succession of microorganisms in the food chains and the interconnected food webs they form, or about the sequence of events in the cycling pathways of soil ecosystem.

The arrival of new substrate in the soil increases bacterial populations that feed on them, thus recycling in the process, nutrients important to both plants and other soil organisms. Bacterial expansion leads to a second event, known as succession, which is the growth of **protozoa** populations that predate bacteria. The expansion of protozoa populations triggers the activity of mites, which feed on protozoans. Substrate arrival triggers as well the activity and expansion of fungi populations, which are also decomposers. Some fungal species compete with other fungal species for the same substrates, such as the *Pisolithus* and the *Fusarium*. Nematodes are triggered into action and feed on both fungi and other species of nematodes. Some fungi are able to entrap and feed on nematodes too. In the rhizospheres, these populations are more active than in other parts of the soil and atmospheric factors may influence rhizospheres biota. An American research

group is studying the response of soil biota in California grasslands to determine the long-term effect of increased levels of carbon dioxide on soil biota dynamics and on plant growth. They found that in a carbon dioxide enriched atmospheric environment, the colonization of plant roots by fungi is augmented, which facilitates carbon and nutrient exchange between the host plants and the fungi (i.e., symbiosis), thus favoring fungi colonies to expand within the soil, as well favoring the growth of grass. Consequently, the number of soil micro arthropods has also increased, since many of them feed on fungi colonies. However, after six years of experimental carbon dioxide atmospheric enrichment, significant increases on bacterial populations were not recorded. Therefore, the experiment succeeded in illustrating one portion of the food chain in grassland soil, and supplied evidence that the induced enhancement of natural-occurring symbiotic relationships in the rhizosphere may be useful for agricultural productive purposes.

See also Bacterial kingdoms; Composting, microbiological aspects; Microbial symbiosis; Microbial taxonomy; Photosynthetic microorganisms; Protozoa; Slime molds

SPACE MICROBIOLOGY · *see* EXTRATERRESTRIAL MICROBIOLOGY

SPECTROPHOTOMETER

A spectrophotometer is an optical device that can determine the concentration of a compound or particles in a solution or suspension.

Light of a pre-selected wavelength is shone through a chamber that houses the sample. The sample particles, **bacteria** for example, will absorb some of the light. The amount of light that is absorbed increases with increasing numbers of bacteria in a predictable way. The relationship between absorbance and the number of absorbing sample molecules is expressed mathematically as the Beer-Lambert Law.

The absorbance of light can also be described as the optical density of the sample solution or suspension.

The percent of light that has been absorbed can be determined and, by comparing this absorption to a graph of the absorption of known numbers of bacteria, the concentration of bacteria in the suspension can be computed. In a microbiology laboratory, such measurements are routinely used in **bacterial growth** studies, to determine the number of bacteria growing in a **culture** at certain times based on the absorbance of the suspension. A standard curve can be constructed that relates the various measured optical densities to the resulting number of living bacteria, as determined by the number of bacteria from a defined portion of the suspensions that grows on **agar** medium.

Some spectrophotometers are equipped with a single measuring chamber. For these so-called single-beam instruments, the absorbance of a sample is taken, followed by the absorbance of a control. Typically, a bacterial control is uninoculated growth medium, so the absorbance should be zero. In typical growth curve studies, the bacterial culture can be grown in a special flask called a side-arm flask. The side arm is a test tube that can be inserted directly into a spectrophotometer.

Double-beam spectrophotometers are also available and are the norm now in research microbiology laboratories. In these instruments the light beam is split into two beams by means of mirrors. One light path goes through the sample chamber and the other light beam passes through what is referred to as the reference cell or chamber. The ration of the absorbance between the two chambers is computed and is used to determine sample concentration.

Depending on the spectrophotometer, absorbance can be taken at a single wavelength, or scanned through a spectrum of wavelengths. The latter can be a useful means of identifying components of the sample, based on their preferential absorption of certain wavelengths of light.

See also Laboratory techniques in microbiology

SPECTROSCOPY

Because organisms present unique spectroscopic patterns, spectroscopic examination (e.g., Raman spectroscopy) of **microorganisms** (e.g., microbial cells) can help to differentiate between species and strains of microbes. Spectroscopic examination can also aid in the identification and measurement of subcellular processes (e.g., CO_2 production) that facilitate the understanding of cell growth, response to environmental stimuli, and drug actions.

The measurement of the absorption, emission, or scattering of electromagnetic radiation by atoms or molecules is referred to as spectroscopy. A transition from a lower energy level to a higher level with transfer of electromagnetic energy to the atom or molecule is called absorption; a transition from a higher energy level to a lower level results in the emission of a photon if energy is transferred to the electromagnetic field; and the redirection of light as a result of its interaction with matter is called scattering.

When atoms or molecules absorb electromagnetic energy, the incoming energy transfers the quantized atomic or molecular system to a higher energy level. Electrons are promoted to higher orbitals by ultraviolet or visible light; vibrations are excited by infrared light, and rotations are excited by microwaves. Atomic-absorption spectroscopy measures the concentration of an element in a sample, whereas atomic-emission spectroscopy aims at measuring the concentration of elements in samples. UV-VIS absorption spectroscopy is used to obtain qualitative information from the electronic absorption spectrum, or to measure the concentration of an analyte molecule in solution. Molecular fluorescence spectroscopy is a technique for obtaining qualitative information from the electronic fluorescence spectrum, or, again, for measuring the concentration of an analyte in solution.

Infrared spectroscopy has been widely used in the study of surfaces. The most frequently used portion of the infrared spectrum is the region where molecular vibrational frequencies occur. This technique was first applied around the turn of the twentieth century in an attempt to distinguish water of crystallization from water of constitution in solids.

Ultraviolet spectroscopy takes advantage of the selective absorbance of ultraviolet radiation by various substances. The technique is especially useful in investigating biologically active substances such as compounds in body fluids, and drugs and narcotics either in the living body (in vivo) or outside it (in vitro). Ultraviolet instruments have also been used to monitor air and **water pollution**, to analyze dyestuffs, to study carcinogens, to identify food additives, to analyze petroleum fractions, and to analyze pesticide residues. Ultraviolet photoelectron spectroscopy, a technique that is analogous to x-ray photoelectron spectroscopy, has been used to study valence electrons in gases.

Microwave spectroscopy, or molecular rotational resonance spectroscopy, addresses the microwave region and the absorption of energy by molecules as they undergo transitions between rotational energy levels. From these spectra, it is possible to obtain information about molecular structure, including bond distances and bond angles. One example of the application of this technique is in the distinction of trans and gauche rotational isomers. It is also possible to determine dipole moments and molecular collision rates from these spectra.

In nuclear magnetic resonance (NMR), resonant energy is transferred between a radio-frequency alternating magnetic field and a **nucleus** placed in a field sufficiently strong to decouple the nuclear spin from the influence of atomic electrons. Transitions induced between substrates correspond to different quantized orientations of the nuclear spin relative to the direction of the magnetic field. Nuclear magnetic resonance spectroscopy has two subfields: broadline NMR and high resolution NMR. High resolution NMR has been used in inorganic and organic chemistry to measure subtle electronic effects, to determine structure, to study chemical reactions, and to follow the motion of molecules or groups of atoms within molecules.

Electron paramagnetic resonance is a spectroscopic technique similar to nuclear magnetic resonance except that microwave radiation is employed instead of radio frequencies. Electron paramagnetic resonance has been used extensively to study paramagnetic species present on various solid surfaces. These species may be metal ions, surface defects, or adsorbed molecules or ions with one or more unpaired electrons. This technique also provides a basis for determining the bonding characteristics and orientation of a surface complex. Because the technique can be used with low concentrations of active sites, it has proven valuable in studies of oxidation states.

Atoms or molecules that have been excited to high energy levels can decay to lower levels by emitting radiation. For atoms excited by light energy, the emission is referred to as atomic fluorescence; for atoms excited by higher energies, the emission is called atomic or optical emission. In the case of molecules, the emission is called fluorescence if the transition occurs between states of the same spin, and phosphorescence if the transition takes place between states of different spin.

In x-ray fluorescence, the term refers to the characteristic x rays emitted as a result of absorption of x rays of higher frequency. In electron fluorescence, the emission of electromagnetic radiation occurs as a consequence of the absorption of energy from radiation (either electromagnetic or particulate), provided the emission continues only as long as the stimulus producing it is maintained.

The effects governing x-ray photoelectron spectroscopy were first explained by Albert Einstein in 1905, who showed that the energy of an electron ejected in photoemission was equal to the difference between the photon and the binding energy of the electron in the target. In the 1950s, researchers began measuring binding energies of core electrons by x-ray photoemission. The discovery that these binding energies could vary as much as 6 eV, depending on the chemical state of the atom, led to rapid development of x-ray photoelectron spectroscopy, also known as Electron Spectroscopy for Chemical Analysis (ESCA). This technique has provided valuable information about chemical effects at surfaces. Unlike other spectroscopies in which the absorption, emission, or scattering of radiation is interpreted as a function of energy, photoelectron spectroscopy measures the kinetic energy of the electrons(s) ejected by x-ray radiation.

Mössbauer spectroscopy was invented in the late 1950s by Rudolf Mössbauer, who discovered that when solids emit and absorb gamma rays, the nuclear energy levels can be separated to one part in 10^{14}, which is sufficient to reflect the weak interaction of the nucleus with surrounding electrons. The Mössbauer effect probes the binding, charge distribution and symmetry, and magnetic ordering around an atom in a solid matrix. An example of the Mössbauer effect involves the Fe-57 nuclei (the absorber) in a sample to be studied. From the ground state, the Fe-57 nuclei can be promoted to their first excited state by absorbing a 14.4-keV gamma-ray photon produced by a radioactive parent, in this case Co-57. The excited Fe-57 nucleus then decays to the ground state via electron or gamma ray emission. Classically, one would expect the Fe-57 nuclei to undergo recoil when emitting or absorbing a gamma-ray photon (somewhat like what a person leaping from a boat to a dock observes when his boat recoils into the lake); but according to quantum mechanics, there is also a reasonable possibility that there will be no recoil (as if the boat were embedded in ice when the leap occurred).

When electromagnetic radiation passes through matter, most of the radiation continues along its original path, but a tiny amount is scattered in other directions. Light that is scattered without a change in energy is called Rayleigh scattering; light that is scattered in transparent solids with a transfer of energy to the solid is called Brillouin scattering. Light scattering accompanied by vibrations in molecules or in the optical region in solids is called Raman scattering.

In vibrational spectroscopy, also known as Raman spectroscopy, the light scattered from a gas, liquid, or solid is accompanied by a shift in wavelength from that of the incident radiation. The effect was discovered by the Indian physicist C. V. Raman in 1928. The Raman effect arises from the inelastic scattering of radiation in the visible region by molecules. Raman spectroscopy is similar to infrared spectroscopy in its ability to provide detailed information about molecular structures. Before the 1940s, Raman spectroscopy was the method of choice in molecular structure determinations, but since that time infrared measurements have largely supplemented it. Infrared absorption requires that a vibration change the dipole moment of a molecule, but Raman spectroscopy is associated with the change in polarizability that accompanies a vibration. As a consequence, Raman spectroscopy provides information about molecular vibrations that is particularly well suited to the structural analysis of covalently bonded molecules, and to a lesser extent, of ionic crystals. Raman spectroscopy is also particularly useful in studying the structure of polyatomic molecules. By comparing spectra of a large number of compounds, chemists have been able to identify characteristic frequencies of molecular groups, e.g., methyl, carbonyl, and hydroxyl groups.

See also Biotechnology; Electron microscope, transmission and scanning; Electron microscopic examination of microorganisms; Electrophoresis; Enzyme-linked immunosorbant assay (ELISA); Epidemiology, tracking diseases with technology; Fluorescence in situ hybridization (FISH); Laboratory techniques in immunology; Laboratory techniques in microbiology; Microscope and microscopy

SPHEROPLASTS · *see* PROTOPLASTS AND SPHEROPLASTS

SPINAE · *see* BACTERIAL APPENDAGES

SPIROCHETES

Spirochetes are a group comprised of six genera of **bacteria** in a family known as *Spirochaete*. They are named because of their spiral shape. Typically, spirochetes are very slender. Their length can vary from about five microns (millionths of an inch) to several hundred microns, depending on the species. Under the light or electron **microscope**, the tight coiling that is characteristic of spirochetes is readily visible. Spirochetes are a significant health threat to humans. Both **syphilis** and **Lyme disease** are caused by spirochetes. Beneficially, spirochetes contribute to digestion in ruminants such as cows.

Besides their shape, another distinctive aspect of spirochetes in the presence of what is essentially internal flagella. These structures, called axial filaments, are embedded in the cell wall of the bacterium. They are constructed very similarly as flagella, having the characteristic arrangement of structures that anchors the filament to the cell membrane. There can be only a few to as many as 200 axial filaments present in a given bacterium. The rigidity of an axial filament allows a bacterium to move in a corkscrew type of motion. Axial filaments are present in all spirochetes except *Treponema*.

Spirochetes have varied habitats and growth requirements. Some of the bacteria require oxygen for their survival, while others do not tolerate the presence of oxygen.

In terms of human health, spirochetes are noteworthy because of the disease causing members of the group. *Treponema pallidum* is the cause of syphilis and *Borrelia burgdorferi* is the cause of Lyme disease, which can produce a chronic infection that can result in arthritis, damage to the central nervous system, and even heart failure. *Borrelia burgdorferi* can convert to a metabolically dormant cyst in natural environments and even in humans. The cyst form allows the bacterium to survive inhospitable conditions and to elude host immune defense mechanisms.

In ruminants, spirochetes are beneficial. Their chemical activities help the cow or other ruminant digest food. Spirochetes also live in harmony with mussels and oysters, where the bacteria help in feeding by acting as cilia to sweep food into the mollusk.

A spirochete known as *Aquaspririllum magneto-tacticum* is of interest to microbiologists because it is one of a number of bacteria that possess magnetic particles. These particles allow a bacterium to orient itself in the water in relation to Earth's magnetic field.

See also Bacteria and bacterial infection; Bacterial movement; Magnetotactic bacteria

SPONTANEOUS GENERATION THEORY · *see* HISTORY OF MICROBIOLOGY

SPOROZOA

The fifth Phylum of the Protist Kingdom, known as Apicomplexa, gathers several species of obligate intracellular protozoan **parasites** classified as Sporozoa or Sporozoans, because they form reproductive cells known as spores. Many sporozoans are parasitic and pathogenic species, such as *Plasmodium (P. falciparum, P. malariae, P. vivax), Toxoplasma gondii, Pneumocysts carinii, Coccidian, Babesia, Cryptosporidum (C. parvum, C. muris),* and *Gregarian.* The Sporozoa reproduction cycle has both asexual and sexual phases. The asexual phase is termed schizogony (from the Greek, meaning generation through division), in which merozoites (daughter cells) are produced through multiple nuclear fissions. The sexual phase is known as sporogony (i.e., generation of spores) and is followed by gametogony or the production of sexually reproductive cells termed gamonts. Each pair of gamonts form a gamontocyst where the division of both gamonts, preceded by repeated nuclear divisions, originates numerous gametes. Gametes fuse in pairs, forming zygotes that undergo meiosis (cell division), thus forming new sporozoites. When sporozoites invade new host cells, the life cycle starts again. This general description of Sporozoan life cycle has some variation among different species and groups.

Sporozoans have no flagellated extensions for locomotion, with most species presenting only gliding motility, except for male gametes in the sexual phase, which have a flagellated stage of motility. All Sporozoa have a cellular structure known as apical complex, which gave origin to the name of the Phylum, i.e., Apicomplexa. Sporozoa cellular organization consists of the apical complex, micropore, longitudinal microtubular cytoskeleton, and cortical alveoli. The apical complex consists of cytoskeletal and secretory structures forming a conoid (a small open cone), polar wings that fix the cytoskeletal microtubules, two apical rings, and secretory vesicles known as micronemes and rhoptries. The apical complex enables Sporozoans to invade the host cells.

Plasmodium species are the causing agents of **malaria** in humans and animals and affects approximately 300 million people around the world, with an estimative of one million new cases each year. They are transmitted by the female anopheles mosquito (infecting vector) that injects *Plasmodium* sporozoites present in the salivary glands of the mosquito into the host's blood stream. Once in the blood stream, *Plasmodium* sporozoites invade erythrocytes (red blood cells) and migrate to the liver to infect the hepatocytes, where their asexual reproductive phase starts. When the merozoite stage is reached, they are released into the circulation again, where they become ring-like trophozoites that undergo schizogony, forming new merozoites that invade the erythrocytes, thus repeating the reproductive cycle. Female anopheles mosquitoes ingest merozoites together with the host's blood. Ingested merozoites form zygotes in the guts of the vector mosquito, later developing into oocysts, from which new sporozoites will be formed and migrate to the anopheles' salivary gland, ready to contaminate the next host. Malaria can also be transmitted through infected blood transfusions.

The vectors for *Babesia* are ticks, causing fever, peripheral capillary hemorrhage, and anemia. Contaminated cats are *Toxoplasma gondii* direct vectors to humans, through the ingestion of oocysts present in cat feces. However, this parasite is also present in birds and other mammals, and humans can be infected by ingesting raw or poorly cooked contaminated meat. Pregnant women may have miscarriages when infected, or can transmit **toxoplasmosis** through the placenta to the fetus, leading to blindness and/or mental retardation of the child. Periodic fecal tests of the house cat and adequate treatment may prevent transmission, as well as avoidance of half-cooked meat in the diet.

Pneumocysts carinii causes interstitial plasma cell **pneumonia** when the cysts containing trophozoites are inhaled. *Cryptosporidium parvum* is usually transmitted through the ingestion of water or foods contaminated with its oocysts, causing intestinal infection and, in immunodepressed patients, diarrhea can be chronic, accompanied by fever. *Coccidian* species infect epithelial tissues of both vertebrates and invertebrates whereas *Gregarian* species are found in the body cavities of invertebrates, such as earthworms.

See also Gastroenteritis; Malaria and the physiology of parasitic infections; Microbial taxonomy

SPORULATION

Sporulation is the formation of nearly dormant forms of **bacteria**. In a limited number of bacteria, spores can preserve the genetic material of the bacteria when conditions are inhospitable and lethal for the normal (vegetative) form of the bacteria. The commitment of a bacterium to the sporulation process sets in motion a series of events that transform the cell.

Sporulation ultimately provides for a multilayered structure can be maintained for a very long time. Relative to the norm life span of the microorganism, spores are designed to protect a bacterium from heat, dryness, and excess radiation for a long time. Endospores of *Bacillus subtilis* have been recovered from objects that are thousands of years old. Furthermore, these are capable of resuscitation into an actively growing and dividing cell. Spores have been recovered from amber that is more than 250 million years old.

Given that resuscitation is possible, sporulation does not result in a completely inert structure. The interior of a spore contains genetic material, **cytoplasm**, and the necessary **enzymes** and other materials to sustain activity. But, this activity occurs at an extremely slow rate; some 10 million times slower than the metabolic rate of a growing bacterium.

The sporulation process has been well studied in *Bacillus subtilis*. The process is stimulated by starvation. Typically, sporulation is a "last resort," when other options fail (e.g., movement to seek new food, production of enzymes to degrade surrounding material, production of antimicrobial agents to wipe out other microbes competing for the food source, etc.). The genetic grounding for the commitment to form a spore is a protein called SpoA. This protein functions to promote the **transcription** of genes that are required for the conversion of the actively growing bacterium to a spore. The formation of an active SpoA protein is controlled by a series of reactions that are themselves responsive to the environmental conditions. Thus, the activation of SpoA comes only after a number of checkpoints have been passed. In this way a bacterium has a number of opportunities to opt out of the sporulation process. Once committed to sporulation, the process is irreversible.

A similar series of reactions has been identified as a means of regulating the degree of host damage caused by a *Bordetella pertussis*, the bacterium that causes **pertussis**, as well as in the response of the **yeast** *Saccharomyces cervesiae* to osmotic pressure.

Sporulation begins with the duplication of the bacterial genome. The second copy and some of the cytoplasm is then enveloped in an in-growth of the membrane that surrounds the bacterium. The result is essentially a little spherical cell inside the larger bacterium. The little cell is referred to as the "daughter cell" and the original bacterium is now called the "mother cell." Another membrane layer is laid down around the daughter cell. Between these two membranes lies a layer of **peptidoglycan** material, the same rigid material that forms the stress-bearing network in the bacterial cell wall. Finally, a coat of proteins is layered around the outside of the daughter cell. The result is a nearly impregnable sphere.

The above spore is technically termed an endospore, because the formation of the membrane-enclosed daughter cell occurs inside the mother cell. In a so-called exospore, the duplicated **DNA** migrates next to a region on the inner surface of the cell membrane and then a bud forms. As the bud protrudes further outward, the DNA is drawn inside the bud. Examples of endospore forming bacteria include those in the genera *Bacillus* and *Clostridium*. Endospore forming bacteria include *Methylosinus*, *Cyanobacteria*, and *Microsporidia*.

When still in the mother cell, the location of the spore (e.g., in the center, near one end or at one pole) is often a distinctive feature for a particular species of bacteria, and can be used as a feature to identify the bacteria.

As the mother cell dies and degrades, the spore will be freed. When conditions become more hospital, the metabolic machinery within the spore will sense the change and a reverse process will be initiated to transform the spore into a vegetative cell.

The type of sporulation described here is different from the sporulation process that occurs in many kinds of **fungi** and in the bacteria called *Actinomyces*. The latter spores are essentially seeds, and are used in the normal reproduction cycle of the **microorganisms**. Bacterial sporulation is an emergency protective and survival strategy.

See also Asexual generation and reproduction; Bacterial adaptation; Bacterial growth and division; Bacterial kingdoms; Bacterial membranes and cell wall; Cell cycle (prokaryotic), genetic regulation of; Desiccation; Extraterrestrial microbiology; Extremophiles; Fossilization of bacteria; Genetic identification of microorganisms; Genetic regulation of prokaryotic cells; Life, origin of; Radiation resistant bacteria

STANLEY, WENDELL MEREDITH (1904-1971)

American biochemist

Wendell Meredith Stanley was a biochemist who was the first to isolate, purify, and characterize the crystalline form of a virus. During World War II, he led a team of scientists in developing a **vaccine** for viral **influenza**. His efforts have paved the way for understanding the molecular basis of heredity and formed the foundation for the new scientific field of **molecular biology**. For his work in crystallizing the **tobacco mosaic virus**, Stanley shared the 1946 Nobel Prize in chemistry with John Howard Northrop and James B. Sumner.

Stanley was born in the small community of Ridgeville, Indiana. His parents, James and Claire Plessinger Stanley, were publishers of a local newspaper. As a boy, Stanley helped the business by collecting news, setting type, and delivering papers. After graduating from high school he enrolled in Earlham College, a liberal arts school in Richmond, Indiana, where he majored in chemistry and mathematics. He played football as an undergraduate, and in his senior year, he became team captain and was chosen to play end on the Indiana All-State team. In June of 1926, Stanley graduated with a Bachelor of Science degree. His ambition was to become a football coach, but the course of his life was changed forever when an Earlham chemistry professor invited him on a trip to Illinois State University. Here, he was introduced to Roger Adams, an organic chemist, who inspired him to seek a career in chemical research. Stanley applied and was accepted as a graduate assistant in the fall of 1926.

In graduate school, Stanley worked under Adams, and his first project involved finding the stereochemical characteristics of biphenyl, a molecule containing carbon and hydrogen atoms. His second assignment was more practical; Adams was interested in finding chemicals to treat **leprosy**, and Stanley set out to prepare and purify compounds that would destroy the disease-causing pathogen. Stanley received his master's degree in 1927 and two years later was awarded his Ph.D. In the summer of 1930, he was awarded a National Research Council Fellowship to do postdoctoral studies with Heinrich Wieland at the University of Munich in Germany. Under Wieland's tutelage, Stanley extended his knowledge of experimental **biochemistry** by characterizing the properties of some **yeast** compounds.

Stanley returned to the United States in 1931 to accept the post of research assistant at the Rockefeller Institute in New York City. Stanley was assigned to work with W. J. V. Osterhout, who was studying how living cells absorb potassium ions from seawater. Stanley was asked to find a suitable chemical model that would simulate how a marine plant called *Valonia* functions. Stanley discovered a way of using a water-insoluble solution sandwiched between two layers of water to model the way the plant exchanged ions with its environment. The work on *Valonia* served to extend Stanley's knowledge of biophysical systems, and it introduced him to current problems in biological chemistry.

In 1932, Stanley moved to the Rockefeller Institute's Division of Plant Pathology in Princeton, New Jersey. He was primarily interested in studying **viruses**. Viruses were known to cause diseases in plants and animals, but little was known about how they functioned. Stanley's assignment was to characterize viruses and determine their composition and structure.

Stanley began work on a virus that had long been associated with the field of **virology**. In 1892, D. Ivanovsky, a Russian scientist, had studied tobacco mosaic disease, in which infected tobacco plants develop a characteristic mosaic pattern of dark and light spots. He found that the tobacco plant juice retained its ability to cause infection even after it was passed through a filter. Six years later M. Beijerinck, a Dutch scientist, realized the significance of Ivanovsky's discovery: the filtration technique used by Ivanovsky would have filtered out all known **bacteria**, and the fact that the filtered juice remained infectious must have meant that something smaller than a bacterium and invisible to the ordinary light **microscope** was responsible for the disease. Beijerinck concluded that tobacco mosaic disease was caused by a previously undiscovered type of infective agent, a virus.

Stanley was aware of recent techniques used to precipitate the tobacco mosaic virus (**TMV**) with common chemicals. These results led him to believe that the virus might be a protein susceptible to the reagents used in protein chemistry. He

set out to isolate, purify, and concentrate the tobacco mosaic virus. He planted Turkish tobacco plants, and when the plants were about 6 in (15 cm) tall, he rubbed the leaves with a swab of linen dipped in TMV solution. After a few days, the heavily infected plants were chopped and frozen. Later, he ground and mashed the frozen plants to obtain a thick, dark liquid. He then subjected the TMV liquid to various **enzymes** and found that some would inactivate the virus and concluded that TMV must be a protein or something similar. After exposing the liquid to more than 100 different chemicals, Stanley determined that the virus was inactivated by the same chemicals that typically inactivated proteins, and this suggested to him, as well as others, that TMV was protein-like in nature.

Stanley then turned his attention to obtaining a pure sample of the virus. He decanted, filtered, precipitated, and evaporated the tobacco juice many times. With each chemical operation, the juice became more clear and the solution more infectious. The result of two-and-one-half years of work was a clear concentrated solution of TMV that began to form into crystals when stirred. Stanley filtered and collected the tiny, white crystals and discovered that they retained their ability to produce the characteristic lesions of tobacco mosaic disease.

After successfully crystallizing TMV, Stanley's work turned toward characterizing its properties. In 1936, two English scientists at Cambridge University confirmed Stanley's work by isolating TMV crystals. They discovered that the virus consisted of 94% protein and 6% nucleic acid, and they concluded that TMV was a nucleoprotein. Stanley was skeptical at first. Later studies, however, showed that the virus became inactivated upon removal of the nucleic acid, and this work convinced him that TMV was indeed a nucleoprotein. In addition to chemical evidence, the first **electron microscope** pictures of TMV were produced by researchers in Germany. The pictures showed the crystals to have a distinct rod-like shape. For his work in crystallizing the tobacco mosaic virus, Stanley shared the 1946 Nobel prize in chemistry with John Howard Northrop and James Sumner.

During World War II, Stanley was asked to participate in efforts to prevent viral diseases, and he joined the Office of Scientific Research and Development in Washington D.C. Here, he worked on the problem of finding a vaccine effective against viral influenza. Such a substance would change the virus so that the body's **immune system** could build up defenses without causing the disease. Using fertilized hen eggs as a source, he proceeded to grow, isolate, and purify the virus. After many attempts, he discovered that formaldehyde, the chemical used as a biological preservative, would inactivate the virus but still induce the body to produce antibodies. The first flu vaccine was tested and found to be remarkably effective against viral influenza. For his work in developing large-scale methods of preparing vaccines, he was awarded the Presidential Certificate of Merit in 1948.

In 1948, Stanley moved to the University of California in Berkeley, where he became director of a new virology laboratory and chair of the department of biochemistry. In five years, Stanley assembled an impressive team of scientists and technicians who reopened the study of **plant viruses** and began an intensive effort to characterize large, biologically important molecules. In 1955 Heinz Fraenkel-Conrat, a protein chemist, and R. C. Williams, an electron microscopist, took TMV apart and reassembled the viral **RNA**, thus proving that RNA was the infectious component. In addition, their work indicated that the protein component of TMV served only as a protective cover. Other workers in the virus laboratory succeeded in isolating and crystallizing the virus responsible for polio, and in 1960, Stanley led a group that determined the complete amino acid sequence of TMV protein. In the early 1960s, Stanley became interested in a possible link between viruses and cancer.

Stanley was an advocate of academic freedom. In the 1950s, when his university was embroiled in the politics of McCarthyism, members of the faculty were asked to sign oaths of loyalty to the United States. Although Stanley signed the oath of loyalty, he publicly defended those who chose not to, and his actions led to court decisions which eventually invalidated the requirement.

Stanley received many awards, including the Alder Prize from Harvard University in 1938, the Nichols Medal of the American Chemical Society in 1946, and the Scientific Achievement Award of the American Medical Association in 1966. He held honorary doctorates from many colleges and universities. He was a prolific author of more than 150 publications and he co-edited a three volume compendium entitled *The Viruses*. By lecturing, writing, and appearing on television he helped bring important scientific issues before the public. He served on many boards and commissions, including the National Institute of Health, the **World Health Organization**, and the National Cancer Institute.

Stanley married Marian Staples Jay on June 25, 1929. The two met at the University of Illinois, when they both were graduate students in chemistry. They co-authored a scientific paper together with Adams, which was published the same year they were married. The Stanleys had three daughters and one son. While attending a conference on biochemistry in Spain, Stanley died from a heart attack at the age of 66.

See also History of immunology; History of microbiology; Viral genetics; Viral vectors in gene therapy; Virology; Virus replication; Viruses and responses to viral infection

STAPHYLOCOCCI AND STAPHYLOCOCCI INFECTIONS

Staphylococci are a group of Gram-positive **bacteria** that are members of the genus *Staphylococcus*. Several infections are caused by staphylococci. In particular, infections associated with methicillin-resistant *Staphylococcus aureus* are an increasing problem in hospitals.

The name staphyloccus is derived from Greek (staphyle—a bunch of grapes). The designation describes the typical grape-like clustered arrangement of staphylococci viewed under a light **microscope**. Staphylococci are divided into two groups based on the presence or absence of the plasma-clotting enzyme called **coagulase**. The coagulase-positive staphylococci consist mainly of *Staphylococcus aureus*

and the coagulase-negative group consists primarily of *Staphylococcus epidermidis* and *Staphylococcus saprophyticus*. Because the treatment of infections caused by these bacteria can be different, the coagulase test provides a rapid means of indicating the identity of the bacteria of concern.

Staphylococci are not capable of movement and do not form spores. They are capable of growth in the presence and absence of oxygen. Furthermore, staphylococci are hardy bacteria, capable of withstanding elevated conditions of temperature, salt concentration, and a wide **pH** range. This hardiness allows them to colonize the surface of the skin and the mucous membranes of many mammals including humans.

Staphylococcus aureus is the cause of a variety of infections in humans. Many are more of an inconvenience than a threat (e.g., skin infection, infection of hair follicles, etc.). However, other infections are serious. One example is a skin infection known as scalded skin syndrome. In newborns and burn victims, scalded skin syndrome can be fatal. Another example is **toxic shock syndrome** that results from the infection of a tampon with a toxin-producing strain (other mechanisms also cause toxic shock syndrome). The latter syndrome can overwhelm the body's defenses, due to the production by the bacteria of what is called a superantigen. This superantigen causes a large proportion of a certain type of immune cells to release a chemical that causes dramatic changes in the physiology of the body.

Staphylococci can also infect wounds. From there, the infection can spread further because some strains of staphylococci produce an arsenal of **enzymes** that dissolve membranes, protein, and degrade both **DNA** and **RNA**. Thus, the bacteria are able to burrow deeper into tissue to evade the host's immune response and antibacterial agents such as **antibiotics**. If the infection spreads to the bloodstream, a widespread **contamination** of the body can result (e.g., **meningitis**, endocarditis, **pneumonia**, bone **inflammation**).

Because staphylococci are resident on the skin of the hands, the bacteria can be easily transferred to objects or people. Within the past few decades the extent to which staphylococci infection of implanted devices is a cause of chronic diseases has become clear. For example, contamination of implanted heart valves and artificial hips joints is now recognized to be the cause of heart damage and infection of the bone.

Additionally, the ready transfer of staphylococci from the skin is an important reason why staphylococci infections are pronounced in settings such as hospitals. *Staphylococcus aureus* is an immense problem as the source of hospital-acquired infections. This is especially true when the strain of bacteria is resistant to the antibiotic methicillin and other common antibiotics. This resistance necessitates more elaborate treatment with more expensive antibiotics. Furthermore, the infection can be more established by the time the **antibiotic resistance** of the bacteria is determined. These so-called methicillin-resistant *Staphylococcus aureus* (MRSA) are resistant to only a few antibiotics currently available. The prevalence of MRSA among all the *Staphylococcus aureus* that is isolated in hospitals in the United States is about 50%. The fear is that the bacteria will acquire resistance to the remaining antibiotics that are currently effective. This fear is

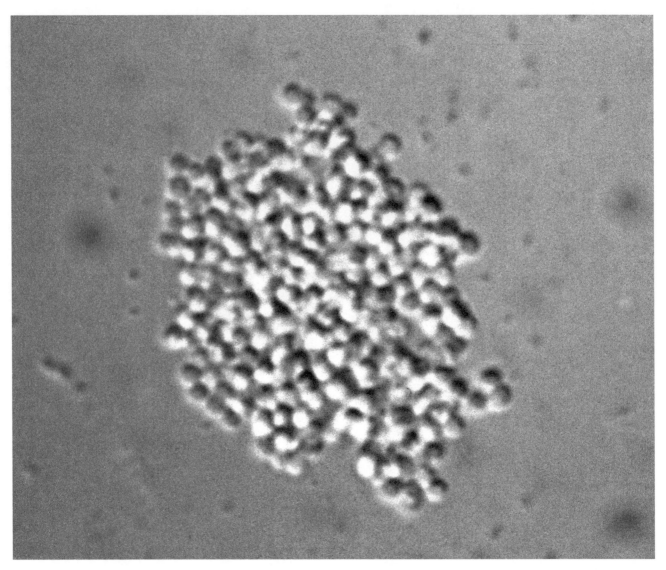

A cluster of Staphylococcus bacteria.

real, since the MRSA is prevalent in an environment (the hospital) where antibiotics are in constant use. Development of a fully resistant strain of *Staphylococcus aureus* would make treatment of MRSA infections extremely difficult, and would severely compromise health care.

Staphylococci are also responsible for the poisoning of foods (e.g., ham, poultry, potato salad, egg salad, custards). The poisoning typically occurs if contaminated food is allowed to remain at a temperature that allows the staphylococci to grow and produce a toxin. Ingestion of the toxin produces an intestinal illness and can affect various organs throughout the body.

The need for more effective prevention and treatment strategies for staphylococcal infections is urgent, given the wide variety of infections that are caused by staphylococci and the looming specter of a completely resistant staphylococcus.

See also Bacteria and bacterial infection; Infection and resistance

STEAM PRESSURE STERILIZER

Steam pressure **sterilization** requires a combination of pressure, high temperatures, and moisture, and serves as one of the most widely used methods for sterilization where these functions will not affect a load. The simplest example of a steam pressure sterilizer is a home pressure cooker, though it is not recommended for accurate sterilization. Its main component is a chamber or vessel in which items for sterilization are sealed and subjected to high temperatures for a specified length of time, known as a cycle.

Steam pressure sterilizer has replaced the term autoclave for all practical purposes, though autoclaving is still used to describe the process of sterilization by steam. The function of the sterilizer is to kill unwanted **microorganisms** on instruments, in cultures, and even in liquids, because the presence of foreign microbes might negatively affect the outcome of a test, or the purity of a sample. A sterilizer also acts as a test vehicle for industrial products such as plastics that must withstand certain pressures and temperatures.

Larger chambers are typically lined with a metal jacket, creating a pocket to trap pressurized steam. This method preheats the chamber to reduce condensation and cycle time. Surrounding the unit with steam-heated tubes produces the same effect. Steam is then introduced by external piping or, in smaller units, by internal means, and begins to circulate within the chamber. Because steam is lighter than air, it quickly builds enough mass to displace it, forcing interior air and any air-steam mixtures out of a trap or drain.

Most sterilization processes require temperatures higher than that of boiling water (212°F, 100°C), which is not sufficient to kill microorganisms, so pressure is increased within the chamber to increase temperature. For example, at 15 psi the temperature rises to 250°F (121°C). Many clinical applications require a cycle of 20 minutes at this temperature for effective sterilization. Cycle variables can be adjusted to meet the requirements of a given application. The introduction of a vacuum can further increase temperature and reduce cycle time by quickly removing air from the chamber. The process of steam sterilization is kept in check by pressure and temperature gauges, as well as a safety valve that automatically vents the chamber should the internal pressure build beyond the unit's capacity.

See also Infection control; Laboratory techniques in microbiology

STENTOR

Stentor is a genus of protozoan that is found in slow moving or stagnant fresh water. The microorganism is named for a Greek hero in the Trojan War, who was renowned for his loud voice, in an analogous way to the sound of a trumpet rising up over the sound of other instruments. The description is fitting the microorganism because the organism is shaped somewhat like a trumpet, with small end flaring out to form a much larger opening at the other end. The narrow end can elaborate a sticky substance that aids the protozoan in adhering to plants. At the other end, fine hair-like extensions called cilia beat rhythmically to drive food into the gullet of the organism. The various species of stentor tend to be brightly colored. For example, *Stentor coeruleus* is blue in color. Other species are yellow, red, and brown.

Stentor are one of the largest **protozoa** found in water. As a protozoan, *Stentor* is a single cell. Nonetheless, a typical organism can be 2 mm in length, making them visible to the unaided eye, and even larger than some multi-celled organisms such as rotifers. This large size and ubiquity in pond water has made the organism a favorite tool for school science classes, particularly as a learning tool for the use of the light

microscope. In particular, the various external and internal features are very apparent under the special type of microscopic illumination called phase contrast. Use of other forms of microscopic illumination, such as bright field, dark field, oblique, and Rheinberg illumination, can each reveal features that together comprise a detailed informational picture of the protozoan. Thus, examination of stentor allows a student to experiment with different forms of light microscopic illumination and to directly compare the effects of each type of illumination of the same sample.

Another feature evident in *Stentor* is known as a contractile vacuole. The vacuole functions to collect and cycle back to the outside of *Stentor* the water that flows in to balance the higher salt concentration inside the protozoan. Careful observation of the individual protozoa usually allows detection of full and collapsed vacuoles.

For the student, fall is a good time to observe *Stentor*. Leaves that have fallen into the water decay and support the growth of large numbers of **bacteria**. These, in turn, support the growth of large numbers of stentor.

See also Microscope and microscopy; Water pollution and purification

STERILIZATION

Sterilization is a term that refers to the complete killing or elimination of living organisms in the sample being treated. Sterilization is absolute. After the treatment the sample is either devoid of life, or the possibility of life (as from the subsequent germination and growth of bacterial spores), or it is not.

There are four widely used means of sterilization. Standard sterilization processes utilize heat, radiation, chemicals, or the direct removal of the **microorganisms**.

The most widely practiced method of sterilization is the use of heat. There are a number of different means by which heat can be applied to a sample. The choice of which method of delivery depends on a number of factors including the type of sample. As an example, when bacterial spores are present the heating conditions must be sufficient to kill even these dormant forms of the **bacteria**.

A common type of heat sterilization that is used many types each day in a microbiology laboratory is known as incineration. Microorganisms are burned by exposing them to an open flame of propane. "Flaming" of inoculating needles and the tops of laboratory glassware before and after sampling are examples of incineration.

Another form of heat sterilization is boiling. Drinking water can be sterilized with respect to potentially harmful microorganisms such as *Escherichia coli* by heating the water to a temperature of 212°F (100°C) for five minutes. However, the dormant cyst form of the protozoan *Giardia lamblia* that can be present in drinking water, can survive this period of boiling. To ensure complete sterility, the 212°F (100°C) temperature must be maintained for 30 minutes. Even then, some bacterial spores, such as those of *Bacillus* or *Clostridium* can survive. To guarantee sterilization, fluids must be boiled for an extended time or intermittent boiling can be done, wherein at least three—and up to 30—periods of boiling are interspersed with time to allow the fluid to cool.

Steam heat (moist heat) sterilization is performed on a daily basis in the microbiology laboratory. The pressure cooker called an autoclave is the typical means of steam heat sterilization. Autoclaving for 15 minutes at 15 pounds of pressure produces a temperature of 250°F (121°C), sufficient to kill bacterial spores. Indeed, part of a quality control regiment for a laboratory should include a regular inclusion of commercially available bacterial spores with the load being sterilized. The spores can then be added to a liquid growth medium and growth should not occur.

Pasteurization is employed to sterilize fluids such as milk without compromising the nutritional or flavor qualities of the fluid.

The final form of heat sterilization is known as dry heat sterilization. Essentially this involves the use of an oven to heat dry objects and materials to a temperature of 320–338°F (160–170°C) for two hours. Glassware is often sterilized in this way.

Some samples cannot be sterilized by the use of heat. Devices that contain rubber gaskets and plastic surfaces are often troublesome. Heat sterilization can deform these materials or make them brittle. Fortunately, other means of sterilization exist.

Chemicals or gas can sterilize objects. Ethylene oxide gas is toxic to many microorganisms. Its use requires a special gas chamber, because the vapors are also noxious to humans. Chemicals that can be used to kill microorganisms include formaldehyde and glutaraldehyde. Ethanol is an effective sterilant of laboratory work surfaces. However, the exposure of the surface to ethanol must be long enough to kill the adherent microorganisms, otherwise survivors may develop resistance to the sterilant.

Another means of sterilization utilizes radiation. Irradiation of foods is becoming a more acceptable means of sterilizing the surface of foods (e.g., poultry). Ultraviolet radiation acts by breaking up the genetic material of microorganisms. The damage is usually too severe to be repaired. The sole known exception is the **radiation-resistant bacteria** of the genus *Deinococcus*.

The final method of sterilization involves the physical removal of microorganisms from a fluid. This is done by the use of filters that have extremely small holes in them. Fluid is pumped through the filter, and all but water molecules are excluded from passage. Filters—now in routine use in the treatment of drinking water—can be designed to filter out very small microorganisms, including many **viruses**.

See also Bacterial growth and division; Bacteriocidal, bacteriostatic; Laboratory techniques in microbiology

STREP THROAT

Streptococcal sore throat, or strep throat as it is more commonly called, is an infection caused by group A *Streptococcus*

bacteria. The main target of the infection is the mucous membranes lining the pharynx. Sometimes the tonsils are also infected (tonsillitis). If left untreated, the infection can develop into rheumatic fever or other serious conditions.

Strep throat is a common malady, accounting for 5–10% of all sore throats. Strep throat is most common in school age children. Children under age two are less likely to get the disease. Adults who smoke, are fatigued, or who live in damp, crowded conditions also develop the disease at higher rates than the general population.

The malady is seasonal. Strep throat occurs most frequently from November to April. In these winter months, the disease passes directly from person to person by coughing, sneezing, and close contact. Very occasionally the disease is passed through food, most often when a food handler infected with strep throat accidentally contaminates food by coughing or sneezing.

Once infected with the *Streptococcus,* a painful sore throat develops from one to five days later. The sore throat can be accompanied by fatigue, a fever, chills, headache, muscle aches, swollen lymph glands, and nausea. Young children may complain of abdominal pain. The tonsils look swollen and are bright red with white or yellow patches of pus on them. Sometimes the roof of the mouth is red or has small red spots. Often a person with strep throat has a characteristic odor to their breath.

Others who are infected may display few symptoms. Still others may develop a fine, rough, sunburn-like rash over the face and upper body, and have a fever of 101–104ºF (38–40ºC). The tongue becomes bright red with a flecked, strawberry-like appearance. When a rash develops, this form of strep throat is called scarlet fever. The rash is a reaction to toxins released by the streptococcus bacteria. Scarlet fever is essentially treated the same way. The rash disappears in about five days. One to three weeks later, patches of skin may peel off, as might occur with a sunburn.

Strep throat can be self-limiting. Symptoms often subside in four or five days. However, in some cases untreated strep throat can cause rheumatic fever. This is a serious illness, although it occurs rarely. The most recent outbreak appeared in the United States in the mid-1980s. Rheumatic fever occurs most often in children between the ages of five and 15, and may have a genetic component, because susceptibility seems to run in families. Although the strep throat that causes rheumatic fever is contagious, rheumatic fever itself is not.

Rheumatic fever begins one to six weeks after an untreated streptococcal infection. The joints, especially the wrists, elbows, knees, and ankles become red, sore, and swollen. The infected person develops a high fever, and possibly a rapid heartbeat when lying down, paleness, shortness of breath, and fluid retention. A red rash over the trunk may come and go for weeks or months. An acute attack of rheumatic fever lasts about three months. Rheumatic fever can cause permanent damage to the heart and heart valves. It can be prevented by promptly treating streptococcal infections with **antibiotics**. It does not occur if all the *Streptococcus* bacteria are killed within the first 10–12 days after infection.

In the 1990s, outbreaks of a virulent strain of group A *Streptococcus* were reported to cause a toxic-shock-like illness and a severe invasive infection called necrotizing fasciitis, which destroys skin and muscle tissue. Although these diseases are caused by group A *Streptococcus*, they rarely begin with strep throat. Usually the *Streptococcus* bacteria enter the body through a skin wound. These complications are rare. However, since the death rate in necrotizing fasciitis is 30–50%, prompt medical attention for any streptococcal infection is prudent.

The *Streptococcus* bacteria are susceptible to antibiotics such as **penicillin**. However, in some 10% of infections, penicillin is ineffective. Then, other antibiotics are used, including amoxicillin, clindamycin, or a cephalosporin.

See also Bacteria and bacterial infection; Streptococci and streptococcal infections

STREPTOCOCCAL ANTIBODY TESTS

Species of Gram positive **bacteria** from the genus *Streptococcus* are capable of causing infections in humans. There are several disease-causing strains of **streptococci**. These strains have been categorized into groups (A, B, C, D, and G), according to their behavior, chemistry, and appearance.

Each group causes specific types of infections and symptoms. For example, group A streptococci are the most virulent species for humans and are the cause of "strep throat," tonsillitis, wound and **skin infections**, blood infections (septicemia), scarlet fever, **pneumonia**, rheumatic fever, Sydenham's chorea (formerly called St. Vitus' dance), and glomerulonephritis.

While the symptoms affected individuals experience may be suggestive of a streptococcal infection, a diagnosis must be confirmed by testing. The most accurate common procedure is to take a sample from the infected area for **culture**, a means whereby the bacteria of interest can be grown and isolated using various synthetic laboratory growth media. This process can take weeks. A more rapid indication of the presence of streptococci can be obtained through the detection of antibodies that have been produced in response to the infecting bacteria. The antibody-based tests can alert the physician to the potential presence of living infectious streptococci.

The presence of streptococci can be detected using antibody-based assays. Three streptococcal **antibody** tests that are used most often are known as the antistreptolysin O titer (ASO), the antideoxyribonuclease-B titer (anti-Dnase-B, or ADB), and the streptozyme test.

The antistreptolysin O titer determines whether an infection with the group A Streptococcus has precluded the development of post-infection complications. The term titer refers to the amount of antibody. Thus, this test is quantitative. That is, the amount of specific antibody in the sample can be deduced. In an infection the amount of antibody will rise, as the **immune system** responds to the invading bacteria. These complications include scarlet fever, rheumatic fever, or a kidney disease termed glomerulonephritis.

The ASO titer is used to demonstrate the body's reaction to an infection caused by group A beta-hemolytic streptococci. The beta-hemolytic designation refers to a reaction produced by the bacteria when grown in the presence of red blood cells. Bacteria of this group are particularly important in suspected cases of acute rheumatic fever (ARF) or acute glomerulonephritis. Group A streptococci produce the enzyme streptolysin O, which can destroy (lyse) red blood cells. Because streptolysin O is antigenic (contains a protein foreign to the body), the body reacts by producing antistreptolysin O (ASO), which is a neutralizing antibody. ASO appears in the blood serum one week to one month after the onset of a strep infection. A high titer (high levels of ASO) is not specific for any type of poststreptococcal disease, but it does indicate if a streptococcal infection is or has been present.

Tests conducted after therapy starts can reveal if an active infection was in progress. This will be evident by a decreasing antibody titer over time, as more and more of the streptococci are killed.

The anti-DNase-B test likewise detects groups A beta-hemolytic Streptococcus. This test is often done at the same time as the ASO titer. This done as the Dnase-based test can produce results that are more variable than those produced by the ASO test. This blanket coverage typically detects some 95% of previous strep infections are detected. If both tests are repeatedly negative, the likelihood is that the patient's symptoms are not caused by a poststreptococcal disease.

The final antibody-based test is a screening test. That is, the test is somewhat broader in scope than the other tests. The streptozyme test is often used as a screening test for antibodies to the streptococcal antigens NADase, DNase, streptokinase, streptolysin O, and hyaluronidase. This test is most useful in evaluating suspected poststreptococcal disease following infection with *Streptococcus pyogenes*, such as rheumatic fever.

The streptozyme assay has certain advantages over the other two tests. It can detect several antibodies in a single assay, is quick and easy to perform, and is unaffected by factors that can produce false-positives in the ASO test. However, the assay does have some disadvantages. While it detects different antibodies, it does not determine which one has been detected, and it is not as sensitive in children as in adults.

See also Antibody and antigen; Antibody formation and kinetics; Bacteria and bacterial infection

STREPTOCOCCI AND STREPTOCOCCAL INFECTIONS

Streptococci are spherical, Gram positive **bacteria**. Commonly they are referred to as strep bacteria. Streptococci are normal residents on the skin and mucous surfaces on or inside humans. However, when strep bacteria normally found on the skin or in the intestines, mouth, nose, reproductive tract, or urinary tract invade other parts of the body—via a cut or abrasion—and contaminate blood or tissue, infection can be the result.

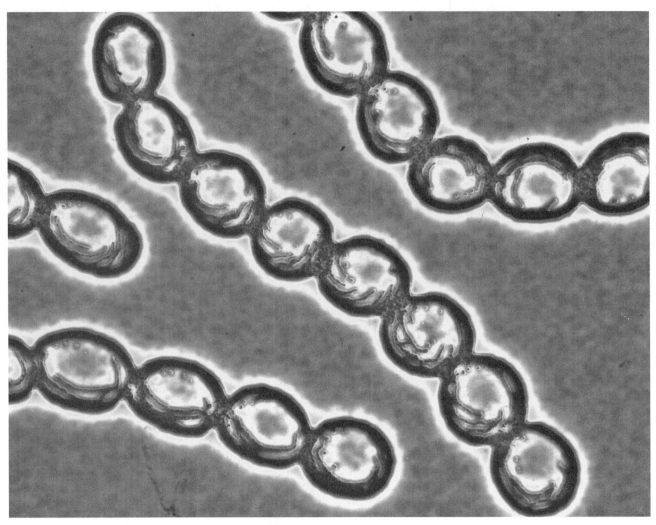

Chains of *Streptococcus pyogenes*.

Numerous strains of strep bacteria have been identified. Those streptococci from groups A, B, C, D, and G are most likely to cause disease. While some of these infections do not produce symptoms, and the infected person can become a carrier of the disease-causing bacteria, other strep infections can be fatal.

Primary strep infections invade healthy tissue, and most often affect the throat. Secondary strep infections invade tissue already weakened by injury or illness. They frequently affect the bones, ears, eyes, joints, or intestines. Both primary and secondary strep infections can travel from affected tissues to lymph glands, enter the bloodstream, and spread throughout the body.

Group A streptococci contains those strep bacteria that are most apt to be associated with serious illness. Between 10,000 and 15,000 infections attributable to group A streptococci occur in the United States every year. Most are mild inflammations of the throat or skin, the environments where the bacteria are normally found. However, other infections can be deadly.

One example of a serious infection is known as necrotizing fasciitis (which is also referred in the popular press as flesh-eating disease). The disease results from the invasion of host tissue cells by the bacteria. There, shielded from the immune responses of the host, toxic bacterial products cause the destruction of muscle tissue and fat. The infection is able to quickly spread outward from the point of origin. Unless intervention is undertaken quickly, which includes antibiotic therapy and, in severe cases where a limb is involved, amputation of the affected limb, the infection can be fatal.

A second example of a serious group A streptococcal infection manifests **toxic shock syndrome**.

Another division of streptococci is known as group B. Infections caused by group B streptococci most often affects pregnant women, infants, the elderly, and chronically ill adults. Group B was designated in the 1970s. The intervening years have revealed group B streptococci to be the primary cause of life-threatening illness and death in newborns. The bacteria reside in the reproductive tract of a quarter of all pregnant women. Only a small percentage of these women develop invasive infection. However, about half of those who are infected will transmit the bacteria to their babies during delivery.

In the United States, about 12,000 newborns will be infected each year. Of these, about 8,000 develop early-onset infection within hours or days of birth. Complications include **inflammation** of the membranes covering the brain and spinal cord (**meningitis**), **pneumonia**, and blood infection (sepsis). In other infants, meningitis will develop in the first three months of life.

The streptococci in group D are a common cause of wound infections in hospital patients. As well, group D streptococci are associated with abnormal growth of tissue in the gastrointestinal tract, urinary tract infection, and infections of the womb in women who have just given birth.

Another group of the streptococci that is of concern to human health is group G. Normally present on the skin, in the mouth and throat, and in the intestines and genital tract, group G streptococci can cause opportunistic infections in people whose immune systems are compromised by disease, therapy, or neglect. Candidates for infection include severe alcoholics, those with cancer, diabetes mellitus, and rheumatoid arthritis. The bacteria of this group can cause a variety of infections, including infection of the bloodstream (bacteremia), inflammation of the connective tissue structure surrounding a joint (bursitis), infection of various regions of the heart and heart valves (endocarditis), meningitis, inflammation of bone and bone marrow (osteomyelitis), and the inflammation of the lining of the abdomen (peritonitis).

The conventional treatment for streptococcal infections is the administration of **antibiotics**. Many strains of strep are still susceptible to **penicillin**. However, strains of *Streptococcus pneumonia* that are resistant to multiple antibiotics are a problem in hospitals world-wide.

Prevention of infection involves keeping wounds clean and good hygienic practices, such as frequent hand washing, especially before eating and after using the bathroom.

See also Bacteria and bacterial infection

STREPTOMYCIN · *see* ANTIBIOTICS

SULFA DRUGS

Sulfa drugs, developed in the 1930s, were the first medications effective against bacterial disease. They appeared as the first "miracle drugs" at a time when death from bacterial infections such as **pneumonia** and blood poisoning were common.

In 1932, German physician and biomedical researcher Gerhard Domagk was working on a project for the German industrial giant I. G. Farbenindustrie to test industrial chemicals for medical utility. One of the chemicals was a dye called Prontosil, or sulfamidochrysoidine. Domagk hypothesized that since the dye worked by binding to the proteins in fabric and leather, it might also bind to the proteins in **bacteria**, thus inhibiting their action. Experiments on laboratory animals

infected with streptococcus were promising, and were soon followed by successful clinical tests.

In 1936, Prontosil was successfully used against puerperal sepsis, or "childbed fever," which was killing thousands of mothers every year. It was also shown to be effective against **meningitis**, pneumonia, and streptococcal infections.

Meanwhile, scientists at the Pasteur Institute in Paris discovered that upon ingestion, the dye molecule was cleaved in two, and that the active part, sulfanilamide, was just as effective on its own. This was important because the smaller molecule was not covered by Farben's patent on Prontosil, and was also less expensive to produce.

There followed a rush by pharmaceutical companies in the United States and Europe to develop sulfa drugs of their own. Among the most effective were sulfapyridine for pneumonia, sulfathiazole against pneumonia and staphylococcus, sulfaguanadine to treat **dysentery**, and sulfadiazine, which worked against pneumonia, strep and staph. Domagk was awarded the Nobel Prize in Medicine in 1939, but World War II prevented him from receiving his medal until 1947.

Investigating the action of the sulfa drugs led to an important new understanding of the action of pharmaceuticals. Sulfanilamides compete with the action of para-aminobenzoic acid (PABA), which bacteria use to produce folic acid. Without folic acid, the bacteria cannot synthesize **DNA**. This is an example of a common drug mechanism called antagonism. A structurally similar molecule can work against a substance necessary to the **metabolism** of a microorganism (or involved in some other disease process) by competitively binding to the same enzyme and thus blocking its action.

A tragic episode involving a sulfa drug was also important in medical history because of its effect on United States law. In 1937, the S. E. Massengill Company released a sulfa medication in liquid form. Unfortunately, a toxic solvent (the medium suspending the sulfa medication) was used, and more than 100 people died. The next year, the Federal Food, Drug and Cosmetics Act was passed, requiring that new drugs be tested for safety.

The ability to fight dysentery and other bacterial diseases with sulfa drugs was important to soldiers in World War II. However, too much sulfa was bad for the kidneys, and by the end of the war, **penicillin** and other newly developed **antibiotics** with fewer side effects became increasingly available and preferred in treatment. In addition, many bacterial strains have developed resistance against sulfa drugs in the decades since they were developed, which has also limited their usefulness. Regardless, they are still effective against some infections, including **leprosy**, and are often used in developing nations because of their low cost.

See also Antibiotic resistance, tests for; Antibiotics; Bacteria and bacterial infection; Bioterrorism, protective measures; History of the development of antibiotics; History of public health; Infection and resistance; Penicillin; Streptococci and streptococcal infections

SULFUR CYCLE IN MICROORGANISMS

Sulfur is a key constituent of certain amino acids, proteins, and other biochemicals of both **eukaryotes** and prokaryotes. For example, sulfur is a component of an enzyme called coenzyme A, which is vital for **respiration** of plant and animal cells.

Plants are not able to directly use elemental sulfur. Instead, they rely on the ability of certain types of **bacteria** to convert elemental sulfur to another form. Bacteria that are known as **chemoautotrophic bacteria** can combine sulfur with water and oxygen to produce hydrogen sulfate. Plants are able to incorporate the sulfate compound into proteins.

Bacteria can participate in the reduction of sulfur, in which the sulfur compounds act as an electron receptor, or in the oxidation of sulfur, in which an electron is removed from the sulfur compound.

Hydrogen sulfide, a gas that has the characteristic smell of rotten eggs, is toxic to air-requiring plant and animal tissue. However, the gas can be utilized by oxygen-requiring bacteria such as *Thiothrix* and *Beggiatoa*, and by the anaerobic purple sulfur bacteria. These bacteria utilize the hydrogen sulfide and carbon dioxide to produce elemental sulfur.

Sulfur can occur in many chemically reduced mineral forms, or sulfides, in association with many metals. The most common metal sulfides in the environment are iron sulfides (called pyrites when they occur as cubic crystals), but all heavy metals can occur in this mineral form. Whenever metal sulfides are exposed to an oxygen-rich environment, certain bacteria begin to oxidize the sulfide, generating sulfate as a product, and tapping energy from the process that is used to sustain their own growth and reproduction. This autotrophic process is called chemosynthesis, and the bacteria involved are named *Thiobacillus thiooxidans*. When a large quantity of sulfide is oxidized in this way, an enormous amount of acidity is associated with the sulfate product. Indeed, *Thiobacillus prosperus* has an optimum **pH** of between pH=1 and pH=4, and *Thiobacillus ferroxidans* has an optimum pH range of between pH=2 and pH=4.

Some species of the genus *Thiobacillus*, including *Thiobacillus thiooxidans* and *Thiobacillus ferroxidans* are able to process elemental sulfur and iron sulfate, respectively.

Within the past several decades, the existence of bacteria that utilize sulfur at **hydrothermal vents** deep within the ocean has been chronicled. These bacteria form the basis of the entire complex ecosystem that springs up, in the total absence of light, around the sulfur-rich emission form the vents. Some of the bacteria live in symbiosis with the so-called tubeworms that thrive in this ecosystem. The worms provide protection and an incoming supply of nutrients to the bacteria. In turn, the bacteria metabolize the sulfur to forms usable to the worms. The discovery of the bacterial basis of this undersea ecosystem greatly increased human awareness of the microbial diversity on Earth.

See also Biogeochemical cycles; Economic uses and benefits of microorganisms

SUPERFUND • *see* BIOREMEDIATION

SWINE FEVER

Swine fever is a viral disease that afflicts swine. The disease is also known as hog cholera. A related form of the disease is called African swine fever.

The virus that causes swine fever is a member of the family Flaviviridae and the genus *Pestivirus*. A virus causes African swine fever from the family Iridovirisae. The virus itself is designated *Asfarviridae*, a name derived from "African Swine Fever and Related Viruses." The virus is so far the sole member of the newly created genus *Asfivirus*.

The two **viruses** are quite different from one another in structure and behavior. Yet, the diseases they cause are very similar with respect to their transmission and the symptoms of infection. Both viruses can be easily passed from an infected pig to a healthy pig. Contact can be direct or via body secretions or feces. The resulting infection can be mild or more severe. Also a long lasting form of infection can result. The more severe form of the infection results in a very high fever that can lead to convulsions. Often the skin appears discolored and pigs will huddle together. Death usually results a week or two weeks after the appearance of symptoms. The chronic form of the infection displays similar but less severe symptoms. The symptoms can persist for months before the swine succumbs. Finally, an infection can display few if any symptoms. However, this mild bout of the disease can caused reduce number of live births.

Swine that survive the infections can be life-long carriers of the viruses.

Distinction of swine fever from African swine fever is only possible by the direct examination of the viruses. The examinations typically involve the isolation of the virus in an appropriate cell **culture** and the use of fluorescent-labeled antibodies and the **enzyme-linked immunosorbant assay** (**ELISA**).

Both viruses are easily spread from hog to hog. Pigs and related animals such as wild boar are the only natural reservoirs of *Pestivirus*. *Asfivirus* can reside in species such as ticks. The viruses can also be accidentally carried from an infected swine to a susceptible swine via humans, animals, and birds. This is in part due to the environmental persistence of the viruses. For example, *Pestivirus* is able to survive cold conditions, and so can survive in a refrigerated carcass during transport. As well, the virus is able to survive some forms of meat processing (e.g., curing and smoking). However, *Pestivirus* is susceptible to various disinfectants (e.g., sodium hydroxide, Formalin, various detergents).

Pestivirus infects the blood and virtually all body fluids of an infected animal. Furthermore, the animal can excrete the virus for months.

The adverse effects to the health of the swine, and to their economic value, has made the eradication of swine fevers a priority in many countries around the world. In the United States, for example, a concerted effort by State and Federal governments and industry over almost two decades has virtually eliminated the disease in the country. However, vigilance is necessary to maintain this record. In Great Britain, where swine fever had been eliminated by 1966, it reappeared in 2000.

Such is not the case around the world. In many countries, swine fever remains a problem. Belgium and France experienced heavy economic losses in 1997, for example. African swine fever is a major problem affecting swine in countries such s Gambia, Ghana, and Madagascar, and there have also been outbreaks in more northern countries (e.g., Italy in 1999 and Portugal in 2000).

In countries such as the United States, swine entering the country are quarantined for 90 days to ensure that the swine do not harbor the virus that has yet to be evident as an infection.

Currently there is no treatment for either swine fever, save slaughter of the infected animals. In this regard, swine fever is similar to foot and mouth disease that afflicts cattle and sheep. The use of a **vaccine** consisting of weakened but living virus has been an effective preventative measure for swine fever. However, unless the **vaccination** involves the total swine population in the target region, the prevention of infection will not be absolute.

See also Virology

SYNCHRONOUS GROWTH

Synchronous growth is the growth of **bacteria** such that all the bacteria are at the same stage in their growth cycle (e.g., exponential phase, stationary phase). Because the same cellular reactions occur simultaneously throughout the bacterial population, synchronous growth permits the detection of events not normally detectable in a single cell or in a population consisting of bacteria in various stages of growth.

In a normal batch **culture** of fluid, or on an **agar** plate, bacteria in the population exhibit a range of sizes, ages, and growth rates. In contrast, the bacteria in a synchronized culture are virtually identical in terms of these parameters.

Synchronized growth is imposed in the laboratory. A population of bacteria can be filtered to obtain bacteria of a certain size range. Usually, the filter that is used has very small holes. All but the smallest bacteria in a population are excluded from passing through the filter. Because the smallest bacteria are frequently the youngest bacteria, the filtering method selects for a population comprised of bacteria that usually have just completed a division event. When the bacteria are suspended in fresh growth medium the population will subsequently grow and then divide at the same rate.

Bacteria of the same size can also be recovered using special techniques of centrifugation, where the bacteria in the fluid that is spinning around in a centrifuge are separated on the basis of their different densities. The smallest bacteria will have the lowest density and so will move furthest down the centrifuge tube.

Another method of obtaining a synchronous bacterial population involves the manipulation of some environmental

factor that the bacteria depend on for growth. Typically, the factor is a nutrient that the bacteria cannot manufacture, and so is required to be present in the medium. In the alternative, an agent (e.g., an antibiotic) can be added that does not kill the bacteria but rather halts their growth at a certain point. Again, once the bacteria are added to fresh medium, the growth of all the bacteria will recommence from the point of blockage in the **cell cycle**.

Synchronous growth can only be maintained for a few rounds of growth and division. Ultimately, the inherent randomness of bacterial population growth again dominates. In other words, not all the bacteria will continue to divide at exactly and differences in size and other attributes will once again appear in the population. For those few generations, however, much useful information can be extracted from a synchronously growing population.

See also Bacterial growth and division; Laboratory techniques in microbiology

SYPHILIS

Syphilis is a chronic, degenerative, sexually transmitted disease caused by the bacterium *Treponema pallidum*. Although modern treatments now control the disease, its incidence remains high worldwide, making it a global **public health** concern. Spread by sexual contact, syphilis begins as a small, hard, painless swelling, called a primary (or Hunter's) chancre. The disease is very contagious in the early stages. The initial sore will usually pass away in about eight weeks, but the disease will then spread through the body and lodge in the lymph nodes, causing a skin rash to appear in two to four months along with fever and headaches. This second stage can last two to six weeks. After a latent period, which can extend for years, the disease can appear in various bodily organs and it can be spread to others.

The earliest records of syphilis are those of Spanish physician Rodrigo Ruiz de Isla, who wrote that he treated syphilis patients in Barcelona in 1493. He further claimed that the soldiers of explorer Christopher Columbus contracted the disease in the Caribbean and brought it back to Europe in 1492. However, others challenge this position. Some medical historians believe that syphilis has been present from ancient times but was often mislabeled or misdiagnosed. Italian physician and writer Girolamo Fracastoro gave the disease its name in his poem "Syphilis sive morbus Gallicus" (Syphilis or the French Disease), published in 1530, during the height of a European epidemic. However, for centuries, the disease was called pox or the great pox. At that time, the treatment was mercury, used in vapor baths, as an ointment, or taken orally. The mercury increased the flow of saliva and phlegm to wash out the poisons, but it also caused discomfort, such as loss of hair and teeth, abdominal pains, and mouth sores. Through the centuries, a milder form of the disease evolved and often became confused with **gonorrhea**. In 1767, physician John Hunter infected himself with fluid from a patient who had gonorrhea to prove these were two different diseases. Unknown to Hunter, the patient also had syphilis. Hunter developed the sore indicative of syphilis that now bears his name.

The distinction between the two diseases was made clear in 1879, when German bacteriologist Albert Neisser isolated the bacterium responsible for gonorrhea. In 1903, Russian biologist Elie Metchnikoff and French scientist Pierre-Paul-Emile Roux demonstrated that syphilis could be transmitted to monkeys and then studied in the laboratory. They also showed that mercury ointment was an effective treatment in the early stages. Two years later, German zoologist Fritz Schaudinn and his assistant Erich Hoffmann discovered the bacterium responsible for syphilis, the spiral-shaped spirochete *Treponema pallidum*. The following year, German physician August von Wassermann (1866–1925) developed the first diagnostic test for syphilis based on new findings in **immunology**. The test involved checking for the syphilis **antibody** in a sample of blood. One drawback was that the test would take two days to complete.

In 1904, German research physician **Paul Ehrlich** began focusing on a safe, effective treatment for syphilis. Ehrlich had spent many years studying the effect of dyes on biological tissues and treatments for tropical diseases. His work in the emerging field of immunology earned him a Nobel Prize in 1908. Ehrlich began working with the arsenic-based compound atoxyl as a possible treatment for syphilis. Japanese bacteriologist Sahachiro Hata came to study syphilis with Ehrlich. Hata tested hundreds of derivatives of atoxyl and finally found one that worked, number 606. Ehrlich called it Salvarsan. Following clinical trials, in 1911 Ehrlich and Hata announced the drug was an effective cure for syphilis. The drug attacked the disease germs but did not harm healthy cells; thus, Salvarsan ushered in the new field of **chemotherapy**. Ehrlich went on to develop two safer forms of the drug, including neosalvarsan in 1912 and sodium salvarsan in 1913.

Penicillin came into widespread use in treating bacterial diseases during World War II. It was first used to against syphilis in 1943 by New York physician John F. Mahoney, and it remains the treatment of choice today. Other **antibiotics** are also effective. Meanwhile, Russian-American researcher Reuben Leon Kahn (1887–1979) developed a modified test for syphilis in 1923 that took only a few minutes to complete. Another test was developed by researchers William A. Hinton (1883–1959) and J. A. V. Davies. Today fluorescent antibody tests are used for detection. Although there is no inoculation for syphilis, the disease can be controlled through education, safe sexual practices, and proper medical treatment.

See also Sexually transmitted diseases

T

T-CELL LEUKEMIA VIRUS • *see* HUMAN T-CELL
LEUKEMIA VIRUS (HTLV)

T CELLS OR T-LYMPHOCYTES

When a vertebrate encounters substances that are capable of causing it harm, a protective system known as the **immune system** comes into play. This system is a network of many different organs that work together to recognize foreign substances and destroy them. The immune system can respond to the presence of a disease-causing agent (pathogen) in two ways. Immune cells called the **B cells** can produce soluble proteins (antibodies) that can accurately target and kill the pathogen. This branch of **immunity** is called "humoral immunity." In cell-mediated immunity, immune cells known as the T cells produce special chemicals that can specifically isolate the pathogen and destroy it.

The T cells and the B cells together are called the lymphocytes. The precursors of both types of cells are produced in the bone marrow. While the B cells mature in the bone marrow, the precursors to the T cells leave the bone marrow and mature in the thymus. Hence the name, "T cells" for thymus-derived cells.

The role of the T cells in the immune response is to specifically recognize the pathogens that enter the body and to destroy them. They do this either by directly killing the cells that have been invaded by the pathogen, or by releasing soluble chemicals called **cytokines**, which can stimulate other killer cells specifically capable of destroying the pathogen.

During the process of maturation in the thymus, the T cells are taught to discriminate between self (an individual's own body cells) and non-self (foreign cells or pathogens). The immature T cells, while developing and differentiating in the thymus, are exposed to the different thymic cells. Only those T cells that are self-tolerant, that is to say, they will not interact with the molecules normally expressed on the different body cells are allowed to leave the thymus. Cells that react with the body's own proteins are eliminated by a process known as "clonal deletion." The process of clonal deletion ensures that the mature T cells, which circulate in the blood, will not interact with or destroy an individual's own tissues and organs. The mature T cells can be divided into two subsets, the T-4 cells (that have the accessory molecule CD4), or the T-8 (that have CD8 as the accessory molecule).

There are millions of T cells in the body. Each T cell has a unique protein structure on its surface known as the T cell receptor (TCR), which is made before the cells ever encounter an **antigen**. The TCR can recognize and bind only to a molecule that has a complementary structure. It is kind of like a lock-and key arrangement. Each TCR has a unique binding site that can attach to a specific portion of the antigen called the epitope. As stated before, the binding depends on the complementarity of the surface of the receptor and the surface of the epitope. If the binding surfaces are complementary, and the T cells can effectively bind to the antigen, then it can set into motion the immunological cascade which eventually results in the destruction of the pathogen.

The first step in the destruction of the pathogen is the activation of the T cells. Once the T-lymphocytes are activated, they are stimulated to multiply. Special cytokines called interleukins that are produced by the T-4 lymphocytes mediate this proliferation. It results in the production of thousands of identical cells, all of which are specific for the original antigen. This process of clonal proliferation ensures that enough cells are produced to mount a successful immune response. The large clone of identical lymphocytes then differentiates into different cells that can destroy the original antigen.

The T-8 lymphocytes differentiate into cytotoxic T-lymphocytes (CTLs) that can destroy the body cells that have the original antigenic epitope on its surface, e.g., bacterial infected cells, viral infected cells, and tumor cells. Some of the T lymphocytes become memory cells. These cells are capable of remembering the original antigen. If the individual is exposed to the same **bacteria** or virus again, these memory

---

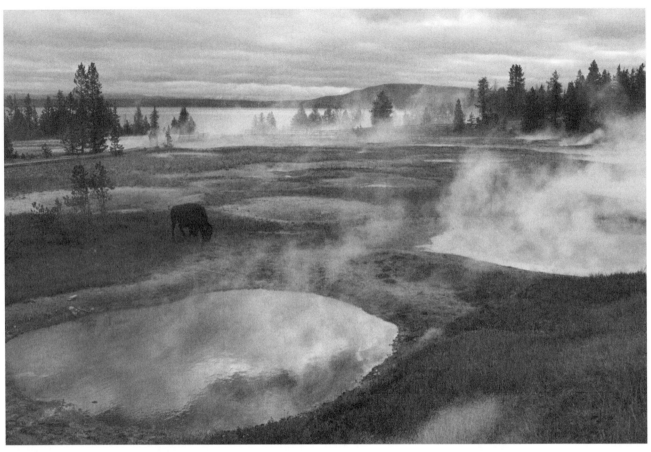

Bison grazing near hot springs. Bacteria growing in hot springs are the source of taq.

cells will initiate a rapid and strong immune response against it. This is the reason why the body develops a permanent immunity after an infectious disease.

Certain other cells known as the T-8 suppressor cells play a role in turning off the immune response once the antigen has been removed. This is one of the ways by which the immune response is regulated.

See also Bacteria and bacterial infection; Immune stimulation, as a vaccine; Immunity, active, passive and delayed; Immunity, cell mediated; Immunity, humoral regulation; Immunochemistry; Immunological analysis techniques; Immunology, nutritional aspects; Viruses and responses to viral infection

TAQ ENZYME

A taq enzyme is a bacterial enzyme that functions in the manufacture of **deoxyribonucleic acid** (**DNA**). The ability of the enzyme to function at higher temperatures than other similarly functioning bacterial **enzymes** has made it valuable in the **polymerase chain reaction**.

The moniker taq denotes the origin of the enzyme. The enzyme is produced by a bacterium known as *Thermus aquati-*

cus. This bacterium was discovered by Thomas Brock in the mid 1970s in the nearly boiling waters of Mushroom pool, a hot spring in Yellowstone National Park

Taq is a DNA polymerase. The enzyme manufactures a strand of DNA that is complimentary to a single strand of DNA. All **bacteria** possess DNA polymerase. The reason that the taq polymerase has become so significant to biotechnological processes is because of the resistance of the enzyme to heat. A **molecular biology** technique known as the polymerase chain reaction relies upon the exposure of DNA to heat in order to separate the two strands of the double helix. Taq can then use both of the single strands as templates for the manufacture of two new strands of DNA. To perform this function, the polymerase is able to recognize the particular building block, or nucleotide, on the DNA single strand and then position a nucleotide that is the complimentary match to the particular target. Binding of the two nucleotides occurs. The polymerase can then move on to the next nucleotide and the process is repeated. When the DNA mixture is allowed to cool the matching strands link together forming two double stranded helices of DNA. If this process is repeated many times, a huge number of copies of the target region of DNA can be manufactured. The heat resistance of taq allows the enzyme to function in the temperature conditions that keep the DNA strands apart from each other. The DNA polymerase from other bacteria, for example from the bacterium *Escherichia coli*, do not function nearly as efficiently in the polymerase chain reaction as the taq polymerase of *Thermus aquaticus*.

Since the discovery of taq enzyme and the development of the polymerase chain reaction, the importance of the enzyme to molecular biology research and commercial applications of **biotechnology** have soared. Taq polymerase is widely used in the molecular diagnosis of maladies and in forensics ("DNA fingerprinting"). These and other applications of taq have spawned an industry worth hundreds of millions of dollars annually.

See also DNA (Deoxyribonucleic acid); DNA hybridization; Extremophiles; Molecular biology and molecular genetics; PCR

TATUM, EDWARD LAWRIE (1909-1975)
American biochemist

Edward Lawrie Tatum's experiments with simple organisms demonstrated that cell processes can be studied as chemical reactions and that such reactions are governed by genes. With George Beadle, he offered conclusive proof in 1941 that each biochemical reaction in the cell is controlled via a catalyzing enzyme by a specific **gene**. The "one gene-one enzyme" theory changed the face of biology and gave it a new chemical expression. Tatum, collaborating with **Joshua Lederberg**, demonstrated in 1947 that **bacteria** reproduce sexually, thus introducing a new experimental organism into the study of **molecular genetics**. Spurred by Tatum's discoveries, other scientists worked to understand the precise chemical nature of the unit of heredity called the gene. This study culminated in 1953, with the description by James Watson and **Francis Crick** of the structure of **DNA**. Tatum's use of **microorganisms** and laboratory **mutations** for the study of biochemical genetics led directly to the **biotechnology** revolution of the 1980s. Tatum and Beadle shared the 1958 Nobel Prize in physiology or medicine with Joshua Lederberg for ushering in the new era of modern biology.

Tatum was born in Boulder, Colorado, to Arthur Lawrie Tatum and Mabel Webb Tatum. He was the first of three children. Tatum's father held two degrees, an M.D. and a Ph.D. in pharmacology. Edward's mother was one of the first women to graduate from the University of Colorado. As a boy, Edward played the French horn and trumpet; his interest in music lasted his whole life.

Tatum earned his A.B. degree in chemistry from the University of Wisconsin in 1931, where his father had moved the family in order to accept as position as professor in 1931. In 1932, Tatum earned his master's degree in microbiology. Two years later, in 1934, he received a Ph.D. in **biochemistry** for a dissertation on the cellular biochemistry and nutritional needs of a bacterium. Understanding the biochemistry of microorganisms such as bacteria, **yeast**, and molds would persist at the heart of Tatum's career.

In 1937, Tatum was appointed a research associate at Stanford University in the department of biological sciences. There he embarked on the *Drosophila* (fruit fly) project with geneticist George Beadle, successfully determining that kynurenine was the enzyme responsible for the fly's eye color, and that it was controlled by one of the eye-pigment genes. This and other observations led them to postulate several theories about the relationship between genes and biochemical reactions. Yet, the scientists realized that *Drosophila* was not an ideal experimental organism on which to continue their work.

Tatum and Beadle began searching for a suitable organism. After some discussion and a review of the literature, they settled on a pink **mold** that commonly grows on bread known as *Neurospora crassa*. The advantages of working with *Neurospora* were many: it reproduced very quickly, its nutritional needs and biochemical pathways were already well known, and it had the useful capability of being able to reproduce both sexually and asexually. This last characteristic made it possible to grow cultures that were genetically identical, and also to grow cultures that were the result of a cross between two different parent strains. With *Neurospora,* Tatum and Beadle were ready to demonstrate the effect of genes on cellular biochemistry.

The two scientists began their *Neurospora* experiments in March 1941. At that time, scientists spoke of "genes" as the units of heredity without fully understanding what a gene might look like or how it might act. Although they realized that genes were located on the **chromosomes**, they didn't know what the chemical nature of such a substance might be. An understanding of DNA (**deoxyribonucleic acid**, the molecule of heredity) was still 12 years in the future. Nevertheless, geneticists in the 1940s had accepted Gregor Mendel's work with inheritance patterns in pea plants. Mendel's theory, rediscovered by three independent investigators in 1900, states that an inherited characteristic is determined by the combination of two hereditary units (genes), one each contributed by the parental cells. A dominant gene is expressed even when it is carried by only one of a pair of chromosomes, while a recessive gene must be carried by both chromosomes to be expressed. With *Drosophila*, Tatum and Beadle had taken genetic **mutants**—flies that inherited a variant form of eye color—and tried to work out the biochemical steps that led to the abnormal eye color. Their goal was to identify the variant enzyme, presumably governed by a single gene that controlled the variant eye color. This proved technically difficult, and as luck would have it, another lab announced the discovery of kynurenine's role before theirs did. With the *Neurospora* experiments, they set out to prove their one gene-one enzyme theory another way.

The two investigators began with biochemical processes they understood well: the nutritional needs of *Neurospora*. By exposing cultures of *Neurospora* to x rays, they would cause genetic damage to some bread mold genes. If their theory was right, and genes did indeed control biochemical reactions, the genetically damaged strains of mold would show changes in their ability to produce nutrients. If supplied with some basic salts and sugars, normal *Neurospora* can make all the amino acids and vitamins it needs to live except for one (biotin).

This is exactly what happened. In the course of their research, the men created, with x-ray bombardment, a number of mutated strains that each lacked the ability to produce a particular amino acid or vitamin. The first strain they identified, after 299 attempts to determine its mutation, lacked the ability to make vitamin B_6. By crossing this strain with a normal strain, the offspring inherited the defect as a recessive gene according to the inheritance patterns described by Mendel. This proved that the mutation was a genetic defect, capable of being passed to successive generations and causing the same nutritional mutation in those offspring. The x-ray bombardment had altered the gene governing the enzyme needed to promote the production of vitamin B_6.

This simple experiment heralded the dawn of a new age in biology, one in which molecular genetics would soon dominate. Nearly 40 years later, on Tatum's death, Joshua Lederberg told the *New York Times* that this experiment "gave impetus and morale" to scientists who strived to understand how genes directed the processes of life. For the first time, biologists believed that it might be possible to understand and quantify the living cell's processes.

Tatum and Beadle were not the first, as it turned out, to postulate the one gene-one enzyme theory. By 1942, the work of English physician Archibald Garrod, long ignored, had been rediscovered. In his study of people suffering from a particular inherited enzyme deficiency, Garrod had noticed the disease seemed to be inherited as a Mendelian recessive. This suggested a link between one gene and one enzyme. Yet Tatum and Beadle were the first to offer extensive experimental evidence for the theory. Their use of laboratory methods, like x rays, to create genetic mutations also introduced a powerful tool for future experiments in biochemical genetics.

During World War II, the methods Tatum and Beadle had developed in their work with pink bread mold were used to produce large amounts of **penicillin**, another mold. In 1945, at the end of the war, Tatum accepted an appointment at Yale University as an associate professor of botany with the promise of establishing a program of biochemical microbiology within that department. In 1946, Tatum did indeed create a new program at Yale and became a professor of microbiology. In work begun at Stanford and continued at Yale, he demonstrated that the one gene-one enzyme theory applied to yeast and bacteria as well as molds.

In a second fruitful collaboration, Tatum began working with Joshua Lederberg in March 1946. Lederberg, a Columbia University medical student 15 years younger than Tatum, was at Yale during a break in the medical school curriculum. Tatum and Lederberg began studying the bacterium *Escherichia coli*. At that time, it was believed that *E. coli* reproduced asexually. The two scientists proved otherwise. When cultures of two different mutant bacteria were mixed, a third strain, one showing characteristics taken from each parent, resulted. This discovery of biparental inheritance in bacteria, which Tatum called genetic **recombination**, provided geneticists with a new experimental organism. Again, Tatum's methods had altered

the practices of experimental biology. Lederberg never returned to medical school, earning instead a Ph.D. from Yale.

In 1948 Tatum returned to Stanford as professor of biology. A new administration at Stanford and its department of biology had invited him to return in a position suited to his expertise and ability. While in this second residence at Stanford, Tatum helped establish the department of biochemistry. In 1956, he became a professor of biochemistry and head of the department. Increasingly, Tatum's talents were devoted to promoting science at an administrative level. He was instrumental in relocating the Stanford Medical School from San Francisco to the university campus in Palo Alto. In that year Tatum also was divorced, then remarried in New York City. Tatum left the West coast and took a position at the Rockefeller Institute for Medical Research (now Rockefeller University) in January 1957. There he continued to work through institutional channels to support young scientists, and served on various national committees. Unlike some other administrators, he emphasized nurturing individual investigators rather than specific kinds of projects. His own research continued in efforts to understand the genetics of *Neurospora* and the nucleic acid **metabolism** of mammalian cells in **culture**.

In 1958, together with Beadle and Lederberg, Tatum received the Nobel Prize in physiology or medicine. The Nobel Committee awarded the prize to the three investigators for their work demonstrating that genes regulate the chemical processes of the cell. Tatum and Beadle shared one-half the prize and Lederberg received the other half for work done separately from Tatum. Lederberg later paid tribute to Tatum for his role in Lederberg's decision to study the effects of x-ray-induced mutation. In his Nobel lecture, Tatum predicted that "with real understanding of the roles of heredity and environment, together with the consequent improvement in man's physical capacities and greater freedom from physical disease, will come an improvement in his approach to, and understanding of, sociological and economic problems."

Tatum's second wife, Viola, died in 1974. Tatum married Elsie Bergland later in 1974 and she survived his death the following year, in 1975. Tatum died at his home on East Sixty-third Street in New York City after an extended illness, at age 65.

See also Fungal genetics; Microbial genetics; Molecular biology and molecular genetics; Molecular biology, central dogma of

TECHNOLOGY AND TECHNIQUES IN IDENTIFICATION OF MICROORGANISMS •
see GENETIC IDENTIFICATION OF MICROORGANISMS

TEM • *see* ELECTRON MICROSCOPE, TRANSMISSION AND SCANNING

TERRORISM, USE OF MICROBIOLOGICAL AGENTS • *see* BIOTERRORISM

TETANUS AND TETANUS IMMUNIZATION

Tetanus is a bacterial disease that affects the nervous system in humans. The disease is caused by the **bacteria** *Clostridium tetani*. This organism, which is a common inhabitant of soil, dust, and manure, can contaminate an abrasion in the skin. Small cuts and pinpoint wounds can be contaminated. Because the organism can survive and grow in the absence of oxygen, deep wounds, such as those caused by puncture with a nail or a deep cut by a knife, are especially susceptible to infections with *Clostridium tetani*. The disease cannot be transmitted from one person to another.

In addition to being able to grow in oxygen-free environments, such as is found in a deep wound, *Clostridium tetani* is able to hibernate in environments such as the soil. This is because the bacteria can convert from an actively growing and dividing state, when conditions are favorable for growth, to a dormant state, when growth conditions are more hostile. Dormancy is achieved by the conversion of the so-called vegetative cell to an endospore. Essentially, an endospore is an armored ball in which the genetic material of the organism can be stored, in a form that resists heat, dryness, and lack of nutrients. When conditions once again become favorable, such as in the nutrient-rich and warm environment of a wound, the dormant bacteria revive and begin to grow and divide once more.

Tetanus is also commonly known as lockjaw, in recognition of the stiffening of the jaw that occurs because of the severe muscle spasms triggered by the infecting bacteria. The muscle paralysis restricts swallowing, and may even lead to death by suffocation. The muscular stiffening of the jaw, along with a headache, are usually the first symptoms of infection. These typically begin about a week after infection has begun. Some people experience symptoms as early as three days or as late as three weeks following the start of an infection. Following the early symptoms, swallowing becomes difficult. Other symptoms include the stiffening of the abdominal muscles, muscle spasms, sweating, and fever.

The muscle contractions can be so severe that, in some cases, they have actually broken bones with which they are associated. Treatment can include drugs to stimulate muscle relaxation, neutralize toxin that has not yet had a chance to react with the nervous system, and the administration of **antibiotics** to fight the **bacterial infection**. In spite of these efforts, three of every 10 people who contract tetanus will die from the effects of the disease. As of 2001, 50–100 cases of tetanus occur each year, usually involving people who either have never taken protective measures against the disease or who have let this protection lapse. In the absence of the protective measures such as **vaccination**, many more people would develop tetanus.

Interestingly, another group who are susceptible to tetanus are heroin addicts who inject themselves with a compound called quinine. This compound is used to dilute the heroin. Available evidence indicates that quinine may actually promote the growth of *Clostridium tetani*, by an as yet unknown mechanism.

For those who survive tetanus, recovery can take months and is not an easy process. Muscle stiffness and weakness may persist.

The molecular basis of the effects of infection by *Clostridium tetani* is a very potent toxin produced and excreted from the bacteria. The toxin is a neurotoxin. That is, the toxin affects neurons that are involved in transmitting signals to and from the brain in order to make possible the myriad of functions of the body. Specifically, in tetanus the neurotoxin blocks the release of neurotransmitters.

Clostridium tetani neurotoxin is composed of two chains of protein that are linked together. An enzyme present in the microorganism cuts these chains apart, which makes the toxin capable of the neurotransmitter inhibitory activity. One of the chains is called tetanospasmin. It binds to the ends of neurons and blocks the transmission of impulses. This blockage results in the characteristic spasms of the infection. The other toxin chain is known as tetanolysin. This chain has a structure that allows it to insert itself into the membrane surrounding the neuron. The inserted protein actually forms a pore, or hole, through the membrane. Molecules can move freely back and forth through the hole, which disrupts the functioning of the membrane.

The devastating effects of tetanus are entirely preventable. Vaccination in childhood, and even in adulthood, can prevent an infection from developing if *Clostridium tetani* should subsequently gain entry to a wound. Indeed, in the United States, laws requiring children to be immunized against tetanus now exist in most states, and all states require children in day care facilities to be immunized against tetanus.

Tetanus vaccination involves the administration of what is called tetanus toxoid. In use since the 1920s, tetanus toxoid is inactivated tetanus toxin. Injection of the toxoid stimulates the production of antibodies that will act to neutralize the active toxin. The toxoid can be given on its own. But typically, the toxoid is administered in combination with vaccines against **diphtheria** and **pertussis** (diphtheria toxoid pertussis, or DTP, **vaccine**). The DTP vaccine is given to children several times (two months after birth, four months, six months, 15 months, and between four and six years of age). Thereafter, a booster injection should be given every 10 years to maintain the **immunity** to tetanus. A lapse in the 10-year cycle of vaccination can leave a person susceptible to infection.

Tetanus toxoid will not provide protection to someone who has already been wounded. There is a substance called tetanus immune globulin that can provide immediate immunity.

The tetanus vaccination can produce side effects, ranging from slight fever and crankiness to severe, but non-lethal convulsions. Very rarely, brain damage has resulted from vaccination. Even though the possibility of the serious side effects is far outweighed by the health risks of foregoing vaccination, controversy exists over the wisdom of tetanus vaccination. Available evidence indicates that tetanus **immunization** is a wise measure.

See also Anaerobes and anaerobic infections

TETRACYCLINES • *see* ANTIBIOTICS

THE INSTITUTE FOR GENOMIC RESEARCH (TIGR)

The Institute for Genomic Research (TIGR) is a non-profit research institute located in Rockville, Maryland. The primary interest of TIGR is the sequencing of the genomes and the subsequent analysis of the sequences in prokaryotic and eukaryotic organisms. J. Craig Venter founded TIGR in 1992 and acted as president until 1998. As of 2002, Venter remained as chairman of the board of trustees for TIGR.

TIGR scientists sequenced the genomes of a number of **viruses**, **bacteria**, archaebacteria, plants, animals, **fungi**, and **protozoa**. The sequences of the bacteria *Haemophilus influenzae* and *Mycoplasma genitalium*, published in 1996, were the first complete bacterial **DNA** sequences ever accomplished. In 1996, the complete sequence of an archaebacteria (*Methanococcus jannaschii*) was published. Since that time, TIGR has sequenced 19 other bacterial genomes. These include the genomes of the bacteria that cause cholera, **tuberculosis**, **meningitis**, **syphilis**, **Lyme disease**, and stomach ulcers. In addition, TIGR sequenced the genome of the protozoan parasite *Plasmodium falciparum*, the cause of **malaria**.

The genesis of TIGR was the automation of the DNA sequencing process. This advance made the idea of large-scale sequencing efforts tangible. At about the same time, Venter was the leader of a section at the National Institute of Neurological Disorders and Stroke. He developed a technique called **shotgun cloning** that could efficiently and rapidly sequence large stretches of DNA. Use of the bacterial artificial **chromosomes** in a sequencing strategy that had been developed by Venter allowed large sections of the human genome to be inserted into the bacterium *Escherichia coli* where many copies of the sequences could be produced for sequence analysis. This technique proved to be much faster than the more conventional sequencing technique that was simultaneously being done by the United States government. The technique involved the creation of many overlapping fragments of the DNA, determination of the sequences, and then, using the common sequences present in the overlapping regions, piecing together the fragments to produce the full sequence of a genome. However, the concept was not readily accepted. At the time, the conventional sequencing strategy was to begin sequencing at one end of the genome and progress through to the other end in a linear manner.

In 1992, Venter left the National Institutes of Health and, with the receipt of a 10-year, $70 million grant from a private company, he founded TIGR in order to utilize the shotgun **cloning** philosophy as applied to the large-scale sequencing of genetic information.

Acceptance of Venter's and TIGR's approach to **gene** sequencing came with the 1995 publication of the genome sequence of the bacterium *Haemophilus influenzae*. This represented the first determination of a genome sequence of a living organism.

Another major research trust at TIGR has been the development of software analysis programs that sift through the vast amounts of sequence information in order to identify probable gene sequences. Also, programs are being developed to permit the analysis of these putative genes and the presentation of the structure of the proteins they code for. A technology known as micro-arraying is being refined. In this technique, thousands of genes can be placed onto a support for simultaneous analysis. This and other initiatives hold the promise of greatly increasing the speed of DNA sequencing.

TIGR also gained widespread public notoriety for its involvement in the sequencing of the human genome. Specifically, TIGR's establishment thrust the issue of corporate ownership of genetic information into the forefront of public awareness. Backed by the financing necessary to begin operations, TIGR partnered with an organization called Human Genome Sciences. The latter company had first opportunity to utilize any sequences emerging from TIGR labs. The specter of genetic information, especially that associated with diseases, being controlled by a private interest was, and remains, extremely controversial.

In 1997, TIGR dissolved the partnership with Human Genome Services. Since then, the genetic sequencing efforts have moved more toward the public domain. For example, now all TIGR gene sequences are posted on the organization's web site and the institute spearheads public forums and symposia.

TIGR is now headquartered on a 17-acre facility on the outskirts of Washington, D.C., and the institute is comprised of nearly 200 research staff.

See also Biotechnology; DNA (Deoxyribonucleic acid); Genetic mapping

THEILER, MAX (1899-1972)
South African virologist

Max Theiler (pronounced Tyler) was a leading scientist in the development of the yellow-fever **vaccine**. His early research proved that yellow-fever virus could be transmitted to mice. He later extended this research to show that mice that were given serum from humans or animals that had been previously infected with **yellow fever** developed **immunity** to this disease. From this research, he developed two different vaccines in the 1930s, which were used to control this incurable tropical disease. For his work on the yellow-fever vaccine, Theiler was awarded the Nobel Prize in medicine or physiology in 1951.

Theiler was born on a farm near Pretoria, South Africa, on January 30, 1899, the youngest of four children of Emma (Jegge) and Sir Arnold Theiler, both of whom had emigrated from Switzerland. His father, director of South Africa's veterinary services, pushed him toward a career in medicine. In part to satisfy his father, he enrolled in a two-year premedical program at the University of Cape Town in 1916. In 1919, soon after the conclusion of World War I, he sailed for England, where he pursued further medical training at St. Thomas's Hospital Medical School and the London School of **Hygiene** and Tropical Medicine, two branches of the

University of London. Despite this rigorous training, Theiler never received the M.D. degree because the University of London refused to recognize his two years of training at the University of Cape Town.

Theiler was not enthralled with medicine and had not intended to become a general practitioner. He was frustrated by the ineffectiveness of most medical procedures and the lack of cures for serious illnesses. After finishing his medical training in 1922, the 23-year-old Theiler obtained a position as an assistant in the Department of Tropical Medicine at Harvard Medical School. His early research, highly influenced by the example and writings of American bacteriologist Hans Zinsser, focused on amoebic **dysentery** and rat-bite fever. From there, he developed an interest in the yellow-fever virus.

Yellow fever is a tropical viral disease that causes severe fever, slow pulse, bleeding in the stomach, jaundice, and the notorious symptom, "black vomit." The disease is fatal in 10–15% of cases, the cause of death being complete shutdown of the liver or kidneys. Most people recover completely, after a painful, extended illness, with complete immunity to reinfection. The first known outbreak of yellow fever devastated Mexico in 1648. The last major breakout in the continental United States claimed 435 lives in New Orleans in 1905. Despite the medical advances of the twentieth century, this tropical disease remains incurable. As early as the eighteenth century, mosquitoes were thought to have some relation to yellow fever. Cuban physician Carlos Finlay speculated that mosquitoes were the carriers of this disease in 1881, but his writings were largely ignored by the medical community. Roughly 20 years later, members of America's Yellow Fever Commission, led by Walter Reed, the famous U.S. Army surgeon, concluded that mosquitoes were the medium that spread the disease. In 1901, Reed's group, using humans as research subjects, discovered that yellow fever was caused by a blood-borne virus. Encouraged by these findings, the Rockefeller Foundation launched a world-wide program in 1916 designed to control and eventually eradicate yellow fever.

By the 1920s, yellow fever research shifted away from an all-out war on mosquitoes to attempts to find a vaccine to prevent the spread of the disease. In 1928, researchers discovered that the Rhesus monkey, unlike most other monkeys, could contract yellow fever and could be used for experimentation. Theiler's first big breakthrough was his discovery that mice could be used experimentally in place of the monkey and that they had several practical research advantages.

One unintended research discovery kept Theiler out of his lab and in bed for nearly a week. In the course of his experiments, he accidentally contracted yellow fever from one of his mice, which caused a slight fever and weakness. Theiler was much luckier than some other yellow-fever researchers. Many had succumbed to the disease in the course of their investigations. However, this small bout of yellow fever simply gave Theiler immunity to the disease. In effect, he was the first recipient of a yellow-fever vaccine.

In 1930, Theiler reported his findings on the effectiveness of using mice for yellow fever research in the respected journal *Science*. The initial response was overwhelmingly negative; the Harvard faculty, including Theiler's immediate

supervisor, seemed particularly unimpressed. Undaunted, Theiler continued his work, moving from Harvard University, to the Rockefeller Foundation in New York City. Eventually, yellow-fever researchers began to see the logic behind Theiler's use of the mouse and followed his lead. His continued experiments made the mouse the research animal of choice. By passing the yellow-fever virus from mouse to mouse, he was able to shorten the incubation time and increase the virulence of the disease, which enabled research data to be generated more quickly and cheaply. He was now certain that an attenuated live vaccine, one weak enough to cause no harm yet strong enough to generate immunity, could be developed.

In 1931, Theiler developed the mouse-protection test, which involved mixing yellow-fever virus with human blood and injecting the mixture into a mouse. If the mouse survived, then the blood had obviously neutralized the virus, proving that the blood donor was immune to yellow fever (and had most likely developed an immunity by previously contracting the disease). This test was used to conduct the first worldwide survey of the distribution of yellow fever.

A colleague at the Rockefeller Foundation, Dr. Wilbur A. Sawyer, used Theiler's mouse strain, a combination of yellow fever virus and immune serum, to develop a human vaccine. Sawyer is often wrongly credited with inventing the first human yellow-fever vaccine. He simply transferred Theiler's work from the mouse to humans. Ten workers in the Rockefeller labs were inoculated with the mouse strain, with no apparent side effects. The mouse-virus strain was subsequently used by the French government to immunize French colonials in West Africa, a hot spot for yellow fever. This so-called "scratch" vaccine was a combination of infected mouse brain tissue and **cowpox** virus and could be quickly administered by scratching the vaccine into the skin. It was used throughout Africa for nearly 25 years and led to the near total eradication of yellow fever in the major African cities.

While encouraged with the new vaccine, Theiler considered the mouse strain inappropriate for human use. In some cases, the vaccine led to encephalitis in a few recipients and caused less severe side effects, such as headache or nausea, in many others. Theiler believed that a "killed" vaccine, which used a dead virus, wouldn't produce an immune effect, so he and his colleagues set out to find a milder live strain. He began working with the Asibi yellow-fever strain, a form of the virus so powerful that it killed monkeys instantly when injected under the skin. The Asibi strain thrived in a number of media, including chicken embryos. Theiler kept this virus alive for years in tissue cultures, passing it from embryo to embryo, and only occasionally testing the potency of the virus in a living animal. He continued making subcultures of the virus until he reached strain number 176. Then, he tested the strain on two monkeys. Both animals survived and seemed to have acquired a sufficient immunity to yellow fever. In March 1937, after testing this new vaccine on himself and others, Theiler announced that he had developed a new, safer, attenuated vaccine, which he called 17D strain. This new strain was much easier to produce, cheaper, and caused very mild side effects.

From 1940 to 1947, with the financial assistance of the Rockefeller Foundation, more than 28 million 17D-strain vaccines were produced, at a cost of approximately two cents per unit, and given away to people in tropical countries and the United States. The vaccine was so effective that the Rockefeller Foundation ended its yellow-fever program in 1949, safe in the knowledge that the disease had been effectively eradicated worldwide and that any subsequent outbreaks could be controlled with the new vaccine. Unfortunately, almost all yellow-fever research ended around this time and few people studied how to cure the disease. For people in tropical climates who live outside of the major urban centers, yellow fever is still a problem. A major outbreak in Ethiopia in 1960–1962 caused 30,000 deaths. The **World Health Organization** still uses Theiler's 17D vaccine and had mounted efforts to inoculate people in remote areas.

The success of the vaccine brought Theiler recognition both in the U.S. Over the next ten years, he received the Chalmer's Medal of the Royal Society of Tropical Medicine and Hygiene (1939), the Lasker Award of the American Public Health Association, and the Flattery Medal of Harvard University (1945).

In 1951, Theiler received the Nobel Prize in medicine or physiology "for his discoveries concerning yellow fever and how to combat it."

After developing the yellow-fever vaccine, Theiler turned his attention to other **viruses**, including some unusual and rare diseases, such as Bwamba fever and Rift Valley fever. His other, less exotic research focused on polio and led to his discovery of a polio-like infection in mice known as encephalomyelitis or Theiler's disease. In 1964, he retired from the Rockefeller Foundation, having achieved the rank of associate director for medical and natural sciences and director of the Virus Laboratories. In that same year, he accepted a position as professor of **epidemiology** and microbiology at Yale University in New Haven, Connecticut. He retired from Yale in 1967.

Theiler married in 1938 and had one daughter. Theiler died on August 11, 1972, at the age of 73.

See also Epidemics, viral; Epidemiology, tracking diseases with technology; History of immunology; History of public health; Immune stimulation, as a vaccine; Viruses and responses to viral infection; Zoonoses

THERMAL DEATH

Thermal death is the death of a population of **microorganisms** due to exposure to an elevated temperature.

The nature of the thermal death varies depending on the source of the heat. The heat of an open flame incinerates the microorganisms. The dry heat of an oven causes the complete removal of water, which is lethal for biological structures. In contrast, the moist heat delivered by a sterilizer such as an autoclave causes the proteins in the sample to coagulate in a way that is analogous to the coagulation of the proteins of an egg to form the familiar cooked egg white.

The coagulation of proteins by heat is a drastic alteration in the three-dimensional shape of these protein mole-

cules. Typically, the alteration is irreversible and renders a protein incapable of proper function.

Thermal death also involves the destruction of the membranes surrounding microorganisms such as **bacteria**. The high temperatures can cause the phospholipid constituents of the membrane to dissolve and thus destroy the membrane structure. Finally, the high heat will also cause the destruction of the nucleic acid of the target microorganism. In the case of double-stranded **DNA**, the heat will result in the disassociation of the two DNA strands.

Thermal death can be related to time. A term known as the thermal death time is defined as the time required to kill a population of the target microorganism in a water-based solution at a given temperature. The thermal death time of microorganisms can vary, depending on the thermal tolerance of the microbes. For example, thermophilic bacteria such as *Thermophilus aquaticus* that can tolerate high temperatures will have a thermal death time that is longer than the more heat-sensitive bacterium *Escherichia coli*.

Another aspect or measure of thermal death is termed the thermal death point. This is defined as the lowest temperature that will completely kill a population of a target microorganism within 10 minutes. This aspect of thermal death is useful in purifying water via boiling. Whereas *Escherichia coli* populations will be readily killed within 10 minutes at 212°F (100°C), spores of bacteria such as *Bacillus subtilus* and *Clostridium perfringens* will have a higher thermal death point, because a higher temperature is required to kill spores within 10 minutes.

Exact temperatures and times are usually used in calculating thermal death variables because terms such as "boiling" are not precise. For example, the boiling point of water (i.e., the temperature of boiling water) depends upon pressure. As altitude above sea level increases, the boiling temperature of water (H_2O) lowers.

See also Laboratory techniques in microbiology; Sterilization

THERMOTOLERANT BACTERIA · *see* EXTREMOPHILES

THIN SECTIONS AND THIN SECTIONING · *see* ELECTRON MICROSCOPIC EXAMINATION OF MICROORGANISMS

THRUSH

Thrush, or oropharyngeal **candidiasis**, is an infection of the mouth and throat caused by the fungus *Candida*, a genus of **yeast**. This microorganism is naturally present on the skin and mucous membranes, but overgrowth can cause disease. Candidiasis is not considered communicable because the microorganism is ubiquitous (common and widespread).

Symptoms of thrush include cottage cheese-like white patches in the mouth and throat, with raw areas underneath.

Esophageal involvement may result in difficulty in swallowing, nausea, vomiting, and chest pain. Candidiasis is confirmed by **culture** from a swab of the infected tissue.

Proliferation of *Candida* is most often the result of a weakened **immune system**. Candidiasis is one of the most common and visible opportunistic infections that strike people with **AIDS, chemotherapy** patients, and other immunocompromised individuals. Many AIDS patients have been first diagnosed after they, or their dentists, noticed a thrush infection. In individuals with normal immune systems, candidiasis may be associated with antibiotic use. Infants, diabetics, smokers, and denture wearers are particularly susceptible to thrush.

In addition to causing thrush, *Candida* may affect the gastrointestinal tract or genitals. The microorganism may also enter the bloodstream, either via surgery or catheterization, or through damage to the skin or mucosa. If the immune system is unable to clear the fungus from the bloodstream, a dangerous systemic infection may occur, resulting in endocarditis, **meningitis**, or other serious problems.

Antifungal medications such as fluconazole and clotrimazole are generally effective in treating candidiasis. However, drug-resistant strains of *Candida* are becoming increasingly prevalent, and recurrence is common. This situation is driving research into new therapies and potential vaccines.

See also Bacteria and bacterial infection; Fungal genetics; Fungi; Fungicide; Immunodeficiency; Immunosuppressant drugs; Infection and resistance; Infection control; Microbial flora of the oral cavity, dental caries; Yeast genetics; Yeast, infectious

TIGR · *see* THE INSTITUTE FOR GENOMIC RESEARCH (TIGR)

TMV · *see* TOBACCO MOSAIC VIRUS (TMV)

TOBACCO MOSAIC VIRUS (TMV)

Tobacco mosaic virus (TMV), also known as tobamovirus, is a rod-shaped virus with **ribonucleic acid (RNA)** surrounded by a coat of protein that causes mosaic-like symptoms in plants. Mosaic-like symptoms are characterized by mottled patches of green or yellow color on the leaves of infected plants. The virus causes abnormal cellular function that usually does not kill the plant but stunts growth. Infected plants may have brittle stems, abnormally small, curled leaves, and unripened fruit.

Tobacco mosaic virus is capable of infecting many kinds of plants, not just tobacco plants. TMV is spread through small wounds caused by handling, insects, or broken leaf hairs that result from leaves rubbing together. The virus attaches to the cell wall, injects its RNA into the host cell, and forces the host cell to produce new viral RNA and proteins. Finally, the viral RNA and proteins assemble into new **viruses** and infect other cells by passing through small openings called plasmodesmata

that connect adjacent plant cells. This process allows the virus to take over metabolic processes without killing cells.

Tobacco mosaic virus is highly infectious and can survive for many years in dried plant parts. Currently, there is no **vaccine** to protect plants from TMV, nor is there any treatment to eliminate the virus from infected plants. However, seeds that carry TMV externally can be treated by acid extraction or trisodium phosphate and seeds that carry the virus internally can receive dry heat treatments.

The discovery of viruses came about in the late 1800's when scientists were looking for the **bacteria** responsible for damaging tobacco plants. During one experiment in 1892, Russian biologist Dimitri Ivanovsky concluded that the disease in tobacco plants could not be caused by bacteria because it passed through a fine-pored filter that is too small for bacteria to pass through. In 1933, American biologist Wendell Stanley of the Rockefeller Institute discovered that the infectious agent formed crystals when purified. The purified extract continued to cause infection when applied to healthy tobacco plants and therefore, could not be a living organism. Soon after, scientists were able to break down the virus into its constituent parts. Today, it is known that the infectious agent that causes the disease in tobacco plants is a virus, not bacteria.

See also Genetic regulation of prokaryotic cells; Plant viruses; Viral genetics; Virus replication

TOXIC SHOCK SYNDROME

Toxic shock syndrome is an illness caused by the bacterium *Staphylococcus aureus*. The syndrome was first recognized in the 1970s when women who were wearing a "superabsorbant" tampon for their menstrual flow developed the illness. The majority of cases occur with this population. Less frequently, toxic shock syndrome can occur in females who do not use tampons, as well as in males.

The symptoms of toxic shock syndrome are caused by a toxin that is produced by *Staphylococcus aureus*. The exact nature of the association of the **bacterial growth** in superabsorbant tampons and the production of the toxin remains unclear. Whatever the exact cause, the cell-density behavior of other **bacteria** lends support to the suggestion that toxin production is triggered by the accumulation of large numbers of the bacteria. In the syndrome occurring in males or women who do not use tampons, there is usually a staphylococcal infection present in the body.

The symptoms of toxic shock syndrome include a sudden high fever, nausea with vomiting, diarrhea, headache, aches all over the body, dizziness and disorientation, a sunburn-like rash on the palms of the hands and the soles of the feet, and a decrease in blood pressure. The latter can send a victim into shock and can result in death. Those who recover may have permanent kidney and liver damage.

These symptoms are produced by the particular toxin that is released by the bacteria. The toxin can enter the bloodstream and move throughout the body. The toxin has been called a "superantigen" because of its potent stimulation of cells of the

immune system. The immune cells release a compound called cytokine. Normally, only a small proportion of the immune cells are releasing cytokine. But the massive cytokine release that occurs in response to the staphylococcal toxin produces the myriad of physiological changes in the body.

Treatment of toxic shock syndrome depends on the prompt recognition of the symptoms and their potential severity. Immediate administration of **antibiotics** is essential.

The number of cases of toxic shock syndrome has been reduced since the suspect superabsorbant tampons were withdrawn from the marketplace.

See also Bacteria and bacterial infection; Enterotoxin and exotoxin; Immune system

TOXOPLASMOSIS

Toxoplasmosis is an infectious disease caused by the protozoan *Toxoplasma gondii*. The infection results from a parasitic association with a human host.

Cats are the primary carrier of the protozoan *Toxoplasma gondii*. In the United States, approximately 30% of cats are at some time infected by *Toxoplasma gondii*. Cattle, sheep, or other livestock can also excrete a form of the protozoan known as an oocyst. Although oocysts are not capable of producing an infection, they are important because they act to preserve the infectious capability of the protozoan during exposure to inhospitable environments. In this capacity they are analogous to the bacterial spore. Oocysts are often capable of resuscitation into the infectious form after prolonged periods of exposure to adverse environments.

Humans can also become infected by eating fruits and vegetables that have themselves become contaminated when irrigated with untreated water contaminated with oocyte-containing feces.

Humans typically contract toxoplasmosis by eating cyst-contaminated raw or undercooked meat, vegetables, or milk products. The protozoan can also be spread from litter boxes or a sandbox soiled with cat feces. In all cases, the agent that is ingested can be the inactive oocyst or the actively growing and infectious egg form of the parasite.

In the human host, the parasite is able to grow and divide. This causes the symptoms of the infection.

Symptoms of toxoplasmosis include a sporadic and reoccurring fever, muscle pain, and a general feeling of malaise. Upon recovery, a life-long **immunity** is conferred. In some people, the disease can become chronic and cause an **inflammation** of the eyes, called retinochoroiditis, that can lead to blindness, severe yellowing of the skin and whites of the eyes (jaundice), easy bruising, and convulsions. As well inflammation of the brain (encephalitis), one-sided weakness or numbness, mood and personality changes, vision disturbances, muscle spasms, and severe headaches can result.

Person to person transmission is not frequent. Such transmission occurs only during pregnancy. Some six out of 1,000 women contract toxoplasmosis during pregnancy. Nearly half of these infections are passed on to the fetus.

Congenital toxoplasmosis afflicts approximately 3,300 newborns in the United States each year. In such children, symptoms may be severe and quickly fatal, or may not appear until several months, or even years, after birth.

As for many other microbial diseases, the observance of good **hygiene** (including appropriate hand washing protocols) is a key means of preventing toxoplasmosis.

See also Immunodeficiency diseases; Protozoa; Zoonoses

TRACKING DISEASES WITH TECHNOLOGY

• *see* EPIDEMIOLOGY, TRACKING DISEASES WITH TECHNOLOGY

TRANSCRIPTION

Transcription is defined as the transfer of genetic information from **deoxyribonucleic acid** (**DNA**) to **ribonucleic acid** (**RNA**). The process of transcription in prokaryotic cells (e.g., **bacteria**) differs from the process in eukaryotic cells (cells with a true **nucleus**) but the underlying result of both transcription processes is the same, which is to provide a template for the formation of proteins.

The use of DNA as a blueprint to manufacture RNA begins with an enzyme called RNA polymerase. The enzyme is guided to a certain region on the DNA, called the promoter, by association with molecules known as sigma factors. There are many promoters on DNA, located just before a region of DNA that codes for a protein. The promoter serves to position the RNA polymerase so that transcription of the full coding region is accomplished.

Once the polymerase has bound to a promoter, the sigma factors detach and can serve another polymerase. The attached polymerase then begins to move along the DNA, unwinding the two strands of DNA that are linked together and using the sequence on one of the strands as the blueprint for RNA manufacture. The strand from which RNA is made is known as the template or the antisense strand, while the other strand to which it is complimentary is called the sense or the coding strand.

As the polymerase moves along the DNA, the strands link back together behind the polymerase. The effect is somewhat similar to a zipper with a bulge, where the two links of the zipper have come apart. The bulging region can move along the zipper, with separation and reannealing of the strands occurring continuously with time. The promoter can accommodate the binding of another polymerase as soon as the region is free. Thus, the same stretch of DNA can be undergoing several rounds of transcription at the same end, with polymerase molecules positioned all along the DNA.

The RNA that is produced is known as messenger RNA (or mRNA). The species derives its name from its function. It is the tangible form of the message that is encoded in the DNA. The mRNA in turn functions as a template for the next step in the genetic process, that of **translation**. In translation the mRNA information is used to manufacture protein.

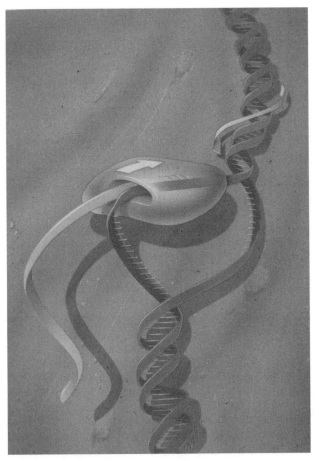

Transcription of a strand of the DNA double helix by DNA polymerase to form messenger RNA.

Termination of transcription occurs when the RNA polymerase reaches a signal on the DNA template strand that signals the polymerase to stop and to end the association with the DNA.

Some **microorganisms** have variations on the basic transcription mechanism. For example, in **yeast** cells the mRNA can be "capped" by the addition of specialized pieces of nucleic acid called telomeres to either end of the transcribed molecule. The telomeres function to extend the life of the mRNA and provide a signal of the importance of the information contained within.

The intricate and coordinated transcription process in bacteria is also a rapid process. For example, measurements in *Escherichia coli* have established that the RNA polymerase moves along the DNA at a speed of 50 nucleotides per second.

See also Bacterial artificial chromosome; Genetic regulation of prokaryotic cells

TRANSDUCTION

Transduction is defined as the transfer of genetic information between cells using a type of virus particle called a **bacterio-phage**. The virus contains genetic material from one cell, which is introduced into the other cell upon virus infection of the second cell. Transduction does not, therefore, require cell to cell contact and is resistant to **enzymes** that can degrade **DNA**.

Bacteriophage can infect the recipient cell and commandeer the host's replication machinery to produce more copies of itself. This is referred to as the lytic cycle. Alternatively, the phage genetic material can integrate into the host DNA where it can replicate undetected along with the host until such time as an activation signal stimulates the production of new virus particles. This is referred to as the lysogenic cycle. Transduction relies on the establishment of the lysogenic cycle, with the bacterial DNA becoming incorporated into the recipient cell chromosome along with the phage DNA. This means of transferring **bacteria** DNA has been exploited for genetic research with bacteria like *Escherichia coli, Salmonella typhimurium,* and *Bacillus subtilis,* which are specifically targeted by certain types of bacteriophage.

There are two types of transduction: generalized transduction and specialized transduction. In generalized transduction, the packaging of bacterial DNA inside the phage particle that subsequently infects another bacterial cell occurs due to error. The error rate is about one phage particle in 1,000. Experimental **mutants** of phage have been engineered where the error rate is higher. Once the bacterial DNA has been injected inside the second bacterium, there is approximately a 10percent change that the DNA will be stably incorporated into the chromosome of the recipient. A successful integration changes the **genotype and phenotype** of the recipient, which is called a transductant. A transductant will arise for about every 10^6 phage particles that contain bacterial DNA.

Specialized transduction utilizes specialized phage, in which some of the phage genetic material has been replaced by other genetic material, typically the bacterial chromosome. All of the phage particles carry the same portion of the bacterial chromosome. The phage can introduce their DNA into the recipient bacterium as above or via **recombination** between the chromosomal DNA carried by the phage and the chromosome itself.

Transduction has proved to be a useful means of transferring genetic traits from one bacterial cell to another.

See also Bacterial ultrastructure; Bacteriophage and bacteriophage typing; Molecular biology and molecular genetics; Viral genetics; Viral vectors in gene therapy; Virus replication; Viruses and responses to viral infection

TRANSFORMATION

Transformation is a process in which exogenous **DNA** is taken up by a (recipient) cell, sphaeroplast, or protoplast. In order to take up DNA, the cells must be competent. Competence is a state of bacterial cells during which the usually rigid cell wall can transport a relatively large DNA macromolecule. This is a highly unusual process, for **bacteria** normally lack the ability to transport macromolecules across the rigid cell wall and through the cyotplasmic membrane. Several bacteria, such as *Bacillus,*

Haemophilis, Neisseria, and *Streptococcus,* possess natural competence because their cells do not require special treatment to take up DNA. This process is transient and occurs only in special growth phases, typically toward the end of log phase.

The demonstration of DNA transformation was a landmark in the history of genetics. In 1944, Oswald Avery, Colin MacLeod, and **Maclyn McCarty** conducted famous *Streptococcus pneumoniae* transformation experiments. Bacterial **pneumonia** is caused by the S strain of *S. pneumoniae*. The S strain synthesizes a slimy capsule around each cell. The capsule is composed of a polysaccharide that protects the bacterium from the immune response of the infected animal and enables the bacterium to cause the disease. The colonies of the S strain appear smooth because of the capsule formation. The strain that does not synthesize the polysaccharide, hence does not have the capsule, is called R strain because the surface of the colonies looks rough. The R strain does not cause the disease. When heat-killed S strain was mixed with live R strain, cultured, and spread on to a solid medium, a few S strain colonies appeared. When S cell extract was treated with RNase or proteinase and mixed with the live R strain, R colonies and a few S colonies appeared. When the S strain cell extract was treated with DNase and mixed with live R strain, there were only R strain colonies growing on the **agar** plates. These experiments proved fundamentally that DNA is the genetic material that carries genes.

Transformation is widely used in DNA manipulation in **molecular biology**. For most bacteria that do not possess natural competency, special treatment, such as calcium chloride treatment, can render the cells competent. This is one of the most important techniques for introducing recombinant DNA molecules into bacteria and **yeast** cells in genetic engineering.

See also Cell membrane transport; Microbial genetics

TRANSGENICS

The term transgenics refers to the process of transferring genetic information from one organism to another. By introducing new genetic material into a cell or individual, a transgenic organism is created that has new characteristics it did not have before. The genes transferred from one organism or cell to another are called transgenes. The development of biotechnological techniques has led to the creation of transgenic **bacteria**, plants, and animals that have great advantages over their natural counterparts and sometimes act as living machines to create pharmaceutical therapies for the treatment of disease. Despite the advantages of transgenics, some people have great concern regarding the use of transgenic plants as food, and with the possibility of transgenic organisms escaping into the environment where they may upset ecosystem balance.

Except for retroviruses that utilize **ribonucleic acid (RNA)**, all of the cells of every living thing on Earth contain **DNA (deoxyribonucleic acid)**. DNA is a complex and long molecule composed of a sequence of smaller molecules, called nucleotides, linked together. Nucleotides are nitrogen-containing molecules, called bases, that are combined with sugar and

phosphate. There are four different kinds of nucleotides in DNA. Each nucleotide has a unique base component. The sequence of nucleotides, and therefore of bases, within an organism's DNA is unique. In other words, no two organisms have exactly the same sequence of nucleotides in their DNA, even if they belong to the same species or are related. DNA holds within its nucleotide sequence information that directs the activities of the cell. Groups, or sets of nucleotide sequences that instruct a single function are called genes.

Much of the genetic material, or DNA, of organisms is coiled into compact forms called **chromosomes**. Chromosomes are highly organized compilations of DNA and protein that make the long molecules of DNA more manageable during cell division. In many organisms, including human beings, chromosomes are found within the **nucleus** of a cell. The nucleus is the central compartment of the cell that houses genetic information and acts as a control center for the cell. In other organisms, such as bacteria, DNA is not found within a nucleus. Instead, the DNA (usually in the form of a circular chromosome) chromosome is free within the cell. Additionally, many cells have extrachromosomal DNA that is not found within chromosomes. The mitochondria of cells, and the chloroplasts of plant cells have extrachromosomal DNA that help direct the activities of these organelles independent from the activities of the nucleus where the chromosomes are found. **Plasmids** are circular pieces of extrachromosomal DNA found in bacteria that are extensively used in transgenics.

DNA, whether in chromosomes or in extrachromosomal molecules, uses the same code to direct cell activities. The **genetic code** is the sequence of nucleotides in genes that is defined by sets of three nucleotides. The genetic code itself is universal, meaning it is interpreted the same way in all living things. Therefore, all cells use the same code to store information in DNA, but have different amounts and kinds of information. The entire set of DNA found within a cell (and all of the identical cells of a multicellular organism) is called the genome of that cell or organism.

The DNA of chromosomes within the cellular genome is responsible for the production of proteins. The universal genetic code simply tells cells which proteins to make. Proteins, in turn have many varied and important functions; and in fact help determine the major characteristics of cells and whole organisms. As **enzymes**, proteins carry out thousands of kinds of chemical reactions that make life possible. Proteins also act as cell receptors and signal molecules, which enable cells to communicate with one another, to coordinate growth and other activities important for wound healing and development. Thus, many of the vital activities and characteristics that define a cell are really the result of the proteins that are present. The proteins, in turn, are determined by the genome of the organism.

Because the genetic code with genes is the same for all known organisms, and because genes determine characteristics of organisms, the characteristics of one kind of organism can be transferred to another. If genes from an insect, for example, are placed into a plant in such a way that they are functional, the plant will gain characteristics of the insect. The insect's DNA provides information on how to make insect proteins within the plant because the genetic code is interpreted in the same way. That is, the insect genes give new characteristics to the plant. This very process has already been performed with firefly genes and tobacco plants. Firefly genes were spliced into tobacco plants, which created new tobacco plants that could glow in the dark. This amazing artificial genetic mixing, called recombinant **biotechnology**, is the crux of transgenics. The organisms that are created from mixing genes from different sources are transgenic. The glow-in-the-dark tobacco plants in the previous example, then, are transgenic tobacco plants.

One of the major obstacles in the creation of transgenic organisms is the problem of physically transferring DNA from one organism or cell into another. It was observed early on that bacteria resistant to **antibiotics** transferred the resistance characteristic to other nearby bacterial cells that were not previously resistant. It was eventually discovered that the resistant bacterial cells were actually exchanging plasmid DNA carrying resistance genes. The **plasmids** traveled between resistant and susceptible cells. In this way, susceptible bacterial cells were transformed into resistant cells.

The permanent modification of a genome by the external application of DNA from a cell of different **genotype** is called **transformation**. Transformed cells can pass on the new characteristics to new cells when they reproduce because copies of the foreign transgenes are replicated during cell division. Transformation can be either naturally occurring or the result of transgenics. Scientists mimic the natural uptake of plasmids by bacterial cells for use in creating transgenic cells. Certain chemicals make transgenic cells more willing to take-up genetically engineered plasmids. Electroporation is a process where cells are induced by an electric current to take up pieces of foreign DNA. Transgenes are also introduced via engineered **viruses**. In a procedure called transfection, viruses that infect bacterial cells are used to inject the foreign pieces of DNA. DNA can also be transferred using microinjection, which uses microscopic needles to insert DNA to the inside of cells. A new technique to introduce transgenes into cells uses liposomes. Liposomes are microscopic spheres filled with DNA that fuse to cells. When liposomes merge with host cells, they deliver the transgenes to the new cell. Liposomes are composed of lipids very similar to the lipids that make up cell membranes, which gives them the ability to fuse with cells.

With the aid of new scientific knowledge, scientists can now use transgenics to accomplish the same results as selective breeding.

By recombining genes, bacteria that metabolize petroleum products are created to clean-up the environment, antibiotics are made by transgenic bacteria on mass industrial scales, and new protein drugs are produced. By creating transgenic plants, food crops have enhanced productivity. Transgenic corn, wheat, and soy with herbicide resistance, for example, are able to grow in areas treated with herbicide that kills weeds. Transgenic tomato plants produce larger, more colorful tomatoes in greater abundance. Transgenics is also used to create **influenza** immunizations and other vaccines.

Despite their incredible utility, there are concerns regarding trangenics. The Human Genome Project is a large collaborative effort among scientists worldwide that announced the determination of the sequence of the entire human genome in 2000. In doing this, the creation of transgenic humans could become more of a reality, which could lead to serious ramifications. Also, transgenic plants used as genetically modified food is a topic of debate. For a variety of reasons, not all scientifically based, some people argue that transgenic food is a consumer safety issue because not all of the effects of transgenic foods have been fully explored.

See also Cell cycle (eukaryotic), genetic regulation of; Cell cycle (prokaryotic), genetic regulation of; Chromosomes, eukaryotic; Chromosomes, prokaryotic; DNA (Deoxyribonucleic acid); DNA hybridization; Molecular biology and molecular genetics

TRANSLATION

Translation is the process in which genetic information, carried by messenger **RNA** (mRNA), directs the synthesis of proteins from amino acids, whereby the primary structure of the protein is determined by the nucleotide sequence in the mRNA. Although there are some important differences between translation in **bacteria** and translation in eukaryotic cells the overall process is similar. Essentially, the same type of translational control mechanisms that exist in eukaryotic cells do not exist in bacteria.

A molecule known as the ribosome is the site of the **protein synthesis**. The ribosome is protein bound to a second species of RNA known as ribosomal RNA (rRNA). Several **ribosomes** may attach to a single mRNA molecule, so that many polypeptide chains are synthesized from the same mRNA. The ribosome binds to a very specific region of the mRNA called the promoter region. The promoter is upstream of the sequence that will be translated into protein.

The nucleotide sequence on the mRNA is translated into the amino acid sequence of a protein by adaptor molecules composed of a third type of RNA known as transfer RNAs (tRNAs). There are many different species of tRNAs, with each species binding a particular type of amino acid. In protein synthesis, the nucleotide sequence on the mRNA does not specify an amino acid directly, rather, it specifies a particular species of tRNA. Complementary tRNAs match up on the strand of mRNA every three bases and add an amino acid onto the lengthening protein chain. The three base sequence on the mRNA are known as "codons," while the complementary sequence on the tRNA are the "anti-codons."

The ribosomal RNA has two subunits, a large subunit and a small subunit. When the small subunit encounters the mRNA, the process of translation to protein begins. There are two sites in the large subunit, an "A" site, and a "P" site. The start signal for translation is the codon ATG that codes for methionine. A tRNA charged with methionine binds to the translation start signal. After the first tRNA bearing the amino acid appears in the "A" site, the ribosome shifts so that the tRNA is now in the "P" site. A new tRNA molecule corresponding to the codon of the mRNA enters the "A" site. A pep-

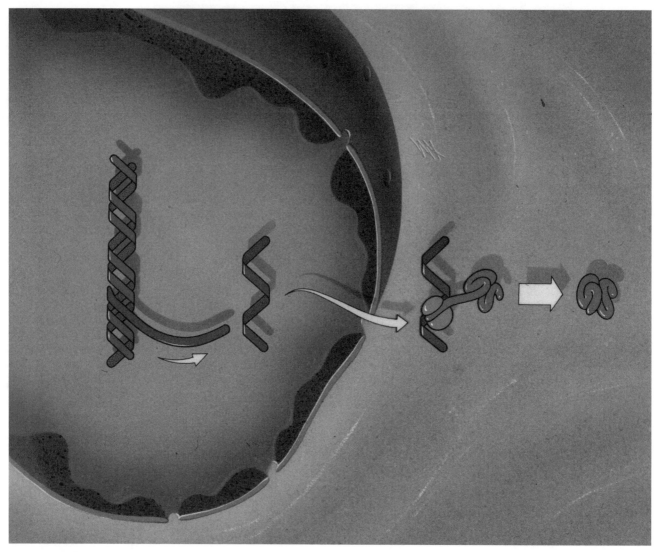

Illustration depicting the transcription of DNA inside the eukaryotic nucleus and the translation of the messenger RNA to form protein that occurs outside the nucleus.

tide bond is formed between the amino acid brought in by the second tRNA and the amino acid carried by the first tRNA. The first tRNA is now released and the ribosome again shifts. The second tRNA bearing two amino acids is now in the "P" site, and a third tRNA can now bind to the "A" site. The process of the tRNA binding to the mRNA aligns the amino acids in a specific order. This long chain of amino acids constitutes a protein. Therefore, the sequence of nucleotides on the mRNA molecule directs the order of the amino acids in a given protein. The process of adding amino acids to the growing chain occurs along the length of the mRNA until the ribosome comes to a sequence of bases that is known as a "stop codon." When that happens, no tRNA binds to the empty "A" site. This is the signal for the ribosome to release the polypeptide chain and the mRNA.

Bacterial ribosomes are smaller than eukaryotic ribosomes. In some cases, bacterial ribosomes contain less than

have the total protein found in eukaryotic ribosomes. Bacteria also respond to fewer initiation factors than do eukaryotic cells.

After being released from the tRNA, some proteins may undergo post-translational modifications. They may be cleaved by a proteolytic (protein cutting) enzyme at a specific site. Alternatively, they may have some of their amino acids biochemically modified. After such modifications, the polypeptide forms into its native shape and starts acting as a functional protein in the cell.

There are four different nucleotides, A, U, G and T. If they are taken three at a time (to specify a codon, and thus, indirectly specify an amino acid), 64 codons could be specified. However, there are only 20 different amino acids. Therefore, several triplets code for the same amino acid; for example UAU and UAC both code for the amino acid tyrosine. In addition, some codons do not code for amino acids, but code for polypeptide chain initiation and termination. The genetic code is non-overlapping, i.e., the nucleotide in one codon is never part of the adjacent codon. The code also seems to be universal in all living organisms.

See also Cell cycle (prokaryotic), genetic regulation of; Chromosomes, prokaryotic; Cytoplasm, prokaryotic; Genetic regulation of prokaryotic cells; Molecular biology and molecular genetics; Protein synthesis; Proteins and enzymes; Ribonucleic acid (RNA)

TRANSMISSION ELECTRON MICROSCOPE (TEM) • *see* ELECTRON MICROSCOPE, TRANSMISSION AND SCANNING

TRANSMISSION OF PATHOGENS

Microorganisms that cause disease in humans and other species are known as pathogens. The transmission of pathogens to a human or other host can occur in a number of ways, depending upon the microorganism.

A common route is via water. The ingestion of contaminated water introduces the microbes into the digestive system. Intestinal upsets can result. As well, an organism may be capable of entering the cells that line the digestive tract and gaining entry to the bloodstream. From there, an infection can become widely dispersed. A prominent example of a water borne pathogen is *Vibrio cholerae*, the bacterium that causes cholera. The contamination of drinking water by this bacterium is still at epidemic proportions in some areas of the world.

Pathogens can also be transmitted via the air. Viruses and bacterial spores are light enough to be lifted on the breeze. These agents can subsequently be inhaled, where they cause lung infections. An example of such as virus is the Hanta virus. A particularly prominent bacterial example is the spore form of the anthrax-causing bacterium *Bacillus anthracis*. The latter has also been identified as a bioterrorist weapon that can, as exemplified in a 2001 terrorist attack on the United States, be transmitted in mail that when opened or touched can result in cutaneous or inhalation anthrax.

Still other microbial pathogens are transmitted from one human to another via body fluids such as the blood. This route is utilized by a number of viruses. The most publicized example is the transmission of Human Immunodeficiency Virus (HIV). HIV is generally regarded to be the cause of acquired immunodeficiency syndrome. As well, viruses that cause hemorrhagic fever (e.g., Ebola) are transmitted in the blood. If precautions are not taken when handling patients, the caregiver can become infected.

Transmission of pathogens can occur directly, as in the above mechanisms. As well, transmission can be indirect. An intermediate host that harbors the microorganism can transfer the microbes to humans via a bite or by other contact. *Coxiella burnetti*, the bacterium that cause Q-fever, is transmitted to humans from the handling of animals such as sheep. As another example, the trypanosome parasite that causes sleeping sick-

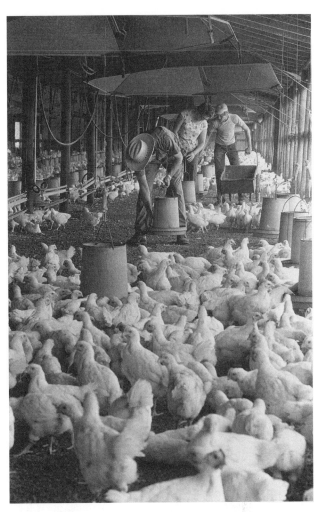

Transmission of pathogens, such as those affecting poultry, can be promoted by crowded living conditions.

ness enters the bloodstream upon the bite of a female mosquito that acts as a vector for the transmission of the parasite.

Finally, some viruses are able to transmit infection over long periods of time by become latent in the host. More specifically, the genetic material of viruses such as the hepatitis viruses and the herpes virus can integrate and be carried for decades in the host genome before the symptoms of infections appear.

See also Anthrax, terrorist use as a biological weapon; Bacteria and bacterial infection; Epidemics and pandemics; Yeast, infectious; Zoonoses

TRANSPLANTATION GENETICS AND IMMUNOLOGY

There are several different types of transplantation. An autograft is a graft from one part of the body to another site on the same individual. An isograft is one between individuals that are genetically alike, as in identical twins. An allograft is a graft between members of the same species but who are not genetically alike. A xenograft is one between members of different species. The allograft we are most familiar with is that of a blood transfusion. Nonetheless, the replacement of diseased organs by transplantation of healthy tissues has frustrated medical science because the **immune system** of the recipient recognizes that the donor organ is not "self" and rejects the new organ.

The ability to discriminate between self and nonself is vital to the functioning of the immune system so it can protect the body from disease and invading **microorganisms**. However, the same immune response that serves well against foreign proteins prevents the use of organs needed for life saving operations. Virtually every cell in the body carries distinctive proteins found on the outside of the cell that identify it as self. Central to this ability is a group of genes that are called the **(MHC)**, or **major histocompatibility complex**. The genes that code for those proteins in humans are called the **HLA** or **Human Leukocyte Antigen**. These are broken down to class I (HLA-A, B, and Cw), class II (HLA-DR, DQ, and DP) and class III (no HLA genes).

The MHC was discovered during tumor transplantation studies in mice by Peter Gorer in 1937 at the Lister Institute, and was so named because "histo" stands for tissue in medical terminology. The genes that compose the MHC are unique in that they rarely undergo **recombination** and so are inherited as a haplotype, one from each parent. They are also highly polymorphic. This means that the genes and the molecules they code for vary widely in their structure from one individual to another and so transplants are likely to be identified as foreign and rejected by the body. Scientists have also noted that this area of the genome undergoes more mutational events then other regions, which probably accounts for some of its high degree of polymorphism. As previously mentioned, there are several classes of the MHC. The role of the MHC Class I is to make those proteins that identify the cells of the body as "self," and they are found on nearly every cell in the body that has **nucleus**. Nonself proteins are called antigens and the body first learns to identify self from nonself just before birth, in a **selection** process that weeds out all the immature T-cells that lack self-tolerance. Normally, this process continues throughout the lifespan of the organism. A breakdown in this process leads to **allergies** and at the extreme, results in such autoimmune diseases as multiple sclerosis, rheumatoid arthritis, and systemic lupus erythematosus. The job of the Class I proteins is to alert killer **T cells** that certain cells in the body have somehow been transformed, either by a viral infection or cancer, and they need to be eliminated. Killer T-cells will only attack cells that have the same Class I glycoproteins that they carry themselves. The Class II MHC molecules are found on another immunocompetant cell called the B-cells. These cells mature into the cells that make antibodies against foreign proteins. The class II molecules are also found on macrophages and other cells that present foreign antigens to T-helper cells. The Class II antigens combine with the foreign **antigen** and form a complex with the **antibody**, which is subsequently recognized and then eliminated by the body.

The ability of killer T-cells to respond only to those transformed cells that carry Class I antigen, and the ability of helper T-cells to respond to foreign antigens that carry Class II antigen, is called MHC restriction. This is what is tested for when tissues are typed for transplantation. Most transplantation occurs with allogeneic organs, which by definition are those that do not share the same MHC locus. The most sensitive type of transplantation with respect to this are those involving the bone marrow (Haematopoietic Stem Cell Transplantation) HLA matching is an absolute requirement so its use is limited to HLA-matched donors, usually a brother or sister. The major complications include graft-versus-host disease (GvHD is an attack of immunocompetant donor cells to immunosuppressed recipient cells) and rejection, which is the reverse of GvHD. The least sensitive are corneal lens transplantation, probably because of lack of vascularisation in the cornea and its relative immunological privilege. Drugs like cyclosporin A have made transplant surgery much easier, although the long term consequences of suppressing immune function are not yet clear. This antirejection drug is widely used in transplant surgery and to prevent and treat rejection and graft-versus-host disease in bone marrow transplant patients by suppressing their normal immune system. Newer strategies, including **gene** therapy, are being developed to prevent the acute and chronic rejection of transplanted tissues by introducing new genes that are important in preventing rejection. One promising aspect is the delivery of genes that encode foreign donor antigens (alloantigens). This might be an effective means of inducing immunological tolerance in the recipient and eliminate the need for whole-body immunosuppression.

See also Antibody and antigen; Immunogenetics; Immunologic therapies; Immunosuppressant drugs; Major histocompatibility complex (MHC)

TRANSPOSITION

A transposition is a physical movement of genetic material (i.e., **DNA**) within a genome or the movement of DNA across genomes (i.e., from one genome to another). Because these segments of genetic material contain genes, transpositions resulting in changes of the loci (location) or arrangements of genes are **mutations**. Transposition mutations occur in a wide range of organisms. **Transposons** occur in **bacteria**, and transposable elements have been demonstrated to operate in higher eukaryotic organisms, including mammalian systems.

Transposition mutations may only occur if the DNA being moved, termed the transposon, contains intact inverted repeats at its ends (terminus). In addition, functional tranposase **enzymes** must be present.

There are two types or mechanisms of transposition. Replicative transpositions involve the copying of the segment of section DNA to be moved (transposable element) before the segment is actually moved. Accordingly, with replicative transposition, the original section of DNA remains at its original location and only the copy is moved and inserted into its new position. In contrast, with conservative transpositions, the segment of DNA to be moved is physically cut from its original location and then inserted into a new location. The DNA from which the tranposon is removed is termed the donor DNA, and the DNA to which the transposon is added is termed the receptor DNA.

Transposons are not passive participants in transposition. Transposons carry the genes that code for the enzymes needed for transposition. In essence, they carry the mechanisms of transposition with them as they move or jump (hence Barbara McClintok's original designation of "jumping genes") throughout or across genomes. Transposons carry special **insertion sequences** (IS elements) that carry the genetic information to code for the enzyme transposase that is required to accomplish transposition mutations. One of the most important mechanisms of transposase is that they are the enzymes responsible for cutting the receptor DNA to allow the insertion of the transposon.

Transitions are a radical mutational mechanism. The physical removal of both DNA and genes can severely damage or impair the function of genes located in the transposons (especially those near either terminus). Correspondingly, the donor molecules suffer a deletion of material that may also render the remaining genes inoperative or highly impaired with regard to function.

McClintok's discovery of transposons, also termed "jumping genes" in the late 1940's (before the formation of the Waston-Crick model of DNA) resulted in her subsequent award of a Nobel Prize for Medicine or Physiology.

Transposition segments termed retrotransposons may also utilize an **RNA** intermediate complimentary copy to accomplish their transposition.

Transposition can radically and seriously affect phenotypic characteristics including transfer of **antibiotic resistance** in bacterium. Following insertion, transposed genetic elements usually generate multiple copies of the genes transferred, further increasing their disruption to both the **genotype** and phenotypic expression.

See also Antibiotics; Microbial genetics

TREPONEMA · *see* SYPHILIS

TRYPANOSOME · *see* CHAGAS' DISEASE

TUBERCULOSIS

Tuberculosis (TB) is an infectious disease of the lungs caused by the bacterium *Mycobacterium tuberculosis*. In the mid-nineteenth century, about one-fourth of the mortality rate was attributable to tuberculosis. It was particularly rampant in early childhood and young adulthood. Its presence was felt throughout the world, but by the 1940s, with the introduction of **antibiotics**, there was a sharp decline of cases in developed countries. For less-developed countries with poor **public health** structures, tuberculosis is still a major problem. Since

1989, however, there has been an increase in reported cases in economically advanced countries due mainly to immunosuppression associated with **AIDS**, and the emergence of antibiotic-resistant strains of TB.

The bacillus infects the lungs of those who inhale the infected droplets formed during coughing by an individual who has an active case of the disease. It can also be transmitted by unpasteurized milk, as animals can be infected with the **bacteria**. The disease is dormant in different parts of the body until it becomes active and attacks the lungs, leading to a chronic infection. Symptoms include fatigue, loss of weight, night fevers and chills, and persistent coughing with sputum-streaked blood. The virulent form of the infection can then spread to other parts of the body. Without treatment, the condition is eventually fatal.

Chest x rays and sputum examinations can show the presence of tuberculosis. Tuberculin, a purified protein taken from the tuberculosis bacilli, is placed under the skin of the forearm during a tuberculosis skin test. In two or three days if there is a red swelling at the site, the test is positive, and indicates TB infection, but not necessarily active TB disease. Early detection of the disease facilitates effective treatment to avoid the possibility of it becoming active later on.

Populations at risk of contracting TB are people with certain medical conditions or those using drugs for medical conditions that weaken the **immune system**. Others at risk are low-income groups, people from undeveloped countries with high TB rates, people who work in or are residents of long-term care facilities (nursing homes, prisons, hospitals), those who are significantly underweight, alcoholics, and intravenous drug users.

Traces of lesions from tuberculosis have been found in the lungs of ancient Egyptian mummies. The recent discovery of a Pre-Columbian mummy has resolved the debate on whether or not European explorers introduced the disease to the New World. Lung samples from a Peruvian woman who lived 500 years before Columbus discovered America show a lump that was identified as tuberculosis by **DNA** testing. Hippocrates, a Greek physician who lived from 460 to 370 B.C., described the disease. The Greek name for the disease was *phthisis,* derived from the verb *phthinein,* meaning to waste away. Tuberculosis was also called consumption because of the wasting away effects (notably, significant losses of weight over a period of time) of the disease.

In 1839, Johann Schonlein is credited with first labeling the disease tuberculosis. In 1882, the tubercle bacillus was discovered by **Robert Koch**, the German physician who pioneered the science of bacteriology. This landmark discovery was followed eight years later by his extraction of a protein from dead bacilli called tuberculin. This protein is still used to test for the presence of TB infection in a dormant or early stage. Another important diagnostic breakthrough came in 1895 with the discovery of Wilhelm Conrad Roentgen's x rays. The presence of TB lesions was detected on x rays.

Two twentieth century French scientists, Albert Calmette and Camille Guerin, developed a **vaccine** against tuberculosis from a weakened strain of bovine bacillus. Called BCG for Bacillus-Calmette-Guerin, this vaccine is the only

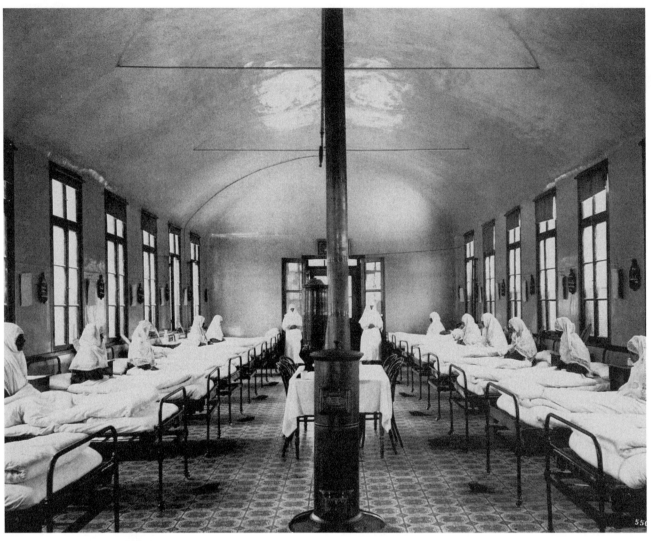

Hospital for tuberculosis patients in Turkey.

one still in use although some scientists question its effectiveness. Despite doubts about the vaccine, it is still widely used, especially in TB endemic countries where other preventive measures are lacking. The U.S. Public Health Service's policy recommends testing and drug therapy for those infected instead of **vaccination**. The two factors responsible for this policy are the low incidence of TB in the United States and the doubts raised about BCG. The **Centers for Disease Control** and Prevention, (CDC), however, in its concern over the rising incidence of TB in the United States and the appearance of multidrug-resistant tuberculosis (MDR TB) which is difficult to treat, reexamined the TB vaccination issue, and released recommendations for its use in limited situations.

The CDC still recommends the use of skin tests and drug therapy as the most important measures in controlling the incidence of TB in the United States. Drug therapy is 90% effective in halting the infection. Since those vaccinated test positive with the skin test, a vaccination program would interfere with skin testing. Mass vaccination would risk giving up

a simple test that provides an early warning. Relying on the drug treatment program to stop TB **epidemics**, however, has one major drawback. The drug therapy takes six months to a year before halting the infection. People infected are often among the homeless, poor, drug addicted, or criminal societies. Unless these people are carefully supervised to make sure they complete a regimen of drug therapy, it is difficult to effect a cure for the disease.

Throughout the nineteenth century and up until the 1960s, physicians sent their TB patients to sanatoriums which were rest homes located in mountains or semi-arid regions such as the American southwest. These locations were supposed to help the breathing process by providing clean and dry air. Physicians assumed that deeper, easier breathing in a work-free environment would help overcome the disease. Prior to the advent of antibiotics, these retreats were the only recourse for chronically ill tubercular patients. Although treatment in sanatoriums did help many, they were phased out before the 1960s, and replaced by antibiotic drug **chemother-**

apy, which could be administered in either a hospital or home environment. Over 90% of TB patients can be cured by a combination of inexpensive antibiotics, but it is necessary they be used for a period of at least six months.

The impact of tuberculosis was evident in the nineteenth and early twentieth centuries in literature, art, and music. Puccini's opera, *La Boheme,* was created around the tragic death of the tubercular heroine, Mimi. Since TB often attacked the young, many poets, artists and musicians fell prey to the disease before they had a chance to fulfill their creative work. Among them, Amedeo Modigliani, John Keats, Frederic Chopin, and Anton Chekhov were claimed by the disease, along with millions of other young people during the period. In the United States, American playwright Eugene O'Neill was one of the fortunate few who did recover in a sanatorium and went on to write his plays. His early play, *The Straw,* written in 1919, dramatically shows what life was like in a sanatorium.

In the past, U.S. city and state governments were actively involved in regulations that controlled infected people from spreading the infection. At present, federal, state, and local agencies must again take a leading role in formulating a public policy on this complicated health problem. Several states are using a program called Directly Observed Therapy (DOT) to combat the rising incidence of TB. This program has met with considerable success in lowering reported cases of TB as much as 15% in New York City during the late 1990s.

DOT is offered at soup kitchens, clinics, hospitals, neighborhood health centers, and drug rehabilitation centers. Outreach workers enable those with TB to get help with the least amount of red tape. The wide array of medicines needed to treat the disease are made available, and ample funding has been provided from federal, state, and local agencies. Apartments are located for homeless patients and special provisions are made to help released prison inmates and those on parole. Guidelines for compassionate, supervised medical services are periodically reviewed for the successful implementation of the DOT program.

Despite such measures, the U.S. Department of Health and Human Services predicts tuberculosis, will spread further by the year 2005. In 1990, there were 7,537,000 TB cases worldwide. That number is expected to rise to 11,875,000 in 2005, a 58% increase. Most of the rise in rate is attributed to demographic factors (77%) while 23% accounts for the epidemiological factors, i.e., the rise in **HIV** infection. Approximately 30 million people around the world will die of TB from 2000 to 2009. These predictions are considered conservative because many cases of TB are never reported.

See also AIDS, recent advances in research and treatment; Bacteria and bacterial infection; Epidemiology, tracking diseases with technology; Public health, current issues

TULAREMIA

Tularemia is a plague-like disease caused by the bacterium *Francisella tularensis* that can transferred to man from animals such as rodents, voles, mice, squirrels, and rabbits.

Reflecting the natural origin of the disease, tularemia is also known as rabbit fever. Indeed, the rabbit is the most common source of the disease. Transfer of the bacterium via contaminated water and vegetation is possible as well.

The disease can easily spread from the environmental source to humans (although direct person-to-person contact has not been documented). This contagiousness and the high death rate among those who contract the disease made the bacterium an attractive bioweapon. Both the Japanese and Western armies experimented with *Francisella tularensis* during World War II. Experiments during and after that war established the devastating effect that aerial dispersion of the **bacteria** could exact on a population. Until the demise of the Soviet Union, its biological weapons development program actively developed strains of the bacterium that were resistant to **antibiotics** and vaccines.

Tularemia naturally occurs over much of North America and Europe. In the United States, the disease is predominant in south-central and western states such as Missouri, Arkansas, Oklahoma, South Dakota, and Montana. The disease almost always occurs in rural regions. The animal reservoirs of the bacterium become infected typically by a bite from a blood-feeding tick, fly, or mosquito.

The causative bacterium, *Francisella tularensis,* is a Gram-negative bacterium that, even though it does not form a spore, can survive for protracted periods of time in environments such as cold water, moist hay, soil, and decomposing carcasses.

The number of cases of tularemia in the world is not known, as accurate statistics have not been kept, and because illnesses attributable to the bacterium go unreported. In the United States, the number of cases used to be high. In the 1950s thousands of people were infected each year. This number has dropped considerable, to less than 200 each year in the 1990s and those who are infected now tend to be those who are exposed to the organism in its rural habitat (e.g., hunters, trappers, farmers, and butchers).

Humans can acquire the infection through breaks in the skin and mucous membranes, by ingesting contaminated water, or by inhaling the organism. An obligatory step in the establishment of an infection is the invasion of host cells. A prime target of invasion is the immune cell known as macrophages. Infections can initially become established in the lymph nodes, lungs, spleen, liver, and kidney. As these infections become more established, the microbe can spread to tissues throughout the body.

Symptoms of tularemia vary depending on the route of entry. Handling an infected animal or carcass can produce a slow-growing ulcer at the point of initial contact and swollen lymph nodes. When inhaled, the symptoms include the sudden development of a headache with accompanying high fever, chills, body aches (particularly in the lower back), and fatigue. Ingestion of the organism produces a sore throat, abdominal pain diarrhea, and vomiting. Other symptoms can include eye infection and the formation of skin ulcers. Some people also develop **pneumonia**-like chest pain. An especially severe pneumonia develops from the inhalation of one type of the organism, which is designated as *Francisella tularensis biovar* *tularensis* (type A). The pneumonia can progress to respiratory failure and death. The symptoms typically tend to appear three to five days after entry of the microbe into the body.

The infection responds to antibiotic treatment and recovery can be complete within a few weeks. Recovery produces a long-term **immunity** to re-infection. Some people experience a lingering impairment in the ability to perform physical tasks. If left untreated, tularemia can persist for weeks, even months, and can be fatal. The severe form of tularemia can kill up to 60% of those who are infected if treatment is not given.

A **vaccine** is available for tularemia. To date this vaccine has been administered only to those who are routinely exposed to the bacterium (e.g., researchers). The potential risks of the vaccine, which is a weakened form of the bacterium, have been viewed as being greater than the risk of acquiring the infection.

See also Bacteria and bacterial infection; Bioterrorism, protective measures; Infection control; Zoonoses

TUMOR VIRUSES

Tumor **viruses** are those viruses that are able to infect cells and cause changes within the cell's operating machinery such that the cell's ability to regulate its growth and division is destroyed and the cells become cancerous.

Human papillomavirus, **hepatitis** B, **Epstein-Barr virus**, **human T-cell leukemia virus**, SV-40, and Rous sarcoma virus are all tumor viruses.

The ability of the Rous sarcoma virus to cause sarcomas (cancers of connective tissue) has been known since 1911, when **Peyton Rous** demonstrated that a sarcoma material from chicken could be filtered and the filtered fluid was still capable of inducing the cancer. The virus was both the first oncogenic (cancer-causing) virus to be discovered and (although not known until much later) the first retrovirus to be discovered. Another, well-known example of a retrovirus is **HIV**.

There are some 90 types of human papillomavirus, based upon the genetic sequence of their genomes. The target of the viral infection is a certain type of epithelial cell known as stratified squamous epithelium. The cells can be located on the surface of the skin, or can be mucosal cells in regions of the body such as the genital tract. For example, two human papillomaviruses are the most common cause of genital warts. While these warts are noncancerous, other types of papillomavirus result in the development of cervical cancer. Furthermore, human papillomavirus types 16 and 18 are the main cause of genital tract malignancies. The virus is transmitted from person to person typically via sexual contact.

How human papillomavirus triggers the uncontrolled growth that is a hallmark of cancerous cells is still unknown. Studies have determined that in cells that have not yet become cancerous, the viral genetic material is not associated with the cell's genetic material, and that production of new virus particles is still occurring. However, in cancerous cells the viral genetic material has been integrated into that of the host and no new virus particles are being made. Whether the integration event is a trigger for cancerous growth is not known.

The hepatitis B virus is associated with liver damage and liver cancer. The virus is transmitted from person to person via contaminated blood (which commonly occurs via sharing of needles), breast milk, and possibly saliva. Over 90% of all hepatitis B infections are cleared as the **immune system** responds to the infection. However, in some 5% of those infected the infection becomes chronic. Infected individuals can be asymptomatic, but remain carriers of the virus and thus able to pass on the virus to others.

Chronic infection with the hepatitis B virus greatly elevates the chances of developing cancer of the liver. Because the virus can be present for decades before the damage of liver cancer is diagnosed, the best strategy is the preemptive use of hepatitis B **vaccine** in those offspring born to mothers who are known to be positive for the virus.

As for human papillomavirus, the molecular mechanism by which hepatitis B virus triggers cancerous growth of cells is unknown. The periodic response of the immune system to the virus may over time favor the expression of genes whose products are involved in overriding growth and division control mechanisms.

The Epstein-Barr virus is linked to two specific cancers. One is called Burkitt's lymphoma, a cancer of the B-cell components of the immune system. The lymphoma is a common cancer of children and occurs almost exclusively in the central region of Africa. The region's high rate of **malaria** may play a role in the prevalence of the lymphoma, as malaria causes an increase in the number of the already-infected B-cells. The rapid increase in the virally infected B-cells might cause a genetic malfunction that leads to tumor development. The second cancer associated with the virus is nasopharyngeal carcinoma. This cancer is restricted to the coastal region of China, for as yet unknown reasons.

Human T-cell leukemia virus causes cancer in the T-cell components of the immune system. Infection is widespread in Japan and areas of Africa, and is spreading to western nations including the United States.

A virus designated SV-40, which is harbored by species of monkeys, is isolated from a sizable number of cancer sufferers.

See also Oncogene; Oncogenetic research

TYPHOID FEVER

Typhoid fever is a severe infection causing a sustained high fever, and caused by the **bacteria** *Salmonella typhi*—similar to the bacteria spread by chicken and eggs resulting in "Salmonella poisoning," or food poisoning. *S. typhi* bacteria, however, do not multiply directly in food, as do the **Salmonella** responsible for food poisoning, nor does it have vomiting and diarrhea as the most prominent symptoms. Instead, persistently high fever is the hallmark of infection with *Salmonella typhi*.

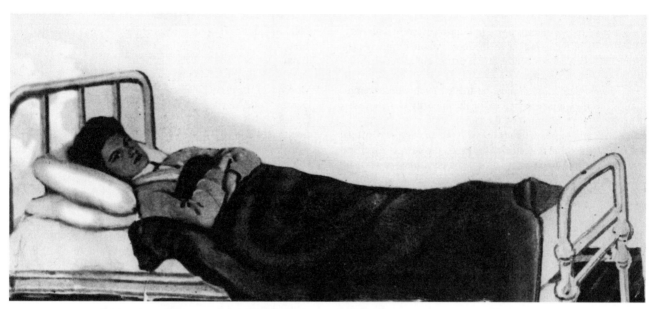

Mary Mallon ("Typhoid Mary") spread the typhoid bacterium before she was quarantined.

S. typhi bacteria are passed into the stool and urine of infected patients, and may continue to be present in the stool of asymptomatic carriers (individuals who have recovered from the symptoms of the disease, but continue to carry the bacteria). This carrier state occurs in about 3% of all individuals recovered from typhoid fever.

The disease is passed between humans, then, through poor **hygiene**, such as deficient hand washing after toileting. Individuals who are carriers of the disease and who handle food can be the source of epidemic spread of typhoid. One such individual was the inspiration for the expression "Typhoid Mary," a name given to someone with whom others wish to avoid all contact. The real "Typhoid Mary" was a cook named Mary Mallon (1855–1938) who lived in New York City around 1900. She was a carrier of typhoid and was the cause of at least 53 outbreaks of typhoid fever.

Typhoid fever is a particularly difficult problem in parts of the world with less-than-adequate sanitation practices. In the United States, many patients who become afflicted with typhoid fever have recently returned from travel to another country, where typhoid is much more prevalent, such as Mexico, Peru, Chile, India, and Pakistan.

To cause disease, the *S. typhi* bacteria must be ingested. This often occurs when a carrier does not wash hands sufficiently well after defecation, and then serves food to others. In countries where open sewage is accessible to flies, the insects land on the sewage, pick up the bacteria, and then land on food to be eaten by humans.

Ingested bacteria travel down the gastrointestinal tract, where they are taken in by cells called mononuclear phagocytes. These phagocytes usually serve to engulf and kill invading bacteria and **viruses**. However, in the case of *S. typhi*, the bacteria survive ingestion by the phagocytes, and multiply within these cells. This period of time, during which the bacteria are multiplying within the phagocytes, is the 10–14 day incubation period. When huge numbers of bacteria fill an individual **phagocyte**, the bacteria are discharged out of the cell and into the bloodstream, where their presence begins to cause symptoms.

The presence of increasingly large numbers of bacteria in the bloodstream (called bacteremia) is responsible for an increasingly high fever, which lasts throughout the four to eight weeks of the disease, in untreated individuals. Other symptoms include constipation (initially), extreme fatigue, headache, a rash across the abdomen known as "rose spots," and joint pain.

The bacteria move from the bloodstream into certain tissues of the body, including the gallbladder and lymph tissue of the intestine (called Peyer's patches). The tissue's inflammatory response to this invasion causes symptoms ranging from **inflammation** of the gallbladder (cholecystitis) to intestinal bleeding and actual perforation of the intestine. Perforation of the intestine refers to an actual hole occurring in the wall of the intestine, with leakage of intestinal contents into the abdominal cavity. This causes severe irritation and inflammation of the lining of the abdominal cavity, called peritonitis, which is frequently a fatal outcome of typhoid fever.

Other complications of typhoid fever include liver and spleen enlargement (sometimes so extreme that the spleen ruptures), anemia (low red blood cell count due to blood loss from the intestinal bleeding), joint infections (especially frequent in patients with sickle cell anemia and **immune system** disorders), **pneumonia** (due to a superimposed infection, usually by Streptococcus pneumoniae), heart infections, **meningitis**, and infections of the brain (causing confusion and even coma). Untreated typhoid fever may take several months to resolve fully.

Samples of a patient's stool, urine, blood, and bone marrow can all be used to **culture** (grow) the *S. typhi* bacteria in a laboratory for identification under a **microscope**. These types of cultures are the most accurate methods of diagnosis.

Chloramphenicol is the most effective drug treatment for *S. typhi*, and symptoms begin to improve slightly after only 24–48 hours of receiving the medication. Another drug, ceftriaxone, has been used recently, and is extremely effective, lowering fever fairly quickly.

Carriers of *S. typhi* must be treated even when asymptomatic, as they are responsible for the majority of new cases of typhoid fever. Eliminating the carrier state is actually a difficult task, and requires treatment with one or even two different medications for four to six weeks. In the case of a carrier with gall stones, surgery may need to be performed to remove the gall bladder, because the *S. typhi* bacteria are often housed in the gall bladder, where they may survive despite antibiotic treatment.

Hygienic sewage disposal systems in a community, as well as hygienic personal practices, are the most important factors in preventing typhoid fever. For travelers who expect to go to countries where *S. typhi* is a known **public health** problem, immunizations are available. Some of these immunizations provide only short-term protection (for a few months), while others may be protective for several years. Immunizations that provide a longer period of protection, with fewer side effects from the **vaccine** itself, are being developed.

See also Antibody formation and kinetics; Bacteria and bacterial infection; Immunity, active, passive and delayed; Immunochemistry; Immunogenetics; Immunology; Vaccination

TYPHUS

Typhus is a disease caused by a group of **bacteria** called **Rickettsia**. Three forms of typhus are recognized: epidemic typhus, a serious disease that is fatal if not treated promptly; rat-flea or endemic typhus, a milder form of the disease; and scrub typhus, another fatal form. The Rickettsia species of bacteria that cause all three forms of typhus are transmitted by insects. The bacteria that cause epidemic typhus, for instance, are transmitted by the human body louse; the bacteria that cause endemic typhus are transmitted by the Oriental rat flea; and bacteria causing scrub typhus are transmitted by chiggers.

Typhus takes its name from the Greek word *typhos* meaning smoke, a description of the mental state of infected persons. Typhus is marked by a severe stupor and delirium, as well as headache, chills, and fever. A rash appears within four to seven days after the onset of the disease. The rash starts on the trunk and spreads to the extremities. In milder forms of typhus, such as endemic typhus, the disease symptoms are not severe. In epidemic and scrub typhus, however, the symptoms are extreme, and death can result from complications such as stroke, renal failure, and circulatory disturbances. Fatality can be avoided in these forms of typhus with the prompt administration of **antibiotics**.

Epidemic typhus is a disease that has played an important role in history. Because typhus is transmitted by the human body louse, **epidemics** of this disease break out when humans are in close contact with each other under conditions in which the same clothing is worn for long periods of time. Cold climates also favor typhus epidemics, as people will be more likely to wear heavy clothing in colder conditions. Typhus seems to be a disease of war, poverty, and famine. In fact, according to one researcher, Napoleon's retreat from Moscow in the early nineteenth century was beset by typhus. During World War I, more than three million Russians died of typhus, and during the Vietnam war, sporadic epidemics killed American soldiers.

Epidemic typhus is caused by *Rickettsia prowazekii*. Humans play a role in the life cycle of the bacteria. Lice become infected with the bacteria by biting an infected human; these infected lice then bite other humans. A distinguishing feature of typhus disease transmission is that the louse bite itself does not transmit the bacteria. The feces of the lice are infected with bacteria; when a person scratches a louse bite, the lice feces that have been deposited on the skin are introduced into the bloodstream.

If not treated promptly, typhus is fatal. Interestingly, a person who has had epidemic typhus can experience a relapse of the disease years after they have been cured of their infection. Called Brill-Zinsser disease, after the researchers who discovered it, the relapse is usually a milder form of typhus, which is treated with antibiotics. However, a person with Brill-Zinsser disease can infect lice, which can in turn infect other humans. Controlling Brill-Zinsser relapses is important in stopping epidemics of typhus before they start, especially in areas where lice infestation is prominent.

Endemic typhus is caused by *R. typhi*. These bacteria are transmitted by the Oriental rat flea, an insect that lives on small rodents. Endemic typhus (sometimes called murine typhus or rat-flea typhus) is found worldwide. The symptoms of endemic typhus are mild compared to those of epidemic typhus. In fact, many people do not seek treatment for their symptoms, as the rash that accompanies the disease may be short-lived. Deaths from endemic typhus have been documented, however; these deaths usually occur in the elderly and in people who are already sick with other diseases.

Scrub typhus is caused by *R. tsutsugamushi*, which is transmitted by chiggers. The term "scrub typhus" comes from the observation that the disease is found in habitats with scrub vegetation, but the name is somewhat of a misnomer. Scrub typhus is found in beach areas, savannas, tropical rains forests, deserts, or anywhere chiggers live. Scientists studying scrub typhus label a habitat that contains all the elements that might prompt an outbreak of the disease a "scrub typhus island." A scrub typhus island contains chiggers, rats, vegetation that will sustain the chiggers, and, of course, a reservoir of *R. tsutsugamushi*. Scrub typhus islands are common in the geographic area that includes Australia, Japan, Korea, India, and Vietnam.

The rash that occurs in scrub typhus sometimes includes a lesion called an eschar. An eschar is a sore that develops around the chigger bite. Scrub typhus symptoms of fever, rash, and chills may evolve into stupor, **pneumonia**, and circulatory failure if antibiotic treatment is not administered. Scrub typhus, like epidemic typhus, is fatal if not treated.

Prevention of typhus outbreaks takes a two-pronged approach. Eliminating the carriers and reservoirs of

Rickettsia is an important step in prevention. Spraying with insecticides, rodent control measures, and treating soil with insect-repellent chemicals have all been used successfully to prevent typhus outbreaks. In scrub typhus islands, cutting down vegetation has been shown to lessen the incidence of scrub typhus. The second preventative prong is protecting the body from insect bites. Wearing heavy clothing when venturing into potentially insect-laden areas is one way to protect against insect bites; applying insect repellent to the skin is another. Proper personal **hygiene**, such as frequent bathing and changing of clothes, will eliminate human body lice and thus prevent epidemic typhus. A typhus **vaccine** is also available; however, this vaccine only lessens the severity and shortens the course of the disease, and does not protect against infection.

See also Bacteria and bacterial infection; Bioterrorism, protective measures; Infection control; Zoonoses

U

ULTRA-VIOLET STERILIZATION • *see* STERILIZATION

UREY, HAROLD (1893-1981)

American biochemist

Already a scientist of great honor and achievement, Harold Urey's last great period of research brought together his interests and experiences in a number of fields of research to which he devoted his life. The subject of that research was the **origin of life** on Earth.

Urey hypothesized that the earth's primordial atmosphere consisted of reducing gases such as hydrogen, ammonia, and methane. The energy provided by electrical discharges in the atmosphere, he suggested, was sufficient to initiate chemical reactions among these gases, converting them to the simplest compounds of which living organisms are made, amino acids. In 1953, Urey's graduate student Stanley Lloyd Miller carried out a series of experiments to test this hypothesis. In these experiments, an electrical discharge passed through a glass tube containing only reducing gases resulted in the formation of amino acids.

The **Miller-Urey experiment** is a classic experiment in biology. The experiment established that the conditions that existed in Earth's primitive atmosphere were sufficient to produce amino acids, the subunits of proteins comprising and required by living organisms. In essence, the Miller-Urey experiment fundamentally established that Earth's primitive atmosphere was capable of producing the building blocks of life from inorganic materials.

The Miller-Urey experiment also remains the subject of scientific debate. Scientists continue to explore the nature and composition of Earth's primitive atmosphere and thus, continue to debate the relative closeness of the conditions of the experimental conditions to Earth's primitive atmosphere.

The Miller-Urey experiment was but one part of a distinguished scientific career for Urey. In 1934, Harold Urey was awarded the Nobel Prize in chemistry for his discovery of deuterium, an isotope, or species, of hydrogen in which the atoms weigh twice as much as those in ordinary hydrogen. Also known as heavy hydrogen, deuterium became profoundly important to future studies in many scientific fields, including chemistry, physics, and medicine. Urey continued his research on isotopes over the next three decades, and during World War II his experience with deuterium proved invaluable in efforts to separate isotopes of uranium from each other in the development of the first atomic bombs. Later, Urey's research on isotopes also led to a method for determining the earth's atmospheric temperature at various periods in past history. This experimentation has become especially relevant because of concerns about the possibility of global climate change.

Harold Clayton Urey was born in Walkerton, Indiana. His father, Samuel Clayton Urey, was a schoolteacher and lay minister in the Church of the Brethren. His mother was Cora Reinoehl Urey. After graduating from high school, Urey hoped to attend college but lacked the financial resources to do so. Instead, he accepted teaching jobs in country schools, first in Indiana (1911–1912) and then in Montana (1912–1914) before finally entering Montana State University in September of 1914 at the age of 21. Urey was initially interested in a career in biology, and the first original research he ever conducted involved a study of **microorganisms** in the Missoula River. In 1917, he was awarded his bachelor of science degree in zoology by Montana State.

The year Urey graduated also marked the entry of the United States into World War I. Although he had strong pacifist beliefs as a result of his early religious training, Urey acknowledged his obligation to participate in the nation's war effort. As a result, he accepted a job at the Barrett Chemical Company in Philadelphia and worked to develop high explosives. In his Nobel Prize acceptance speech, Urey said that this experience was instrumental in his move from industrial chemistry to academic life.

At the end of the war, Urey returned to Montana State University where he began teaching chemistry. In 1921 he decided to resume his college education and enrolled in the doctoral program in physical chemistry at the University of California at Berkeley. His faculty advisor at Berkeley was the great physical chemist Gilbert Newton Lewis. Urey received his doctorate in 1923 for research on the calculation of heat capacities and entropies (the degree of randomness in a system) of gases, based on information obtained through the use of a spectroscope. He then left for a year of postdoctoral study at the Institute for Theoretical Physics at the University of Copenhagen where Niels Bohr, a Danish physicist, was researching the structure of the atom. Urey's interest in Bohr's research had been cultivated while studying with Lewis, who had proposed many early theories on the nature of chemical bonding.

Upon his return to the United States in 1925, Urey accepted an appointment as an associate in chemistry at the Johns Hopkins University in Baltimore, a post he held until 1929. He interrupted his work at Johns Hopkins briefly to marry Frieda Daum in Lawrence, Kansas, in 1926. Daum was a bacteriologist and daughter of a prominent Lawrence educator. The Ureys later had four children.

In 1929, Urey left Johns Hopkins to become associate professor of chemistry at Columbia University, and in 1930, he published his first book, *Atoms, Molecules, and Quanta,* written with A. E. Ruark. Writing in the *Dictionary of Scientific Biography,* Joseph N. Tatarewicz called this work "the first comprehensive English language textbook on atomic structure and a major bridge between the new quantum physics and the field of chemistry." At this time he also began his search for an isotope of hydrogen. Since Frederick Soddy, an English chemist, discovered isotopes in 1913, scientists had been looking for isotopes of a number of elements. Urey believed that if an isotope of heavy hydrogen existed, one way to separate it from the ordinary hydrogen isotope would be through the vaporization of liquid hydrogen. Urey's subsequent isolation of deuterium made Urey famous in the scientific world, and only three years later he was awarded the Nobel Prize in chemistry for his discovery.

During the latter part of the 1930s, Urey extended his work on isotopes to other elements besides hydrogen. Urey found that the mass differences in isotopes can result in modest differences in their reaction rates

The practical consequences of this discovery became apparent during World War II. In 1939, word reached the United States about the discovery of nuclear fission by the German scientists Otto Hahn and Fritz Strassmann. The military consequences of the Hahn-Strassmann discovery were apparent to many scientists, including Urey. He was one of the first, therefore, to become involved in the U.S. effort to build a nuclear weapon, recognizing the threat posed by such a weapon in the hands of Nazi Germany. However, Urey was deeply concerned about the potential destructiveness of a fission weapon. Actively involved in political topics during the 1930s, Urey was a member of the Committee to Defend America by Aiding the Allies and worked vigorously against the fascist regimes in Germany, Italy, and Spain. He explained

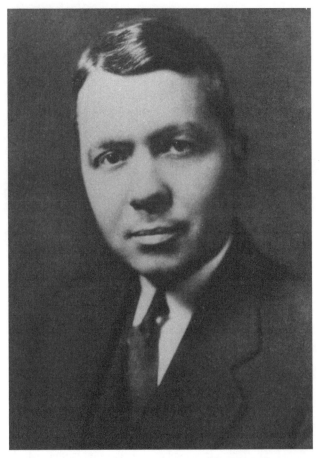

Harold Urey won the 1934 Nobel Prize in Chemistry for his discovery of heavy hydrogen (deuterium).

the importance of his political activism by saying that "no dictator knows enough to tell scientists what to do. Only in democratic nations can science flourish."

Urey worked on the Manhattan Project to build the nation's first atomic bomb. As a leading expert on the separation of isotopes, Urey made critical contributions to the solution of the Manhattan Project's single most difficult problem, the isolation of ^{235}uranium.

At the conclusion of World War II, Urey left Columbia to join the Enrico Fermi Institute of Nuclear Studies at the University of Chicago where Urey continued to work on new applications of his isotope research. During the late 1940s and early 1950s, he explored the relationship between the isotopes of oxygen and past planetary climates. Since isotopes differ in the rate of chemical reactions, Urey said that the amount of each oxygen isotope in an organism is a result of atmospheric temperatures. During periods when the earth was warmer than normal, organisms would take in more of a lighter isotope of oxygen and less of a heavier isotope. During cool periods, the differences among isotopic concentrations would not be as great. Over a period of time, Urey was able to develop a scale, or an "oxygen thermometer," that related the relative concentrations of oxygen isotopes in the shells of sea animals with atmospheric temperatures. Some of those studies continue to be highly relevant in current research on the possibilities of global climate change.

In the early 1950s, Urey became interested in yet another subject: the chemistry of the universe and of the formation of the planets, including Earth. One of his first papers on this topic attempted to provide an estimate of the relative abundance of the elements in the universe. Although these estimates have now been improved, they were remarkably close to the values modern chemists now accept.

In 1958, Urey left the University of Chicago to become Professor at Large at the University of California in San Diego at La Jolla. At La Jolla, his interests shifted from original scientific research to national scientific policy. He became extremely involved in the U.S. space program, serving as the first chairman of the Committee on Chemistry of Space and Exploration of the Moon and Planets of the National Academy of Science's Space Sciences Board. Even late in life, Urey continued to receive honors and awards from a grateful nation and admiring colleagues.

See also Cell cycle and cell division; Evolution and evolutionary mechanisms; Evolutionary origin of bacteria and viruses

V

VACCINATION

Vaccination refers to a procedure in which the presence of an **antigen** stimulates the formation of antibodies. The antibodies act to protect the host from future exposure to the antigen. Vaccination is protective against infection without the need of suffering through a bout of a disease. In this artificial process an individual receives the antibody-stimulating compound either by injection or orally.

The technique of vaccination has been practiced since at least the early decades of the eighteenth century. Then, a common practice in Istanbul was to retrieve material from the surface sores of a **smallpox** sufferer and rub the material into a cut on another person. In most cases, the recipient was spared the ravages of smallpox. The technique was refined by **Edward Jenner** into a **vaccine** for **cowpox** in 1796.

Since Jenner's time, vaccines for a variety of bacterial and viral maladies have been developed. The material used for vaccination is one of four types. Some vaccines consist of living but weakened **viruses**. These are called attenuated vaccines. The weakened virus does not cause an infection but does illicit an immune response. An example of a vaccination with attenuated material is the **measles**, **mumps**, and rubella (MMR) vaccine. Secondly, vaccination can involve killed viruses or **bacteria**. The biological material must be killed such that the surface is not altered, in order to preserve the true antigenic nature of the immune response. Also, the vaccination utilizes agents, such as alum, that act to enhance the immune response to the killed target. Current thought is that such agents operate by "presenting" the antigen to the **immune system** in a more constant way. The immune system "sees" the target longer, and so can mount a more concerted response to it. A third type of vaccination involves an inactivated form of a toxin produced by the target bacterium. Examples of such so-called toxoid vaccines are the **diphtheria** and **tetanus** vaccines. Lastly, vaccination can also utilize a synthetic conjugate compound constructed from portions of two antigens. The Hib vaccine is an example of such a biosynthetic vaccine.

During an infant's first two years of life, a series of vaccinations is recommended to develop protection against a number of viral and bacterial diseases. These are **hepatitis** B, polio, measles, mumps, rubella (also called German measles), **pertussis** (also called whooping cough), diphtheriae, tetanus (lockjaw), *Haemophilus influenzae* type b, pneumococcal infections, and chickenpox. Typically, vaccination against a specific microorganism or groups of organisms is repeated three or more times at regularly scheduled intervals. For example, vaccination against diphtheria, tetanus, and pertussis is typically administered at two months of age, four months, six months, 15–18 months, and finally at four to six years of age.

Often, a single vaccination will not suffice to develop **immunity** to a given target antigen. For immunity to develop it usually takes several doses over several months or years. A series of vaccinations triggers a greater production of **antibody** by the immune system, and primes the antibody producing cells such that they retain the memory (a form of protein coding and **antibody formation**) of the stimulating antigen for along time. For some diseases, this memory can last for a lifetime following the vaccination schedule. For other diseases, such as tetanus, adults should be vaccinated every ten years in order to keep their body primed to fight the tetanus microorganism. This periodic vaccination is also referred to as a booster shot. The use of booster vaccinations produces a long lasting immunity.

Vaccination acts on the lymphocyte component of the immune system. Prior to vaccination there are a myriad of lymphocytes. Each one recognizes only a single protein or bit of the protein. No other lymphocyte recognizes the same site. When vaccination occurs, a lymphocyte will be presented with a recognizable protein target. The lymphocyte will be stimulated to divide and some of the daughter cells will begin to produce antibody to the protein target. With time, there will be many daughter lymphocytes and much antibody circulating in the body.

With the passage of more time, the antibody production ceases. But the lymphocytes that have been produced still retain the memory of the target protein. When the target is pre-

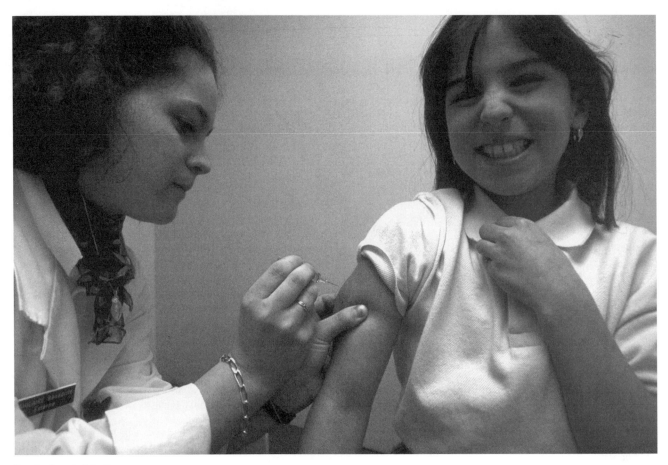

Vaccination via injection.

sented again to the lymphocytes, as happens in the second vaccination in a series, the many lymphocytes are stimulated to divide into daughter cells, which in turn form antibodies. Thus, the second time around, a great deal more antibody is produced. The antibody response also becomes highly specific for the target. For example, if the target is a virus that causes polio, then a subsequent entry of the virus into the body will trigger a highly specific and prompt immune response, which is designed to quell the invader.

Most vaccinations involve the injection of the immune stimulant. However, oral vaccination has also proven effective and beneficial. The most obvious example is the oral vaccine to polio devised by **Albert Sabin**. Oral vaccination is often limited by the passage of the vaccine through the highly acidic stomach. In the future it is hoped that the bundling of the vaccine in a protective casing will negate the damage caused by passage trough the stomach. Experiments using bags made out of lipid molecules (liposomes) have demonstrated both protection of the vaccine and the ability to tailor the liposome release of the vaccine.

The nature of vaccination, with the use of living or dead material that stimulates the immune system, holds the potential for side effects. For some vaccines, the side effects are minor. For example, a person may develop a slight ache and redness at the site of injection. In some very rare cases, however, more severe reactions can occur, such as convulsions and high fever. However, while there will always be a risk of an adverse reaction from any vaccination, the risk of developing disease is usually far greater than the probability of experiencing severe side effects.

See also Adjuvant; Anti-adhesion methods; Immune stimulation, as a vaccine

VACCINE

A vaccine is a medical preparation given to provide **immunity** from a disease. Vaccines use a variety of different substances ranging from dead **microorganisms** to genetically engineered antigens to defend the body against potentially harmful microorganisms. Effective vaccines change the **immune system** by promoting the development of antibodies that can quickly and effectively attack a disease causing microorganism when it enters the body, preventing disease development.

The development of vaccines against diseases ranging from polio and **smallpox** to **tetanus** and **measles** is considered among one of the great accomplishments of medical science.

Contemporary researchers are continually attempting to develop new vaccinations against such diseases as Acquired Immune Deficiency Syndrome (**AIDS**), cancer, **influenza**, and other diseases.

Physicians have long observed that individuals who were exposed to an infectious disease and survived were somehow protected against that disease in the future. Prior to the invention of vaccines, however, infectious diseases swept through towns, villages, and cities with a horrifying vengeance.

The first effective vaccine was developed against small-pox, an international peril that killed thousands of its victims and left thousands of others permanently disfigured. The disease was so common in ancient China that newborns were not named until they survived the disease. The development of the vaccine in the late 1700s followed centuries of innovative efforts to fight smallpox.

The ancient Chinese were the first to develop an effective measure against smallpox. A snuff made from powdered smallpox scabs was blown into the nostrils of uninfected individuals. Some individuals died from the therapy; however, in most cases, the mild infection produced offered protection from later, more serious infection.

By the late 1600s, some European peasants employed a similar method of immunizing themselves against smallpox. In a practice referred to as "buying the smallpox," peasants in Poland, Scotland, and Denmark reportedly injected the smallpox virus into the skin to obtain immunity. At the time, conventional medical doctors in Europe relied solely on isolation and quarantine of people with the disease.

Changes in these practices took place, in part, through the vigorous effort of Lady **Mary Wortley Montague**, the wife of the British ambassador to Turkey in the early 1700s. Montague said the Turks injected a preparation of small pox scabs into the veins of susceptible individuals. Those injected generally developed a mild case of smallpox from which they recovered rapidly, Montague wrote.

Upon her return to Great Britain, Montague helped convince King George I to allow trials of the technique on inmates in Newgate Prison. Success of the trials cleared the way for variolation, or the direct injection of smallpox, to become accepted medical practice in England until a **vaccination** was developed later in the century. Variolation also was credited with protecting United States soldiers from smallpox during the Revolutionary War.

Regardless, doubts remained about the practice. Individuals were known to die after receiving the smallpox injections.

The next leap in the battle against smallpox occurred when **Edward Jenner** (1749–1823) acted on a hunch. Jenner observed that people who were in contact with cows often developed **cowpox**, which caused pox but was not life threatening. Those people did not develop smallpox. In 1796, Jenner decided to test his hypothesis that cowpox could be used to protect humans against smallpox. Jenner injected a healthy eight-year-old boy with cowpox obtained from a milkmaid's sore. The boy was moderately ill and recovered. Jenner then injected the boy twice with the smallpox virus, and the boy did not get sick.

Jenner's discovery launched a new era in medicine, one in which the intricacies of the immune system would become increasingly important. Contemporary knowledge suggests that cowpox was similar enough to smallpox that the **antigen** included in the vaccine stimulated an immune response to smallpox. Exposure to cowpox antigen transformed the boy's immune system, generating cells that would remember the original antigen. The smallpox vaccine, like the many others that would follow, carved a protective pattern in the immune system, one that conditioned the immune system to move faster and more efficiently against future infection by smallpox.

The term vaccination, taken from the Latin for cow (*vacca*) was developed by **Louis Pasteur** (1822–1895) a century later to define Jenner's discovery. The term also drew from the word vaccinia, the virus drawn from cowpox and developed in the laboratory for use in the smallpox vaccine. In spite of Jenner's successful report, critics questioned the wisdom of using the vaccine, with some worrying that people injected with cowpox would develop animal characteristics, such as women growing animal hair. Nonetheless, the vaccine gained popularity, and replaced the more risky direct inoculation with smallpox. In 1979, following a major cooperative effort between nations and several international organizations, world health authorities declared smallpox the only infectious disease to be completely eliminated.

The concerns expressed by Jenner's contemporaries about the side effects of vaccines would continue to follow the pioneers of vaccine development. Virtually all vaccinations continue to have side effects, with some of these effects due to the inherent nature of the vaccine, some due to the potential for impurities in a manufactured product, and some due to the potential for human error in administering the vaccine.

Virtually all vaccines would also continue to attract intense public interest. This was demonstrated in 1885 when Louis Pasteur (1822–1895) saved the life of Joseph Meister, a nine year old who had been attacked by a rabid dog. Pasteur's series of experimental **rabies** vaccinations on the boy proved the effectiveness of the new vaccine.

Until development of the rabies vaccine, Pasteur had been criticized by the public, though his great discoveries included the development of the **food preservation** process called **pasteurization**. With the discovery of a rabies vaccine, Pasteur became an honored figure. In France, his birthday declared a national holiday, and streets renamed after him.

Pasteur's rabies vaccine, the first human vaccine created in a laboratory, was made of an extract gathered from the spinal cords of rabies-infected rabbits. The live virus was weakened by drying over potash. The new vaccination was far from perfect, causing occasional fatalities and temporary paralysis. Individuals had to be injected 14–21 times.

The rabies vaccine has been refined many times. In the 1950s, a vaccine grown in duck embryos replaced the use of live virus, and in 1980, a vaccine developed in cultured human cells was produced. In 1998, the newest vaccine technology—genetically engineered vaccines—was applied to rabies. The new **DNA** vaccine cost a fraction of the regular vaccine. While only a few people die of rabies each year in the United States, more than 40,000 die worldwide, particularly in Asia and Africa. The less expensive vaccine will make vaccination far more available to people in less developed nations.

The story of the most celebrated vaccine in modern times, the polio vaccine, is one of discovery and revision. While the **viruses** that cause polio appear to have been present for centuries, the disease emerged to an unusual extent in the early 1900s. At the peak of the epidemic, in 1952, polio killed 3,000 Americans and 58,000 new cases of polio were reported. The crippling disease caused an epidemic of fear and illness as Americans—and the world—searched for an explanation of how the disease worked and how to protect their families.

The creation of a vaccine for **poliomyelitis** by **Jonas Salk** (1914–1995) in 1955 concluded decades of a drive to find a cure. The Salk vaccine, a killed virus type, contained the three types of polio virus which had been identified in the 1940s.

In 1955, the first year the vaccine was distributed, disaster struck. Dozens of cases were reported in individuals who had received the vaccine or had contact with individuals who had been vaccinated. The culprit was an impure batch of vaccine that had not been completely inactivated. By the end of the incident, more than 200 cases had developed and 11 people had died.

Production problems with the Salk vaccine were overcome following the 1955 disaster. Then in 1961, an oral polio vaccine developed by Albert B. Sabin (1906–1993) was licensed in the United States. The continuing controversy over the virtues of the Sabin and Salk vaccines is a reminder of the many complexities in evaluating the risks versus the benefits of vaccines.

The Sabin vaccine, which used weakened, live polio virus, quickly overtook the Salk vaccine in popularity in the United States, and is currently administered to all healthy children. Because it is taken orally, the Sabin vaccine is more convenient and less expensive to administer than the Salk vaccine.

Advocates of the Salk vaccine, which is still used extensively in Canada and many other countries, contend that it is safer than the Sabin oral vaccine. No individuals have developed polio from the Salk vaccine since the 1955 incident. In contrast, the Sabin vaccine has a very small but significant rate of complications, including the development of polio. However, there has not been one new case of polio in the United States since 1975, or in the Western Hemisphere since 1991. Though polio has not been completely eradicated, there were only 144 confirmed cases worldwide in 1999.

Effective vaccines have limited many of the life-threatening infectious diseases. In the United States, children starting kindergarten are required to be immunized against polio, **diphtheria**, tetanus, and several other diseases. Other vaccinations are used only by populations at risk, individuals exposed to disease, or when exposure to a disease is likely to occur due to travel to an area where the disease is common. These include influenza, **yellow fever**, typhoid, cholera, and **Hepatitis** A and B.

The influenza virus is one of the more problematic diseases because the viruses constantly change, making development of vaccines difficult. Scientists grapple with predicting what particular influenza strain will predominate in a given year. When the prediction is accurate, the vaccine is effective. When they are not, the vaccine is often of little help.

The classic methods for producing vaccines use biological products obtained directly from a virus or a **bacteria**. Depending on the vaccination, the virus or bacteria is either used in a weakened form, as in the Sabin oral polio vaccine; killed, as in the Salk polio vaccine; or taken apart so that a piece of the microorganism can be used. For example, the vaccine for Streptococcus pneumoniae uses bacterial polysaccharides, carbohydrates found in bacteria which contain large numbers of monosaccharides, a simple sugar. These classical methods vary in safety and efficiency. In general, vaccines that use live bacterial or viral products are extremely effective when they work, but carry a greater risk of causing disease. This is most threatening to individuals whose immune systems are weakened, such as individuals with leukemia. Children with leukemia are advised not to take the oral polio vaccine because they are at greater risk of developing the disease. Vaccines which do not include a live virus or bacteria tend to be safer, but their protection may not be as great.

The classical types of vaccines are all limited in their dependence on biological products, which often must be kept cold, may have a limited life, and can be difficult to produce. The development of recombinant vaccines—those using chromosomal parts (or DNA) from a different organism—has generated hope for a new generation of man-made vaccines. The hepatitis B vaccine, one of the first recombinant vaccines to be approved for human use, is made using recombinant **yeast** cells genetically engineered to include the **gene** coding for the hepatitis B antigen. Because the vaccine contains the antigen, it is capable of stimulating **antibody** production against hepatitis B without the risk that live hepatitis B vaccine carries by introducing the virus into the blood stream.

As medical knowledge has increased—particularly in the field of DNA vaccines—researchers have set their sights on a wealth of possible new vaccines for cancer, melanoma, AIDS, influenza, and numerous others. Since 1980, many improved vaccines have been approved, including several genetically engineered (recombinant) types which first developed during an experiment in 1990. These recombinant vaccines involve the use of so-called "naked DNA." Microscopic portions of a viruses' DNA are injected into the patient. The patient's own cells then adopt that DNA, which is then duplicated when the cell divides, becoming part of each new cell. Researchers have reported success using this method in laboratory trials against influenza and **malaria**. These DNA vaccines work from inside the cell, not just from the cell's surface, as other vaccines do, allowing a stronger cell-mediated fight against the disease. Also, because the influenza virus constantly changes its surface proteins, the immune system or vaccines cannot change quickly enough to fight each new strain. However, DNA vaccines work on a core protein, which researchers believe should not be affected by these surface changes.

Since the emergence of AIDS in the early 1980s, a worldwide search against the disease has resulted in clinical trials for more than 25 experimental vaccines. These range from whole-inactivated viruses to genetically engineered types. Some have focused on a therapeutic approach to help infected individuals to fend off further illness by stimulating components of the immune system; others have genetically engineered a protein on the surface of **HIV** to prompt immune response against the virus; and yet others attempted to protect uninfected individuals. The challenges in developing a protective vaccine include the fact that HIV appears to have multiple viral strains and mutates quickly.

In January 1999, a promising study was reported in Science magazine of a new AIDS vaccine created by injecting a healthy cell with DNA from a protein in the AIDS virus that is involved in the infection process. This cell was then injected with genetic material from cells involved in the immune response. Once injected into the individual, this vaccine "catches the AIDS virus in the act," exposing it to the immune system and triggering an immune response. This discovery offers considerable hope for development of an effective vaccine. As of June 2002, a proven vaccine for AIDS had not yet been proven in clinical trials.

Stimulating the immune system is also considered key by many researchers seeking a vaccine for cancer. Currently numerous clinical trials for cancer vaccines are in progress, with researchers developing experimental vaccines against cancer of the breast, colon, and lung, among other areas. Promising studies of vaccines made from the patient's own tumor cells and genetically engineered vaccines have been reported. Other experimental techniques attempt to penetrate the body in ways that could stimulate vigorous immune responses. These include using bacteria or viruses, both known to be efficient travelers in the body, as carriers of vaccine antigens. Such bacteria or viruses would be treated or engineered to make them incapable of causing illness.

Current research also focuses on developing better vaccines. The Children's Vaccine Initiative, supported by the **World Health Organization**, the United Nation's Children's Fund, and other organizations, are working diligently to make vaccines easier to distribute in developing countries. Although more than 80% of the world's children were immunized by 1990, no new vaccines have been introduced extensively since then. More than four million people, mostly children, die needlessly every year from preventable diseases. Annually, measles kills 1.1 million children worldwide; whooping cough (**pertussis**) kills 350,000; hepatitis B 800,000; **Haemophilus** influenzae type b (Hib) 500,000; tetanus 500,000; rubella 300,000; and yellow fever 30,000. Another 8 million die from diseases for which vaccines are still being developed. These include pneumococcal **pneumonia** (1.2 million); acute respiratory virus infections (400,000), malaria (2 million); AIDS (2.3 million); and rotavirus (800,000). In August, 1998, the Food and Drug Administration approved the first vaccine to prevent rotavirus—a severe diarrhea and vomiting infection.

The measles epidemic of 1989 was a graphic display of the failure of many Americans to be properly immunized. A total of 18,000 people were infected, including 41 children who died after developing measles, an infectious, viral illness whose complications include pneumonia and encephalitis. The epidemic was particularly troubling because an effective, safe vaccine against measles has been widely distributed in the United States since the late 1960s. By 1991, the number of

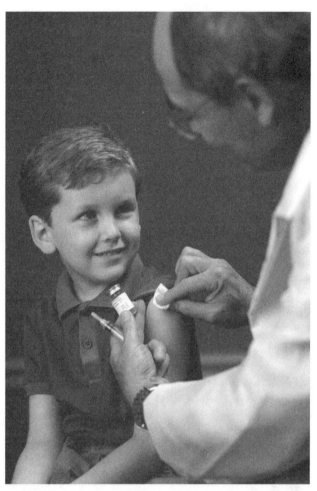
Vaccines stimulate the production of antibodies that provide immunity from disease.

new measles cases had started to decrease, but health officials warned that measles remained a threat.

This outbreak reflected the limited reach of vaccination programs. Only 15% of the children between the ages of 16 and 59 months who developed measles between 1989 and 1991 had received the recommended measles vaccination. In many cases parent's erroneously reasoned that they could avoid even the minimal risk of vaccine side effects "because all other children were vaccinated."

Nearly all children are immunized properly by the time they start school. However, very young children are far less likely to receive the proper vaccinations. Problems behind the lack of **immunization** range from the limited health care received by many Americans to the increasing cost of vaccinations. Health experts also contend that keeping up with a vaccine schedule, which requires repeated visits, may be too challenging for Americans who do not have a regular doctor or health provider.

Internationally, the challenge of vaccinating large numbers of people has also proven to be immense. Also, the reluctance of some parents to vaccinate their children due to potential side effects has limited vaccination use. Parents in the United States and several European countries have balked at vaccinating their children with the pertussis vaccine due to the development of neurological complications in a small number of children given the vaccine. Because of incomplete immunization, whooping cough remains common in the United States, with 30,000 cases and about 25 deaths due to complications annually. One response to such concerns has been testing in the United States of a new pertussis vaccine that has fewer side effects.

Researchers look to genetic engineering, gene discovery, and other innovative technologies to produce new vaccines.

See also AIDS, recent advances in research and treatment; Antibody formation and kinetics; Bacteria and bacterial infection; Bioterrorism, protective measures; Immune stimulation, as a vaccine; Immunity, active, passive and delayed; Immunity, cell mediated; Immunity, humoral regulation; Immunochemistry; Immunogenetics; Immunologic therapies; Immunology; Interferon actions; Poliomyelitis and polio; Smallpox, eradication, storage, and potential use as a bacteriological weapon

VARICELLA

Varicella, commonly known as chickenpox, is a disease characterized by skin lesions and low-grade fever, and is common in the United States and other countries located in areas with temperate climates. The incidence of varicella is extremely high; almost everyone living in the United States is exposed to the disease, usually during childhood, but sometimes in adulthood. In the United States, about 3.9 million people a year contract varicella. A highly contagious disease, varicella is caused by Varicella-Zoster virus (VZV), the same virus that causes the skin disease shingles. For most cases of varicella, no treatment besides comfort measures and management of itching and fever is necessary. In some cases, however, varicella may evolve into more serious conditions, such as **bacterial infection** of the skin lesions or **pneumonia**. These complications tend to occur in persons with weakened immune systems, such as children receiving **chemotherapy** for cancer, or people with Acquired Immune Deficiency Syndrome (**AIDS**). A **vaccine** for varicella is now receiving widespread use.

There are two possible origins for the colloquialism "chickenpox." Some think that "chicken" comes from the French word chiche (chick-pea) because at one stage of the disease, the lesions may resemble chick-peas. Others think that "chicken" may have evolved from the Old English word gigan (to itch). Interestingly, the term "varicella" is a diminutive form of the term "variola," the Latin word for **smallpox**. Although both varicella and smallpox are viral diseases that cause skin lesions, smallpox is more deadly and its lesions cause severe scarring.

Varicella is spread by breathing in respiratory droplets spread through the air by a cough or sneeze of an infected individual. Contact with the fluid from skin lesions can also spread the virus. The incubation period, or the time from expo-

sure to VZV to the onset of the disease, is about 14–15 days. The most contagious period is just prior to the appearance of the rash, and early in the illness, when fresh vesicles are still appearing. The first sign of varicella in children is often the appearance of the varicella rash. Adults and some children may have a prodrome, or series of warning symptoms. This prodrome is typical of the flu, and includes headache, fatigue, backache, and a fever. The onset of the rash is quite rapid. First, a diffuse, small, red dot-like rash appears on the skin. Soon, a vesicle containing clear fluid appears in the center of the dots. The vesicle rapidly dries, forming a crust. This cycle, from the appearance of the dot to the formation of the crust, can take place within eight to 12 hours. As the crust dries, it falls off, leaving a slight depression that eventually recedes. Significant scarring from varicella is rare.

Over the course of a case of varicella, an individual may develop between 250 and 500 skin lesions. The lesions occur in waves, with the first set of lesions drying up just as successive waves appear. The waves appear over two to four days. The entire disease runs its course in about a week, but the lesions continue to heal for about two to three weeks. The lesions first appear on the scalp and trunk. Most of the lesions in varicella are found at the center of the body; few lesions form on the soles and palms. Lesions are also found on the mucous membranes, such as the respiratory tract, the gastrointestinal tract, and the urogenital tract. Researchers think that the lesions on the respiratory tract may help transmit the disease. If a person with respiratory lesions coughs, they may spray some of the vesicle fluid into the atmosphere, to be breathed by other susceptible persons.

Although the lesions may appear alarming, varicella in children is usually a mild disease with few complications and a low fever. Occasionally, if the rash is severe, the fever may be higher. Varicells is more serious in adults, who usually have a higher fever and general malaise. The most common complaint about varicella from both children and adults is the itching caused by the lesions. It is important not to scratch the lesions, as scratching may cause scarring.

Because varicella is usually a mild disease, no drug treatment is normally prescribed. For pain or fever relief associated with varicella, physicians recommended avoiding salicylate, or aspirin. Salicylate may contribute to Reye's syndrome, a serious neurological condition that is especially associated with aspirin intake and varicella; in fact, 20–30% of the total cases of Reye's syndrome occur in children with varicella.

Varicella, although not deadly for most people, can be quite serious in those who have weakened immune systems, and drug therapy is recommended for these cases. **Antiviral drugs** (such as acyclovir) have been shown to lessen the severity and duration of the disease, although some of the side effects, such as gastrointestinal upset, can be problematic.

If the lesions are severe and the person has scratched them, bacterial infection of the lesions can result. This complication is managed with antibiotic treatment. A more serious complication is pneumonia. Pneumonia is rare in otherwise healthy children and is more often seen in older patients or in children who already have a serious disease, such as cancer. Pneumonia is also treated with **antibiotics**. Another complication of varicella is shingles. Shingles are painful outbreaks of skin lesions that occur some years after a bout with varicella. Shingles are caused by VZV left behind in the body that eventually reactivates. Shingles causes skin lesions and burning pain along the region served by a specific nerve. It is not clear why VZV is reactivated in some people and not in others, but many people with compromised immune systems can develop severe, even life-threatening cases of shingles.

Pregnant women are more susceptible to varicella, which also poses a threat to both prenatal and newborn children. If a woman contracts varicella in the first trimester (first three months) of pregnancy, the fetus may be at increased risk for birth defects such as eye damage. A newborn may contract varicella in the uterus if the mother has varicella five days before birth. Newborns can also contract varicella if the mother has the disease up to two days after birth. Varicella can be a deadly disease for newborns; the fatality rate from varicella in newborns up to five days old approaches 30%. For this reason, women contemplating pregnancy may opt to be vaccinated with the new VZV vaccine prior to conception if they have never had the disease. If this has not been done, and a pregnant woman contracts varicella, an injection of varicella-zoster immunoglobulin can lessen the chance of complications to the fetus.

Researchers have long noted the seasonality of varicella. According to their research, varicella cases occur at their lowest rate during September. Numbers of cases increase throughout the autumn, peak in March and April, and then fall sharply once summer begins. This cycle corresponds to the typical school year in the United States. When children go back to school in the fall, they begin to spread the disease; when summer comes and school ends, cases of varicella diminish. Varicella can spread quickly within a school when one child contracts varicella. This child rapidly infects other susceptible children. Soon, all the children who had not had varicella contract the disease within two or three cycles of transmission. It is not uncommon for high numbers of children to be infected during a localized outbreak; one school with 69 children reported that the disease struck 67 of these students.

Contrary to popular belief, it is possible to get varicella a second time. If a person had a mild case during childhood, his or her **immunity** to the virus may be weaker than that of someone who had a severe childhood case. In order to prevent varicella, especially in already-ill children and immunocompromised patients, researchers have devised a VZV vaccine, consisting of live, attenuated (modified) VZV. **Immunization** recommendations of the American Academy of Pediatrics state that children between 12 and 18 months of age who have not yet had varicella should receive the vaccine. Immunization can be accomplished with a single dose. Children up to the age of 13 who have had neither varicella nor the immunization, should also receive a single dose of the vaccine. Children older than age 13 who have never had either varicella or the vaccine should be immunized with two separate doses, given about a month apart. The vaccine provokes immunity against the virus. Although some side effects have been noted, including a mild rash and the reactivation of shingles, the vaccine is considered safe and effective.

See also Immunity, active, passive and delayed; Immunity, cell mediated; Viruses and responses to viral infection

VARICELLA ZOSTER VIRUS

Varicella zoster virus is a member of the alphaherpesvirus group and is the cause of both chickenpox (also known as varicella) and shingles (**herpes** zoster).

The virus is surrounded by a covering, or envelope, that is made of lipid. As such, the envelope dissolves readily in solvents such as alcohol. Wiping surfaces with alcohol is thus an effective means of inactivating the virus and preventing spread of chickenpox. Inside the lipid envelope is a protein shell that houses the **deoxyribonucleic acid**.

Varicella zoster virus is related to Herpes Simplex **viruses** types 1 and 2. Indeed, nucleic acid analysis has revealed that the genetic material of the three viruses is highly similar, both in the genes present and in the arrangement of the genes.

Chickenpox is the result of a person's first infection with the virus. Typically, chickenpox occurs most often in children. From 75% to 90% of the cases of chickenpox occur in children under five years old. Acquisition of the virus is usually via inhalation of droplets containing the virus. From the lung the virus migrates to the blood stream. Initially a sore throat leads to a blister-like rash that appears on the skin and the mucous membranes, as the virus is carried through the blood stream to the skin. The extent of the rash varies, from minimal to all over the body. The latter is also accompanied by fever, itching, abdominal pain, and a general feeling of tiredness. Recovery is usually complete within a week or two and **immunity** to another bout of chickenpox is life-long.

In terms of a health threat, childhood chickenpox is advantageous. The life-long immunity conferred to the child prevents adult onset infections that are generally more severe. However, chickenpox can be dangerous in infants, whose immune systems are undeveloped. Also chickenpox carries the threat of the development of sudden and dangerous liver and brain damage. This condition, called Reye's Syndrome, seems related to the use of aspirin to combat the fever associated with chickenpox (as well as other childhood viruses). When adults acquire chickenpox, the symptoms can be much more severe than those experienced by a child. In immunocompromised people, or those suffering from leukemia, chickenpox can be fatal. The disease can be problematic in pregnant women in terms of birth defects and the development of **pneumonia**.

Treatment for chickenpox is available. A drug called acyclovir can slow the replication of the virus. Topical lotions can ease the itching associated with the disease. However, in mild to moderate cases, intervention is unnecessary, other than keeping the affected person comfortable. The life-long immunity conferred by a bout of chickenpox is worth the temporary inconvenience of the malady. The situation is different for adults. Fortunately for adults, a **vaccine** to chickenpox exists for those who have not contracted chickenpox in their childhood.

Naturally acquired immunity to chickenpox does not prevent individuals from contracting shingles years, even decades later. Shingles occurs in between 10% and 20% of those who have had chickenpox. In the United States, upwards of 800,000 people are afflicted with shingles each year. The annual number of shingles sufferers worldwide is in the millions. The disease occurs most commonly in those who are over 50 years of age.

As the symptoms of chickenpox fade, varicella zoster virus is not eliminated from the body. Rather, the virus lies dormant in nerve tissue, particularly in the face and the body. The roots of sensory nerves in the spinal cord are also a site of virus hibernation. The virus is stirred to replicate by triggers that are as yet unclear. Impairment of the **immune system** seems to be involved, whether from **immunodeficiency diseases** or from cancers, the effect of drugs, or a generalized debilitation of the body with age. Whatever forces of the immune system that normally operate to hold the hibernating virus in check are abrogated.

Reactivation of the virus causes pain and a rash in the region that is served by the affected nerves. The affected areas are referred to as dermatomes. These areas appear as a rash or blistering of the skin. This can be quite painful during the one to two weeks they persist. Other complications can develop. For example, shingles on the face can lead to an eye infection causing temporary or even permanent blindness. A condition of muscle weakness or paralysis, known as Guillan-Barre Syndrome, can last for months after a bout of shingles. Another condition known as postherpetic neuralgia can extend the pain of shingles long after the visible symptoms have abated.

See also Immunity, active, passive and delayed; Infection and resistance; Latent viruses and diseases

VARIOLA VIRUS

Variola virus (or variola major virus) is the virus that causes **smallpox**. The virus is one of the members of the poxvirus group (Family *Poxviridae*). The virus particle is brick shaped and contains a double strand of **deoxyribonucleic acid**. The variola virus is among the most dangerous of all the potential biological weapons.

Variola virus infects only humans. The virus can be easily transmitted from person to person via the air. Inhalation of only a few virus particles is sufficient to establish an infection. Transmission of the virus is also possible if items such as contaminated linen are handled. The various common symptoms of smallpox include chills, high fever, extreme tiredness, headache, backache, vomiting, sore throat with a cough, and sores on mucus membranes and on the skin. As the sores burst and release pus, the afflicted person can experience great pain. Males and females of all ages are equally susceptible to infection. At the time of smallpox eradication approximately one third of patients died—usually within a period of two to three weeks following appearance of symptoms.

The origin of the variola virus in not clear. However, the similarity of the virus and **cowpox** virus has prompted the suggestion that the variola virus is a mutated version of the cowpox virus. The mutation allowed to virus to infect humans. If such a mutation did occur, then the adoption of farming activities by people, instead of the formally nomadic existence, would have been a selective pressure for a virus to adopt the capability to infect humans.

Vaccination to prevent infection with the variola virus is long established. In the 1700s, English socialite and **public health** advocate Lady **Mary Wortley Montague** popularized the practice of injection with the pus obtained from smallpox sores as a protection against the disease. This technique became known as variolation. Late in the same century, **Edward Jenner** successfully prevented the occurrence of smallpox by an injection of pus from cowpox sores. This represented the start of vaccination.

Vaccination has been very successful in dealing with variola virus outbreaks of smallpox. Indeed, after two decades of worldwide vaccination programs, the virus has been virtually eliminated from the natural environment. The last recorded case of smallpox infection was in 1977 and vaccination against smallpox is not practiced anymore.

In the late 1990s, a resolution was passed at the World Health Assembly that the remaining stocks of variola virus be destroyed, to prevent the re-emergence of smallpox and the misuse of the virus as a biological weapon. At the time only two high-security laboratories were thought to contain variola virus stock (**Centers for Disease Control** and Prevention in Atlanta, Georgia, and the Russian State Centre for Research on **Virology** and **Biotechnology**, Koltsovo, Russia). However, this decision was postponed until 2002, and now the United States government has indicated its unwillingness to comply with the resolution for security issues related to potential **bioterrorism**. Destruction of the stocks of variola virus would deprive countries of the material needed to prepare **vaccine** in the event of the deliberate use of the virus as a biological weapon. This scenario has gained more credence in the past decade, as terrorist groups have demonstrated the resolve to use biological weapons, including smallpox. In addition, intelligence agencies in several Western European countries issued opinions that additional stocks of the variola virus exist in other than the previously authorized locations.

See also Bioterrorism, protective measures; Bioterrorism; Centers for Disease Control (CDC); Smallpox, eradication, storage, and potential use as a bacteriological weapon; Viral genetics; Virology; Virus replication; Viruses and responses to viral infection

VENTER, JOHN CRAIG (1946-)
American molecular biologist

John Craig Venter, who until January 2002 was the President and Chief Executive Officer of Celera Genomics, is one of the central figures in the Human Genome Project. Venter cofounded Celera in 1998, and he directed its research and operations while he and the company's other scientists completed a draft of the human genome. Using a fast sequencing technique, Venter and his colleagues were able to sequence the human genome, and the genomes of other organisms, including the bacterium *Haemophilus infuenzae,*.

Venter was born in Salt Lake City, Utah. After high school he seemed destined for a career as a surfer rather than as a molecular biologist. But a tour of duty in Vietnam as a hospital corpsman precipitated a change in the direction of his life. He returned from Vietnam and entered university, earning a doctorate in physiology and pharmacology from the University of California at San Diego. After graduation he took a research position at the National Institutes of Health. While at NIH, Venter became frustrated at the then slow pace of identifying and sequencing genes. He began to utilize a technology that decodes only a portion of the **DNA** from normal copies of genes made by living cells. These partial transcripts, called expressed sequence tags, could then be used to identify the gene-coding regions on the DNA from which they came. The result was to speed up the identification of genes. Hundreds of genes could be discovered in only weeks using the method.

Supported by venture capital, Venter started a nonprofit company called **The Institute for Genomic Research** (**TIGR**) in the mid-1990s. TIGR produced thousands of the expressed sequence tag probes to the human genome.

Venter's success and technical insight attracted the interest of PE Biosystems, makers of automated DNA sequencers. With financial and equipment backing from PE Biosystems, Venter left TIGR and formed a private for-profit company, Celera (meaning 'swift' in Latin). The aim was to decode the human genome faster than the government effort that was underway. Celera commenced operations in May 1998.

Another of Venter's accomplishments was to use a non-traditional approach to quickly sequence DNA. At that time, DNA was typically sequenced by dividing it into several large pieces and then decoding each piece. Venter devised the so-called shotgun method, in which a genome was blown apart into many small bits and then to sequence them without regard to their position. Following sequencing, supercomputer power would reassemble the bits of sequence into the intact genome sequence. The technique, which was extremely controversial, was tried first on the genome of the fruit fly *Drosophila*. In only a year the fruit fly genome sequence was obtained. The sequencing of the genome of the bacterium *H. influenzae* followed this.

Although the privatization of human genome sequence data remains highly controversial, Venter's accomplishments are considerable, both technically and as a force within the scientific community to spur genome sequencing.

See also DNA (Deoxyribonucleic acid); DNA hybridization; Economic uses and benefits of microorganisms; Genetic code; Genetic identification of microorganisms; Genetic mapping; Genetic regulation of eukaryotic cells; Genetic regulation of prokaryotic cells; Genotype and phenotype; Immunogenetics; Molecular biology and molecular genetics

VETERINARY MICROBIOLOGY

Veterinary microbiology is concerned with the **microorganisms**, both beneficial and disease causing, to non-human animal life. For a small animal veterinarian, the typical animals of concern are domesticated animals, such as dogs, cats, birds, fish, and reptiles. Large animal veterinarians focus on animals of economic importance, such as horses, cows, sheep, and poultry.

The dogs and cats that are such a familiar part of the household environment are subject to a variety of microbiological origin ailments. As with humans, **vaccination** of young dogs and cats is a wise precaution to avoid microbiological diseases later in life.

Cats can be infected by a number of **viruses** and **bacteria** that cause respiratory tract infections. For example the bacterium *Bordetella pertussis*, the common cause of kennel cough in dogs, also infects cats, causing the same persistent cough. Another bacteria called *Chlamydia* causes another respiratory disease, although most of the symptoms are apparent in the eyes. **Inflammation** of the mucous covering of the eyelids (conjunctivitis) can be so severe that the eyes swell shut.

Cats are prone to viral infections. Coronavirus is common in environments such as animal shelters, where numbers of cats live in close quarters. The virus causes an infection of the intestinal tract. Feline panleukopenia is a very contagious viral disease that causes a malaise and a decrease in the number of white blood cells. The immune disruption can leave the cat vulnerable to other infections and can be lethal. Fortunately, a protective **vaccine** exists. Like humans, cats are also prone to **herpes** virus infections. In cats the infection is in the respiratory tract and eyes. Severe infections can produce blindness. Another respiratory disease, reminiscent of a **cold** in humans, is caused by a calicivirus. **Pneumonia** can develop and is frequently lethal. Finally the feline leukemia virus causes cancer of the blood. The highly contagious nature of this virus makes vaccination prudent for young kittens.

Dogs are likewise susceptible to bacterial and viral infections. A virus known as parainfluenzae virus also causes kennel cough. Dogs are also susceptible to coronavirus. Members of the bacterial genus called *Leptospira* can infect the kidneys. This infection can be passed to humans and to other animals. A very contagious viral infection, which typically accompanies bacterial infections, is called canine distemper. Distemper attacks many organs in the body and can leave the survivor permanently disabled. A vaccine against distemper exists, but must be administered periodically throughout the dog's life to maintain the protection. Another virus called parvovirus produces a highly contagious, often fatal, infection. Once again, vaccination needs to be at regular (usually yearly) intervals. Like humans, dogs are susceptible to **hepatitis**, a destructive viral disease of the liver. In dogs that have not been vaccinated, the liver infection can be debilitating. Finally, dogs are also susceptible to the viral agent of **rabies**. The virus, often passed to the dog via the bite of another rabid animal, can in turn be passed onto humans. Fortunately again, vaccination can eliminated the risk of acquiring rabies.

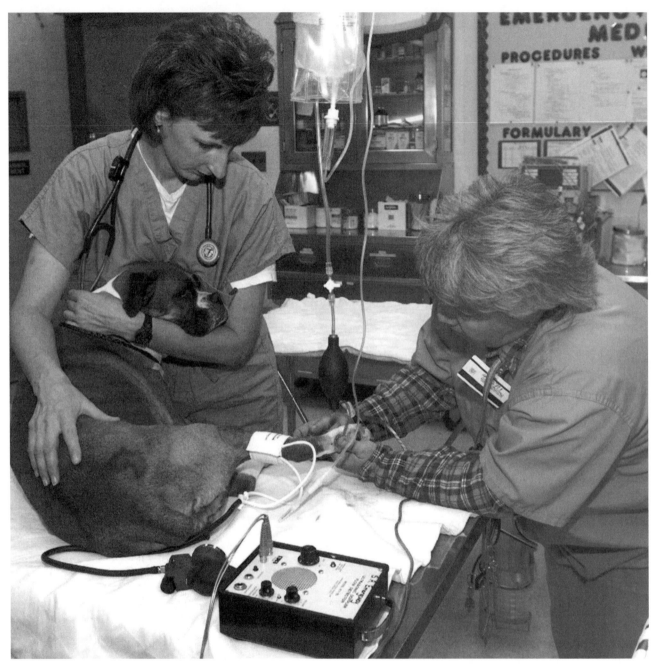

Two veterinarians treat a dog with an infected leg.

Microbiological infections of farm animals and poultry is common. For example, studies have shown that well over half the poultry entering processing plants are infected with the bacterium *Campylobacter jejuni*. Infection with members of the bacterial genus *Salmonella* are almost as common. Fecal **contamination** of poultry held in close quarters is responsible. Similarly the intestinal bacterium **Escherichia coli** is spread from bird to bird. Improper processing can pass on these bacteria to humans, where they cause intestinal maladies.

Chickens and turkeys are also susceptible to a bacterial respiratory disease caused by *Mycoplasma spp.* The "air sac disease" causes lethargy, weight loss, and decreased egg production. Poultry can also acquire a form of cholera, which is caused by *Pasteurella multocida*. Examples of some other bacteria of note in poultry are species of *Clostridium* (intestinal tract infection and destruction of tissue), *Salmonella pullorum* (intestinal infection that disseminates widely throughout the body), *Salmonella gallinarum* (typhoid), and *Clostridium botulinum* (**botulism**).

•

Cattle and sheep are also susceptible to microbiological ailments. Foot and mouth disease is a prominent example. This contagious and fatal disease can sweep through cattle and sheep populations, causing financial ruin for ranchers. Moreover, there is now evidence that bovine spongiform encephalopathy, a disease caused by an infectious agent termed a prion, may be transmissible to humans, where it is manifest as the always lethal brain deterioration called Creutzfeld-Jacob disease.

See also Zoonoses

VIABLE BUT NONCULTURABLE BACTERIA

Viable but nonculturable **bacteria** are bacteria that are alive, but which are not growing or dividing. Their metabolic activity is almost nonexistent.

This state was recognized initially by microbial ecologists examining bacterial populations in natural sediments. Measurements of the total bacterial count, which counts both living and dead bacteria, are often far higher than the count of the living bacteria. At certain times of year, generally when nutrients are plentiful, the total and living numbers match more closely. These observations are not the result of seasonal "die-off," but reflect the adoption of an almost dormant mode of existence by a sizable proportion of some bacterial populations.

A viable but nonculturable bacteria cannot be cultured on conventional laboratory growth media but can be demonstrated to be alive by other means, such as the uptake and **metabolism** of radioactively labeled nutrients. Additionally, the microscopic examination of populations shows the bacteria to be intact. When bacteria die they often lyse, due to the release of **enzymes** that disrupt the interior and the cell wall of the bacteria.

The viable but nonculturable state is reversible. Bacterial that do not form spores can enter the state when conditions become lethal for their continued growth. The state is a means of bacterial survival to stresses that include elevated salt concentration, depletion of nutrients, depletion of oxygen, and exposure to certain wavelengths of light. When the stress is removed, bacteria can revive and resume normal growth.

The shift to the nonculturable state triggers the expression of some 40 genes in bacteria. As well, the composition of the cell wall changes, becoming enhanced in fatty acid constituents, and the genetic material becomes coiled more tightly.

The entry of a bacterium into the nonculturable state varies from days to months. Younger bacterial cells are capable of a more rapid transition than are older cells. In general, however, the transition to a nonculturable state seems to be in response to a more gradual change in the environment than other bacterial stress responses, (e.g., spore formation, **heat shock response**).

In contrast to the prolonged entry into the quiescent phase, the exit from the viable but nonculturable state is quite rapid (within hours for *Vibrio vulnificus*). Other bacteria, such as *Legionella pneumophila*, the causative agent of Legionnaires' disease, revive much more slowly. The adoption

of this mode of survival by disease-causing bacteria further complicates strategies to detect and eradicate them.

See also Bacteria and bacterial infection; Bacterial adaptation

VIRAL EPIDEMICS • *see* EPIDEMICS, VIRAL

VIRAL GENETICS

Viral genetics, the study of the genetic mechanisms that operate during the life cycle of **viruses**, utilizes biophysical, biological, and genetic analyses to study the viral genome and its variation. The virus genome consists of only one type of nucleic acid, which could be a single or double stranded **DNA** or **RNA**. Single stranded RNA viruses could contain positive-sense (+RNA), which serves directly as mRNA or negative-sense RNA (–RNA) that must use an RNA polymerase to synthesize a complementary positive strand to serve as mRNA. Viruses are obligate **parasites** that are completely dependant on the host cell for the replication and **transcription** of their genomes as well as the **translation** of the mRNA transcripts into proteins. Viral proteins usually have a structural function, making up a shell around the genome, but may contain some **enzymes** that are necessary for the **virus replication** and life cycle in the host cell. Both bacterial virus (bacteriophages) and animal viruses play an important role as tools in molecular and cellular biology research.

Viruses are classified in two families depending on whether they have RNA or DNA genomes and whether these genomes are double or single stranded. Further subdivision into types takes into account whether the genome consists of a single RNA molecule or many molecules as in the case of segmented viruses. Four types of bacteriophages are widely used in biochemical and genetic research. These are the T phages, the temperate phages typified by **bacteriophage** lambda, the small DNA phages like M13, and the RNA phages. Animal viruses are subdivided in many classes and types. Class I viruses contain a single molecule of double stranded DNA and are exemplified by adenovirus, simian virus 40 (SV40), **herpes** viruses and human papilloma viruses. Class II viruses are also called parvoviruses and are made of single stranded DNA that is copied in to double stranded DNA before transcription in the host cell. Class III viruses are double stranded RNA viruses that have segmented genomes which means that they contain 10–12 separate double stranded RNA molecules. The negative strands serve as template for mRNA synthesis. Class IV viruses, typified by poliovirus, have single plus strand genomic RNA that serves as the mRNA. Class V viruses contain a single negative strand RNA which serves as the template for the production of mRNA by specific virus enzymes. Class VI viruses are also known as **retroviruses** and contain double stranded RNA genome. These viruses have an enzyme called reverse transcriptase that can both copy minus strand DNA from genomic RNA catalyze the synthesis of a complementary plus DNA strand. The resulting double stranded DNA is integrated in the host chromosome and is transcribed by the host own machinery. The resulting transcripts are either used to synthesize proteins or produce new viral particles. These new viruses are released by budding, usually without killing the host cell. Both **HIV** and **HTLV** viruses belong to this class of viruses.

Virus genetics are studied by either investigating genome **mutations** or exchange of genetic material during the life cycle of the virus. The frequency and types of genetic variations in the virus are influenced by the nature of the viral genome and its structure. Especially important are the type of the nucleic acid that influence the potential for the viral genome to integrate in the host, and the segmentation that influence exchange of genetic information through assortment and **recombination**.

Mutations in the virus genome could either occur spontaneously or be induced by physical and chemical means. Spontaneous mutations that arise naturally as a result of viral replication are either due to a defect in the genome replication machinery or to the incorporation of an analogous base instead of the normal one. Induced virus **mutants** are obtained by either using chemical mutants like nitrous oxide that acts directly on bases and modify them or by incorporating already modified bases in the virus genome by adding these bases as substrates during virus replication. Physical agents such as ultra-violet light and x rays can also be used in inducing mutations. Genotypically, the induced mutations are usually point mutations, deletions, and rarely insertions. The **phenotype** of the induced mutants is usually varied. Some mutants are conditional lethal mutants. These could differ from the wild type virus by being sensitive to high or low temperature. A low temperature mutant would for example grow at 88°F (31°C) but not at 100°F (38°C), while the wild type will grow at both temperatures. A mutant could also be obtained that grows better at elevated temperatures than the wild type virus. These mutants are called hot mutants and may be more dangerous for the host because fever, which usually slows the growth of wild type virus, is ineffective in controlling them. Other mutants that are usually generated are those that show drug resistance, enzyme deficiency, or an altered pathogenicity or host range. Some of these mutants cause milder symptoms compared to the parental virulent virus and usually have potential in **vaccine** development as exemplified by some types of **influenza** vaccines.

Besides mutation, new genetic variants of viruses also arise through exchange of genetic material by recombination and reassortment. Classical recombination involves the breaking of covalent bonds within the virus nucleic acid and exchange of some DNA segments followed by rejoining of the DNA break. This type of recombination is almost exclusively reserved to DNA viruses and retroviruses. RNA viruses that do not have a DNA phase rarely use this mechanism. Recombination usually enables a virus to pick up genetic material from similar viruses and even from unrelated viruses and the eukaryotic host cells. Exchange of genetic material with the host is especially common with retroviruses. Reassortment is a non-classical kind of recombination that occurs if two variants of a segmented virus infect the same cell. The resulting progeny virions may get some segments from one parent and some from the other. All known segmented virus that infect humans are RNA viruses. The process of reassortment is very efficient in the exchange of genetic material and is used in the generation of viral vaccines especially in the case of influenza live vaccines. The ability of viruses to exchange genetic information through recombination is the basis for virus-based vectors in recombinant DNA technology and hold great promises in the development of **gene** therapy. Viruses are attractive as vectors in gene therapy because they can be targeted to specific tissues in the organs that the virus usually infect and because viruses do not need special chemical reagents called transfectants that are used to target a plasmid vector to the genome of the host.

Genetic variants generated through mutations, recombination or reassortment could interact with each other if they infected the same host cell and prevent the appearance of any **phenotype**. This phenomenon, where each mutant provide the missing function of the other while both are still genotypically mutant, is known as complementation. It is used as an efficient tool to determine if mutations are in unique or in different genes and to reveal the minimum number of genes affecting a function. Temperature sensitive mutants that have the same mutation in the same gene will for example not be able to **complement** each other. It is important to distinguish complementation from multiplicity reactivation where a higher dose of inactivated mutants will be reactivated and infect a cell because these inactivated viruses cooperate in a poorly understood process. This reactivation probably involves both a complementation step that allows defective viruses to replicate and a recombination step resulting in new genotypes and sometimes regeneration of the wild type. The viruses that need complementation to achieve an infectious cycle are usually referred to as defective mutants and the complementing virus is the helper virus. In some cases, the defective virus may interfere with and reduce the infectivity of the helper virus by competing with it for some factors that are involved in the viral life cycle. These defective viruses called "defective interfering" are sometimes involved in modulating natural infections. Different wild type viruses that infect the same cell may exchange coat components without any exchange of genetic material. This phenomenon, known as phenotypic mixing is usually restricted to related viruses and may change both the morphology of the packaged virus and the tropism or tissue specificity of these infectious agents.

See also Viral vectors in gene therapy; Virology; Virus replication; Viruses and responses to viral infection

VIRAL INFECTIONS · *see* VIRUSES AND RESPONSES TO VIRAL INFECTION

VIRAL VECTORS IN GENE THERAPY

Gene therapy is the introduction of a gene into cells to reverse a functional defect caused by a defect in a host genome (the set of genes present in an organism).

The use of **viruses** quickly became an attractive possibility once the possibility of gene therapy became apparent. Viruses require other cells for their replication. Indeed, an essential feature of a **virus replication** cycle is the transfer of their genetic material (**deoxyribonucleic acid, DNA**; or **ribonucleic acid, RNA**) into the host cell, and the replication of that material in the host cell. By incorporating other DNA or RNA into the virus genome, the virus then becomes a vector for the transmission of that additional genetic material. Finally, if the inserted genetic material is the same as a sequence in the host cell that is defective, then the expression of the inserted gene will provide the product that the defective host genome does not. As a result, host defective host genetic function and the consequences of the defects can be reduced or corrected.

Retroviruses contain RNA as the genetic material. A viral enzyme called reverse transcriptase functions to manufacture DNA from the RNA, and the DNA can then become incorporated into the host DNA. Despite the known involvement of some retroviruses in cancer, these viruses are attractive for gene therapy because of their pronounced tendency to integrate the viral DNA into the host genome. Retroviruses used as gene vectors also have had the potential cancer-causing genetic information deleted. The most common retrovirus that has been used in experimental gene therapy is the Moloney murine leukaemia virus. This virus can infect cells of both mice and humans. This makes the results obtained from mouse studies more relevant to humans.

Adenoviruses are another potential gene vector. Once they have infected the host cell, many rounds of DNA replication can occur. This is advantageous, as much of the therapeutic product could be produced. However, because integration of the virally transported gene does not occur, the expression of the gene only occurs for a relatively short time. To produce levels of the gene product that would have a substantial effect on a patient, the virus vector needs to administered repeatedly. As for retroviruses, the adenoviruses used as vectors need to be crippled so as to prevent the production of new viruses.

Adenovirus vector has been used to correct **mutations** the gene that is defective in cystic fibrosis. However, as of May 2002, the success rate in human trials remained low. In addition, the immune response to the high levels of the vector that are needed can be problematic.

Another important aspect of gene therapy concerns the target of the viral vectors. The viruses need to be targeted at host cells that are actively dividing, because only in cells in which DNA replication is occurring will the inserted viral genetic material be replicated. This is one reason why cancers are a conceptually attractive target of virus-mediated gene therapy, as cancerous cells are dangerous by virtue of their rapid and uncontrolled division.

Cancerous cells arise by some form of mutation. Therefore, therapy to replace defective genes with functional genes holds promise for cancer researchers. The target of gene therapy can vary, as many cancers have mutations that direct a normal cell towards acquiring the potential to become cancerous, and other mutations that inactivate mechanisms that function to regulate growth control. Furthermore, gene therapy can be directed at the **immune system** rather than directly at the cancerous cell. An example of this strategy is known as immunopotentiation (the enhancement of the immune response to cancers).

A risk of viral gene therapy, in those viruses that operate by integrating genetic material into the host genome, is the possibility of damage to the host DNA by the insertion. Alteration of some other host gene could have unforeseen and undesirable side effects. The elimination of this possibility will require further technical refinements. Adenoviruses are advantageous in this regard as the replication of their DNA in the host cell does not involve insertion of the viral DNA into the host DNA. Accordingly, the possibility of mutations due to insertion do not exist.

The September 1999 death of an 18 year old patient with a rare metabolic condition, who died while receiving viral gene therapy, considerably slowed progress on clinical applications of viral gene therapy.

See also Biotechnology

VIROLOGY, VIRAL CLASSIFICATION, TYPES OF VIRUSES

Virology is the discipline of microbiology that is concerned with the study of **viruses**. Viruses are essentially nonliving repositories of nucleic acid that require the presence of a living prokaryotic or eukaryotic cell for the replication of the nucleic acid.

Scientists who make virology their field of study are known as virologists. Not all virologists study the same things, as viruses can exist in a variety of hosts. Viruses can infect animals (including humans), plants, **fungi**, birds, aquatic organisms, **protozoa**, **bacteria**, and insects. Some viruses are able to infect several of these hosts, while other viruses are exclusive to one host.

All viruses share the need for a host in order to replicate their **deoxyribonucleic acid** (**DNA**) or **ribonucleic acid** (**RNA**). The virus commandeers the host's existing molecules for the nucleic acid replication process. There are a number of different viruses. The differences include the disease symptoms they cause, their antigenic composition, type of nucleic acid residing in the virus particle, the way the nucleic acid is arranged, the shape of the virus, and the fate of the replicated DNA. These differences are used to classify the viruses and have often been the basis on which the various types of viruses were named.

The classification of viruses operates by use of the same structure that governs the classification of bacteria. The International Committee on Taxonomy of Viruses established the viral classification scheme in 1966. From the broadest to the narrowest level of classification, the viral scheme is: Order, Family, Subfamily, Genus, Species, and Strain/type. To use an example, the virus that was responsible for an outbreak of Ebola hemorrhagic fever in a region of Africa called Kikwit is classified as Order Mononegavirales, Family *Filoviridae*, Genus *Filovirus*, and Species **Ebola virus** Zaire.

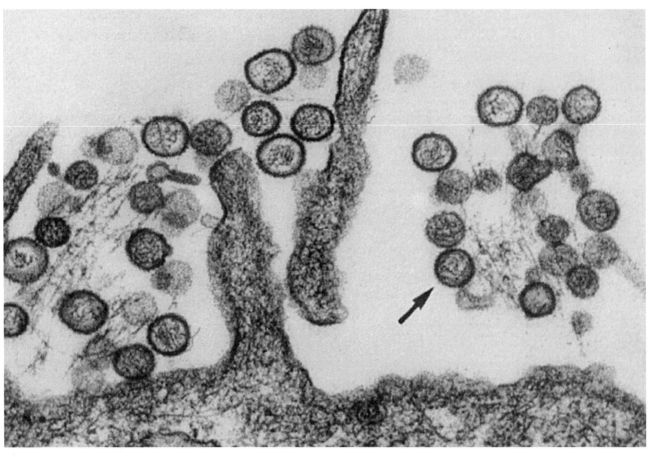

Thin section electron micrograph of adenoviruses.

In the viral classification scheme, all families end in the suffix **viridae**, for example Picornaviridae. Genera have the suffix **virus**. For example, in the family Picornaviridae there are five genera: enterovirus, cardiovirus, rhinovirus, apthovirus, and hepatovirus. The names of the genera typically derive from the preferred location of the virus in the body (for those viral genera that infect humans). As examples, rhinovirus is localized in the nasal and throat passages, and hepatovirus is localized in the liver. Finally, within each genera there can be several species.

As noted above, there are a number of criteria by which members of one grouping of viruses can be distinguished from those in another group. For the purposes of classification, however, three criteria are paramount. These criteria are the host organism or organisms that the virus utilizes, the shape of the virus particle, and the type and arrangement of the viral nucleic acid.

An important means of classifying viruses concerns the type and arrangement of nucleic acid in the virus particle. Some viruses have two strands of DNA, analogous to the double helix of DNA that is present in prokaryotes such as bacteria and in eukaryotic cells. Some viruses, such as the **Adenoviruses**, replicate in the **nucleus** of the host using the replication machinery of the host. Other viruses, such as the poxviruses, do not integrate in the host genome, but replicate

in the **cytoplasm** of the host. Another example of a double-stranded DNA virus are the Herpesviruses.

Other viruses only have a single strand of DNA. An example is the Parvoviruses. Viruses such as the Parvoviruses replicate their DNA in the host's nucleus. The replication involves the formation of what is termed a negative-sense strand of DNA, which is a blueprint for the subsequent formation of the RNA and DNA used to manufacture the new virus particles.

The genome of other viruses, such as Reoviruses and Birnaviruses, is comprised of double-stranded RNA. Portions of the RNA function independently in the production of a number of so-called messenger RNAs, each of which produces a protein that is used in the production of new viruses.

Still other viruses contain a single strand of RNA. In some of the single-stranded RNA viruses, such as Picornaviruses, Togaviruses, and the **Hepatitis** A virus, the RNA is read in a direction that is termed "+ sense." The sense strand is used to make the protein products that form the new virus particles. Other single-stranded RNA viruses contain what is termed a negative-sense strand. Examples are the Orthomyxoviruses and the Rhabdoviruses. The negative strand is the blueprint for the formation of the messenger RNAs that are required for production of the various viral proteins.

Still another group of viruses have + sense RNA that is used to make a DNA intermediate. The intermediate is used to manufacture the RNA that is eventually packaged into the new virus particles. The main example is the **Retroviruses** (the Human **Immunodeficiency** Viruses belong here). Finally, a group of viruses consist of double-stranded DNA that is used to produce a RNA intermediate. An example is the **Hepadnaviruses**.

An aspect of virology is the identification of viruses. Often, the diagnosis of a viral illness relies, at least initially, on the visual detection of the virus. For this analysis, samples are prepared for electron microscopy using a technique called negative staining, which highlights surface detail of the virus particles. For this analysis, the shape of the virus is an important feature.

A particular virus will have a particular shape. For example, viruses that specifically infect bacteria, the so-called bacteriophages, look similar to the Apollo lunar landing spacecraft. A head region containing the nucleic acid is supported on a number of spider-like legs. Upon encountering a suitable bacterial surface, the virus acts like a syringe, to introduce the nucleic acid into the cytoplasm of the bacterium.

Other viruses have different shapes. These include spheres, ovals, worm-like forms, and even irregular (pleomorphic) arrangements. Some viruses, such as the **influenza** virus, have projections sticking out from the surface of the virus. These are crucial to the infectious process.

As new species of eukaryotic and prokaryotic organisms are discovered, no doubt the list of viral species will continue to grow.

See also Viral genetics; Virus replication

VIRULENCE • *see* MICROBIOLOGY, CLINICAL

VIRUS REPLICATION

Viral replication refers to the means by which virus particles make new copies of themselves.

Viruses cannot replicate by themselves. They require the participation of the replication equipment of the host cell that they infect in order to replicate. The molecular means by which this replication takes place varies, depending upon the type of virus.

Viral replication can be divided up into three phases: initiation, replication, and release.

The initiation phase occurs when the virus particle attaches to the surface of the host cell, penetrates into the cell and undergoes a process known as uncoating, where the viral genetic material is released from the virus into the host cell's **cytoplasm**. The attachment typically involves the recognition of some host surface molecules by a corresponding molecule on the surface of the virus. These two molecules can associate tightly with one another, binding the virus particle to the surface. A well-studied example is the haemagglutinin receptor of the influenzae virus. The receptors of many other viruses have also been characterized.

A virus particle may have more than one receptor molecule, to permit the recognition of different host molecules, or of different regions of a single host molecule. The molecules on the host surface that are recognized tend to be those that are known as glycoproteins. For example, the **human immunodeficiency virus** recognizes a host glycoprotein called CD4. Cells lacking CD4 cannot, for example, bind the **HIV** particle.

Penetration of the bound virus into the host interior requires energy. Accordingly, penetration is an active step, not a passive process. The penetration process can occur by several means. For some viruses, the entire particle is engulfed by a membrane-enclosed bag produced by the host (a vesicle) and is drawn into the cell. This process is called endocytosis. Polio virus and orthomyxovirus enters a cell via this route. A second method of penetration involves the fusion of the viral membrane with the host membrane. Then the viral contents are directly released into the host. HIV, paramyxoviruses, and **herpes** viruses use this route. Finally, but more rarely, a virus particle can be transported across the host membrane. For example, poliovirus can cause the formation of a pore through the host membrane. The viral **DNA** is then released into the pore and passes across to the inside of the host cell.

Once inside the host, the viruses that have entered via endocytosis or transport across the host membrane need to release their genetic material. With poxvirus, viral proteins made after the entry of the virus into the host are needed for uncoating. Other viruses, such as **adenoviruses**, herpesviruses, and papovaviruses associate with the host membrane that surrounds the **nucleus** prior to uncoating. They are guided to the nuclear membrane by the presence of so-called nuclear localization signals, which are highly charged viral proteins. The viral genetic material then enters the nucleus via pores in the membrane. The precise molecular details of this process remains unclear for many viruses.

For animal viruses, the uncoating phase is also referred to as the eclipse phase. No infectious virus particles can be detected during that 10–12 hour period of time.

In the replication, or synthetic, phase the viral genetic material is converted to **deoxyribonucleic acid** (DNA), if the material originally present in the viral particle is **ribonucleic acid (RNA)**. This so-called reverse **transcription** process needs to occur in **retroviruses**, such as HIV. The DNA is imported into the host nucleus where the production of new DNA, RNA, and protein can occur. The replication phase varies greatly from virus type to virus type. However, in general, proteins are manufactured to ensure that the cell's replication machinery is harnessed to permit replication of the viral genetic material, to ensure that this replication of the genetic material does indeed occur, and to ensure that this newly made material is properly packaged into new virus particles.

Replication of the viral material can be a complicated process, with different stretches of the genetic material being transcribed simultaneously, with some of these **gene** products required for the transcription of other viral genes. Also replication can occur along a straight stretch of DNA, or when the DNA is circular (the so-called "rolling circle" form). RNA-containing viruses must also undergo a reverse transcription

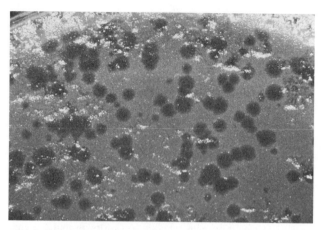

Growth of virus causes clearing (plaques) in lawn of *Escherichia coli* culture on agar.

from DNA to RNA prior to packaging of the genetic material into the new virus particles.

In the final stage, the viral particles are assembled and exit the host cell. The assembly process can involve helper proteins, made by the virus or the host. These are also called **chaperones**. Other viruses, such as **tobacco mosaic virus**, do not need these helper chaperones, as the proteins that form the building blocks of the new particles spontaneously self-assemble. In most cases, the assembly of viruses is symmetrical; that is, the structure is the same throughout the viral particle. For example, in the tobacco mosaic virus, the proteins constituents associate with each other at a slight angle, producing a symmetrical helix. Addition of more particles causes the helix to coil "upward" forming a particle. An exception to the symmetrical assembly is the **bacteriophage**. These viruses have a head region that is supported by legs that are very different in structure. Bacteriophage assembly is very highly coordinated, involving the separate manufacture of the component parts and the direct fitting together of the components in a sequential fashion.

Release of viruses can occur by a process called budding. A membrane "bleb" containing the virus particle is formed at the surface of the cell and is pinched off. For herpes virus this is in fact how the viral membrane is acquired. In other words, the viral membrane is a host-derived membrane. Other viruses, such as bacteriophage, may burst the host cell, spewing out the many progeny virus particles. But many viruses do not adopt such a host destructive process, as it limits the time of an infection due to destruction of the host cells needed for future replication.

See also Herpes and herpes virus; Human immunodeficiency virus (HIV); Invasiveness and intracellular infection

VIRUSES AND RESPONSES TO VIRAL INFECTION

There are a number of different viruses that challenge the human **immune system** and that may produce disease in

humans. In common, viruses are small, infectious agents that consist of a core of genetic material—either **deoxyribonucleic acid (DNA)** or **ribonucleic acid** (RNA)—surrounded by a shell of protein. Although precise mechanisms vary, viruses cause disease by infecting a host cell and commandeering the host cell's synthetic capabilities to produce more viruses. The newly made viruses then leave the host cell, sometimes killing it in the process, and proceed to infect other cells within the host. Because viruses invade cells, drug therapies have not yet been designed to kill viruses, although some have been developed to inhibit their growth. The human immune system is the main defense against a viral disease.

Bacterial viruses, called bacteriophages, infect a variety of **bacteria**, such as *Escherichia coli*, a bacteria commonly found in the human digestive tract. Animal viruses cause a variety of fatal diseases. **Acquired Immunodeficiency Syndrome (AIDS)** is caused by the **Human Immunodeficiency Virus (HIV)**; **hepatitis** and **rabies** are viral diseases; and **hemorrhagic fevers**, which are characterized by severe internal bleeding, are caused by filoviruses. Other animal viruses cause some of the most common human diseases. Often these diseases strike in childhood. **Measles**, **mumps**, and chickenpox are viral diseases. The common **cold** and **influenza** are also caused by viruses. Finally, some viruses can cause cancer and tumors. One such virus, **Human T-cell Leukemia Virus (HTLV)**, was only recently discovered and its role in the development of a particular kind of leukemia is still being elucidated.

Although viral structure varies considerably between the different **types of viruses**, all viruses share some common characteristics. All viruses contain either **RNA** or DNA surrounded by a protective protein shell called a capsid. Some viruses have a double strand of DNA, others a single strand of DNA. Other viruses have a double strand of RNA or a single strand of RNA. The size of the genetic material of viruses is often quite small. Compared to the 100,000 genes that exist within human DNA, viral genes number from 10 to about 200 genes.

Viruses contain such small amounts of genetic material because the only activity that they perform independently of a host cell is the synthesis of the protein capsid. In order to reproduce, a virus must infect a host cell and take over the host cell's synthetic machinery. This aspect of viruses—that the virus does not appear to be "alive" until it infects a host cell—has led to controversy in describing the nature of viruses. Are they living or non-living? When viruses are not inside a host cell, they do not appear to carry out many of the functions ascribed to living things, such as reproduction, **metabolism**, and movement. When they infect a host cell, they acquire these capabilities. Thus, viruses are both living and non-living. It was once acceptable to describe viruses as agents that exist on the boundary between living and non-living; however, a more accurate description of viruses is that they are either active or inactive, a description that leaves the question of life behind altogether.

All viruses consist of genetic material surrounded by a capsid; but variations exist within this basic structure. Studding the envelope of these viruses are protein "spikes." These spikes are clearly visible on some viruses, such as the influenza viruses; on other enveloped viruses, the spikes are extremely difficult to see. The spikes help the virus invade host cells. The influenza virus, for instance, has two types of spikes. One type, composed of **hemagglutinin** protein (HA), fuses with the host cell membrane, allowing the virus particle to enter the cell. The other type of spike, composed of the protein neuraminidase (NA), helps the newly formed virus particles to bud out from the host cell membrane.

The capsid of viruses is relatively simple in structure, owing to the few genes that the virus contains to encode the capsid. Most viral capsids consist of a few repeating protein subunits. The capsid serves two functions: it protects the viral genetic material and it helps the virus introduce itself into the host cell. Many viruses are extremely specific, targeting only certain cells within the plant or animal body. HIV, for instance, targets a specific immune cell, the T helper cell. The cold virus targets respiratory cells, leaving the other cells in the body alone. How does a virus "know" which cells to target? The viral capsid has special receptors that match receptors on their targeted host cells. When the virus encounters the correct receptors on a host cell, it "docks" with this host cell and begins the process of infection and replication.

Most viruses are rod-shaped or roughly sphere-shaped. Rod-shaped viruses include **tobacco mosaic virus** and the filoviruses. Although they look like rods under a **microscope**, these viral capsids are actually composed of protein molecules arranged in a helix. Other viruses are shaped somewhat like spheres, although many viruses are not actual spheres. The capsid of the adenovirus, which infects the respiratory tract of animals, consists of 20 triangular faces. This shape is called an icosahedron. HIV is a true sphere, as is the influenza virus.

Some viruses are neither rod- nor sphere-shaped. The poxviruses are rectangular, looking somewhat like bricks. Parapoxviruses are ovoid. Bacteriophages are the most unusually shaped of all viruses. A **bacteriophage** consists of a head region attached to a sheath. Protruding from the sheath are tail fibers that dock with the host bacterium. Bacteriophage structure is eminently suited to the way it infects cells. Instead of the entire virus entering the bacterium, the bacteriophage injects its genetic material into the cell, leaving an empty capsid on the surface of the bacterium.

Viruses are obligate intracellular **parasites**, meaning that in order to replicate, they need to be inside a host cell. Viruses lack the machinery and **enzymes** necessary to reproduce; the only synthetic activity they perform on their own is to synthesize their capsids.

The infection cycle of most viruses follows a basic pattern. Bacteriophages are unusual in that they can infect a bacterium in two ways (although other viruses may replicate in these two ways as well). In the lytic cycle of replication, the bacteriophage destroys the bacterium it infects. In the lysogenic cycle, however, the bacteriophage coexists with its bacterial host and remains inside the bacterium throughout its life, reproducing only when the bacterium itself reproduces.

An example of a bacteriophage that undergoes lytic replication inside a bacterial host is the T4 bacteriophage, which infects *E. coli*. T4 begins the infection cycle by docking with an *E. coli* bacterium. The tail fibers of the bacteriophage

make contact with the cell wall of the bacterium, and the bacteriophage then injects its genetic material into the bacterium. Inside the bacterium, the viral genes are transcribed. One of the first products produced from the viral genes is an enzyme that destroys the bacterium's own genetic material. Now the virus can proceed in its replication unhampered by the bacterial genes. Parts of new bacteriophages are produced and assembled. The bacterium then bursts, and the new bacteriophages are freed to infect other bacteria. This entire process takes only 20–30 minutes.

In the lysogenic cycle, the bacteriophage reproduces its genetic material but does not destroy the host's genetic material. The bacteriophage called lambda, another *E. coli*-infecting virus, is an example of a bacteriophage that undergoes lysogenic replication within a bacterial host. After the viral DNA has been injected into the bacterial host, it assumes a circular shape. At this point the replication cycle can become either lytic or lysogenic. In a lysogenic cycle the circular DNA attaches to the host cell genome at a specific place. This combination host-viral genome is called a prophage. Most of the viral genes within the prophage are repressed by a special repressor protein, so they do not encode the production of new bacteriophages. However, each time the bacterium divides, the viral genes are replicated along with the host genes. The bacterial progeny are thus lysogenically infected with viral genes.

Interestingly, bacteria that contain prophages can be destroyed when the viral DNA is suddenly triggered to undergo lytic replication. Radiation and chemicals are often the triggers that initiate lytic replication. Another interesting aspect of prophages is the role they play in human diseases. The bacteria that cause **diphtheria** and **botulism** both harbor viruses. The viral genes encode powerful toxins that have devastating effects on the human body. Without the infecting viruses, these bacteria may well be innocuous. It is the presence of viruses that makes these bacterial diseases so lethal.

Scientists have classified viruses according to the type of genetic material they contain. Broad categories of viruses include double-stranded DNA viruses, single-stranded DNA viruses, double-stranded RNA viruses, and single stranded RNA viruses. For the description of virus types that follows, however, these categories are not used. Rather, viruses are described by the type of disease they cause.

Poxviruses are the most complex kind of viruses known. They have large amounts of genetic material and fibrils anchored to the outside of the viral capsid that assist in attachment to the host cell. Poxviruses contain a double strand of DNA.

Viruses cause a variety of human diseases, including **smallpox** and **cowpox**. Because of worldwide **vaccination** efforts, smallpox has virtually disappeared from the world, with the last known case appearing in Somalia in 1977. The only places on Earth where smallpox virus currently exists are two labs: the **Centers for Disease Control** in Atlanta and the Research Institute for Viral Preparation in Moscow. Prior to the eradication efforts begun by the **World Health Organization** in 1966, smallpox was one of the most devastating of human diseases. In 1707, for instance, an outbreak of smallpox killed 18,000 of Iceland's 50,000 residents. In Boston in 1721, smallpox struck 5,889 of the city's 12,000 inhabitants, killing 15% of those infected.

Edward Jenner (1749–1823) is credited with developing the first successful **vaccine** against a viral disease, and that disease was smallpox. A vaccine works by eliciting an immune response. During this immune response, specific immune cells, called memory cells, are produced that remain in the body long after the foreign microbe present in a vaccine has been destroyed. When the body again encounters the same kind of microbe, the memory cells quickly destroy the microbe. Vaccines contain either a live, altered version of a virus or bacteria, or they contain only parts of a virus or bacteria, enough to elicit an immune response.

In 1797, Jenner developed his smallpox vaccine by taking infected material from a cowpox lesion on the hand of a milkmaid. Cowpox was a common disease of the era, transmitted through contact with an infected cow. Unlike smallpox, however, cowpox is a much milder disease. Using the cowpox pus, he inoculated an eight-year-old boy. Jenner continued his vaccination efforts through his lifetime. Until 1976, children were vaccinated with the smallpox vaccine, called vaccinia. Reactions to the introduction of the vaccine ranged from a mild fever to severe complications, including (although very rarely) death. In 1976, with the eradication of smallpox complete, vaccinia vaccinations for children were discontinued, although vaccinia continues to be used as a carrier for recombinant DNA techniques. In these techniques, foreign DNA is inserted in cells. Efforts to produce a vaccine for HIV, for instance, have used vaccinia as the vehicle that carries specific parts of HIV.

Herpesviruses are enveloped, double-stranded DNA viruses. Of the more than 50 **herpes** viruses that exist, only eight cause disease in humans. These include the human herpes virus types 1 and 2 that cause cold sores and genital herpes; human herpes virus 3, or varicella-zoster virus (VZV), that causes chickenpox and shingles; cytomegalovirus (CMV), a virus that in some individuals attacks the cells of the eye and leads to blindness; human herpes virus 4, or **Epstein-Barr virus** (EBV), which has been implicated in a cancer called Burkitt's lymphoma; and human herpes virus types 6 and 7, newly discovered viruses that infect white blood cells. In addition, herpes B virus is a virus that infects monkeys and can be transmitted to humans by handling infected monkeys.

Adenoviruses are viruses that attack respiratory, intestinal, and eye cells in animals. More than 40 kinds of human adenoviruses have been identified. Adenoviruses contain double-stranded DNA within a 20-faceted capsid. Adenoviruses that target respiratory cells cause bronchitis, **pneumonia**, and tonsillitis. Gastrointestinal illnesses caused by adenoviruses are usually characterized by diarrhea and are often accompanied by respiratory symptoms. Some forms of appendicitis are also caused by adenoviruses. Eye illnesses caused by adenoviruses include conjunctivitis, an infection of the eye tissues, as well as a disease called pharyngoconjunctival fever, a disease in which the virus is transmitted in poorly chlorinated swimming pools.

Human papoviruses include two groups: the papilloma viruses and the polyomaviruses. Human papilloma viruses (HPV) are the smallest double-stranded DNA viruses. They replicate within cells through both the lytic and the lysogenic replication cycles. Because of their lysogenic capabilities, HPV-containing cells can be produced through the replication of those cells that HPV initially infects. In this way, HPV infects epithelial cells, such as the cells of the skin. HPVs cause several kinds of benign (non-cancerous) warts, including plantar warts (those that form on the soles of the feet) and genital warts. However, HPVs have also been implicated in a form of cervical cancer that accounts for 7% of all female cancers.

HPV is believed to contain oncogenes, or genes that encode for growth factors that initiate the uncontrolled growth of cells. This uncontrolled proliferation of cells is called cancer. When the HPV oncogenes within an epithelial cell are activated, they cause the epithelial cell to proliferate. In the cervix (the opening of the uterus), the cell proliferation manifests first as a condition called cervical neoplasia. In this condition, the cervical cells proliferate and begin to crowd together. Eventually, cervical neoplasia can lead to full-blown cancer.

Polyomaviruses are somewhat mysterious viruses. Studies of blood have revealed that 80% of children aged five to none years have antibodies to these viruses, indicating that they have at some point been exposed to polyomaviruses. However, it is not clear what disease this virus causes. Some evidence exists that a mild respiratory illness is present when the first antibodies to the virus are evident. The only disease that is certainly caused by polyomavirses is called progressive multifocal leukoencephalopathy (PML), a disease in which the virus infects specific brain cells called the oligodendrocytes. PML is a debilitating disease that is usually fatal, and is marked by progressive neurological degeneration. It usually occurs in people with suppressed immune systems, such as cancer patients and people with AIDS.

The **hepadnaviruses** cause several diseases, including hepatitis B. Hepatitis B is a chronic, debilitating disease of the liver and immune system. The disease is much more serious than hepatitis A for several reasons: it is chronic and long-lasting; it can cause cirrhosis and cancer of the liver; and many people who contract the disease become carriers of the virus, able to transmit the virus through body fluids such as blood, semen, and vaginal secretions.

The hepatitis B virus (HBV) infects liver cells and has one of the smallest viral genomes. A double-stranded DNA virus, HBV is able to integrate its genome into the host cell's genome. When this integration occurs, the viral genome is replicated each time the cell divides. Individuals who have integrated HBV into their cells become carriers of the disease. Recently, a vaccine against HBV was developed. The vaccine is especially recommended for health care workers who through exposure to patient's body fluids are at high risk for infection.

Parvoviruses are icosahedral, single-stranded DNA viruses that infect a wide variety of mammals. Each type of parvovirus has its own host. For instance, one type of parvovirus causes disease in humans; another type causes disease in cats; while still another type causes disease in dogs. The disease caused by parvovirus in humans is called erythremia infectiosum, a disease of the red blood cells that is relatively rare except for individuals who have the inherited disorder sickle cell anemia. Canine and feline parvovirus infections are fatal, but a vaccine against parvovirus is available for dogs and cats.

Orthomyxoviruses cause influenza ("flu"). This highly contagious viral infection can quickly assume epidemic proportions, given the right environmental conditions. An influenza outbreak is considered an epidemic when more than 10% of the population is infected. Antibodies that are made against one type of rhinovirus are often ineffective against other types of viruses. For this reason, most people are susceptible to colds from season to season.

These helical, enveloped, single-stranded RNA viruses cause pneumonia, croup, measles, and mumps in children. A vaccine against measles and mumps has greatly reduced the incidence of these diseases in the United States. In addition, a paramyxovirus called respiratory syncytial virus (RSV) causes bronchiolitis (an infection of the bronchioles) and pneumonia.

Flaviviruses (from the Latin word meaning "yellow") cause insect-carried diseases including **yellow fever**, an often-fatal disease characterized by high fever and internal bleeding. Flaviviruses are single-stranded RNA viruses.

The two filoviruses, **Ebola virus** and Marburg virus, are among the most lethal of all human viruses. Both cause severe fevers accompanied by internal bleeding, which eventually kills the victim. The fatality rate of Marburg is about 60%, while the fatality rate of Ebola virus approaches 90%. Both are transmitted through contact with body fluids. Marburg and Ebola also infect primates.

Rhabdoviruses are bullet-shaped, single-stranded RNA viruses. They are responsible for rabies, a fatal disease that affects dogs, rodents, and humans.

Retroviruses are unique viruses. They are double-stranded RNA viruses that contain an enzyme called reverse transcriptase. Within the host cell, the virus uses reverse transcriptase to make a DNA copy from its RNA genome. In all other organisms, RNA is synthesized from DNA. Cells infected with retroviruses are the only living things that reverse this process.

The first retroviruses discovered were viruses that infect chickens. The Rous sarcoma virus, discovered in the 1950s by **Peyton Rous** (1879–1970), was also the first virus that was linked to cancer. However, it was not until 1980 that the first human retrovirus was discovered. Called Human T-cell Leukemia Virus (HTLV), this virus causes a form of leukemia called adult T-cell leukemia. In 1983, another human retrovirus, Human **Immunodeficiency** Virus, the virus responsible for AIDS, was discovered independently by two researchers. Both HIV and HTLV are transmitted in body fluids.

See also Bacteria and bacterial infection; Epidemics, viral; Immune stimulation, as a vaccine; Immunity, active, passive, and delayed; Immunology; Virology; Virus replication

VITAL STAINS • *see* LABORATORY TECHNIQUES IN MICROBIOLOGY

VOZROZHDENIYE ISLAND

Vozrozhdeniye island is located in the Aral Sea approximately 1,300 miles (2,092 km) to the east of Moscow. The island was used as biological weapons test site for the former Soviet Union. Now decommissioned, the island has served for decades as the repository of a large quantity of spores of *Bacillus anthracis*, the bacterial agent of **anthrax**, and other disease-causing **bacteria** and **viruses**.

Vozrozhdeniye island translates as Renaissance island. The island was used for open-air testing of bioweapons. The sparse vegetation on the island, remote location, and summer temperatures that reach 140°F (60°C) reduced the chances that escaping bioweapons would survive. Besides the testing of anthrax bioweapons, Soviet archives indicate that the microbial agents of **tularemia**, plague, typhoid, and possibly **smallpox** were used for experimentation.

The **biological warfare** agents buried on the island were supposed to have been destroyed following the signing of a treaty with the Soviet Union banning the manufacture and use of such weapons. Similar weapons manufactured for the same reason by the United States were reportedly destroyed in 1972. The bioweapons were manufactured by Soviet Union as part of their Cold War–inspired biological warfare program. They were buried on the island in 1988. The island has been abandoned since 1991 by the Russian government.

Vozrozhdeniye island has remained unguarded since that time. The main reason has been the isolated location of the facility in the middle of the Aral Sea. Over the past two decades, irrigation demands for water have depleted the freshwater sea to such an extent that the sea is becoming smaller. Many scientists now fear that Vozrozhdeniye Island might soon be directly connected to the mainland, making the stockpiled weapons more vulnerable to bioterrorist theft.

Additionally, indications are that some of the buried bioweapons are migrating towards the surface. Once exposed, some of the materials could be aerosolized and spread by the wind, or transported by birds.

The anthrax buried on the island was designed especially for the lethal use on humans in the time of war. The powder is a freeze-dried form of the bacteria called a spore. The spore is a dormant form of the bacterium that allows the persistence of the genetic material for very long periods of time. Resuscitation of the spore requires only suspension in growth media having the appropriate nutrients and incubation of the suspension at a temperature that is hospitable for the **bacterial growth**. Direct inhalation of the spores produces a lethal form of anthrax.

See also Bioterrorism, protective measures; Containment and release prevention protocol

W

WAKSMAN, SELMAN ABRAHAM
(1888-1973)
Russian-born American microbiologist

Selman Waksman discovered life-saving antibacterial compounds and his investigations spawned further studies for other disease-curing drugs. Waksman isolated streptomycin, the first chemical agent effective against **tuberculosis**. Prior to Waksman's discovery, tuberculosis was often a lifelong debilitating disease, and was fatal in some forms. Streptomycin effected a powerful and wide-ranging cure, and for this discovery, Waksman received the 1952 Nobel Prize in physiology or medicine. In pioneering the field of antibiotic research, Waksman had an inestimable impact on human health.

The only son of a Jewish furniture textile weaver, Selman Abraham Waksman was born in the tiny Russian village of Novaya Priluka on July 22, 1888. Life was hard in late-nineteenth-century Russia. Waksman's only sister died from **diphtheria** when he was nine. There were particular tribulations for members of a persecuted ethnic minority. As a teen during the Russian revolution, Waksman helped organize an armed Jewish youth defense group to counteract oppression. He also set up a school for underprivileged children and formed a group to care for the sick. These activities prefaced his later role as a standard-bearer for social responsibility.

Several factors led to Waksman's immigration to the United States. He had received his diploma from the *Gymnasium* in Odessa and was poised to attend university, but he doubtless recognized the very limited options he held as a Jew in Russia. At the same time, in 1910, his mother died, and cousins who had immigrated to New Jersey urged him to follow their lead. Waksman did so, and his move to a farm there, where he learned the basics of scientific farming from his cousin, likely had a pivotal influence on Waksman's later choice of field of study.

In 1911 Waksman enrolled in nearby Rutgers College (later University) of Agriculture, following the advice of fellow Russian immigrant Jacob Lipman, who led the college's bacteriology department. He worked with Lipman, developing a fascination with the **bacteria** of soil, and graduated with a B.S. in 1915. The next year he earned his M.S. degree. Around this time, he also became a naturalized United States citizen and changed the spelling of his first name from Zolman to Selman. Waksman married Bertha Deborah Mitnik, a childhood sweetheart and the sister of one of his childhood friends, in 1916. Deborah Mitnik had come to the United States in 1913, and in 1919 she bore their only child, Byron Halsted Waksman, who eventually went on to a distinguished career at Yale University as a pathology professor.

Waksman's intellect and industry enabled him to earn his Ph.D. in less than two years at the University of California, Berkeley. His 1918 dissertation focused on proteolytic **enzymes** (special proteins that break down proteins) in **fungi**. Throughout his schooling, Waksman supported himself through various scholarships and jobs. Among the latter were ranch work, caretaker, night watchman, and tutor of English and science.

Waksman's former advisor invited him to join Rutgers as a lecturer in soil bacteriology in 1918. He was to stay at Rutgers for his entire professional career. When Waksman took up the post, however, he found his pay too low to support his family. Thus, in his early years at Rutgers he also worked at the nearby Takamine Laboratory, where he produced enzymes and ran toxicity tests.

In the 1920s Waksman's work gained recognition in scientific circles. Others sought out his keen mind, and his prolific output earned him a well-deserved reputation. He wrote two major books during this decade. *Enzymes: Properties, Distribution, Methods, and Applications,* coauthored with Wilburt C. Davison, was published in 1926, and in 1927 his thousand-page *Principles of Soil Microbiology* appeared. This latter volume became a classic among soil bacteriologists. His laboratory produced more than just books. One of Waksman's students during this period was **René Dubos**, who would later discover the antibiotic gramicidin, the first chemotherapeutic

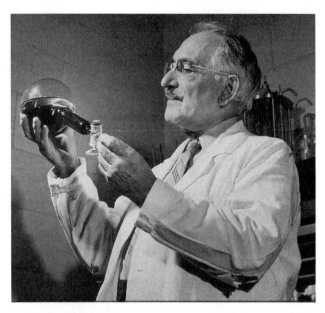

Selman Waksman won the 1952 Nobel prize in Physiology or Medicine for his discovery of streptomycin, the first antibiotic effective against the bacterium that causes tuberculosis.

agent effective against gram-positive bacteria (bacteria that hold dye in a stain test named for Danish bacteriologist Hans Gram). Waksman became an associate professor at Rutgers in the mid–1920s and advanced to the rank of full professor in 1930.

During the 1930s Waksman systematically investigated the complex web of microbial life in soil, humus, and peat. He was recognized as a leader in the field of soil microbiology, and his work stimulated an ever-growing group of graduate students and postdoctoral assistants. He continued to publish widely, and he established many professional relationships with industrial firms that utilized products of microbes. These companies that produced enzymes, pharmaceuticals, vitamins, and other products were later to prove valuable in Waksman's researches, mass-producing and distributing the products he developed. Among his other accomplishments during this period was the founding of the division of Marine Bacteriology at Woods Hole Oceanographic Institution in 1931. For the next decade he spent summers there and eventually became a trustee, a post he filled until his death.

In 1939, Waksman was appointed chair of the U.S. War Committee on Bacteriology. He derived practical applications from his earlier studies on soil **microorganisms**, developing antifungal agents to protect soldiers and their equipment. He also worked with the Navy on the problem of bacteria that attacked ship hulls. Early that same year Dubos announced his finding of two antibacterial substances, tyrocidine, and gramicidin, derived from a soil bacterium (*Bacillus brevis*). The latter compound, effective against gram-positive bacteria, proved too toxic for human use but did find widespread employment against various bacterial infections in veterinary medicine. The discovery of gramicidin also evidently inspired Waksman to dedicate himself to focus on the medicinal uses of antibacterial soil microbes. It was in this period that he

began rigorously investigating the antibiotic properties of a wide range of soil fungi.

Waksman set up a team of about 50 graduate students and assistants to undertake a systematic study of thousands of different soil fungi and other microorganisms. The rediscovery at this time of the power of **penicillin** against gram-positive bacteria likely provided further incentive to Waksman to find an antibiotic effective against gram-negative bacteria, which include the kind that causes tuberculosis.

In 1940, Waksman became head of Rutgers' department of microbiology. In that year too, with the help of Boyd Woodruff, he isolated the antibiotic actinomycin. Named for the actinomycetes (rod- or filament-shaped bacteria) from which it was isolated, this compound also proved too toxic for human use, but its discovery led to the subsequent finding of variant forms (actinomycin A, B, C, and D), several of which were found to have potent anti-cancer effects. Over the next decade Waksman isolated 10 distinct **antibiotics**. It is Waksman who first applied the term antibiotic, which literally means against life, to such drugs.

Among these discoveries, Waksman's finding of streptomycin had the largest and most immediate impact. Not only did streptomycin appear nontoxic to humans, however, it was highly effective against gram-negative bacteria. (Prior to this time, the antibiotics available for human use had been active only against the gram-positive strains.) The importance of streptomycin was soon realized. Clinical trials showed it to be effective against a wide range of diseases, most notably tuberculosis.

At the time of streptomycin's discovery, tuberculosis was the most resistant and irreversible of all the major infectious diseases. It could only be treated with a regime of rest and nutritious diet. The tuberculosis bacillus consigned its victims to a lifetime of invalidism and, when it invaded organs other than the lungs, often killed. Sanatoriums around the country were filled with persons suffering the ravages of tuberculosis, and little could be done for them.

Streptomycin changed all of that. From the time of its first clinical trials in 1944, it proved to be remarkably effective against tuberculosis, literally snatching sufferers back from the jaws of death. By 1950, streptomycin was used against seventy different germs that were not treatable with penicillin. Among the diseases treated by streptomycin were bacterial **meningitis** (an **inflammation** of membranes enveloping the brain and spinal cord), endocarditis (an inflammation of the lining of the heart and its valves), pulmonary and urinary tract infections, **leprosy**, **typhoid fever**, bacillary **dysentery**, cholera, and **bubonic plague**.

Waksman arranged to have streptomycin produced by a number of pharmaceutical companies, since demand for it soon skyrocketed beyond the capacity of any single company. Manufacture of the drug became a $50-million-per-year industry. Thanks to Waksman and streptomycin, Rutgers received millions of dollars of income from the royalties. Waksman donated much of his own share to the establishment of an Institute of Microbiology there. He summarized his early researches on the drug in *Streptomycin: Nature and Practical Applications* (1949). Streptomycin ultimately proved to have some human toxicity and was supplanted by other antibiotics, but its discovery changed the course of modern medicine. Not only did it directly save countless lives, but its development stimulated scientists around the globe to search the microbial world for other antibiotics and medicines.

In 1949, Waksman isolated neomycin, which proved effective against bacteria that had become resistant to streptomycin. Neomycin also found a broad niche as a topical antibiotic. Other antibiotics soon came forth from his Institute of Microbiology. These included streptocin, framicidin, erlichin, candidin, and others. Waksman himself discovered eighteen antibiotics during the course of his career.

Waksman served as director of the Institute for Microbiology until his retirement in 1958. Even after that time, he continued to supervise research there. He also lectured widely and continued to write at the frenetic pace established early in his career. He eventually published more than twenty-five books, among them the autobiography *My Life with the Microbes,* and hundreds of articles. He was author of popular pamphlets on the use of thermophilic (heat-loving) microorganisms in composting and on the enzymes involved in jelly-making. He wrote biographies of several noted microbiologists, including his own mentor, Jacob Lipman. These works are in addition to his numerous publications in the research literature.

On August 16, 1973, Waksman died suddenly in Hyannis, Massachusetts, of a cerebral hemorrhage. He was buried near the institute to which he had contributed so much over the years. Waksman's honors over his professional career were many and varied. In addition to the 1952 Nobel Prize, Waksman received the French Legion of Honor, a Lasker award for basic medical science, elected a fellow of the American Association for the Advancement of Science, and received numerous commendations from academies and scholarly societies around the world.

See also Antibiotic resistance, tests for; Bacteria and bacterial infection; Streptococci and streptococcal infections

VON WASSERMAN, AUGUST PAUL
(1866-1925)
German bacteriologist

August Paul von Wasserman was a German physician and bacteriologist. He is most noteworthy in the **history of microbiology** for his invention of the first test for the sexually transmitted disease of **syphilis**. The test is known as the **Wasserman test**.

Wasserman was born in 1866 in Bamberg, Germany. His entire education was received in that country. Wasserman received his undergraduate bacteriology degree and medical training at the universities of Erlanger, Vienna, Munich, and Strasbourg. He graduated from Strasbourg in 1888. Beginning in 1890, Wasserman joined **Robert Koch** at the latter's Institute for Infectious Diseases in Berlin. He became head of the institute's Department of Therapeutics and Serum research in 1907. In 1913, Wasserman left the Koch institute and joined the fac-

ulty at the Kaiser Wilhelm Institute, where he served as the Director of Experimental Therapeutics until his death in 1925.

Wasserman is remembered for a number of bacteriological accomplishments. He devised a test for **tuberculosis** and developed an antitoxin that was active against **diphtheria**. But his most noteworthy accomplishment occurred while he was still at the Institute for Infectious Diseases. In 1906, he developed a test for the presence of *Treponema pallidum* in humans. The bacterium is a spirochaete and is the cause of syphilis. The test became known as the Wasserman test.

The basis of the test is the production of antibodies to the syphilis bacterium and the ability of those antibodies to combine with known antigens in a solution. The antibody-antigen combination prevents a component called **complement** from subsequently destroying red blood cells. Clearing of the test solution (e.g., destruction of the red blood cells) is diagnostic for the absence of antibodies to *Treponema pallidum*.

The Wasserman test represents the first so-called complement test. In the decades since its introduction the Wasserman's test for syphilis has been largely superseded by other methods. But, the test is still reliable enough to be performed even to the present day in the diagnosis of syphilis.

See also Complement; Sexually transmitted diseases

WASSERMAN TEST

The Wasserman test is used to diagnose the illness known as **syphilis**. The test is named after its developer, the German bacteriologist August Wasserman (1866–1925). The Wasserman test was devised in 1906.

The Wasserman test is used to detect the presence of the bacterium that causes syphilis, the spirochete (spiral-shaped microorganism) *Treponema pallidum*. The basis of the test is the reaction of the **immune system** to the presence of the bacterium. Specifically, the test determines the presence or absence of an **antibody** that is produced in response to the presence of a constituent of the membrane of *Treponema pallidum*. The particular constituent is the membrane phospholipid.

The Wasserman test represents one of the earliest applications of an immunological reaction that is termed **complement** fixation. In the test, a patient's serum is heated to destroy a molecule called complement. A known amount of complement (typically from a guinea pig) is then added to the patient's serum. Next, the **antigen** (the bacterial phospholipid) is added along with red blood cells from sheep. The natural action of complement is to bind to the red blood cells and cause them to lyse (burst). Visually, this is evident as a clearing of the red-colored suspension. However, if the added antigen has bound to antibody that is present in the suspension, the complement becomes associated with the antigen-antibody complex. In technical terms, the complement is described being "fixed." Thus, if lysis of the red blood cells does not occur, then antibody to *Treponema pallidum* is present in the patient's serum, and allows a positive diagnosis for syphilis.

The Wasserman test is still used in the diagnosis of syphilis. However, the test has been found to be limiting, as antibodies to the bacterium are not prevalent in the early stages of the disease. Thus, a patient who had contracted syphilis—but who is in the earliest stages of infection—could produce a negative Wasserman test. This can compromise patient health and treatment, as syphilis becomes more serious as the disease progresses with time.

See also Bacteria and bacterial infection; Laboratory techniques in immunology

WASTEWATER TREATMENT

Wastewater includes the sewage-bearing water that is flushed down toilets as well as the water used to wash dishes and for bathing. Processing plants use water to wash raw material and in other stages of the wastewater treatment production process. The treatment of water that exits households, processing plants and other institutions is a standard, even mandated, practice in many countries around the world. The purpose of the treatment if to remove compounds and **microorganisms** that could pollute the water to which the wastewater is discharged. Particularly with respect to microorganisms, the sewage entering a treatment plant contains extremely high numbers of **bacteria**, **viruses**, and **protozoa** that can cause disease if present in drinking water. Wastewater treatment lowers the numbers of such disease-causing microbes to levels that are deemed to be acceptable from a health standpoint. As well, organic matter, solids, and other pollutants are removed.

Wastewater treatment is typically a multi-stage process. Typically, the first step is known as the preliminary treatment. This step removes or grinds up large material that would otherwise clog up the tanks and equipment further on in the treatment process. Large matter can be retained by screens or ground up by passage through a grinder. Examples of items that are removed at this stage are rags, sand, plastic objects, and sticks.

The next step is known as primary treatment. The wastewater is held for a period of time in a tank. Solids in the water settle out while grease, which does not mix with water, floats to the surface. Skimmers can pass along the top and bottom of the holding tank to remove the solids and the grease. The clarified water passes to the next treatment stage, which is known as secondary treatment.

During secondary treatment, the action of microorganisms comes into play. There are three versions of secondary treatment. One version, which was developed in the mid-nineteenth century, is called the fixed film system. The fixed film in such a system is a film of microorganisms that has developed on a support such as rocks, sand, or plastic. If the film is in the form of a sheet, the wastewater can be overlaid on the fixed film. The domestic septic system represents such a type of fixed film. Alternatively, the sheets can be positioned on a rotating arm, which can slowly sweep the microbial films through the tank of wastewater. The microorganisms are able to extract organic and inorganic material from the wastewater to use as nutrients for growth and reproduction. As the microbial film thickens and matures, the metabolic activity of the film increases. In this way, much of the organic and inorganic load in the wastewater can be removed.

Another version of secondary treatment is called the suspended film. Instead of being fixed on a support, microorganisms are suspended in the wastewater. As the microbes acquire nutrients and grow, they form aggregates that settle out. The settled material is referred to as sludge. The sludge can be scrapped up and removed. As well, some of the sludge is added back to the wastewater. This is analogous to inoculating growth media with microorganisms. The microbes in the sludge now have a source of nutrients to support more growth, which further depletes the wastewater of the organic waste. This cycle can be repeated a number of times on the same volume of water.

Sludge can be digested and the methane that has been formed by bacterial **fermentation** can be collected. Burning of the methane can be used to produce electricity. The sludge can also be dried and processed for use as compost.

A third version of secondary treatment utilizes a specially constructed lagoon. Wastewater is added to a lagoon and the sewage is naturally degraded over the course of a few months. The algae and bacteria in the lagoon consume nutrients such as phosphorus and nitrogen. Bacterial activity produces carbon dioxide. Algae can utilize this gas, and the resulting algal activity produces oxygen that fuels bacterial activity. A cycle of microbiological activity is established.

Bacteria and other microorganisms are removed from the wastewater during the last treatment step. Basically, the final treatment involves the addition of disinfectants, such as chlorine compounds or ozone, to the water, passage of the water past ultraviolet lamps, or passage of the water under pressure through membranes whose very small pore size impedes the passage of the microbes. In the case of ultraviolet irradiation, the wavelength of the lamplight is lethally disruptive to the genetic material of the microorganisms. In the case of disinfectants, neutralization of the high concentration of the chemical might be necessary prior to discharge of the treated water to a river, stream, lake, or other body of water. For example, chlorinated water can be treated with sulfur dioxide.

Chlorination remains the standard method for the final treatment of wastewater. However, the use of the other systems is becoming more popular. Ozone treatment is popular in Europe, and membrane-based or ultraviolet treatments are increasingly used as a supplement to chlorination.

Within the past several decades, the use of sequential treatments that rely on the presence of living material such as plants to treat wastewater by filtration or metabolic use of the pollutants has become more popular. These systems have been popularly dubbed "living machines." Restoration of wastewater to near drinking **water quality** is possible.

Wastewater treatment is usually subject to local and national standards of operational performance and quality in order to ensure that the treated water is of sufficient quality so as to pose no threat to aquatic life or settlements downstream that draw the water for drinking.

See also Biodegradable substances; Biofilm formation and dynamic behavior; Disinfection and disinfectants; Disposal of

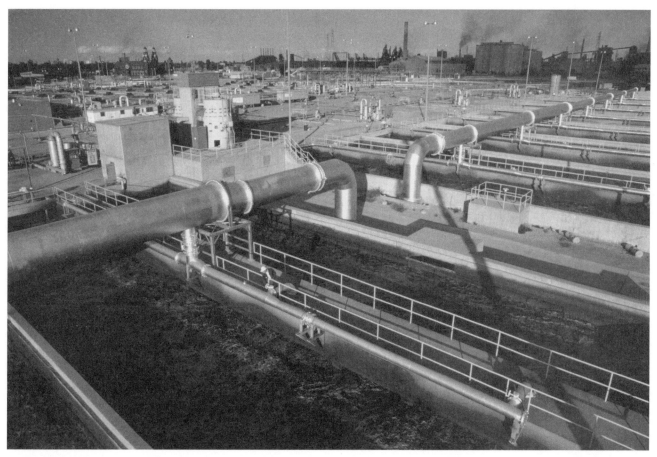

A wastewater treatment plant in Detroit, Michigan.

infectious microorganisms; Economic uses and benefits of microorganisms; Growth and growth media; Public health, current issues; Radiation mutagenesis; Water pollution and purification; Water quality

WATER POLLUTION AND PURIFICATION

With respect to **microorganisms**, water pollution refers to the presence in water of microbes that originated from the intestinal tract of humans and other warm-blooded animals. Water pollution can also refer to the presence of compounds that promote the growth of the microbes. The remediation of polluted water—the removal of the potentially harmful microorganisms—or the reduction of their numbers to levels considered to be acceptable for whatever purpose the water is used, represents the purification of water.

Microorganisms that reside in the intestinal tract find their way into fresh and marine water when feces contaminate the water. Examples of **bacteria** that can pollute water in this way are *Escherichia coli*, *Salmonella*, *Shigella*, and *Vibrio cholerae*. Warm-blooded animals other than humans can also contribute protozoan **parasites** to the water via their feces. The two prominent examples of health relevance to humans are

Cryptosporidium parvum and *Giardia lamblia*. The latter two species are becoming more prominent. They are also resistant to chlorine, the most popular purification chemical.

Normally, the intestinal bacteria do not survive long in the inhospitable world of the water. But, if they are ingested while still living, they can cause maladies, ranging from inconvenient intestinal upset to life-threatening infections. A prominent example of the latter is *Escherichia coli O157:H7*. Pollution of the water with this strain can cause severe intestinal damage, life long damage to organs such as the kidney and—especially in the young, elderly and those whose immune systems are compromised—death.

There are several common ways in which microorganisms can pollute water. Runoff from agricultural establishments, particularly where livestock is raised, is one route of **contamination**. Seasonal runoff can occur, especially in the springtime when rainfall is more pronounced. The feeding of birds (e.g., ducks) is now recognized as a contributing factor. For example, a large numbers of ducks that congregate can contribute large quantities of fecal material to localized ponds and lakes.

Once in the water, the growth of microorganisms can be exacerbated by environmental factors such as the water temperature, and by the chemical composition of the water. For

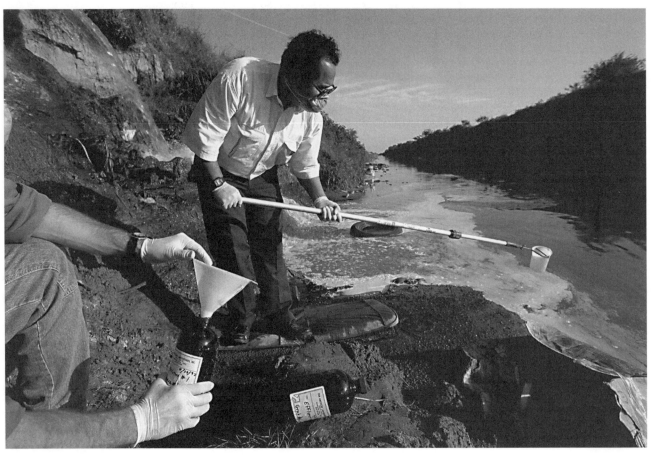

Sampling polluted water.

example, runoff of fertilizers from suburban properties can infuse watercourses with nitrogen, potassium, and phosphorus. All these are desirable nutrients for **bacterial growth**.

Water purification seeks to convert the polluted water into water that is acceptable for drinking, for recreation, or for some other purpose. Techniques such as filtration and exposure to agents or chemicals that will kill the microorganisms in the water are common means of purification. The use of **chlorination** remains the most widely used purification option. Others approaches are the use of ultraviolet radiation, filters of extremely small pore size (such that even **viruses** are excluded), and the use of a chemical known as ozone. Depending on the situation and the intended use of the finished water, combinations of these techniques can be used.

Purification of drinking water aims to remove as many bacteria as possible, and to completely eliminate those bacteria of intestinal origin. Recreational waters need not be that pristine. But bacterial numbers need to be below whatever standard has been deemed permissible for the particular local.

Another microbiological aspect of water pollution that has become recognized only within the past several years has been the presence in water of agents used to treat bacteria in other environments. For example in the household a number of disinfectant compounds are routinely employed in the cleaning of household surfaces. In the hospital, the use of

antibiotics to kill bacteria is an everyday occurrence. Such materials have been detected in water both before and after municipal **wastewater treatment**. The health effect of these compounds is not known at the present time. However, by analogy with other systems, the low concentration of such compounds might provide selective pressure for the development of resistant bacterial populations.

See also Chlorination; Waste water treatment; Water quality

WATER QUALITY

Water is the universal solvent. Many compounds that can dissolve in water are used as food sources by a variety of microbiological life forms. These **microorganisms** are themselves water-based and their constituent molecules are designed to function in aqueous environments. Thus, water can widely support the growth of microorganisms.

Some of this growth is advantageous. For example, the strains of **yeast** whose fermentative abilities make possible the brewing of beer, the production of wine, and the baking of bread. In addition, the growth of **bacteria** in polluted water is used as a means of decontaminating the water. The bacteria

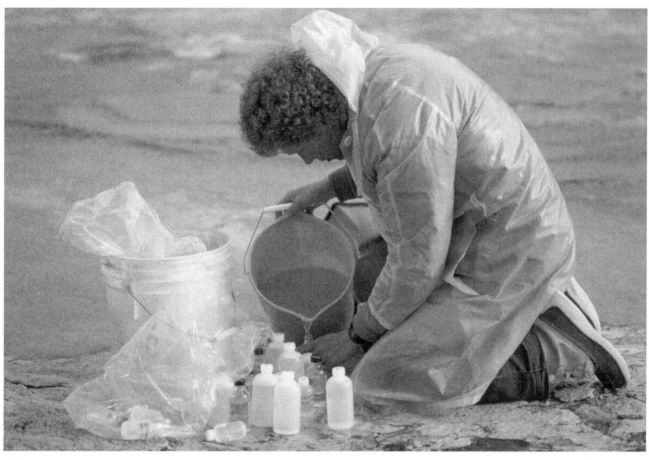

Collecting water for analysis.

are able to use the pollutant compound as a food source. In contrast, some forms of microbial growth can detrimental to products being produced or dangerous to the health of people consuming the water. Ensuring the quality of water from a microbiological standpoint is thus of extreme importance.

The main concern surrounding water quality is the freedom of the water from microorganisms that can cause disease. Typically, these agents are associated with the intestinal tract of warm-blooded animals including humans. Examples of disease causing bacteria are those in the genera of *Salmonella*, *Shigella*, and *Vibrio*. As well certain types of the intestinal bacterium *Escherichia coli* can cause infections. *Escherichia coli* O157:H7 has become prominent in the past decade. **Contamination** of drinking water with O157:H7 can be devastating. An infamous example of this is the contamination of the municipal water supply of Walkerton, Ontario, Canada in the summer of 2000. Several thousand people became ill, and seven people died as a direct result of the O157:H7 infection.

The contamination of the well water in Walkerton occurred because of run-off from adjacent cattle farms. This route of water contamination is common. For this reason, the surveillance of wells for the presence of bacteria is often done more frequently following a heavy rain, or at times of the year when precipitation is marked.

The intestinal tract also harbors **viruses** that can contaminate water and cause disease. Some examples of these viruses are rotavirus, enteroviruses, and coxsackievirus.

A number of protozoan microorganisms are also problematic with respect to water quality. The two most prominent protozoans are in the genera *Giardia* and *Cryptosporidium*. These microorganisms are resident in the intestinal tract of animals such as beaver and deer. Their increasing prevalence in North America is a consequence of the increasing encroachment of civilized areas on natural areas.

Municipal drinking water is usually treated in order to minimize the risk of the contamination of the water with the above microbes. Similarly, the protection of water quality by the boiling of the water has long been known. Even today, so-called "boil water orders" are issued in municipalities when the water quality is suspect. The addition of disinfectant compounds, particularly chlorine or derivatives of chlorine, is a common means utilized to kill bacteria in water. Other treatments that kill bacteria include the use of a gaseous ozone, and irradiation of water with ultraviolet light to disrupt bacterial genetic material. In more recent decades, the filtering of water has been improved so that now filters exist that can exclude even particles as tiny as viruses from the treated (or "finished") water. The killing of the protozoan microorganisms has proved to be challenging, as both *Giardia* and *Cryptosporidium* form dormant and chemically resistant structures called cysts during their life cycles. The cyst forms are resistant to the killing action of chlorine and can pass through the filters typically used in water treatment plants. Contamination of the water supply of Milwaukee, Wisconsin with *Cryptosporidium* in 1993 sickened over 400,000 people and the deaths of at least 47 people were subsequently attributed to the contamination.

Water quality testing often involves the use of a test that measures the turbidity of the water. Turbidity gives an indication of the amount of particulate material in the water. If the water is contaminated with particles as small as bacteria and viruses, the turbidity of the water will increase. Thus, the turbidity test can be a quick means of assessing if water quality is deteriorating and whether further action should be taken to enhance the quality of the water supply.

Water quality is also addressed in many countries by regulations that require the sampling and testing of drinking water for microorganisms. Testing is typically for an "indicator" of fecal pollution of the water. *Escherichia coli* is often the most suitable indicator organism. The bacterium is present in the intestinal tract in greater numbers than the disease-causing bacteria and viruses. Thus, the chances of detecting the indicator organism is better than detecting the actual pathogen. Additionally, the indicator does not usually multiply in the water (except in tropical countries), so its presence is indicative of recent fecal pollution. Finally, *Escherichia coli* can be detected using tests that are inexpensive and easy to perform.

Because the prevention of water borne disease rests on the adequate treatment of the water, underdeveloped regions of the world continue to experience the majority of water borne diseases. For example, in India the prevalence of cholera is so great that the disease is considered to be epidemic. But, as exemplified by communities like Walkerton and Milwaukee, even developed countries having an extensive water treatment infrastructure can experience problems if the treatment barriers are breached by the microorganisms.

See also Bacteria and bacterial infection; Bioremediation; Epidemics and pandemics; Water purification

WATSON, JAMES D. (1928-   )
American molecular biologist

James D. Watson won the 1962 Nobel Prize in physiology and medicine along with **Francis Crick** and Maurice Wilkins for discovering the structure of **DNA**, or **deoxyribonucleic acid**, the molecular carrier of genetic information. Watson and Crick had worked as a team since meeting in the early 1950s, and their research ranks as a fundamental advance in **molecular biology**.

James Dewey Watson was born in Chicago, Illinois, on April 6, 1928, to James Dewey and Jean (Mitchell) Watson. He was educated in the Chicago public schools, and during his adolescence became one of the original Quiz Kids on the radio show of the same name. Shortly after this experience in 1943, Watson entered the University of Chicago at the age of 15.

Watson graduated in 1946, but stayed on at Chicago for a bachelor's degree in zoology, which he attained in 1947. During his undergraduate years Watson studied neither genetics nor biochemistry—his primary interest was in the field of ornithology. In 1946, Watson spent a summer working on advanced ornithology at the University of Michigan's summer research station at Douglas Lake. During his undergraduate career at Chicago, Watson had been instructed by the well-known population geneticist Sewall Wright, but he did not become interested in the field of genetics until he read Erwin Schrödinger's influential book *What Is Life?* It was then, Horace Judson reports in *The Eighth Day of Creation: Makers of the Revolution in Biology,* that Watson became interested in finding out the secret of the **gene**.

Watson enrolled at Indiana University to perform graduate work in 1947. Indiana had several remarkable geneticists who could have been important to Watson's intellectual development, but he was drawn to the university by the presence of the Nobel laureate Hermann Joseph Muller, who had demonstrated 20 years earlier that x rays cause mutation. Nonetheless, Watson chose to work under the direction of the Italian biologist Salvador Edward Luria, and it was under Luria that he began his doctoral research in 1948.

Watson's thesis was on the effect of x rays on the rate of phage lysis (a phage, or **bacteriophage**, is a bacterial virus). The biologist Max Delbrück and Luria—as well as a number of others who formed what was to be known as "the phage group"—demonstrated that phages could exist in a number of mutant forms. A year earlier Luria and Delbrück had published one of the landmark papers in **phage genetics**, in which they established that one of the characteristics of phages is that they can exist in different genetic states so that the lysis (or bursting) of bacterial host cells can take place at different rates. Watson's Ph.D. degree was received in 1950, shortly after his twenty-second birthday.

Watson was next awarded a National Research Council fellowship grant to investigate the molecular structure of proteins in Copenhagen, Denmark. While Watson was studying enzyme structure in Europe, where techniques crucial to the study of macromolecules were being developed, he was also attending conferences and meeting colleagues.

From 1951 to 1953, Watson held a research fellowship under the support of the National Foundation for Infantile Paralysis at the Cavendish Laboratory in Cambridge, England. Those two years are described in detail in Watson's 1965 book, *The Double Helix: A Personal Account of the Discovery of the Structure of DNA.* An autobiographical work, *The Double Helix* describes the events—both personal and professional—that led to the discovery of DNA. Watson was to work at the Cavendish under the direction of Max Perutz, who was engaged in the x-ray crystallography of proteins. However, he soon found himself engaged in discussions with Crick on the structure of DNA. Crick was 12 years older than Watson and, at the time, a graduate student studying protein structure.

Intermittently over the next two years, Watson and Crick theorized about DNA and worked on their model of DNA structure, eventually arriving at the correct structure by recognizing the importance of x-ray diffraction photographs produced by Rosalind Franklin at King's College, London. Both were certain that the answer lay in model-building, and Watson was particularly impressed by Nobel laureate Linus Pauling's use of model-building in determining the alpha-helix structure of protein. Using data published by Austrian-born American biochemist Erwin Chargaff on the symmetry between the four constituent nucleotides (or bases) of DNA molecules, they concluded that the building blocks had to be arranged in pairs. After a great deal of experimentation with their models, they found that the double helix structure corresponded to the empirical data produced by Wilkins, Franklin, and their colleagues. Watson and Crick published their theoretical paper in the journal *Nature* in 1953 (with Watson's name appearing first due to a coin toss), and their conclusions were supported by the experimental evidence simultaneously published by Wilkins, Franklin, and Raymond Goss. Franklin died in 1958. Wilkins shared the Nobel Prize with Watson and Crick in 1962.

After the completion of his research fellowship at Cambridge, Watson spent the summer of 1953 at Cold Spring Harbor, New York, where Delbrück had gathered an active group of investigators working in the new area of molecular biology. Watson then became a research fellow in biology at the California Institute of Technology, working with Delbrück and his colleagues on problems in phage genetics. In 1955, he joined the biology department at Harvard and remained on the faculty until 1976. While at Harvard, Watson wrote *The Molecular Biology of the Gene* (1965), the first widely used university textbook on molecular biology. This text has gone through seven editions, and now exists in two large volumes as a comprehensive treatise of the field. In 1968, Watson became director of Cold Spring Harbor, carrying out his duties there while maintaining his position at Harvard. He gave up his faculty appointment at the university in 1976, however, and assumed full-time leadership of Cold Spring Harbor. With John Tooze and David Kurtz, Watson wrote *The Molecular Biology of the Cell,* originally published in 1983.

In 1989, Watson was appointed the director of the Human Genome Project of the National Institutes of Health, but after less than two years he resigned in protest over policy differences in the operation of this massive project. He continues to speak out on various issues concerning scientific research and is a strong presence concerning federal policies in supporting research. In addition to sharing the Nobel Prize, Watson has received numerous honorary degrees from institutions and was awarded the Presidential Medal of Freedom in 1977 by President Jimmy Carter. In 1968, Watson married Elizabeth Lewis. They have two children.

In his book, *The Double Helix*, Watson confirms that never avoided controversy. His candor about his colleagues and his combativeness in public forums have been noted by critics. On the other hand, his scientific brilliance is attested to by Crick, Delbrück, Luria, and others. The importance of his role in the DNA discovery has been well supported by Gunther Stent—a member of the Delbrück phage group—in an essay that discounts many of Watson's critics through well-reasoned arguments.

Most of Watson's professional life has been spent as a professor, research administrator, and public policy

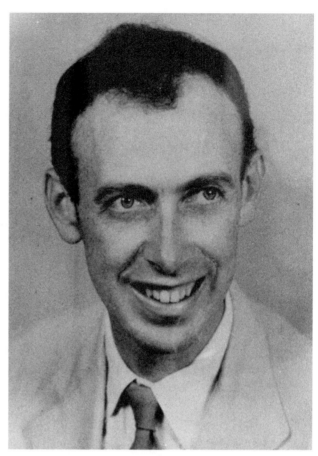

James Watson, co-discoverer of the structure of the DNA double helix.

spokesman for research. More than any other location in Watson's professional life, Cold Spring Harbor (where he is still director) has been the most congenial in developing his abilities as a scientific catalyst for others. Watson's work there has primarily been to facilitate and encourage the research of other scientists.

See also Cell cycle (eukaryotic), genetic regulation of; Cell cycle (prokaryotic), genetic regulation of; DNA (Deoxyribonucleic acid); DNA chips and micro arrays; DNA hybridization; Genetic code; Genetic identification of microorganisms; Genetic mapping; Genetic regulation of eukaryotic cells; Genetic regulation of prokaryotic cells; Genotype and phenotype; Molecular biology and molecular genetics

WELCH, WILLIAM HENRY (1850-1934)

American pathologist

William Henry Welch was a senior pathologist at Johns Hopkins University and its hospital. He researched numerous diseases, including **pneumonia** and **diphtheria**, but is most renowned for his discovery of the *Bacillus welchii*, a bacterium that causes gangrene. Throughout his career, Welch advocated asepsis and other general reforms in American hospitals to control disease and advance medical care.

Welch was born in Norfolk, Connecticut in 1850. He attended Yale and graduated in 1870. He then studied to be a surgeon at Columbia University, earning his M.D. in 1875. Welch then pursued advanced studies in Europe. He studied at several universities, but was perhaps most influenced by his time in Berlin. He returned to the United States in 1878 and was a professor and physician at Bellevue Hospital and Medical College in New York.

Welch conducted most of his career research as a professor and pathologist-in-chief at Johns Hopkins University and hospital. He accepted a position at the emerging hospital and medical school in 1884. His commitment to hospital reform and **public health** led to his discovery of the cause of gas gangrene. Later, Welch was named the director of the School of **Hygiene** and Public Health.

Welch's commitment to public health, as well as clinical medicine, garnered several awards, including the U.S. Army Distinguished Service Medal and Citation. Because gangrene was not only a serious surgical risk, but also an endemic problem with battle wounds, Welch's identification of *Bacillus welchii* was of military and medical interest.

In addition to his academic appointments, Welch held several offices in professional organizations. He founded the *Journal of Experimental Medicine* in 1896. Welch served on the Maryland State Board of Health for 31 years. He was president of the American Medical Association in 1910.

Welch died in 1934, while still serving on several medical boards.

See also Bacteria and bacterial infection; History of microbiology

WELLER, THOMAS (1915-)

American physician

Thomas Weller was corecipient, with **John F. Enders** and Frederick Robbins, of the Nobel Prize in physiology or medicine in 1954. This award was given for the trio's successful growth of the **poliomyelitis** (polio) virus in a non-neural tissue **culture**. This development was significant in the fight against the crippling disease polio, and eventually led to the development, by **Jonas Salk** in 1953, of a successful **vaccination** against the virus. It also revolutionized viral work in the laboratory and aided the recognition of many new **types of viruses**. Weller also distinguished himself with his studies of human **parasites** and the **viruses** that cause rubella and chickenpox.

Thomas Huckle Weller was born June 15, 1915, in Ann Arbor, Michigan. His parents were Elsie A. (Huckle) and Dr. Carl V. Weller. He received his B.S. in 1936 and M.S. in 1937, both from the University of Michigan, where his father was chair of the pathology department. He continued his studies at Harvard Medical School, where he met and roomed with his future Nobel corecipient Robbins. In 1938, Weller received a fellowship from the international health division of the Rockefeller Foundation, which allowed him to study **public**

health in Tennessee and **malaria** in Florida, topics which first interested him during his undergraduate years.

Weller graduated from Harvard with magna cum laude honors in parasitology, receiving his M.D. in 1940. He also received a fellowship in tropical medicine and a teaching fellowship in bacteriology. He completed an internship in pathology and bacteriology (1941) at Children's Hospital in Boston. He then began a residency at Children's, with the intention of specializing in pediatrics, before enlisting in the U.S. Army during World War II.

Weller served in the Army Medical Corps from 1942 to 1945. He was initially given teaching assignments in tropical medicine, but he was soon made officer in charge of bacteriology and **virology** work in San Juan, Puerto Rico. His major research there related to **pneumonia** and the parasitic disease schistosomiasis, an infection that is centered in the intestine and damages tissue and the circulatory system. Before his military service ended, he moved to the Army Medical School in Washington D.C. Upon his discharge in 1945, Weller was married to Kathleen Fahey, with whom he had two sons and two daughters. Returning to Boston's Children's Hospital, he finished his residency and began a post-doctoral year working with Enders.

During 1948, Weller was working with the **mumps** virus, which Enders had been researching since the war. After one experiment, Weller had a few tubes of human embryonic tissue left over, so he and Enders decided to see what the virus poliomyelitis might do in them. A small amount of success prompted the duo, who had been joined in their research by Robbins, to try growing the virus in other biological mediums, including human foreskin and the intestinal cells of a mouse. The mouse intestine did not produce anything, but the trio finally had significant viral growth with human intestinal cells. This was the first time poliomyelitis had been grown in human or simian tissue other than nerve or brain. Using **antibiotics** to ward off unwanted bacterial invasion, the scientists were able to isolate the virus for study.

Once poliomyelitis was grown and isolated in tissue cultures it was possible to closely study the nature of the virus, which in turn made it possible for Salk to create a **vaccine** in 1953. Besides leading to an inhibitor against a debilitating disease, a major result of the trio's development was a decrease in the need for laboratory animals. As Weller was quoted saying in the *Journal of Infectious Diseases,* "In the instance of poliomyelitis, one culture tube of human or monkey cells became the equivalent of one monkey." In times prior, viruses had to be injected into living animals to monitor their potency. Now, with tissue culture growth, cell changes were apparent under the **microscope**, showing the action of the virus and eliminating the need for the animals. The techniques for growing cells in tissue cultures developed by Weller and his associates were not only applicable to the poliomyelitis virus, however. They were soon copied by many other labs and scientists and quickly led to the identification, control, and study of several previously unrecognized virus types. For their work, and the improvements in scientific research it made possible, Weller, Enders, and Robbins shared the 1954 Nobel Prize in physiology or medicine.

Concurrent with his work with Enders and Robbins, Weller was named assistant director of the research division of infectious diseases at Children's Hospital in 1949. He held this position until 1954. At the same time, he began teaching at Harvard in tropical medicine and tropical public health, moving from instructor to associate professor. In 1953, Weller and Robbins shared the Mead Johnson Prize for their contributions to pediatric research. Then, in 1954, Weller was named Richard Pearson Strong Professor of Tropical Public Health and chair of the public health department at Harvard. As a consequence, he moved his research facilities to the Harvard Medical School. Later, he was appointed director of the Center for Prevention of Infectious Diseases at the Harvard School of Public Health.

From the end of World War II until 1982, Weller also continued his research on two types of helminths, *trichinella spiralis* and *schistosoma mansoni*. Helminths are intestinal parasites, and these two cause, respectively, trichinosis, which can also severely affect the human musculature, and schistosomiasis. Weller was concerned with the parasites' basic biology and performed various diagnostic studies on them. His contributions to current understanding of these parasites are significant, advancing an understanding of the ailments they cause.

Weller spent a portion of the same period (1957 to 1973) establishing the basic available knowledge concerning cytomegalovirus (commonly known as CMV), which causes cell enlargement in various organs. Weller's most important finding in this area regarded congenital transmission of both CMV and rubella, a virus also known as German **measles**. A pregnant woman infected with either of these viruses may pass the infection on to her fetus. Weller showed that infected newborns excreted viral strains in their feces, providing another source for the spread of the diseases. His findings became significant when it was also learned that children born to infected mothers often risked birth defects.

In 1962, Weller, along with Franklin Neva, was able to grow and study German Measles in tissue cultures. These two also went on to grow and isolate the chickenpox virus. Subsequently, Weller was the first to show the common origin of the **varicella** virus, which causes chicken pox, and the **herpes** zoster virus, which causes shingles. In 1971, Weller was the first to prove the airborne transmission of *pneumocystis carinii*, a form of pneumonia that later appeared as a frequent side effect of the **human immunodeficiency virus** commonly known as **HIV**.

Weller was elected to the National Academy of Sciences in 1964. In addition, he served on advisory committees of the **World Health Organization**, the Pan American Health Organization, the Agency for International Development, and the National Institute of Allergy and Infectious Disease. He continued his position at Harvard until 1985, when he became professor emeritus. While at Harvard, he helped establish the Public Health Department's international reputation. In 1988, Weller gave the first John F. Enders Memorial Lecture to the Infectious Disease Society of America. In addition to his Nobel Prize, Weller was the recipient of many awards and honorary degrees during his career.

See also Laboratory techniques in immunology; Virology; Virus replication; Viruses and responses to viral infection

WEST NILE VIRUS

The West Nile virus is a member of the family Flaviviridae, a virus that has become more prominent in Europe and North America in the past decade. The virus, which is closely related to the St. Louis encephalitis virus found in the United States, causes an encephalitis (swelling of the brain) in domestic animals (such as horses, dogs, cats), wild animals, and wild birds. When transferred from an infected animal to a human, the viral infection can produce encephalitis as well as **inflammation** of nerve cells of the spinal cord (**meningitis**).

In 1937, the virus was isolated from a woman in the West Nile District of Uganda. This locale was the basis for the designation of the virus as the West Nile virus. During the 1950s, the ability of the virus to cause the serious and life-threatening human disease was recognized. In the 1960s, the virus was established as a cause of equine encephalitis.

Whether the virus has spread geographically from Uganda, or whether increased surveillance has detected the virus in hitherto unsuspected regions is not clear. However, the pattern of detection has been that of a global dissemination. Long found in humans, animals, and birds in Africa, Eastern Europe, West Asia, and the Middle East, the virus was first detected in North America in 1999.

The virus has come to prominent attention in North America following its 1999 appearance on the continent. That year, 62 cases of the disease were reported in New York City. Seven people died. The following year 21 more cases occurred, and two of the people died. In 1999 and 2000, the West Nile virus was confined to the northeastern coastal states of the United States. However, an inexorable spread to other regions of the country and the continent has begun. In the summer of 2001, dead birds that tested positive for the virus were found as far north as Toronto, Canada, as far south as the northern portion of Florida, and as far west as Milwaukee, Wisconsin. Scientists anticipate that the virus will continue to disseminate. During the summer of 2002, more than 300 cases and at least 14 deaths were reported—with a continued spread of the virus into the western United States. By August 2002, West Nile virus was reported in 41 states.

The mosquitoes are the prime vector of the West Nile virus. When mosquitoes obtain a blood meal from an infected animal or a bird, they acquire the virus. The virus resides in the salivary glands of the mosquito, to be passed on to a human when the mosquito seeks another blood meal. The cases in New York City, especially those in 2000, are thought to have been caused by the bite of virus-infected mosquitoes that survived the cold winter months. The emergence of the mosquito in the spring can facilitate the re-emergence of the virus. For example in North America, there were large die-offs of crow populations due to West Nile virus in the Spring of 2000 and then again in the Spring of 2001.

Upon entry to a host's bloodstream, multiplication of the virus in the blood occurs. Then, by a mechanism that is not yet deciphered, the virus crosses the barrier between the blood and the brain. Subsequent multiplication of the virus in brain tissue causes nervous system malfunction and inflammation of the infected brain tissue.

Although a large population of mosquitoes may be present, the chances of acquiring West Nile virus via a mosquito bite is small. Data from the examination of mosquito populations indicates that less than one percent of mosquitoes carry the virus, even in areas where the virus is known to be present.

The mosquito to human route of infection is the only route known thus far. The virus is known to infect certain species of ticks. However, as of early 2002, tick-borne outbreak of the disease has not been documented in humans. Person to person contact cannot occur. Even exchange of body fluids between an infected human and an uninfected person will not transmit the virus.

Currently no human **vaccine** to the West Nile virus exists. Prevention of infection consists of repelling mosquitoes by conventional means, such as the use of repellent sprays or creams, protective clothing, and avoiding locations or times of the day or season when mosquitoes might typically be encountered.

See also Viruses and responses to viral infection; Zoonoses

WET MOUNT · *see* MICROSCOPE AND MICROSCOPY

WHOOPING COUGH · *see* PERTUSSIS

WILKINS, MAURICE HUGH FREDERICK (1916-)
New Zealand English biophysicist

Maurice Hugh Frederick Wilkins is best known for his work regarding the discovery of the structure of **deoxyribonucleic acid (DNA)**. Along with American molecular biologist **James D. Watson** (1924–) and English molecular biologist **Francis Crick** (1916–), Wilkins received the 1962 Nobel Prize in physiology or medicine for his contributions to the discovery of the molecular mechanisms underlying the transmission of genetic information. Specifically, Wilkins' contribution involved discerning the structure of DNA through the use of x–ray diffraction techniques.

Wilkins was born in Pongaroa, New Zealand to Irish immigrants Edgar Henry, a physician, and Eveline Constance Jane (Whittaker) Wilkins. Euperior education began at an early age for Wilkins, who began attending King Edward's School in Birmingham, England, at age six. He later received his B.A. in physics from Cambridge University in 1938. After graduation, he joined the Ministry of Home Security and Aircraft Production and was assigned to conduct graduate research on radar at the University of Birmingham. Wilkins' research centered on improving the accuracy of radar screens.

Soon after earning his Ph.D. in 1940, Wilkins, still with the Ministry of Home Security, was relocated to a new team of British scientists researching the application of uranium isotopes to atomic bombs. A short time later Wilkins became part of another team sent to the United States to work on the Manhattan Project—the military effort to develop the atomic bomb—with other scientists at the University of California at

Berkeley. He spent two years there researching the separation of uranium isotopes.

Wilkins' interest in the intersection of physics and biology emerged soon after his arrival to the United States. He was significantly influenced by a book by Erwin Schrödinger, a fellow physicist, entitled *What is Life? The Physical Aspects of the Living Cell*. The book centers on the possibility that the science of quantum physics could lead to the understanding of the essence of life itself, including the process of biological growth. In addition to Schrödinger's book, the undeniable and undesirable ramifications of his work on the atomic bomb also played a role in Wilkins' declining interest in the field of nuclear physics and emerging interest in biology.

After the war, the opportunity arose for Wilkins to begin a career in biophysics. In 1945, Wilkins' former graduate school professor, Scottish physicist John T. Randall, invited him to become a physics lecturer at St. Andrews University, Scotland, in that school's new biophysics research unit. Later, in 1946, Wilkins and Randall moved on to a new research pursuit combining the sciences of physics, chemistry, and biology to the study of living cells. Together they established the Medical Research Council Biophysics Unit at King's College in London. Wilkins was, for a time, informally the second in command. He officially became deputy director of the unit in 1955 and was promoted to director in 1970, a position he held until 1972.

It was at this biophysics unit, in 1946, that Wilkins soon concentrated his research on DNA, shortly after scientists at the Rockefeller Institute (now Rockefeller University) in New York announced that DNA is the constituent of genes. Realizing the enormous importance of the DNA molecule, Wilkins became excited about uncovering its precise structure. He was prepared to attack this project by a number of different methods. However, he fortuitously discovered that the particular makeup of DNA, specifically the uniformity of its fibers, made it an excellent specimen for x–ray diffraction studies. x–ray diffraction is an extremely useful method for photographing atom arrangements in molecules. The regularly–spaced atoms of the molecule actually diffract the x rays, creating a picture from which the sizing and spacing of the atoms within the molecule can be deduced. This was the tool used by Wilkins to help unravel the structure of DNA.

Physical chemist Rosalind Franklin joined Wilkins in 1951. Franklin, who had been conducting research in Paris, was adept in x–ray diffraction. Together they were able to retrieve some very high quality DNA patterns. One initial and important outcome of their research was that phosphate groups were located outside of the structure, which overturned Linus Pauling's theory that they were on the inside. In another important finding, Wilkins thought the photographs suggested a helical structure, although Franklin hesitated to draw that conclusion. Subsequently, Wilkins passed on to Watson one of the best x–ray pictures Franklin had taken of DNA. These DNA images provided clues to Watson and Crick, who used the pictures to solve the last piece of the DNA structure puzzle.

Consequently, in 1953, Watson and Crick were able to reconstruct the famous double–helix structure of DNA. Their model shows that DNA is composed of two strands of alternating units of sugar and phosphate on the outside, with pairs of bases—including the molecular compounds adenine, thymine, guanine, and cytosine—inside, bonded by hydrogen. It is important to note that while Wilkins' contribution to the discernment DNA's structure is undeniable, controversy surrounds how Watson and Crick obtained Franklin's photographs and the fact that Franklin was not recognized for this scientific breakthrough, particularly in terms of the Nobel Prize. Because the Nobel Prize is not awarded posthumously, Franklin, who died of cancer in 1958, did not receive the same recognition as did Watson, Crick, and Wilkins.

The knowledge of the DNA structure, which has been described as resembling a spiral staircase, has provided the impetus for advanced research in the field of genetics. For example, scientists can now determine predispositions for certain diseases based on the presence of certain genes. Also, the exciting but sometimes controversial area of genetic engineering has developed.

Wilkins, Watson, and Crick were awarded the 1962 Nobel Prize for physiology or medicine for their work which uncovered the structure of hereditary material DNA. After winning the Nobel Prize, Wilkins focused next on elucidating the structure of ribonucleic acids (RNA)—a compound like DNA associated with the control of cellular chemical activities—and, later, nerve cell membranes. In 1962, Wilkins was able to show that **RNA** also had a helical structure somewhat similar to that of DNA. Besides his directorship appointments at the Medical Research Council's Biophysics Unit, Wilkins was also appointed director of the Council's Neurobiology Unit, a post he held from 1974 to 1980. Additionally, he was a professor at King's College, teaching **molecular biology** from 1963 to 1970, and then biophysics as the department head from 1970 to 1982. In 1981, he was named professor emeritus at King's College. Utilizing some of his professional expertise for social causes, Wilkins has maintained membership in the British Society for Social Responsibility in Science (of which he is president), the Russell Committee against Chemical Weapons, and Food and Disarmament International.

Wilkins is an honorary member of the American Society of Biological Chemists and the American Academy of Arts and Sciences. He was also honored with the 1960 Albert Lasker Award of the American Public Health Association (given jointly to Wilkins, Watson, and Crick), and was named Fellow of the Royal Society of King's College in 1959.

See also DNA (Deoxyribonucleic acid); DNA chips and micro arrays; Gene; Genetic mapping; Molecular biology and molecular genetics

WINE MAKING

Along with bread making, the use of the **microorganisms** called yeasts to produce wine from grapes is one of the oldest uses of microorganisms by man. The origins of wine making date from antiquity. Before 2000 B.C. the Egyptians would store crushed fruit in a warm place in order to produce a liquid whose consumption produced feelings of euphoria. The manufacture and consumption of wine rapidly became a part of daily life in many areas of the Ancient world and eventually became a well-established part of Classical civilization. For centuries, wine making has been an important economic activity. In certain areas of the world, such as France, Italy, and Northern California, wine making on a commercial scale is a vital part of the local economy.

The agent of the formation of wine is **yeast**. Yeasts are small, single-celled **fungi** that belong to the genus Ascomycota. Hallmarks of yeast are their ability to reproduce by the methods of fission or budding, and their ability to utilize compounds called carbohydrates (specifically the sugar glucose) with the subsequent production of alcohol and the gas carbon dioxide. This chemical process is called **fermentation**.

Yeast cells are able to carry out fermentation because of **enzymes** they possess. The conversion of sugar to alcohol ultimately proves lethal to the yeast cells, which cannot tolerate the increasing alcohol levels. Depending on the type of yeast used, the alcohol content of the finished product can vary from around 5% to over 20%, by volume.

The scientific roots of fermentation experimentation date back to the seventeenth century. In 1680 **Anton van Leeuwenhoek** used his hand-built light microscopes to detect yeast. Almost one hundred years later the French chemist Antoine Laurent Lavoisier proposed that yeast was the agent of the fermentation of sugar. This was confirmed in 1935 by the examination of yeast vats with the greatly improved microscopes of that day.

In the nineteenth century the role of yeasts as a catalyst (that is, as an agent that accelerates a chemical process without itself being changed in the process) was recognized by the Swedish chemist Jons Berzelius. In the 1860s the renowned microbiologist **Louis Pasteur** discovered that yeast fermentation could proceed in the absence of oxygen. In 1878 Wilhelm Kuhne recognized that the yeast catalyst was contained inside the cell. He coined the term "enzyme" for the catalyst.

In fact more than two dozen yeast enzymes participate in the degradation of glucose. The degradation is a pathway, with one reaction being dependent on the occurrence of a prior reaction, and itself being required for a subsequent reaction. In total some 30 chemical reactions are involved. These reactions require the function of the various enzymes. The yeast cell is the biological machine that creates the enzymes. Once the enzymes are present, alcoholic fermentation can proceed in the absence of living yeast. Enzymes, however, have only a finite period of activity before they themselves degrade. Hence a continual supply of fresh enzymes requires living yeast.

Many types of yeast exist. The stable types suitable for making wine (and bread and beer) are the seven species of yeast belonging to the genus Saccharomyces. The name comes from the Greek words for sugar (sacchar) and fungus (Mykes). The predominant species in wine making is *Saccharomyces cerevisiae*. There are multiple strains of this species that produce wine. The **selection** of yeast type is part of the art of wine making; the yeast is matched to the grape and the fermentation conditions to produce—the wine maker hopes—a finished product of exceptional quality.

The natural source of yeast for wine making is often the population that becomes dominant in the vineyard. Less

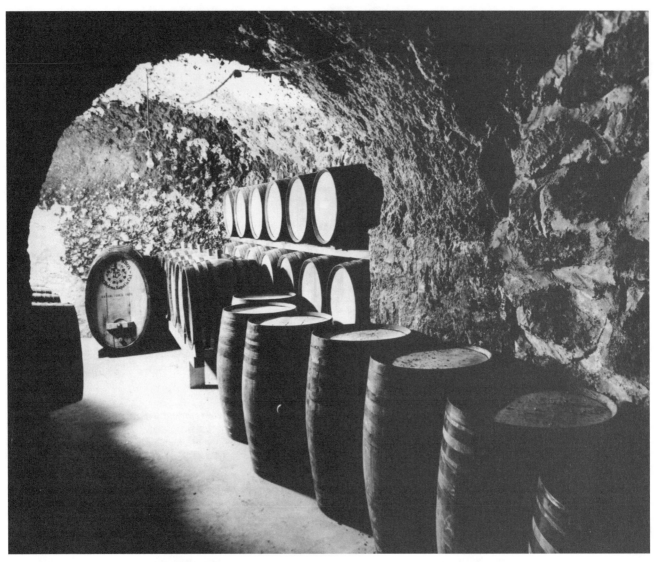

Barrels used to age wine in the wine making process.

mature local vineyards, especially those established in North America, rely on yeast strains that are injected into the crushed grape suspension. The growth of the yeast will then occur in the nutrient-rich mixture of the suspension.

The fermentation process begins when the yeast is added to the juice that is obtained following the crushing of the grapes. This process can be stunted or halted by the poor growth of the yeast. This can occur if conditions such as temperature and light are not favorable. Also, contaminating microorganisms can outgrow the yeast and out compete the yeast cells for the nutrients. Selective growth of *Sacchromyces cerevisiae* can be encouraged by maintaining a temperature of between 158 and 167°F (70 and 75°C). The **bacteria** that are prone to develop in the fermenting suspension do not tolerate such an elevated temperature. Yeast other than *Sacchromyces cerevisiae* are not as tolerant of the presence of sulfur dioxide.

Thus the addition of compounds containing sulfur dioxide to fermenting wine is a common practice.

The explosion in popularity of home-based wine making has streamlined the production process. Home vintners can purchase so-called starter yeast, which is essentially a powder consisting of a form of the yeast that is dormant. Upon the addition of the yeast powder to a solution of grape essence and sugar, resuscitation of the yeast occurs, growth resumes, and fermentation starts. In another modification to this process, the yeast starter can be added to a liquid growth source for a few days. Then this new **culture** of yeast can be used to inoculate the grape essence and sugar solution. The advantage of the second approach is that the amount of yeast, which is added, can be better controlled, and the addition of liquid culture encourages a more efficient dispersion of the yeast cells throughout the grape solution.

The many varieties of wine, including champagne, are the results of centuries of trial and error involving the myriad varieties of grape and yeast.

See also Economic uses and benefits of microorganisms; Fermentation

WINOGRADSKY COLUMN

In a Winogradsky column the conditions change from oxygen-rich (aerobic) at the top of the column to oxygen-deficient (anaerobic) at the bottom. Different **microorganisms** develop in the various environmental niches throughout the column. The products of one microbe's metabolic activities support the growth of another microbe. The result is that the column becomes a self-supporting ecosystem, which is driven only by the energy received from the incoming sunlight. Winogradsky columns are easily constructed, and are often used in classroom experiments and demonstrations.

The Winogradsky column is named after Sergius Winogradsky, a Russian microbiologist who was one of the pioneers of the study of the diversity of the metabolic activities of microorganisms.

To set up a Winogradsky column, a glass or clear plastic tube is filled one-third full with a mixture of mud obtained from a river bottom, cellulose, sodium sulphate, and calcium carbonate. The remaining two-thirds of the tube is filled with lake or river water. The capped tube is placed near a sunlit window.

Over a period of two to three months, the length of the tube becomes occupied by a series of microbial communities. Initially, the cellulose provides nutrition for a rapid increase in bacterial numbers. The growth uses up the available oxygen in the sealed tube. Only the top water layer continues to contain oxygen. The sediment at the bottom of the tube, which has become completely oxygen-free, supports the growth only of those **bacteria** that can grow in the absence of oxygen. Desulfovibrio and Clostridium will predominate in the sediment.

Diffusion of hydrogen sulfide produced by the anaerobic bacteria, from the sediment into the water column above supports the growth of anaerobic photosynthetic bacteria such as green sulfur bacteria and purple sulfur bacteria. These bacteria are able to utilize sunlight to generate energy and can use carbon dioxide in a oxygen-free reaction to produce compounds needed for growth.

The diminished hydrogen sulfide conditions a bit further up the tube then support the development of purple sulfur bacteria such as Rhodopseudomonas, Rhodospirillum, and Rhodomicrobium.

Towards the top of the tube, oxygen is still present in the water. Photosynthetic cyanobacteria will grow in this region, with the surface of the water presenting an atmosphere conducive to the growth of **sheathed bacteria**.

The Winogradsky column has proved to be an excellent learning tool for generations of microbiology students, and a classic demonstration of how carbon and energy specifics result in various niches for different microbes, and of the recycling of sulfur, nitrogen, and carbon.

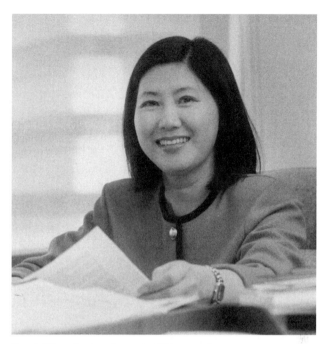

Flossie Wong-Staal, a pioneer in AIDS research.

See also Chemoautotrophic and chemolithotrophic bacteria; Methane oxidizing and producing bacteria

WONG-STAAL, FLOSSIE (1947-)
Chinese American virologist

Although Flossie Wong-Staal is considered one of the world's top experts in **viruses** and a codiscoverer of the **human immunodeficiency virus** (**HIV**) that causes **AIDS**, her interest in science did not come naturally.

Born as Yee Ching Wong in communist mainland China, she fled with her family in 1952 to Hong Kong, where she entered an all-girls Catholic school. When students there achieved high grades, they were steered into scientific studies. The young Wong had excellent marks, but initially had no plans of becoming a scientist. Against her expectations, she gradually became enamored with science. Another significant result of attending the private school was the changing of her name. The school encouraged Wong to adopt an English name. Her father, who did not speak English, chose the name Flossie from newspaper accounts of Typhoon Flossie, which had struck Hong Kong the previous week.

Even though none of Wong's female relatives had ever gone to college or university, her family enthusiastically supported her education and in 1965, she went to the United States to study at the University of California at Los Angeles. In 1968, Wong graduated magna cum laude with a B.S. in bacteriology, also obtaining a doctorate in **molecular biology** in 1972.

During postgraduate work at the university's San Diego campus in 1971–72, Wong married and added Staal to her name. The marriage eventually ended in divorce. In 1973,

Wong-Staal moved to Bethesda, Maryland, where she worked at the National Cancer Institute (NCI) with AIDS pioneer Robert Gallo, studying **retroviruses**, the mysterious family of viruses to which HIV belongs. Searching for a cause for the newly discovered AIDS epidemic, Gallo, Wong-Staal, and other NCI colleagues identified HIV in 1983, simultaneously with a French researcher. In 1985, Wong-Stall was responsible for the first **cloning** of HIV. Her efforts also led to the first **genetic mapping** of the virus, allowing eventual development of tests that screen patients and donated blood for HIV.

In 1990, the Institute for Scientific Information declared Wong-Staal as the top woman scientist of the previous decade. That same year, Wong-Staal returned to the University of California at San Diego to continue her AIDS research. Four years later, the university created a new Center for AIDS Research; Wong-Staal became its chairman. There, she works to find both vaccines against HIV and a cure for AIDS, using the new technology of **gene** therapy.

See also AIDS, recent advances in research and treatment

WOODWARD, ROBERT B. (1917-1979)
American biochemist

Robert B. Woodward was arguably the greatest organic synthesis chemist of the twentieth century. He accomplished the total synthesis of several important natural products and pharmaceuticals. Total synthesis means that the molecule of interest—no matter how complex—is built directly from the smallest, most common compounds and is not just a derivation of a related larger molecule. In order to accomplish his work, Woodward combined physical chemistry principles, including quantum mechanics, with traditional reaction methods to design elaborate synthetic schemes. With Nobel Laureate Roald Hoffmann, he designed a set of rules for predicting reaction outcomes based on stereochemistry, the study of the spatial arrangements of molecules. Woodward won the Nobel Prize in chemistry in 1965.

Robert Burns Woodward was born in Boston on April 10, 1917, to Arthur and Margaret (Burns) Woodward. His father died when he was very young. Woodward obtained his first chemistry set while still a child and taught himself most of the basic principles of the science by doing experiments at home. By the time he graduated at the age of 16 from Quincy High School in Quincy, Massachusetts, in 1933, his knowledge of chemistry exceeded that of many of his instructors. He entered the Massachusetts Institute of Technology (MIT) the same year but nearly failed a few months later, apparently impatient with the rules and required courses.

The MIT chemistry faculty, however, recognized Woodward's unusual talent and rescued him. They obtained funding and a laboratory for his work and allowed him complete freedom to design his own curriculum, which he made far more rigorous than the required one. Woodward obtained his doctorate degree from MIT only four years later, at the age of 20, and then joined the faculty of Harvard University after a year of postdoctoral work there.

Woodward spent virtually all of his career at Harvard but also did a significant amount of consulting work with various corporations and institutes around the world. As is true in most modern scientific endeavors, Woodward's working style was characterized by collaboration with many other researchers. He also insisted on utilizing the most up-to-date instrumentation, theories.

The design of a synthesis, the crux of Woodward's work, involves much more than a simple list of chemicals or procedures. Biochemical molecules exhibit not only a particular bonding pattern of atoms, but also a certain arrangement of those atoms in space. The study of the spatial arrangements of molecules is called stereochemistry, and the individual configurations of a molecule are called its stereoisomers. Sometimes the same molecule may have many different stereoisomers; only one of those, however, will be biologically relevant. Consequently, a synthesis scheme must consider the basic reaction conditions that will bond two atoms together as well as determine how to ensure that the reaction orients the atoms properly to obtain the correct stereoisomer.

Physical chemists postulate that certain areas around an atom or molecule are more likely to contain electrons than other areas. These areas of probability, called orbitals, are described mathematically but are usually visualized as having specific shapes and orientations relative to the rest of the atom or molecule. Chemists visualize bonding as an overlap of two partially full orbitals to make one completely full molecular orbital with two electrons. Woodward and Roald Hoffmann of Cornell University established the Woodward-Hoffmann rules based on quantum mechanics, which explain whether a particular overlap is likely or even possible for the orbitals of two reacting species. By carefully choosing the shape of the reactant species and reaction conditions, the chemist can make certain that the atoms are oriented to obtain exactly the correct stereochemical configuration. In 1970, Woodward and Hoffmann published their classic work on the subject, *The Conservation of Orbital Symmetry;* Woodward by that time had demonstrated repeatedly by his own startling successes at synthesis that the rules worked.

Woodward and his colleagues synthesized a lengthy list of difficult molecules over the years. In 1944 their research, motivated by wartime shortages of the material and funded by the Polaroid Corporation, prompted Woodward—only 27 years old at the time—and William E. Doering to announce the first total synthesis of quinine, important in the treatment of **malaria**. Chemists had been trying unsuccessfully to synthesize quinine for more than a century.

In 1947, Woodward and C. H. Schramm, another organic chemist, reported that they had created an artificial protein by bonding amino acids into a long chain molecule, knowledge that proved useful to both researchers and workers in the plastics industry. In 1951, Woodward and his colleagues (funded partly by Merck and the Monsanto Corporation) announced the first total synthesis of cholesterol and cortisone, both biochemical steroids. Cortisone had only recently been identified as an effective drug in the treatment of rheumatoid arthritis, so its synthesis was of great importance.

Woodward's other accomplishments in synthesis include strychnine (1954), a poison isolated from *Strychnos* species and often used to kill rats; colchicine (1963), a toxic natural product found in autumn crocus; and lysergic acid (1954) and reserpine (1956), both psychoactive substances. Reserpine, a tranquilizer found naturally in the Indian snake root plant *Rauwolfia,* was widely used to treat mental illness and was one of the first genuinely effective psychiatric medicines. In 1960, after four years of work, Woodward synthesized **chlorophyll**, the light energy capturing pigment in green plants, and in 1962 he accomplished the total synthesis of a tetracycline antibiotic.

Total synthesis requires the design and then precise implementation of elaborate procedures composed of many steps. Each step in a synthetic procedure either adds or subtracts chemical groups from a starting molecule or rearranges the orientation or order of the atoms in the molecule. Since it is impossible, even with the utmost care, to achieve one hundred percent conversion of starting compound to product at any given step, the greater the number of steps, the less product is obtained.

Woodward and Doering produced approximately a half a gram of quinine from about five pounds of starting materials; they began with benzaldehyde, a simple, inexpensive chemical obtained from coal tar, and designed a 17-step synthetic procedure. The 20-step synthesis that led to the first steroid **nucleus** required 22 lb (10 kg) of starting material and yielded less than a twentieth of an ounce of product. The best synthesis schemes thus have the fewest number of steps, although for some very complicated molecules, "few" may mean several dozen. When Woodward successfully synthesized chlorophyll (which has an elaborate interconnected ring structure), for example, he required 55 steps for the synthesis.

Woodward's close friend, Nobel Laureate Vladimir Prelog, helped establish the CIBA-Geigy Corporation-funded Woodward Institute in Zurich, Switzerland, in the early 1960s. There, Woodward could work on whatever project he chose, without the intrusion of teaching or administrative duties. Initially, the Swiss Federal Institute of Technology had tried to hire Woodward away from Harvard; when it failed, the Woodward Institute provided an alternative way of ensuring that Woodward visited and worked frequently in Switzerland. In 1965, Woodward and his Swiss collaborators synthesized Cephalosporin C, an important antibiotic. In 1971 he succeeded in synthesizing vitamin B$_{12}$, a molecule bearing some chemical similarity to chlorophyll, but with cobalt instead of magnesium as the central metal atom. Until the end of his life, Woodward worked on the synthesis of the antibiotic erythromycin.

Woodward, who received a Nobel Prize in 1965, helped start two organic chemistry journals, *Tetrahedron Letters* and *Tetrahedron,* served on the boards of several science organizations, and received awards and honorary degrees from many countries. Some of his many honors include the Davy Medal (1959) and the Copley Medal (1978), both from the Royal Society of Britain, and the United States' National Medal of Science (1964). He reached full professor status at Harvard in 1950 and in 1960 became the Donner Professor of Science. Woodward supervised more than three hundred graduate students and postdoctoral students throughout his career.

Woodward married Irji Pullman in 1938 and had two daughters. He was married for the second time in 1946 to Eudoxia Muller, who had also been a consultant at the Polaroid Corporation. The couple had two children. Woodward died at his home of a heart attack on July 8, 1979, at the age of 62.

See also Biochemical analysis techniques; Biochemistry; History of the development of antibiotics

WORLD HEALTH ORGANIZATION (WHO)

The World Health Organization (WHO) is the principle international organization managing **public health** related issues on a global scale. Headquartered in Geneva, the WHO is comprised of 191 member states (e.g., countries) from around the globe. The organization contributes to international public health in areas including disease prevention and control, promotion of good health, addressing diseases outbreaks, initiatives to eliminate diseases (e.g., **vaccination** programs), and development of treatment and prevention standards.

The genesis of the WHO was in 1919. Then, just after the end of World War I, the League of Nations was created to promote peace and security in the aftermath of the war. One of the mandates of the League of Nations was the prevention and control of disease around the world. The Health Organization of the League of Nations was established for this purpose, and was headquartered in Geneva. In 1945, the United Nations Conference on International Organization in San Francisco approved a motion put forth by Brazil and China to establish a new and independent international organization devoted to public health. The proposed organization was meant to unite the number of disparate health organizations that had been established in various countries around the world.

The following year this resolution was formally enacted at the International Health Conference in New York, and the Constitution of the World Health organization was approved. The Constitution came into force on April 7, 1948. The first Director General of WHO was Dr. Brock Chisholm, a psychiatrist from Canada. Chisholm's influence was evident in the Constitution, which defines health as not merely the absence of disease. A definition that subsequently paved the way for WHO's involvement in the preventative aspects of disease.

From its inception, WHO has been involved in public health campaigns that focus on the improvement of sanitary conditions. In 1951, the Fourth World Health Assembly adopted a WHO document proposing new international sanitary regulations. Additionally, WHO mounted extensive vaccination campaigns against a number of diseases of microbial origin, including **poliomyelitis, measles, diphtheria**, whooping cough, **tetanus, tuberculosis**, and **smallpox**. The latter campaign has been extremely successful, with the last known natural case of smallpox having occurred in 1977. The elimination of poliomyelitis is expected by the end of the first decade of the twenty-first century.

Another noteworthy initiative of WHO has been the Global Programme on **AIDS**, which was launched in 1987. The participation of WHO and agencies such as the **Centers for Disease Control** and Prevention is necessary to adequately address AIDS, because the disease is prevalent in under-developed countries where access to medical care and health promotion is limited.

Today, WHO is structured as eight divisions. The themes that are addressed by individual divisions include communicable diseases, noncommunicable diseases and mental health, family and community health, sustainable development and health environments, health technology and pharmaceuticals, and policy development. These divisions support the four pillars of WHO: worldwide guidance in health, worldwide development of improved standards of health, cooperation with governments in strengthening national health programs, and development of improved health technologies, information, and standards.

See also History of public heath; Public health, current issues

WRIGHT, ALMROTH EDWARD

(1861-1947)

English bacteriologist and immunologist

Almroth Edward Wright is best known for his contributions to the field of **immunology** and the development of the autogenous **vaccine**. Wright utilized **bacteria** that were present in the host to create his vaccines. He also developed an anti-typhoid inoculation composed of heat-killed **typhus** specific bacilli. Wright was a consistent advocate for vaccine and inoculation therapies, and at the onset of World War I convinced the British military to inoculate all troops against typhus. However, Wright was also interested in bacteriological research. Wright conducted several studies on bacteriological infections in post-surgical and accidental wounds.

Wright was born in Yorkshire, England. He studied medicine at Trinity College Dublin, graduating in 1884. He then studied medicine in France, Germany, and Australia for few years before returning home to accept a position in London. He conducted most of his research at the Royal Victoria Hospital where he was Chair of Pathology at the Army Medical School. In 1899, Wright lobbied to have all of the troops departing to fight in the Boer War in Africa inoculated against typhus. The government permitted Wright to institute a voluntary program, but only a small fraction of troops participated. Typhus was endemic among the soldiers in Africa, and accounted for over 9,000 deaths during the war. Following the return of the troops, the Army conducted a study into the efficacy of the inoculation and for unknown reasons, decided to suspend the inoculation program. Wright was infuriated and resigned his post.

Wright then took a position at St. Mary's Hospital in London. He began a small **vaccination** and inoculation clinic

that later became the renowned Inoculation Department. Convinced that his anti-typhus inoculation worked, he arranged for a second study of his therapy on British troops stationed in India. The results were promising, but the Army largely ignored the new information. Before the eve of World War I, Wright once again appealed to military command to inoculate troops against typhus. Wright petitioned Lord Kitchener in 1914. Kitchener agreed with Wright's recommendation and ordered a mandatory inoculation program.

Most likely owing to his often sparse laboratory settings, Wright revised several experimental methods, publishing them in various journals. One of his most renowned contributions was a reform of common blood and fluid collection procedures. Common practice was to collect samples from capillaries with pipettes, not from veins with a syringe. Like modern syringes, pipettes required suction. This was usually supplied by mouth. Wright attached a rubberized teat to the **pipette**, permitting for a cleaner, more aseptic, collection of blood and fluid samples. He also developed a disposable capsule for the collection, testing, and storage of blood specimens. In 1912, Wright published a compendium of several of his reformed techniques.

Wright often had to endure the trials of critical colleagues and **public health** officials who disagreed with some of his innovations in the laboratory and his insistence on vaccine therapies. Wright usually prevailed in these clashes. However, Wright stood in opposition to the most formidable medical movement of his early days, antisepsis. Antiseptic surgical protocols called for the **sterilization** of all instruments and surgical surfaces with a carbolic acid solution. However, some surgeons and proponents of the practice advocated placing bandages soaked in a weaker form of the solution directly on patient wounds. Wright agreed with the practice of instrument sterilization, but claimed that antiseptic wound care killed more leukocytes, the body's natural defense against bacteria and infection, than harmful bacteria. Wright's solution was to treat wounds with a saline wash and let the body fight infection with its own defenses. Not until the advancement of asepsis, the process of creating a sterile environment within the hospital, and the discovery of **antibiotics** was Wright's claim re-evaluated.

Wright had a distinguished career in his own right, but is also remembered as the teacher of **Alexander Fleming**, who later discovered **penicillin** and antibiotics. During Wright's campaign to inoculate troops before World War I, and throughout the course of his research on wound care, Fleming was Wright's student and assistant. Fleming's later research vindicated many of Wright's theories on wound care, but also lessened the significance of autogenous vaccine therapies. The Inoculation Department in which both Wright and Fleming worked was later renamed in honor of the two scientists.

Wright died, while still actively working at his laboratory in Buckinghamshire, at the age of 85.

See also Immune stimulation, as a vaccine; Immune system; Immunity, active, passive and delayed; Immunity, cell mediated; Immunity, humoral regulation; Immunization

X

XANTHOPHYLLS

Photosynthesis is the conversion of light energy into chemical energy utilized by plants, many algae, and cyanobacteria. However, each photosynthetic organism must be able to dissipate the light radiation that exceeds its capacity for carbon dioxide fixation before it can damage the photosynthetic apparatus (i.e., the **chloroplast**). This photoprotection is usually mediated by oxygenated carotenoids, i.e., a group of yellow pigments termed xanthophylls, including violaxanthin, antheraxanthin, and zeaxanthin, which dissipate the thermal radiation from the sunlight through the xanthophyll cycle.

Xanthophylls are present in two large protein-cofactor complexes, present in photosynthetic membranes of organisms using Photosystem I or Photosystem II. Photosystem II uses water as electron donors, and pigments and quinones as electron acceptors, whereas the Photosystem I uses plastocyanin as electron donors and iron-sulphur centers as electron acceptors. Photosystem I in thermophilic Cyanobacteria, for instance, is a crystal structure that contains 12 protein subunits, 2 phylloquinones, 22 carotenoids, 127 cofactors constituting 96 chlorophylls, besides calcium cations, **phospholipids**, three iron-sulphur groups, water, and other elements. This apparatus captures light and transfers electrons to pigments and at the same time dissipates the excessive excitation energy via the xanthophylls.

Xanthophylls are synthesized inside the plastids and do not depend on light for their synthesis as do chlorophylls. From dawn to sunset, plants and other photosynthetic organisms are exposed to different amounts of solar radiation, which determine the xanthophyll cycle. At dawn, a pool of diepoxides termed violaxanthin is found in the plastids, which will be converted by the monoepoxide antheraxanthin into zeaxanthin as the light intensity gradually increases during the day. Zeaxanthin absorbs and dissipates the excessive solar radiation that is not used by **chlorophyll** during carbon dioxide fixation. At the peak hours of sunlight exposition, almost all xanthophyll in the pool is found under the form of zeaxanthin,

which will be gradually reconverted into violaxanthin as the solar radiation decreases in the afternoon to be reused again in the next day.

See also Autotrophic bacteria; Photosynthetic microorganisms

XANTHOPHYTA

The yellow-green algae are photosynthetic species of organisms belonging to the Xanthophyta Phylum, which is one of the phyla pertaining to the Chromista Group in the Protista Kingdom. Xanthophyta encompasses 650 living species so far identified. Xanthophyta live mostly in freshwater, although some species live in marine water, tree trunks, and damp soils. Some species are unicellular organisms equipped with two unequal flagella that live as free-swimming individuals, but most species are filamentous. Filamentous species may be either siphonous or coenocytic. Coenocytes are organized as a single-cell multinucleated thallus that form long filaments without septa (internal division walls) except in the specialized structures of some species. Siphonous species have multiple tubular cells containing several nuclei.

Xanthophyta synthesize **chlorophyll** a and smaller amounts of chlorophyll c, instead of the chlorophyll b of plants; and the cellular structure usually have multiple chloroplasts without nucleomorphs. The plastids have four membranes and their yellow-green color is due to the presence of beta-carotene and xanthins, such as vaucheriaxanthin, diatoxanthin, diadinoxanthin, and heretoxanthin, but not fucoxanthin, the brown pigment present in other Chromista. Because of the presence of significant amounts of chlorophyll a, Xanthophyceae species are easily mistaken for green algae. They store polysaccharide under the form of chrysolaminarin and carbohydrates as oil droplets.

One example of a relatively common Xanthophyta is the class Vaucheria that gathers approximately 70 species, whose structure consists of several tubular filaments, sharing its nuclei and chloroplasts without septa. They live mainly in freshwater, although some species are found in seawater spreading along the bottom like a carpet. Other Xanthophyceae Classes are Tribonema, whose structure consists of unbranched filaments; Botrydiopsis, such as the species *Botrydium* with several thalli, each thallus formed by a large aerial vesicle and rhizoidal filaments, found in damp soil; Olisthodiscus, such as the species *Ophiocytium* with cylindrical and elongated multinucleated cells and multiple chloroplasts.

See also Photosynthetic microorganisms; Protists

Y

YALOW, ROSALYN SUSSMAN (1921-   )

American medical physicist

Rosalyn Sussman Yalow was co-developer of radioimmunoassay (RIA), a technique that uses radioactive isotopes to measure small amounts of biological substances. In widespread use, the RIA helps scientists and medical professionals measure the concentrations of hormones, vitamins, **viruses**, **enzymes**, and drugs, among other substances. Yalow's work concerning RIA earned her a share of the Nobel Prize in physiology or medicine in the late 1970s. At that time, she was only the second woman to receive the Nobel Prize in medicine. During her career, Yalow also received acclaim for being the first woman to attain a number of other scientific achievements.

Yalow was born on July 19, 1921, in The Bronx, New York, to Simon Sussman and Clara Zipper Sussman. Her father, owner of a small business, had been born on the Lower East Side of New York City to Russian immigrant parents. At the age of four, Yalow's mother had journeyed to the United States from Germany. Although neither parent had attended high school, they instilled a great enthusiasm for and respect of education in their daughter. Yalow also credits her father with helping her find the confidence to succeed in school, teaching her that girls could do just as much as boys. Yalow learned to read before she entered kindergarten, although her family did not own many books. Instead, Yalow and her older brother, Alexander, made frequent visits to the public library.

During her youth, Yalow became interested in mathematics. At Walton High School in the Bronx, her interest turned to science, especially chemistry. After graduation, Yalow attended Hunter College, a women's school in New York that eventually became part of the City University of New York. She credits two physics professors, Dr. Herbert Otis and Dr. Duane Roller, for igniting her penchant for physics. This occurred in the latter part of the 1930s, a time when many new discoveries were made in nuclear physics. It was this field that Yalow ultimately chose for her major. In

1939, she was further inspired after hearing American physicist Enrico Fermi lecture about the discovery of nuclear fission, which had earned him the Nobel Prize the previous year.

As Yalow prepared for her graduation from Hunter College, she found that some practical considerations intruded on her passion for physics. In fact, Yalow's parents urged her to pursue a career as an elementary school teacher. Yalow herself also thought it unrealistic to expect any of the top graduate schools in the country to accept her into a doctoral program or offer her the financial support that men received. "However, my physics professors encouraged me and I persisted," she explained in *Les Prix Nobel 1977*.

Yalow made plans to enter graduate school via other means. One of her earlier college physics professors, who had left Hunter to join the faculty at the Massachusetts Institute of Technology, arranged for Yalow to work as secretary to Dr. Rudolf Schoenheimer, a biochemist at Columbia University in New York. According to the plan, this position would give Yalow an opportunity to take some graduate courses in physics, and eventually provide a way for her to enter a graduate a school and pursue a degree. But Yalow never needed her plan. The month after graduating from Hunter College in January 1941, she was offered a teaching assistantship in the physics department of the University of Illinois at Champaign-Urbana.

Gaining acceptance to the physics graduate program in the College of Engineering at the University of Illinois was one of many hurdles that Yalow had to cross as a woman in the field of science. For example, when she entered the University in September 1941, she was the only woman in the College of Engineering's faculty, which included 400 professors and teaching assistants. She was the first woman in more than two decades to attend the engineering college. Yalow realized that she had been given a space at the prestigious graduate school because of the shortage of male candidates, who were being drafted into the armed services in increasing numbers as America prepared to enter World War II.

Yalow's strong work orientation aided her greatly in her first year in graduate school. In addition to her regular course load and teaching duties, she took some extra undergraduate courses to increase her knowledge. While in graduate school she also met Aaron Yalow, a fellow student and the man she would eventually marry. The pair met the first day of school and wed about two years later on June 6, 1943. Yalow received her master's degree in 1942 and her doctorate in 1945. She was the second woman to obtain a Ph.D. in physics at the University.

After graduation the Yalows moved to New York City, where they worked and eventually raised two children, Benjamin and Elanna. Yalow's first job after graduate school was as an assistant electrical engineer at Federal Telecommunications Laboratory, a private research lab. Once again, she found herself the sole woman as there were no other female engineers at the lab. In 1946, she began teaching physics at Hunter College. She remained a physics lecturer from 1946 to 1950, although by 1947, she began her long association with the Veterans Administration by becoming a consultant to Bronx VA Hospital. The VA wanted to establish some research programs to explore medical uses of radioactive substances. By 1950, Yalow had equipped a radioisotope laboratory at the Bronx VA Hospital and decided to leave teaching to devote her attention to full-time research.

That same year, Yalow met Solomon A. Berson, a physician who had just finished his residency in internal medicine at the hospital. The two would work together until Berson's death in 1972. According to Yalow, the collaboration was a complementary one. In Olga Opfell's *Lady Laureates,* Yalow is quoted as saying, "[Berson] wanted to be a physicist, and I wanted to be a medical doctor." While her partner had accumulated clinical expertise, Yalow maintained strengths in physics, math, and chemistry. Working together, Yalow and Berson discovered new ways to use radioactive isotopes in the measurement of blood volume, the study of iodine **metabolism**, and the diagnosis of thyroid diseases. Within a few years, the pair began to investigate adult-onset diabetes using radioisotopes. This project eventually led them to develop the groundbreaking radioimmunoassay technique.

In the 1950s, some scientists hypothesized that in adult-onset diabetes, insulin production remained normal, but a liver enzyme rapidly destroyed the peptide hormone, thereby preventing normal glucose metabolism. This contrasted with the situation in juvenile diabetes, where insulin production by the pancreas was too low to allow proper metabolism of glucose. Yalow and Berson wanted to test the hypothesis about adult-onset diabetes. They used insulin "labeled" with ^{131}iodine (that is, they attached, by a chemical reaction, the radioactive isotope of iodine to otherwise normal insulin molecules.) Yalow and Berson injected labeled insulin into diabetic and non-diabetic individuals and measured the rate at which the insulin disappeared.

To their surprise and in contradiction to the liver enzyme hypothesis, they found that the amount of radioactively labeled insulin in the blood of diabetics was higher than that found in the control subjects who had never received insulin injections before. As Yalow and Berson looked into this finding further, they deduced that diabetics were forming antibodies to the animal insulin used to control their disease.

These antibodies were binding to radiolabeled insulin, preventing it from entering cells where it was used in sugar metabolism. Individuals who had never taken insulin before did not have these antibodies and so the radiolabeled insulin was consumed more quickly.

Yalow and Berson's proposal that animal insulin could spur **antibody formation** was not readily accepted by immunologists in the mid–1950s. At the time, most immunologists did not believe that antibodies would form to molecules as small as the insulin peptide. Also, the amount of insulin antibodies was too low to be detected by conventional immunological techniques. Yalow and Berson set out to verify these minute levels of insulin antibodies using radiolabeled insulin as their marker. Their original report about insulin antibodies, however, was rejected initially by two journals. Finally, a compromise version was published that omitted "insulin antibody" from the paper's title and included some additional data indicating that an **antibody** was involved.

The need to detect insulin antibodies at low concentrations led to the development of the radioimmunoassay. The principle behind RIA is that a radiolabeled **antigen**, such as insulin, will compete with unlabeled antigen for the available binding sites on its specific antibody. As a standard, various mixtures of known amounts of labeled and unlabeled antigen are mixed with antibody. The amounts of radiation detected in each sample correspond to the amount of unlabeled antigen taking up antibody binding sites. In the unknown sample, a known amount of radiolabeled antigen is added and the amount of radioactivity is measured again. The radiation level in the unknown sample is compared to the standard samples; the amount of unlabeled antigen in the unknown sample will be the same as the amount of unlabeled antigen found in the standard sample that yields the same amount of radioactivity. RIA has turned out to be so useful because it can quickly and precisely detect very low concentrations of hormones and other substances in blood or other biological fluids. The principle can also be applied to binding interactions other than that between antigen and antibody, such as between a binding protein or tissue receptor site and an enzyme. In Yalow's Nobel lecture, recorded in *Les Prix Nobel 1977,* she listed more than 100 biological substances—hormones, drugs, vitamins, enzymes, viruses, non-hormonal proteins, and more—that were being measured using RIA.

In 1968, Yalow became a research professor at the Mt. Sinai School of Medicine, and in 1970, she was made chief of the Nuclear Medicine Service at the VA hospital. Yalow also began to receive a number of prestigious awards in recognition of her role in the development of RIA. In 1976, she was awarded the Albert Lasker Prize for Basic Medical Research. She was the first woman to be honored this laurel—an award that often leads to a Nobel Prize. In Yalow's case, this was true, for the very next year, she shared the Nobel Prize in physiology or medicine with Andrew V. Schally and Roger Guillemin for their work on radioimmunoassay. Schally and Guillemin were recognized for their use of RIA to make important discoveries about brain hormones.

Berson had died in 1972, and so did not share in these awards. According to an essay in The Lady Laureates, she remarked that the "tragedy" of winning the Nobel Prize "is that Dr. Berson did not live to share it." Earlier Yalow had paid tribute to her collaborator by asking the VA to name the laboratory, in which the two had worked, the Solomon A. Berson Research Laboratory. She made the request, as quoted in *Les Prix Nobel 1977*, "so that his name will continue to be on my papers as long as I publish and so that his contributions to our Service will be memorialized."

Yalow has received many other awards, honorary degrees, and lectureships, including the Georg Charles de Henesy Nuclear Medicine Pioneer Award in 1986 and the Scientific Achievement Award of the American Medical Society. In 1978, she hosted a five-part dramatic series on the life of French physical chemist Marie Curie, aired by the Public Broadcasting Service (PBS). In 1980, she became a distinguished professor at the Albert Einstein College of Medicine at Yeshiva University, leaving to become the Solomon A. Berson Distinguished Professor at Large at Mt. Sinai in 1986. She also chaired the Department of Clinical Science at Montefiore Hospital and Medical Center in the early- to mid-1980s.

The fact that Yalow was a trailblazer for women scientists was not lost on her. At a lecture before the Association of American Medical Colleges, as quoted in *Lady Laureates*, Yalow opined: "We cannot expect that in the foreseeable future women will achieve status in academic medicine in proportion to their numbers. But if we are to start working towards that goal we must believe in ourselves or no one else will believe in us; we must match our aspirations with the guts and determination to succeed; and for those of us who have had the good fortune to move upward, we must feel a personal responsibility to serve as role models and advisors to ease the path for those who come afterwards."

See also Laboratory techniques in immunology; Radioisotopes and their uses in microbiology and immunology

YEAST

Yeasts are single-celled **fungi**. Yeast species inhabit diverse habitats, including skin, marine water, leaves, and flowers.

Some yeast are beneficial, being used to produce bread or allow the **fermentation** of sugars to ethanol that occurs during beer and wine production (e.g., *Saccharomyces cerevisiae*). Other species of yeasts are detrimental to human health. An example is *Candida albicans*, the cause of vaginal infections, diaper rash in infants, and **thrush** in the mouth and throat. The latter infection is fairly common in those whose **immune system** is compromised by another infection such as acquired **immunodeficiency** syndrome.

The economic benefits of yeast have been known for centuries. *Saccharomyces carlsbergensis*, the yeast used in the production of various types of beer that result from "bottom fermentation," was isolated in 1888 by Dr. Christian Hansen at the Carlsberg Brewery in Copenhagen. During fermentation, some species of yeast are active at the top of the brew while others sink to the bottom. In contrast to *Saccharomyces carls-*

bergensis, *Saccharomyces cerevisiae* produces ales by "top fermentation." In many cases, the genetic manipulation of yeast has eliminated the need for the different yeast strains to produce beer or ale. In baking, the fermentation of sugars by the bread yeast *Ascomycetes* produces bubbles in the dough that makes the bread dough rise.

Yeasts are a source of B vitamins. This can be advantageous in diets that are low in meat. In the era of **molecular biology**, yeasts have proved to be extremely useful research tools. In particular, *Saccharomyces cerevisiae* has been a model system for studies of genetic regulation of cell division, **metabolism**, and the incorporation of genetic material between organisms. This is because the underlying molecular mechanisms are preserved in more complicated **eukaryotes**, including humans, and because the yeast cells are so easy to grow and manipulate. As well, *Ascomycetes* are popular for genetics research because the genetic information contained in the spores they produce result from meiosis. Thus, the four spores that are produced can contain different combinations of genetic material. This makes the study of genetic inheritance easy to do.

Another feature of yeast that makes them attractive as models of study is the ease by which their genetic state can be manipulated. At different times in the **cell cycle** yeast cells will contain one copy of the genetic material, while at other times two copies will be present. Conditions can be selected that maintain either the single or double-copy state. Furthermore, a myriad of yeast **mutants** have been isolated or created that are defective in various aspects of the cell division cycle. These mutants have allowed the division cycle to be deduced in great detail.

The division process in yeast occurs in several different ways, depending upon the species. Some yeast cells multiply by the formation of a small bud that grows to be the size of the parent cell. This process is referred to as budding. *Saccharomyces* reproduces by budding. The budding process is a sexual process, meaning that the genetic material of two yeast cells is combined in the offspring. The division process involves the formation of spores.

Other yeasts divide by duplicating all the cellular components and then splitting into two new daughter cells. This process, called binary fission, is akin to the division process in **bacteria**. The yeast genus *Schizosaccharomyces* replicates in this manner. This strain of yeast is used as a teaching tool because the division process is so easy to observe using an inexpensive light **microscope**.

The growth behavior of yeast is also similar to bacteria. Yeast cells display a lag phase prior to an explosive period of division. As some nutrient becomes depleted, the increase in cell number slows and then stops. If refrigerated in this stationary phase, cells can remain alive for months. Also like bacteria, yeast are capable of growth in the presence and the absence of oxygen.

The life cycle of yeast includes a step called meiosis. In meiosis pairs of **chromosomes** separate and the new combinations that form can give rise to new genetic traits in the daughter yeast cells. Meiosis is also a sexual feature of genetic replication that is common to all higher eukaryotes as well.

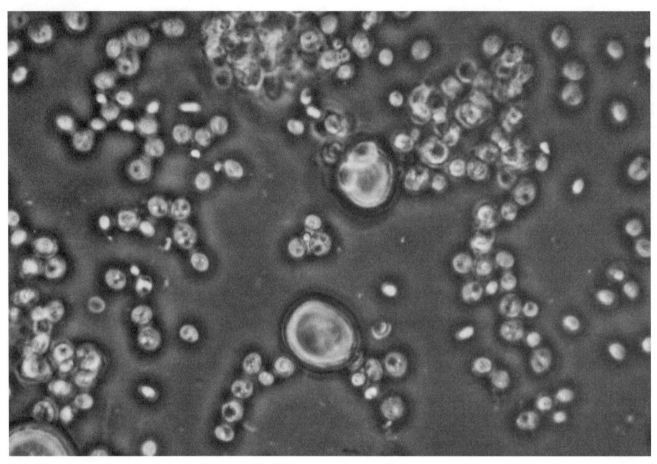

Light micrograph of baker's yeast.

Another feature of the sexual reproduction process in yeast is the production of pheromones by the cells. Yeast cells respond to the presence of the chemicals by changing their shape. The peanut-like shape they adopt has been dubbed "shmoos," after a character in the "Li'l Abner" comic strip. This shape allows two cells to associate very closely together.

See also Cell cycle (eukaryotic), genetic regulation of; Chromosomes, eukaryotic; Economic uses and benefits of microorganisms; Yeast artificial chromosome; Yeast, infectious

YEAST ARTIFICIAL CHROMOSOME (YAC)

The **yeast** artificial chromosome, which is often shortened to YAC, is an artificially constructed system that can undergo replication. The design of a YAC allows extremely large segments of genetic material to be inserted. Subsequent rounds of replication produce many copies of the inserted sequence, in a genetic procedure known as **cloning**.

The reason the cloning vector is called a yeast artificial chromosome has to do with the structure of the vector. The YAC is constructed using specific regions of the yeast chro-

mosome. Yeast cells contain a number of **chromosomes**; organized collections of **deoxyribonucleic acid (DNA)**. For example, the yeast *Saccaromyces cerevisae* contains 16 chromosomes that contain varying amounts of DNA. Each chromosome consists of two arms of DNA that are linked by a region known as the centromere. As the DNA in each arm is duplicated, the centromere provides a region of common linkage. This common area is the region to which components of the replication machinery of the cell attach and pull apart the chromosomes during the cell division process. Another region of importance is called the telomere. The end of each chromosome arm contains a region of DNA called the telomere. The telomere DNA does not code for any product, but serves as a border to define the size of the chromosome. Finally, each chromosome contains a region known as the origin of replication. The origin is where a molecule called DNA polymerase binds and begins to produce a copy of each strand of DNA in the double helix that makes up the chromosome.

The YAC was devised and first reported in 1987 by David Burke, who then also reported the potential to use the construct as a cloning vehicle for large pieces of DNA. Almost immediately, YACs were used in large-scale determination of genetic sequences, most prominently the Human Genome Project.

YAC contains the telomere, centromere, and origin of replication elements. If these elements are spliced into DNA in the proper location and orientation, then a yeast cell will replicate the artificial chromosome along with the other, natural chromosomes. The target DNA is flanked by the telomere regions that mark the ends of the chromosome, and is interspersed with the centromere region that is vital for replication. Finally, the start site for the copying process is present. In essence, the yeast is fooled into accepted genetic material that mimics a chromosome.

The origin of the DNA that is incorporated into a YAC is varied. DNA from prokaryotic organisms such as bacterial or from **eukaryotes** such a humans can be successfully used. The power of YACs is best explained by the size of the DNA that can be copied. **Bacteria** are also capable of cloning DNA from diverse sources, but the length of DNA that a bacterium can handle is up to 20 times less than that capable of being cloned using a YAC.

The engineered YAC is put back into a yeast cell by chemical means that encourage the cell to take up the genetic material. As the yeast cell undergoes rounds of growth and division, the artificial chromosome is replicated as if it were a natural chromosomal constituent of the cell. The result is a **colony** of many genetically identical yeast cells, each containing a copy of the target DNA. The target DNA has thus been amplified in content. Through a subsequent series of procedures, DNA can then be isolated from the rest of the DNA inside the yeast cells.

Use of different regions of DNA in different YACs allows the rapid determination of the sequence, or order of the constituents, of the DNA. YACs were invaluable in this regard in the sequencing of the human genome, which was completed in preliminary form in 2001 The human genome was broken into pieces using various **enzymes**. Each piece could be used to construct a YAC. Then, sufficient copies of each piece of the human genome could be generated so that automatic sequencing machines would have enough material to sequence the DNA.

Commonly, the cutting enzymes are selected so that the fragments of DNA that are generated contain overlapping regions. Once the sequences of all the DNA regions are obtained the common overlapping regions allow the fragment sequences to be chemically bonded so that the proper order and the proper orientation is generated. For example, if no overlapping regions were present, then one sequence could be inserted backwards with respect to the orientation of its neighbouring sequence.

See also Chromosomes, prokaryotic; Gene amplification; Yeast genetics

YEAST, ECONOMIC USES AND BENEFITS ·

see ECONOMIC USES AND BENEFITS OF MICROORGANISMS

YEAST GENETICS

Yeast genetics provides an excellent model for the study of the genetics of growth in animal and plant cells. The yeast *Saccharomyces cerevisiae* is similar to animal cells (e.g., similar length to the phases of its **cell cycle**, similarity of the chromosomal structures called telomeres). Another yeast, *Saccharomyces pombe* is rather more similar to plant cells (e.g., similarities in their patterns of division, and in organization of their genome).

As well as being a good model system to study the mechanics of eukaryotic cells, yeast is well suited for genetic studies. Yeasts are easy to work with in the laboratory. They have a rapid growth cycle (1.5 to two hours), so that many cycles can be studied in a day. Yeasts that are not a health threat are available, so the researcher is usually not in danger when handling the organisms. Yeasts exist that can be maintained with two copies of their genetic material (diploid state) or one copy (haploid state). Haploid strains can be mated together to produce a diploid that has genetic traits of both "parents." Finally, it is easy to introduce new **DNA** sequences into the yeast.

Genetic studies of the yeast cell cycle, the cycle of growth and reproduction, are particularly valuable. For example, the origin of a variety of cancers is a malfunction in some aspect of the cell cycle. Various strains of *Saccharomyces cerevisiae* and *Saccharomyces pombe* provide useful models of study because they are also defective in some part of their cell division cycle. In particular, cell division cycle (cdc) **mutants** are detected when the point in the cell cycle is reached where the particular protein coded for by the defective **gene** is active. These points where the function of the protein is critical have been dubbed the "execution points." **Mutations** that affect the cell division cycle tend to be clustered at two points in the cycle. One point is at the end of a phase known as G1. At the end of G1 a yeast cell becomes committed to the manufacture of DNA in the next phase of the cell cycle (S phase). The second cluster of mutations occurs at the beginning of a phase called the M phase, where the yeast cell commits to the separation of the chromosomal material in the process of mitosis.

Lee Hartwell of the University of Washington at Seattle spearheaded the analysis of the various cdc mutants in the 1960s and 1970s. His detailed examination of the blockage of the cell cycle at certain points—and the consequences of the blocks on later events—demonstrated, for example, that the manufacture of DNA was an absolute prerequisite for division of the nuclear material. In contrast the formation of the bud structures by *Saccharomyces pombe* can occur even when DNA replication is blocked.

Hartwell also demonstrated that the cell cycle depends on the completion of a step that was termed "start." This step is now known to be a central control point, where the cell essentially senses materials available to determine whether the growth rate of the cell will be sufficient to accumulate enough material to permit cell division to occur. Depending on the information, a yeast cell either commits to another cycle of cell growth and division or does not. These events have been confirmed by the analysis of a yeast cell mutant called cdc28. The cdc28 mutant is blocked at start and so does not enter S phase where the synthesis of DNA occurs.

Analysis of this and other cdc mutations has found a myriad of functions associated with the genetic mutations. For example, in yeast cells defective in a gene dubbed cdc2, the protein coded for by the cdc2 gene does not modify various proteins. The absence of these modifications causes defects in the aggregation of the chromosomal material prior to mitosis, the change in the supporting structures of the cell that are necessary for cell division, and the ability of the cell to change shape.

Studies of such cdc mutants has shown that virtually all eukaryotic cells contain a similar control mechanism that governs the ability of a cell to initiate mitosis. This central control point is affected by the activities of other proteins in the cell. A great deal of research effort is devoted to understanding this master control, because scientists presume that knowledge of its operation could help thwart the development of cancers related to a defect in the master control.

See also Cell cycle (eukaryotic), genetic regulation of; Genetic regulation of eukaryotic cells; Molecular biology and molecular genetics

YEAST, INFECTIOUS

Yeast are single-cell **fungi** with ovoid or spherical shapes, which are grouped according to the cell division process into budding yeast (e.g., the species and strains of *Saccharomyces cerevisiae* and *Blastomyces dermatitidis*), or fission yeast (e.g., *Schizosaccharomyces*) species.

Yeast species are present in virtually all natural environments such as fresh and marine water, soil, plants, animals, and in houses, hospitals, schools, etc. Some species are symbiotic, while others are parasitic. Parasitic species may be pathogenic (i.e., cause disease) either because of the toxins they release in the host organism or due to the direct destruction of living tissues such as skin, internal mucosa of the mouth, lungs, gastrointestinal, genital and urinary tracts of animals, along with plant flowers, fruits, seeds, and leaves. They are also involved in the deterioration and **contamination** of stored grains and processed foods.

Yeast and other fungal infections may be superficial (skin, hair, nails); subcutaneous (dermis and surrounding structures); systemic (affecting several internal organs, blood, and internal epithelia); or opportunistic (infecting neutropenic patients, such as cancer patients, transplant patients, and other immunocompromised patients). Opportunistic infections acquired by patients inside hospitals, or due to medical procedures such as catheters are termed **nosocomial infections**, and they are a major concern in **public health**, because they increase both mortality and the period of hospitalization. An epidemiological study, with data collected between 1997 and 2001 in 72 different hospitals in the United States, showed that 7–8% of the nosocomial blood-stream infections were due to a *Candida* species of yeast, especially *Candida albicans*. About 80% of *Candida* infections are nosocomial in the

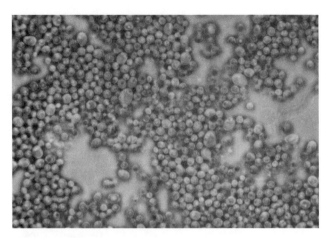

Light micrograph of *Candida albicans*.

United States, and approximately 50% of them are acquired in intensive care units. A national **epidemiology** of mycoses survey in the early 1990s showed that in neonatal ICUs *C. albicans* was the cause of about 75% of infections and *Candida parapsilosis* accounted for the remaining 25%. *Candida albicans* frequently infects infants during birth, due to its presence in the mother's vaginal mucosa, whereas *C. parapsilosis* was found in the hands of healthcare professionals of the neonatal ICUs. In surgical ICUs, *C. albicans* was implicated in 50% of infections while *Candida glabrata* responded for another 25% of the cases. The most frequently community-acquired yeast infections are the superficial mycoses, and among other pathogenic fungi, *Candida albicans* is the cause of mouth **thrush**, and vaginitis. Gastrointestinal yeast infections are also transmitted by contaminated saliva and foods.

Although immunocompetent individuals may host *Candida* species and remain asymptomatic for many years, the eventual occurrence of a debilitating condition may trigger a systemic **candidiasis**. Systemic candidiasis is a chronic infection that usually starts in the gastrointestinal tract and gradually spreads to other organs and tissues, and the *Candida* species commonly involved is *C. albicans*. They release about 79 different toxins in the hosts' organism, and the lesions they cause in the intestinal membranes compromise nutrient absorption by reducing it to about 50% of the normal capacity. *C. albicans* intestinal colonization and lesions expose internal tissues and capillary vessels to contamination by **bacteria** present in fecal material. The elderly, cancer patients, and infants are especially susceptible to *Candida* infections, as are **AIDS** patients. In the long run, systemic candidiasis may lead to a variety of symptoms, such as chronic fatigue, **allergies**, cystitis, endometriosis, diarrhea, colitis, respiratory disorders, dry mouth, halitosis (bad breath), emotional disorders, etc.

The indiscriminate prescription and intake of **antibiotics** usually kills bacteria that are essential for normal digestion and favors the opportunistic spread of *Candida* species on the walls of the digestive tract, which can be worsened when associated with a diet rich in sugars and carbohydrates. Once yeast species colonize the intestinal walls, treatment becomes difficult and is usually followed by recurrence. Another challenge when yeast systemic infection is involved is that they are not detected by standard blood tests. However, laboratorial analysis of collected samples of mucus and affected tissue may detect yeast infection and identify the implicated species.

Another yeast infection, known as blastomycosis, is caused by the species *Blastomyces dermatitidis,* a spherical budding yeast. The main targets of this pathogen are the lung alveoli (60%). Pulmonary blastomycosis is not easily diagnosed because its symptoms are also present in other lung infections, such as cough, chest pain, hemoptysis, and weight loss. Pulmonary lesions may include nodules, cavities, and infiltration, with the severe cases presenting pleuritis. Blastomycosis may also be disseminated to other organs, such as liver, central nervous system, adrenal glands, pancreas, bones, lymph nodes, and gastrointestinal and genitourinary tracts. Osteomyelitis (bone infection) and arthritis may also be caused by this yeast, and about 33% of the patients were diagnosed with skeletal blastomycosis as well. Although the cutaneous chronic infection is curable, the systemic form of the disease has a poor prognosis.

See also Food preservation; Food safety; Mycology; Nosocomial infections; Parasites; Yeast artificial chromosome (YAC); Yeast genetics

YELLOW FEVER

Yellow fever is the name given to a disease that is caused by the yellow fever virus. The virus is a member of the flavivirus group. The name of the disease is derived from the appearance of those infected, who usually present a jaundiced appearance (yellow-tinted skin).

The agent of infection of yellow fever is the mosquito. The agent was first identified in 1900 when the United States Army Yellow Fever Commission (also referred to as the Reed Commission after its leader, Walter Reed) proved that the mosquito species *Aedes aegypti* was responsible for spreading the disease. Until then, yellow fever was regarded as requiring direct person-to-person contact or contact with a contaminated object.

The disease has caused large outbreaks involving many people in North America, South America, and Africa, stretching back at least to the 1700s. At that time the disease was often fatal. The availability of a **vaccine** reduced the incidence and mortality of the disease considerably in the latter part of the twentieth century. However, since 1980 the number of cases of the disease has begun to rise again.

There are now about 200,000 estimated cases of yellow fever in the world each year. Of these, some 30,000 people die. Most researchers and health officials regard these numbers as underestimates, due to underreporting and because in the initial stages yellow fever can be misdiagnosed.

The yellow fever virus infects humans and monkeys—no other hosts are known. Humans become infected when the virus is transmitted from monkeys to humans by mosquitoes. This is referred to as horizontal transmission. Several different species of mosquito are capable of transmitting the virus.

Mosquitoes can also pass the virus to their own offspring via infected eggs. This form of transmission is called vertical transmission. When the offspring hatch they are already infected and can transmit the virus to humans when they have a blood meal. Vertical transmission can be particularly insidious as the eggs are very hardy and can resist dry conditions, hatching when the next rainy season occurs. Thus the infection can be continued from one year to the next even when there is no active infection occurring in a region.

The different habitats of the mosquitoes ensures a wide distribution of the yellow fever virus. Some of the mosquito species breed in urban areas while others are confined to rural regions. The latter types were associated with the outbreak of yellow fever that struck workers during the construction of the Panama Canal in Central America in the nineteenth century. In South America a concerted campaign to control mosquito populations up until the 1970s greatly reduced the number of cases of yellow fever. However, since that time the control programs have lapsed and yellow fever has increased as the mosquito populations have increased.

Infection with the yellow fever virus sometimes produced no symptoms whatsoever. However, in many people, so-called acute (rapid-onset, intense) symptoms appear about three to six days after infection. The symptoms include fever, muscle pain (particularly in the back), headache, chills, nausea, and vomiting. In this early stage the disease is easily confused with a number of other diseases, including **malaria**, **typhoid fever**, **hemorrhagic fevers** such as Lassa fever, and viral **hepatitis**. Diagnosis requires the detection of an **antibody** to the virus in the blood. Such diagnosis is not always possible in underdeveloped regions or in rural areas that are distant from medical facilities and trained laboratory personnel.

In many people the acute symptoms last only a few days and recovery is complete. However, in about 15% of those infected, the disease enters what is termed the toxic phase: a fever reappears and several regions of the body become infected as the virus disseminates from the point of the mosquito bite. Disruption of liver function produces jaundice. Kidney function can also be damaged and even totally shut down. Recovery from this more serious phase of the infection can be complete; although half of those who are afflicted die.

Yellow fever appears in human populations in different ways. One pattern of appearance is called sylvatic (or jungle) yellow fever. As the name implies, this form is restricted to regions that are largely uninhabited by humans. The virus cycles between the indigenous monkey population and the mosquitoes that bite them. Humans that enter the region, such as loggers, can become infected.

Another cycle of infection is referred to as intermediate yellow fever. This infection is found in semi-urban areas, such as where villages are separated by intervening areas of farmland or more natural areas. Infections can spring up in several areas simultaneously. Migration of people from the infected areas to larger population centers can spread the infection. This is the most common pattern of yellow fever occurring in present day Africa.

The final pattern of yellow fever is that which occurs in fully urban settings. The large population base can produce a large epidemic. The infection is spread exclusively by mosquitoes feeding on one person then on another. Control of these **epidemics** concentrates on eradicating the mosquito populations.

Treatment for yellow fever consists primarily of keeping the patient hydrated and comfortable. Prevention of the infection, via **vaccination**, is the most prudent course of action. The current vaccine (which consists of living but weakened virus) is safe and provides long-lasting **immunity**. While side effects are possible, the risks of not vaccinating far outweigh the risk of the adverse vaccine reactions. For a vaccination campaign to be effective, over 80% of the people in a suspect region need to be vaccinated. Unfortunately few countries in Africa have achieved this level of coverage. Another course of action is the control of mosquito populations, typically by spraying with a compound that is toxic to mosquito larvae during breeding season. Once again, this coverage must be extensive to be successful. Breeding areas missed during spraying ensure the re-emergence of mosquitoes and, hence, of the yellow fever virus.

See also Transmission of pathogens; Zoonoses

Z

ZIEHL-NEELSEN STAIN • *see* LABORATORY TECH-
NIQUES IN MICROBIOLOGY

ZOBELL, CLAUDE EPHRAIM (1904-1989)
American microbiologist and marine biologist

Claude Ephraim ZoBell's research confirmed several behavioral characteristics of water and ocean-borne **bacteria**. ZoBell researched the special adhesive properties of organisms to surfaces, and experimented with mean of controlling such populations. He also was one of the pioneering scientists to study marine pollution. His work continues to be utilized by marine biologists, petroleum engineers, and the shipping industry.

ZoBell was born in Provo, Utah, but his family moved to Rigby, Idaho, when he was young. He pursued studies in biology and bacteriology at the University of California at Berkeley. By the time he was awarded his Ph.D. in 1931, he had already conducted several studies on the **biochemistry** of various bacteria and developed his interest in marine biology.

ZoBell's first position was as Instructor of **Marine Microbiology** at the Scripps Institute of Oceanography. He was made a full professor in 1948 after conducting research in environmental biology. While at the Scripps Institute, ZoBell left his research in medical microbiology in favor of pursuing his interests in marine life. Thus, ZoBell was among the first generations of modern marine biologists.

Most of ZoBell's career defining research was conducted while at Scripps. ZoBell noted that most of the research done at the institute focused on relationships between various groups of organisms, instead of trying to isolate various organisms in a specific environment. Also, he quickly found that he, as well as other marine scientists, were frustrated by difficulties in reproducing marine conditions and organism behavior and growth in the lab.

ZoBell and his colleagues devised a number of technical innovations and methodological procedures that help to overcome such obstacles to their research. For example, ZoBell designed a slide carrier that could be lowered into the water to study the attachment of organisms to surfaces, thus eliminating the need to **culture** or breed organisms in the lab. Organisms that colonized the slide carrier were removed from the water and instantly processed for microscopic observation. The device proved successful, eliminating the need for a multitude of culture media in the lab. This microscopic observation of cultured slides became known as biofilm microbiology.

ZoBell and his colleagues also conducted experiments on bacteria and organism levels in seawater. The scientists lowered a series of sterile glass bottles into the water, permitted water to flow in and out of the bottles for several days, and then raised the bottles. ZoBell found that bacterial levels were higher on the glass than in the liquid. Thus, ZoBell devised that certain organisms have a certain "sticking power" and prefer to colonize surfaces rather than remain free-floating. The experiment was repeated in the lab using seawater specimens, with similar results. The exact nature of this sticking power, be it with barnacles or bacteria, remains alusive.

After receiving several rewards for his research at the Scripps Institute for Oceanography, ZoBell briefly researched and taught at Princeton University, in Europe, and spent time at several other oceanographic research institutes. He returned to the Scripps Institute and turned his attention to the effects of pollution and petroleum drilling on marine environments. He remained a passionate advocate for marine preservation and research until his death.

See also Biofilm formation and dynamic behavior

ZOONOSES

Zoonoses are diseases of microbiological origin that can be transmitted from animals to people. The causes of the diseases can be **bacteria**, **viruses**, **parasites**, and **fungi**.

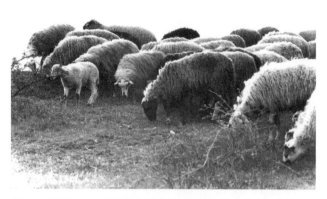

Sheep can act as host for a number of zoonotic disease pathogens.

Zoonoses are relevant for humans because of their species-jumping ability. Because many of the causative microbial agents are resident in domestic animals and birds, agricultural workers and those in food processing plants are at risk. From a research standpoint, zoonotic diseases are interesting as they result from organisms that can live in a host innocuously while producing disease upon entry into a different host environment.

Humans can develop zoonotic diseases in different ways, depending upon the microorganism. Entry through a cut in the skin can occur with some bacteria. Inhalation of bacteria, viruses, and fungi is also a common method of transmission. As well, the ingestion of improperly cooked food or inadequately treated water that has been contaminated with the fecal material from animals or birds present another route of disease transmission.

A classic historical example of a zoonotic disease is **yellow fever**. The construction of the Panama Canal took humans into the previously unexplored regions of the Central American jungle. Given the opportunity, transmission from the resident animal species to the newly arrived humans occurred. This phenomenon continues today. Two examples are illustrative of this. First, the clearing of the Amazonian rain forest to provide agricultural land has resulted in the emergence of Mayaro and Oropouche virus infections in the woodcutters. Second, in the mid 1990s, fatalities in the Southwestern United States were traced to the hanta virus that has been transmitted from rodents to humans.

A number of bacterial zoonotic diseases are known. A few examples are **Tularemia**, which is caused by *Francisella tulerensis*, Leptospirosis (*Leptospiras spp.*), **Lyme disease** (*Borrelia burgdorferi*), Chlaydiosis (*Chlamydia psittaci*), Salmonellosis (*Salmonella spp.*), **Brucellosis** (*Brucella melitensis, suis,* and *abortus*), Q-fever (*Coxiella burnetti*), and **Campylobacteriosis** (*Campylobacter jejuni*).

Zoonoses produced by fungi, and the organism responsible, include Aspergillosis (*Aspergillus fumigatus*). Well-known viral zoonoses include **rabies** and encephalitis. The **microorganisms** called Chlamydia cause a **pneumonia**-like disease called psittacosis.

Within the past two decades two protozoan zoonoses have definitely emerged. These are **Giardia** (also commonly known as "beaver fever"), which is caused by *Giardia lamblia* and **Cryptosporidium**, which is caused by *Cryptosporidium parvum*. These protozoans reside in many vertebrates, particularly those associated with wilderness areas. The increasing encroachment of human habitations with wilderness is bringing the animals, and their resident microbial flora, into closer contact with people.

Similarly, human encroachment is thought to be the cause for the emergence of devastatingly fatal viral **hemorrhagic fevers**, such as Ebola and Rift Valley fever. While the origin of these agents is not definitively known, zoonotic transmission is assumed.

In the present day, outbreaks of hoof and mouth disease among cattle and sheep in the United Kingdom (the latest being in 2001) has established an as yet unproven, but compelling, zoonotic link between these animals and humans, involving the disease causing entities known as **prions**. While the story is not fully resolved, the current evidence supports the transmission of the prion agent of mad cow disease to humans, where the similar brain degeneration disease is known as Creutzfeld-Jacob disease.

The increasing incidence of these and other zoonotic diseases has been linked to the increased ease of global travel. Microorganisms are more globally portable than ever before. This, combined with the innate ability of microbes to adapt to new environments, has created new combinations of microorganism and susceptible human populations.

See also Animal models of infection; Bacteria and bacterial infection

ZOOPLANKTON

Zooplankton are small animals that occur in the water column of either marine or freshwater ecosystems. Zooplankton are a diverse group defined on the basis of their size and function, rather than on their taxonomic affinities.

Most species in the zooplankton community fall into three major groups—Crustacea, Rotifers, and Protozoas. Crustaceans are generally the most abundant, especially those in the order Cladocera (waterfleas), and the class Copepoda (the copepods), particularly the orders Calanoida and Cyclopoida. Cladocerans are typically most abundant in fresh water, with common genera including Daphnia and Bosmina. Commonly observed genera of marine calanoid copepods include Calanus, Pseudocalanus, and Diaptomus, while abundant cyclopoid copepods include Cyclops and Mesocyclops. Other crustaceans in the zooplankton include species of opossum shrimps (order Mysidacea), amphipods (order Amphipoda), and fairy shrimp (order Anostraca). Rotifers (phylum Rotifera) are also found in the zooplankton, as are protozoans (kingdom Protista). Insects may also be important, especially in fresh waters close to the shoreline.

Most zooplankton are secondary consumers, that is, they are herbivores that graze on phytoplankton, or on unicellular or colonial algae suspended in the water column. The productivity of the zooplankton community is ultimately limited by the productivity of the small algae upon which they feed. There are times when the biomass of the zooplankton at any given time may be similar to, or even exceed, that of the phytoplankton. This occurs because the animals of the zooplankton are relatively long-lived compared with the algal cells upon which they feed, so the turnover of their biomass is much less rapid. Some members of the zooplankton are detritivores, feeding on suspended organic detritus. Some species of zooplankton are predators, feeding on other species of zooplankton, and some spend part of their lives as **parasites** of larger animals, such as fish.

Zooplankton are important in the food webs of open-water ecosystems, in both marine and fresh waters.

Zooplankton are eaten by relatively small fish (called planktivorous fish), which are then eaten by larger fish. Zooplankton are an important link in the transfer of energy from the algae (the primary producers) to the ecologically and economically important fish community (the consumers).

Species of zooplankton vary in their susceptibility to environmental stressors, such as exposure to toxic chemicals, acidification of the water, eutrophication and oxygen depletion, or changes in temperature. As a result, the species assemblages (or communities) of zooplankton are indicators of environmental quality and ecological change.

See also Bioremediation; Indicator species; Water pollution and purification

Sources Consulted

Books

Abbas, A. K., A. H. Lichtman, and J. S. Pober. *Cellular and Molecular Immunology.* Philadelphia: W. B. Saunders Co., 1997.

Ackermann U. *Essentials of Human Physiology.* St. Louis: Mosby Year Book, Inc., 1992.

Ahmadjian, V. *The Lichen Symbiosis.* New York: John Wiley & Sons, 1993.

Alberts, B., et al. *Molecular Biology of the Gene,* 2nd ed. New York: Garland Publishing, Inc., 1989.

————. *Molecular Biology of the Cell.* 3rd ed. NewYork: Garland Publishing, Inc., 1994.

Alexopoulos, C. J., et. al. *Introductory Mycology.* New York: John Wiley & Sons, 1996.

Allen, Garland E., William E. Castle, Charles C. Gillispie, eds. *Dictionary of Scientific Biography,* Vol. 3. New York: Scribner, 1971.

American Water Works Association. *Water Quality and Treatment,* 5th ed. Denver: American Water Works Association, 1999.

Atherton, J. C., and M. J. Blaser. "Helicobacter Infections." In *Harrison's Principles of Internal Medicine,* 14th ed., edited by Anthony S. Fauci, et al. New York: McGraw-Hill, 1998.

Audesirk, T., and G. Audesirk. *Biology: Life on Earth,* 4th ed. New Jersey: Prentice Hall Publishing, Inc.,1996.

Baltzer, F. *Theodor Boveri: Life and Work of a Great Biologist.* Berkeley, CA: University of California Press, 1967.

Barlett, D. H. *Molecular Marine Microbiology.* Oxford: Horizon Books, 2000.

Baum, Stuart J., and Charles W. J. Scaife. *Chemistry: A Life Science Approach.* New York: Macmillan Publishing Company, Inc., 1975.

Beers, M. H. and R. Berkow, eds. *The Merck Manual of Diagnosis and Therapy.* Whitehouse Station, New Jersey: Merck & Co., Inc., 2002.

Benenson, A. S. Giardiasis *Control of Communicable Diseases Manual.* Washington: American Public Health Association, 1995.

Bennett, J. C., and F. Plum, Cecil. *Textbook of Medicine.* Philadelphia: W. B. Saunders Co., 1996.

Bennish, M. L., and C. Seas. *Current Diagnosis,* Vol. 9. Philadelphia: W. B. Saunders Company, 1997.

Berkow, Robert, and Andrew J. Fletcher. *The Merck Manual of Diagnosis and Therapy.* Rahway, New Jersey: Merck Research Laboratories, 1992.

Berkow, Robert, ed. *Merck Manual of Medical Information.* Whitehouse Station, NJ: Merck Research Laboratories, 1997.

Beurton, Peter, Raphael Falk, Hans-Jørg Rheinberger., eds. *The Concept of the Gene in Development and Evolution.* Cambridge, UK: Cambridge University Press, 2000.

Beveridge, T. J., and S. F. Koval. *Advances in Bacterial Paracrystalline Surface Layers.* New York: Plenum Press, 1993.

Bierman W. and D. Pearlman, eds. *Allergic Diseases from Infancy to Adulthood.* Reprint. Philadelphia: W. B. Saunders, 1987.

Bodmer, W. F., L. L. Cavalli-Sforza. *Genetics, Evolution and Man.* San Francisco: W. D. Freeman, 1976.

Bolin, B., and R. B. Cook. *The Major Biogeochemical Cycles and Their Interactions.* New York:John Wiley & Sons, 1983.

Bonner, J. T. *First Signals: The Evolution of Multicellular Development.* Princeton, N. J. : Princeton University Press, 2000.

————. *The Ideas of Biology.* New York: Harper & Row, 1962.

Borgstrom, Georg. *Principles of Food Science.* Vol. I. New York: The Macmillan Company, 1969.

Bourrelly, P. *Les Algues D'Eau Douce.* Vol. II. Paris: Editions N. Boubee & Cie., 1968.

Bowler, Peter J. *The Mendelian Revolution: The Emergence of Hereditarian Concepts in Modern Science and Society.* Baltimore: Johns Hopkins University Press, 1989.

Boylan, M. *Method and Practice in Aristotle's Biology.* Lanham, MD: University Press of America, 1983.

Brady, James E., and John R. Holum. *Fundamentals of Chemistry.* 2nd ed. New York: John Wiley & Sons, 1984.

Branden, C., and J. Tooze. *Introduction to Protein Structure,* 2nd ed. London: Garland Publishing, Inc., 1999.

Brandt, Allan M. *No Magic Bullet: A Social History of Venereal Disease in the United States Since 1880.* New York: Oxford University Press, 1987.

Brooker, R. *Genetics Analysis and Principals.* Menlo Park: Benjamin Cummings, 1999.

Brown, Harold, and Franklin Neva. *Basic Clinical Parasitology.* Norwalk, CT: Appleton-Century-Crofts, 1983.

Buchanan, R. E., and N. E. Gibbons. *Bergey's Manual of Determinative Bacteriology,* 8th ed. Baltimore: The Williams & Wilkins Company, 1974.

Cahill. M. *Handbook of Diagnostic Tests.* Springhouse: Springhouse Company, 1995.

Campbell, N., J. Reece, and L. Mitchell. *Biology,* 5th ed. Menlo Park: Benjamin Cummings, Inc. 2000.

Carlson, E. A. *The Gene: A Critical History.* Philadelphia: Saunders, 1966

Carter, Richard. *Breakthrough: The Saga of Jonas Salk.* Naples, FL: Trident Press, 1966.

Caul, E. O. *Immunofluorescence.* London: Public Health laboratory Service, 1992.

Charlebois, R. *Organization of the Prokaryotic Genome.* Washington, D. C. : American Society for Microbiology, 1999.

Clarke, C. A. *Human Genetics and Medicine,* 3rd ed. Baltimore, MD: E. Arnold, 1987.

Clydesdale, Fergus, ed. *Food Science and Nutrition: Current Issues and Answers.* Englewood Cliffs, N. J. : Prentice-Hall, 1979.

Cole, Leonard A. *The Eleventh Plague: The Politics of Biological and Chemical Warfare.* New York: WH Freeman and Company, 1996.

Collier, L., A. Balows, and M. Sussman. Topley and Wilson's Microbiology and Microbial Infections, 9th ed. NewYork: Arnold Publishing, Inc., 1998.

Colliers, A,. et al. *Microbiology and Microbiological Infections,* vol. 3. London: Edward Arnold Press, 1998.

Colwell R. R., D. G. Swartz, M. T. McDonald, eds. *Biomolecular Data: A Resource in Transition.* Oxford: Oxford University Press, 1989.

Connor, J., and C. Baxter. *Kelp Forests.* Monterey, CA: Monterey Bay Aquarium Foundation, 1980.

Conway, P. L., and A. Henriksson. *Human Health: The Contribution of Microorganisms.* Berlin: Springer-Verlag, 1994.

Cooper, Geoffrey M. *The Cell: A Molecular Approach.* Washington DC: ASM Press, 1997.

Cormican, M. G. and M. A. Pfaller. "Molecular Pathology of Infectious Diseases," in *Clinical Diagnosis and Management by Laboratory Methods,* 20th ed., J. B. Henry, ed. Philadelphia: W. B. Saunders, 2001.

Crosby, A. *America's Forgotten Pandemic: The Influenza of 1918.* Cambridge: Cambridge University Press, 1989.

Curson, Marjorie. *Jonas Salk.* New Jersey: Silver Burdett, 1990.

Daintith, John and D. Gjertsen, eds. *A Dictionary of Scientists.* New York: Oxford University Press, 1999.

Dando, Malcolm. *Biological Warfare in the 21st Century.* New York: Macmillan, 1994.

Darnell, J., H. Lodish, and D. Baltimore. *Molecular Cell Biology.* New York: Scientific American Books Inc., 1986

Darwin, C. R. *The Origin of the Species.* London: John Murray, 1859.

Davies, Robert and Susan Ollier. *Allergy: The Facts.* Oxford: Oxford University Press, 1989.

Davis, R. H. *Neurospora—Contributions of a Model Organism.* Oxford: Oxford University Press, 2000.

Dawes, C. J. *Biological Techniques in Electron Microscopy.* NewYork: Barnes and Noble, 1979.

Dawkins, R. *The Selfish Gene.* Oxford: Oxford University Press. 1989.

DeGrood, David H. *Haeckel's Theory of the Unity of Nature: A Monograph in the History of Philosophy.* Boston: Christopher, 1965.

Doyle, M. P., and V. S. Padhye. *Escherichia coli In Foodborne Bacterial Pathogens.* NewYork: Marcel Dekker, Inc., 1989.

Drew, W. Lawrence. "Chlamydia." *Sherris Medical Microbiology: An Introduction to Infectious Diseases,* 3rd ed. Ed. Kenneth J. Ryan. Norwalk, CT: Appleton & Lange, 1994.

Droegemueller, William. "Infections of the Lower Genital Tract." In *Comprehensive Gynecology,* edited by Arthur L. Herbst, et. al., pp. 633–90. St. Louis: Mosby Year Book, 1992.

Edwards, L. E. "Dinoflagellates" *Fossil Prokaryotes and Protists.* Lipps, J. H., ed. Boston: Blackwell Scientific Publications, 1993.

Ehrlich, H. L. *Geomicrobiology,* 2nd ed. New York: Marcel Dekker, Inc. 1996.

Elseth, G. D., and K. D. Baumgardner. *Principles of Modern Genetics.* Minnesota: West Publishing Co., 1995.

Embree, Harland D. *Brief Course: Organic Chemistry.* Glenview, IL: Scott, Foresman, 1983.

Emde, Robert N., and John K. Hewitt, eds. *Infancy to Early Childhood: Genetic and Environmental Influences on Developmental Change.* New York: Oxford University Press, 2001.

Emery, A. E. H. *Neuromuscular Disorders: Clinical and Molecular Genetics.* Chicester: John Wiley & Sons, 1998.

Engs, R. C., ed. *Controversies in the Addiction's Field.* Dubuque: Kendal-Hunt, 1990.

Estuarine Microbial Ecology. Columbia: University of South Carolina Press, 1973.

Fauci, A., ed. *Harrison's Principles of Internal Medicine,* 14th ed. NewYork: McGraw-Hill, 1997.

Fleming, D. O., and D. L. Hunt. *Biological Safety: Principles and Practices,* 3rd ed. Washington: American Society for Microbiology, 2000.

Flint, S. J., et al. *Principles of Virology: Molecular Biology, Pathogenesis, and Control.* Washington: American Society for Microbiology, 1999.

Foo, E. L., et al. *The Lactic Acid Bacteria.* Norfolk: Horizon Scientific Press, 1997.

Foster, M. S., and D. R. Scheil. *The Ecology of Giant Kelp Forests in California: A Community Pprofile.* U. S. Fish and Wildlife Service, 1985.

Freedman, B. *Environmental Ecology,* 2nd ed. New York: Academic Press, 1994.

Friedman, J., F. Dill, M. Hayden, B. McGillivray. *Genetics.* Maryland: Williams & Wilkins, 1996.

Fruton, J. S. *Molecules and Life. Historical Essays on the Interplay of Chemistry and Biology.* New York: Wiley-Interscience, 1972.

Futuyama, D. J. *Evolutionary Biology.* Sunderland, MA: Sinauer Associates, Inc., 1979.

Ganong W. F. *Review of Medical Physiology,* 16th ed. Prentice-Hall International, Inc., 1993.

Gardner, Joan F. and Peel Margaret M. *Introduction to Sterilization and Disinfection.* Melbourne: Churchill Livingstone, 1986.

Garrett, L. *The Coming Plague: Newly Emerging Diseases in a World out of Balance.* New York: Penguin Books, 1995.

Gaskings, E. *Investigations into Generation 1651–1828.* Baltimore, MD: Johns Hopkins University Press, 1967.

Gasman, Daniel. *Haeckel's Monism and the Birth of Fascist Ideology.* New York: Peter Lang, 1998.

Gasman, Daniel. *The Scientific Origins of National Socialism: Social Darwinism in Ernst Haeckel and the German Monist League.* London: Macdonald, 1971.

Geison G. L. *The Private Science of Louis Pasteur.* Princeton: Princeton University Press, 1995.

Gilbert, S. F., ed. *A Conceptual History of Modern Embryology.* Baltimore, MD: Johns Hopkins Press, 1991.

Gould, Stephen Jay. *Ever Since Darwin: Reflections in Natural History.* New York: W. W. Norton & Co., 1977.

Griffiths, A. et al. *Introduction to Genetic Analysis,* 7th ed. New York, W. H. Freeman and Co., 2000.

Gronowicz, Antoni. *Bela Schick and the World of Children.* New York: Abelard-Shuman, 1954.

Guyton & Hall. *Textbook of Medical Physiology,* 10th ed. New York: W. B. Saunders Company, 2000.

Hamburger, V. *Heritage of Experimental Embryology.* New York: Oxford University Press, 1988.

Harden, Victoria Angela. *Rocky Mountain Spotted Fever: History of a Twentieth-Century Disease.* Baltimore: Johns Hopkins University Press, 1990.

Hardy, Anne. *The Epidemic Streets: Infectious Diseases and the Rise of Preventive Medicine, 1956–1900.* New York: Oxford University Press, 1993.

Hargrove, Jim. *The Story of Jonas Salk and the Discovery of the Polio Vaccine.* Children's Press, 1990.

Harper, David R. and Andrea S. Meyer. *Of Mice, Men, and Microbes: Hantavirus.* San Diego: Academic Press., 1999.

Hendin, David. *The Life Givers.* New York: Wm. Morrow & Co., 1976.

Herskowitz, I. H. *Genetics, 2nd ed. Boston: Little, Brown and Company, 1965.*

•

Hintzsche, Erich. "Rudolf Albert von Koelliker." *Dictionary of Scientific Biography.* , vol. 7 (1973): 437-440.

Hobot, J. A. . *Bacterial Ultrastructure.* London: San Diego: Academic Press, 2001.

Hoehling, A. A. *The Great Epidemic.* Boston: Little, Brown and Company, 1961.

Hopkins, Donald R. *Princes and Peasants, Smallpox in History.* Chicago: The University of Chicago Press, 1983.

Hopla, C. E., and A. K. Hopla. "Tularemia" *Handbook of Zoonoses.* Boca Raton: CRC Press, 1994.

Horder, T. J., J. A. Witkowski, and C. C. Wylie, eds. *A History of Embryology.* New York: Cambridge University Press, 1986.

Hughes, Arthur. *A History of Cytology.* London: Abelard-Schuman, 1959.

Hughes, S. *The Virus: A History of the Concept.* New York: Science History Publications, 1977.

Hurst, C. J., R. L. Crawford, G. R. Knudsen, M. J. McInerney, and L. D. Stetzenbach. *Manual of Environmental Microbiology,* 2nd ed. Washington: American Society for Microbiology, 2001.

Ingraham, C. A., and J. L. Ingraham. *Introduction to Microbiology,* 2nd ed. Pacific Grove: Brooks/Cole Publishing Co., 1999.

Ingram, V. M. *Hemoglobins in Genetics & Evolution.* New York: Columbia University Press, 1963.

Irion, C. W. *Home Winemaking Chem. 101.* Philadelphia: Xlibris Corporation, 2000.

Isenberg, H. D. *Clinical Microbiology Procedures Handbook.* Washington: American Society for Microbiology, 1992.

Isselbacher, Kurt J., et al. *Harrison's Principles of Internal Medicine.* New York: McGraw Hill, 1994.

Jacob, François *The Logic of Life: A History of Heredity.* New York: Pantheon, 1973.

Jacobs, D. S. *Laboratory Test Handbook,* 4th ed. Cleveland: Lexi-Comp, Inc., 1996.

Jacobson, Michael F. *Eater's Digest: The Consumer's Factbook of Food Additives.* Garden City, NY: Doubleday and Company, Inc., 1972.

Jenkins, John B. *Human Genetics,* 2nd ed. New York: Harper & Row, 1990.

Johnson, George, and Peter Raven. *Biology: Principles & Explorations.* Austin: Holt, Rinehart, and Winston, Inc., 1996.

Joklik, Wolfgang K., et al. Zinsser *Microbiology,* 20th ed. Norwalk, Conn. : Appleton and Lange, 1992.

Jones, E. W., J. R. Pringle, and J. R. Broach. *The Molecular and Cellular Biology of the Yeast* Saccharomyces cere-

visiae:. Gene Expression. Cold Spring Harbor: Cold Spring Harbor Press, 1992.

Jorde, L. B., J. C. Carey, M. J. Bamshad, and R. L. White. *Medical Genetics,* 2nd ed. Mosby-Year Book, Inc., 2000.

Julich, W. *Color Atlas of Micromycetes.* New York: VCH Publishers, 1993.

Kass-Simon, G., and P. Farnes. *Women of Science.* Bloomington: Indiana University Press, 1990.

Katsaros, P. *Illustrated Guide to Common Slime Molds.* Eureka, CA: Mad River Press, 1989.

Kay, L. E. *Who Wrote the Book of Life? A History of the Genetic Code.* Stanford: Stanford University Press.

Keenan, Katherine. "Lilian Vaughan Morgan (1870–1952)." *Women in the Biological Sciences: A Biobibliographic Sourcebook.* Ed. Grinstein, Louise A., Carol A. Biermann, and Rose K. Rose. Westport, CT: Greenwood Press, 1997.

Kendrew, J., et al. *The Encyclopedia of Molecular Biology.* Oxford: Blackwell Science Ltd., 1994.

Keusch, Gerald T. "Diseases Caused by Gram-Negative Bacteria" *Harrison's Principles of Internal Medicine.* New York: McGraw-Hill, 1998.

Klaassen, Curtis D. *Casarett and Doull's Toxicology* . 6 th ed. Columbus: McGraw-Hill, Inc. 2001.

Koch, A. L. *Bacterial Growth and Form.* Dordrecht: Kluwer Academic Publishers, 2001.

Koneman, E., et al., eds. *Color Atlas and Textbook of Diagnostic Microbiology,* 4th ed. Philadelphia: J. B. Lippincott, 1992.

Krasner, R. I. *The Microbial Challenge: Human-Microbe Interactions.* Washington: American Society for Microbiology, 2002.

Krug, R. M., J. S. Flint, L. W. Enquist, V. R. Racaniello, and A. M. Skalka. *Principles of Virology.* Washington: American Society for Microbiology, 1999.

Krugman, Saul, et al. *Infectious Diseases of Children.* St. Louis: Mosby-Year Book, Inc., 1992.

Kupchella, C. E. *Environmental Science: Living within the System of Nature,* 3rd ed. Boston: Allyn and Bacon, 1993.

Labuza, Theodore P. *Food and Your Well-Being.* St. Paul, MN: West Publishing Company, 1977.

Lechevalier, Herbert A., and Solotorovsky, Morris, eds. *Modern Scientists and Engineers,* Vol. 1 Columbus: McGraw-Hill, 1980.

Lechevalier, Herbert A., and Solotorovsky, Morris, eds. *Three Centuries of Microbiology.* Columbus: McGraw-Hill, 1965.

Lee, J. J., S. H. Hutner, and E. C. Bovee, eds. *An Illustrated Guide to the Protozoa.* Lawrence, Kansas:Society of Protozoologists, 1985.

Lewin, B. *Genes VII*. New York, Oxford University Press Inc., 2000

Lewis, Ricki. *Human Genetics: Concepts and Applications*. 2nd ed. IA: William C. Brown, Publishers, 1997.

Lide, D. R., ed. *CRC Handbook of Chemistry and Physics*. Boca Raton: CRC Press, 2001.

Lobban C. S., and P. J. Harrison. *Seaweed Ecology and Physiology*. Cambridge: Cambridge University Press, 1996.

Loomis, William F. *Dictyostelium Discoideum -A Developmental System*. San Diego: Academic Press, 1975.

Louro, Iuri D., Juan C. Llerena, Jr., Mario S. Vieira de Melo., Patricia Ashton-Prolla, Gilberto Schwartsmann, Nivea Conforti-Froes, eds. *Genética Molecular do Cancer*. Sao Paulo: MSG Produçao Editorial Ltda., 2000.

Lyons, Albert S. and R. Joseph Petrucelli, II. *Medicine: An Illustrated History*. New York: Harry N. Abrams, Inc., 1987.

Madigan, M. M., J. Martinko, and J. Parker. *Brock Biology of Microorganisms,* 8th ed. Upper Saddle River: Prentice-Hall, 2000.

Magner, L. *A History of the Life Sciences*. New York: Marcel Dekker, Inc., 1994

Magner, Lois N. "Syphilis, the Scourge of the Renaissance" *In A History of Medicine*. New York: Marcel Dekker, 1992.

Mandell, Douglas, et al. *Principles and Practice of Infectious Diseases*. New York: Churchill Livingstone, 1995.

Mange, E. and A. Mange. *Basic Human Genetics*. 2nd ed. Massachusetts: Sinauer Associates, Inc., 1999.

Margulis, L., and K. V. Schwartz. *Five Kingdoms*. San Francisco, W. H. Freeman, 1988.

Martini, F. H., et al. *Fundamentals of Anatomy and Physiology,* 3rd ed. New jersey: Prentice Hall, Inc., 1995.

Mayr, E. *The Growth of Biological Thought*. Cambridge, MA: Harvard University Press, 1982.

——, and P. D. Ashlock. *Principles of Systematic Zoology,* 2nd ed. New York: McGraw-Hill, Inc., 1991.

McCarty, M. *Biographical Memoirs, National Academy of Sciences*. Volume 57, 1987, pp. 226–46.

McClatchey, K. *Clinical Laboratory Medicine*. Baltimore: Williams & Wilkins, 1994.

McPeak, R. and Amber Forest. *The Beauty and Biology of California's Submarine Forest*. CA: Watersport Publishers, 1988.

McRee, D. E. *Practical Protein Crystallography*. San Diego: Academic Press, 1993.

Mertz, L.,*Recent Advances and Issues in Biology*. Phoenix, Arizona: Oryx Press, 2000.

Meyer, A. W. *An Analysis of William Harvey's Generation of Animals*. Stanford, CA: Stanford University Press.

Miller, G. T., Jr. *Living in the Environment, .* 7th ed. Belmont, CA: Wadsworth Publishing Company, 1992.

Moore, F. *Give and Take: The Development of Tissue Transplantation,* New York: Saunders, 1964.

Morgan, Thomas Hunt. *The Theory of The Gene*. New Haven: Yale University Press, 1926.

Nataro, J. P., M. J. Blaser, and S. Cunningham-Rundles. *Persistent Bacterial Infections*. Washington: American Society for Microbiology, 2000.

National Institute of Allergy and Infectious Diseases. *Facts About STDS*. Bethesda: National Institutes of Health, 1992.

Nei, M. *Molecular Evolutionary Genetics*. New York: Columbia University Press, 1987.

Nelkin, D., and M. S. Lindee. *The DNA Mystique*. New York: Freeman, 1995.

Nelson, K. E., C. M. Williams, and N. M. H. Graham. *Infectious Disease Epidemiology: Theory and Practice*. Gaithersburg: Aspen Publishers, 2001.

Nishioka, K., et al. *Viral Hepatitis and Liver Disease*. New York: Springer- Verlag, 1993.

O'Hern, E. M. *Profiles of Pioneer Women Scientists*. Washington: Acropolis Books, 1985.

Okaichi, T., D. M. Anderson, and T. Nemoto, eds. Red Tides: *Biology, Environmental Science, and Toxicology*. New York: Elsevier, 1989.

Olbright, Susan M., et al. *Manual of Clinical Problems in Dermatology*. Boston: Little, Brown and Co.,1992.

Olby, R. *The Path to the Double Helix*. Seattle, WA: University of Washington Press, 1974.

——. *Origins of Mendelism,* 2nd ed. Chicago: University of Chicago Press, 1985.

Oliver, J. D. "Formation of Viable but Nonculturable Cells" *Starvation in Bacteria*. NewYork: Plenum Press, 1993.

Oppenheimer, J. M. *Essays in the History of Embryology and Biology*. Cambridge, MA: MIT Press, 1967.

Ottaway, J. H., D. K. Apps. *Biochemistry*. 4th ed. Edinburgh: Baillier Tindall, 1986.

Pagana, K. D., *Mosby's Manual of Diagnostic and Laboratory Tests*. St. Louis: Mosby, Inc., 1998.

Perkins, J. J. *Principles and Methods of Sterilization in Health Sciences,* 2nd ed. Springfield: Charles C. Thomas Publishers, 1969.

Pinto-Correia, C. *The Ovary of Eve: Egg and Sperm and Preformation.* Chicago, IL: University of Chicago Press, 1997.

Portugal, F. H. and J. S. Cohen. *A Century of DNA.* Cambridge, MA: The MIT Press.

Powell,J. A., G. R. Schnitzler, et al. "Spatial and Temporal Regulation of *1Dictyostelium.* Development Through Signal Transduction Pathways" *Evolutionary Conservation of Developmental Mechanisms.* A. C. Spradling, ed. New York: Wiley-Liss, 1993.

Prescott, L., J. Harley, and D. Klein. *Microbiology,* 5th ed. NewYork: McGraw-Hill, 2002.

Primrose, S. P. *Principles of Genome Analysis.* Oxford: Blackwell, 1995.

Prusiner, S. B., J. Collinge, J. Powell and B. Anderson. *Prion Diseases Of Humans And Animals.* Crystal City: Ellis Horwood, 1992.

Richardson, D. H. S. *Pollution Monitoring With Lichens.* United Kingdom: Richmond, 1992.

Richman, D. D., and R. J. Whitley. *Clinical Virology,* 2nd ed. Washington: American Society for Microbiology, 2002.

Rieger, R, A. Michaelis, and M. M. Green. *Glossary of Genetics and Cytogenetics.* 4th ed. Berlin: Springer Verlag, 1976.

Rifkin, J. *The Biotech Century.* Putnam Publishing Group. 1998.

Ritter, B., et al. *Biology,* B. C. ed. Scarborough: Nelson Canada, 1996.

Roberts, Brad. *Biological Weapons: Weapons of the Future?.* Wahington, D. C. : Center for Strategic and International Studies, 1993.

Roe, S. A. *Matter, Life, and Generation. Eighteenth Century Embryology and the Haller-Wolff Debate.* New York: Cambridge University Press.

Roit, I. M. *Roit's Essential Immunology.* Oxford: Blackwell Science Ltd., 1997.

Ron, E. Z., et al. "Regulation of Heat-Shock Response in Bacteria" `1Microbial Biosystems: New Frontiers. *Proceedings of the 8th International Symposium on Microbial Ecology*, Bell, C. R., M. Brylinsky, and P. Johnson-Green, eds. Halifax: Atlantic Canada Society for Microbial Ecology, 1999.

Rose, N. R. *Manual of Clinical Laboratory Immunology,* 4th ed. Washington: American Society for Microbiology, 2002.

Rosebury, Theodor. *Microbes and Morals. The Strange Story of Venereal Disease.* New York: Viking, 1971.

Rothwell, Norman V. *Human Genetics.* New Jersey: Prentice-Hall, 1977.

———. *Understanding Genetics.* 4th ed. New York: Oxford University Press, 1988.

Round, F. E. et al. *Diatoms: Biology and Morphology of the Genera.* Cambridge: Cambridge University Press, 1990.

Rowland, John. *The Polio Man: The Story of Dr. Jonas Salk.* Roy Publishing, 1961.

Russell, P. J. *Genetics,* 3rd ed. New York: Harper Collins, 1992.

Ryan, Frank. *The Forgotten Plague: How the Battle Against Tuberculosis Was Won-and Lost.* Boston: Little Brown, 1993.

Sagan, D., and L. Margulis. *Garden of Microbial Delights.* Boston: Harcourt, Brace, Jovanovich, 1988.

Sager, R. and F. J. Ryan. *Cell Heredity.* New York: John Wiley & Sons, 1961.

Salvato, M. S. *The Arenaviridae.* New York: Plenum, 1993.

Salyers, A. A., and D. D. Whitt. *Bacterial Pathogenesis, a Molecular Approach,* 2nd ed. Washington: American Society for Microbiology, 2001.

Sambrook, J., E. F. Fritsch, and T. Maniatis. *Molecular Cloning: a Laboratory Manual,* 2nd ed. New York: Cold Spring Harbor Press, 1989.

Sayre, A. *Rosalind Franklin & DNA.* New York: Norton, 1975.

Schottenfeld, D., and J. F. Fraumeni Jr., eds. *Cancer Epidemiology and Prevention.* New York: Oxford University Press, 1996.

Scriver, Charles R et al. *The Metabolic and Molecular Bases of Inherited Disease,* 8th ed. New York: McGraw-Hill Professional Book Group, 2001.

Seashore, M. and R. Wappner. *Genetics in Primary Care & Clinical Medicine.* Stamford: Appleton and Lange, 1996.

Sell, A. *Immunology, immunopathology, and immunity,* 6th ed. Washington: American Society for Microbiology, 2001.

Sherris, John C., et al. *Medical Microbiology.* Norwalk, CT: Appleton & Lange, 1994.

Shulman, S. T., et al. *The Biologic and Clinical Basis of Infectious Diseases,* 5th ed. Philadelphia: W. B. Saunders Co., 1997.

Siegel, J. P., and R. T. Finley. *Women in the Scientific Search.* Scarecrow, 1985.

Simpson, G. G. *Principles of Animal Taxonomy.* New York: Columbia University Press, 1961.

Singer, M. and P. Berg. *Genes and Genomes.* Mill Valley, CA: University Science Books, 1991.

Smith, A. D., et al. *Oxford Dictionary of Biochemistry and Molecular Biology.* New York: Oxford University Press, Inc., 1997.

Smith, Jane S. *Patenting the Sun*. New York: William Morrow and Company, Inc., 1990.

Snustad, D. Peter, Michael J. Simmons, and John B. Jenkins. *Principles of Genetics*. New York: John Wiley, 1997.

Solomon, Eldra Pearl, Linda R. Berg, and Diana W. Martin. *Biology,* 5th ed. New York: Saunders College Publishing, 1999.

Spector, D. L., R. D. Goldman, and L. A. Leinwand. *Cells: A Laboratory Manual*. Plainview, N. Y. : Cold Spring Harbor Laboratory Press, 1998.

Spudich, James A. *Dictyostelium Discoideum: Molecular Approaches to Cell Biology*. New Jersey: Academic Press, 1987.

Staben, C. A. "Evolutionary Conservation of Developmental Mechanisms- The Neurospora Mating Type Locus" *Evolutionary Conservation of Developmental Mechanisms*. A. C. Spradling, ed. Wiley-Liss, 1993.

Stanier, R. Y., J. L. Ingraham, M. L. Wheelis, P. R. Painter. *General Microbiolgy,* 5th ed. U. K. : Macmillan Press Ltd., 1993.

Stent, G. S., ed. *The Double Helix. A Personal Account of the Discovery of the Structure of DNA*. New York: Norton, 1980.

Stoermer, Eugene F. and John P. Smol. *The Diatoms: Applications for the Environmental and Earth Sciences*. New York: Cambridge University Press, 1999.

Stoffman, Phyllis. *The Family Guide to Preventing and Treating 100 Infectious Diseases*. New York: John Wiley & Sons, 1995.

Strachan, T. and A. Read. *Human Molecular Genetics*. New York: Bios Scientific Publishers, 1998.

Stryer. L. *Biochemistry,* 4th ed. New York: W. H. Freeman and Co., 1995.

Sturtevant, A. H. *A History of Genetics*. New York: Harper & Row, 1965.

Sze, S. *The Origins of the World Health Organization: a Personal Memoir*. Boca Raton: LISZ Publications, 1982.

Territo, J., and D. V. Lang. *Coping With Lyme Disease: A Practical Guide to Dealing With Diagnosis and Treatment*. New York: Henry Holt, 1997.

Thimm, Bernhard M. *Brucellosis: Distribution in Man, Domestic, and Wild Animals*. Berlin: Springer-Verlag, 1982.

Thompson, M., et al. *Genetics in Medicine*. Philadelphia : Saunders, 1991.

Tortora G., and S. Grabowski. *Principles of Anatomy and Physiology,* 7th ed. New York: Harper Collins College Publishers, 1993.

Truant, A. L. *Manual of Commercial Methods in Clinical Microbiology*. Washington: American Society for Microbiology, 2001.

Vanderhoof-Forschne, K. *Everything You Need to Know About Lyme Disease and Other Tick-Borne Disorders*. New York: John Wiley & Sons, 1997.

Vassiliki, Betty Smocovitis. *Unifying Biology: The Evolutionary Synthesis and Evolutionary Biology*. Princeton, NJ: Princeton University Press, 1996.

Virella, Gabriel. *Introduction to Medical Immunology*. New York: Marcel Dekker, Inc., 1993.

Voet D. and Voet J. *Biochemistry*. , 2nd ed. New York: John Wiley & Sons, Inc., 1995.

Vogelstein, B & Kinzler, K., eds. *The Genetic Basis of Human Cancer* New York: McGraw-Hill, 1998.

Volk, W., ed. *Basic Microbiology,* 7th ed. New York: Harper Collins, 1992.

Waterson, A. and L. Wilkinson. *An Introduction of the History of Virology*. Cambridge: Cambridge University Press, 1978.

Watson, J. D., et al. *Recombinant DNA*. 2nd ed. New York: Scientific American Books, Inc., 1992.

Webster, John G., ed. *Encyclopedia of Medical Devices and Instrumentation*. New York: John Wiley & Sons, 1988.

Willier, B. H. and J. M. Oppenheimer, eds. *Foundations of Experimental Embryology*. New York: Hafner Press, 1974.

Wilson, E. O. *The Diversity of Life*. Cambridge, MA: The Belknap Press of Harvard University Press, 1992.

Wyngaarden, J. B., L. H. Smith, Jr., and J. C. Bennett. *Cecil Textbook of Medicine,* 19th ed. Philadelphia: W. B. Saunders, 1992.

Zak, O. *Handbook of Animal Models of Infection: Experimental Models in Antimicrobial Chemotherapy*. San Diego: Academic Press, 1999.

Periodicals

Alger, L. S. "Toxoplasmosis and Parvovirus B19." *Infectious Disease Clinics of North America*, no. 11 (March 1997): 55-75.

Allen, U. "The Battle Against Influenza: The Role of Neuraminidase Inhibitors in Children." *Paediatrics and Child Health,* no. 8 (November/December 2000): 457–60.

Alouf, J. E. "From Diphtheritic Poison to Molecular Toxicology." *American Society for Microbiology News* 53, no. 10 (1987): 547–51.

Alper, T., et al. "Does the Agent of Scrapie Replicate Without Nucleic Acid?" *Nature* 214 (1967):764–66.

Anderson, C. L., and W. S. Stillman. "Raji Cell Assay for Immune Complexes: Evidence for Detection of Raji-directed Immunoglobulin G Antibody in Sera from Patients with Systemic Lupus Erythematosus." *Journal of Clinical Investigation,* no. 66 (1980): 353–60.

Andreansky, S. S., et al. "The Application of Genetically Engineered Herpes Simplex Viruses to the Treatment of Experimental Brain Tumors." *Proceedings of the National Academy of Sciences USA,* no. 93 (1996): 11313–18.

Andrews, Joan Kostick. "Lady With A Mission." *Natural Science* (May 1991): 304–10.

Aral, Sevgi O., and King K. Holmes. "Sexually Transmitted Diseases in the AIDS Era." *Scientific American* (February 1991): 62–9.

Bachmaier, K., A. Hessel, J. M. Penninger, et al. "Chlamydia Infections and Heart Disease Linked Through Antigenic Mimicry." *Science,* no. 283 (February 26, 1999): 1335–39.

Bachmaier, K., J. Le, and J. M. Penninger. "'Catching Heart Disease': Antigenic Mimicry and Bacterial Infections." *Nature Medicine,* no. 6 (August 2000): 841–42.

Baddour, L. M. "Staphylococcal infections." *Postgraduate Medicine,* no. 4 (October 2001): 1–3.

Bass, C. J., H. M. Lappin-Scott, and P. F. Saunders. "Bacteria that sour reservoirs." *Journal of Offshore Technology,* no. 1 (January 1993): 31–36.

Berg, P., et al. "Asilomar Conference on Recombinant DNA Molecules." *Science,* no. 188 (6 June 1975): 991–94.

Beveridge, T. J. "The Bacterial Surface: General Considerations Towards Design and Function." *Canadian Journal of Microbiology,* no. 34 (April 1988): 363–72.

Bhagavati, S., et al. "Detection of Human T-cell Lymphoma/Leukemia Virus Type I DNA and Antigen in Spinal Fluid and Blood of Patients with Chronic Progressive Myelopathy." *New England Journal of Medicine,* no. 318 (1988): 1141–47.

Billingham, R. E., L. Brent, and P. B. Medawar. "Actively Acquired Tolerance of Foreign Cells." *Nature,* no. 172 (1953): 603–06.

"Biotechnology in the Marine Sciences." *Science* (October 7, 1983): 19–24.

Birke, D. T., G. F. Carle, and M. V. Olson. "Cloning of Large Segments of Exogenous DNA into Yeast by Means of Artificial Chromosome Vectors." *Science,* no. 236 (1987): 806–12.

Bishop, Jerry E. "A 'Naked' DNA Vaccine Shows Promise in Combating Malaria in Mice Tests." *The Wall Street Journal* (October 11, 1994).

Blakemore, R. "Magnetotactic Bacteria." *Science,* no. 190 (1975): 377–79.

Bloomfield, S. F., et al. "The Viable but Nonculturable Phenomenon Explained?" *Microbiology,* no. 144 (1998): 1–3.

Boguski, M. S. "The Turning Point in Genome Research." *Trends in Biochemical Sciences* 20 (August 1995): 295–96.

Borel, J. F., C. Feurer, H. U. Gubler, and H. Staehelin. "Biological Effects of Cyclosporin A: A New Antilymphocytic Agent." *Agents and Actions,* no. 4 (June 1976):458–75.

Breo, Dennis L. "The US Race to 'Cure' AIDS—At '4' on a Scale of Ten, Says Dr. Fauci." *Journal of the American Medical Association* (June 9, 1993): 2898–900.

Brown, D. R. "BSE: A Post-Industrial Disease?" *Chemistry and Industry* (February 2001): 73–6.

Brown, K. S. "Scientists Find Jobs Turning 'Extremozymes' into Industrial Catalysts." *The Scientist* 19, no. 10 (September 30, 1996): 1–5.

Bryant, R. S. "Potential Uses of Microorganisms in Petroleum Recovery Technology." *Proceedings of the Oklahoma Academy of Science,* no. 67 (1987): 97–104.

Buchanan, K. L., and J. W. Murphy. "What Makes *Cryptococcus Neoformans* a Pathogen?" *Emerging Infectious Diseases,* no. 4 (January-March 1998): 1–18.

Bunk, S. "New Weapon Attacks Latent HIV Reservoirs." *The Scientist,* no. 5 (December 1998): 5.

Buret, A., et al. "Pathophysiology of Small Intestinal Malabsorption in Gerbils Infected with *Giardia lamblia*." *Gastroenterology,* no. 103 (1992): 506–16.

Burkhart, N. W., E. J. Burkes, and E. J. Burker. "Meeting the Educational Needs of Patients with Oral Lichen Planus." *General Dentistry,* 45 (1997): 126–32.

Campagna, A. C. "Pulmonary Toxoplasmosis." *Seminars in Respiratory Infections,* no. 12 (June 1997): 98–105.

Caplan, A. L. "If Gene Therapy Is the Cure, What Is the Disease?" *Gene mapping* (1992): 128–41.

Casjeans, S. "The Diverse and Dynamic Structure of Bacterial Genomes." *Annual Review of Genetics,* no. 32 (January 1998): 339–77.

CDC. "Case-Control Study of HIV Seroconversion in Health-Care Workers after Percutaneous Exposure to HIV-Infected Blood—France, United Kingdom, and United States, January 1988—August 1994." *Morbidity and Mortality Weekly Report,* no. 44 (December 1995): 929–33.

Chakravarti, A. "To a Future of Genetic Medicine." *Nature* 409 (2001): 822–23.

Chan, K. C., A. Csikasz-Nagy, et al. "Kinetic Analysis of a Molecular Model of the Budding Yeast Cell Cycle." *Molecular Biology of Cell* 11 (2000): 369–91.

Chapelle, F. H., et al. "A Hydrogen-based Subsurface Microbial Community Dominated by Methanogens." *Nature,* no. 15 (2002): 312–15.

Cimons, M. "New Prospects on the HIV Vaccine Scene." *ASM News,* no. 68 (January 2002): 19–22.

Clark, B. C. "Planetary Interchange of Bioactive Material: Probability Factors and Implications." *Origins of Life and Evolution of the Biosphere,* no. 31 (2001): 185–97.

Cohen, Jon. "Cancer Vaccines Get a Shot in the Arm." *Science* (November 5, 1993).

Collins F. S., and V. A. McKusick. "Implications of the Human Genome Project for Medical Science." *JAMA* 285 (7 February 2001): 540–44.

Compton, A. "Professor Félix d'Hérelle." *Naure* (June 25, 1949): 984–85.

Cooper, S. "Size, Volume, Length, and the Control of the Bacterial Division Cycle." *Microbiology,* no. 147 (October 2001): 2629–30.

Cowan, S. W., et al. "Crystal Structures Explain Functional Properties of two *E. coli* Porins." *Nature,* no. 358 (1992): 727–33.

Crick, F. H. C. "The Origin of the Genetic Code." *Journal of Molecular Biology* 38 (1968): 367–79.

Crowe, J. H., and A. F. Cooper., Jr. "Cryptobiosis." *Scientific American,* no. 225 (1971): 30–36.

Dalhoff, Klaus, and Matthias Maass. "Chlamydia Pneumoniae Pneumonia in Hospitalized Patients: Clinical Characteristics and Diagnosis." *Chest* 110, no. 2 (Aug. 1996): 351.

Darnell, J. E., Jr. "The Processing of RNA." *Scientific American* 249 (1983): 90–100.

Della Penna, D. "Nutritional Genomics: Manipulating Plant Micronutrients to Improve Human Health." *Science,* no. 285 (July 1999): 375–79.

Demmig-Adams, B., W. W. Adams III. "Photosynthesis: Harvesting Sunlight Safely." *Nature* 403 (January 2000): 371–74.

Dempsey, D. A., H. Silva, and D. F. Klessig. "Engineering Disease and Pest Resistance in Plants." *Trends in Microbiology,* no. 6 (June 1998): 54–61.

Dennis, D. T., et al. "Tularemia as a Biological Weapon." *Journal of the American Medical Association,* no. 285 (June 2001): 2763–73.

Diaz-Mitoma, F., S. Paton, and A. Giulivi. "Hospital Infection Control and Bloodborne Infective Agents." *Canada Communicable Disease Report,* no. 27S3 (September 2001): 40-45.

Dire, D. J., and T. W. McGovern. "CBRNE—Biological Warfare Agents." *eMedicine Journal,* no. 4 (April 2002): 1–39.

Donnenberg, M. S., J. B. Kaper, and B. B. Finlay. "Interactions between Enteropathogenic *Escherichia coli* and Host Epithelial Cells. *Trends in Microbiology,* no. 5 (1997): 109–14.

Doolittle, W. F. "Phylogentic Classification and the Universal Tree." *Science,* no. 284 (2000): 2124–29.

Douglas, S., S. Zauner, M. Fraunholz, et. al. "The Highly Reduced Genome of an Enslaved Algal Nucleus." *Nature* 410 (April 2001): 1091–96.

Doyle, D. A., et al. "The Structure of the Potassium Channel: Molecular Basis of K^+ Conduction and Selectivity." *Science,* no. 280 (1998): 69–77.

Dumler, Stephen J., et al. "Clinical and Laboratory Features of Murine Typhus in South Texas, 1980 through 1987." *The Journal of the American Medical Association.* 266 (11 September 1991): 1365–70.

Dunny, G. M., et al. "Cell-cell Communication in Gram-positive Bacteria." *Annual Review of Microbiology* (1997): 527–64.

Dybul, M., T. K. Chun, C. Yoder, et al. "Short-cycle Structured Intermittent Treatment of Chronic HIV Infection with Highly Effective Antiretroviral Therapy: Effects on Virologic, Immunologic, and Toxicity Parameters." *Proceedings of the National Academy of Sciences,* no. 98 (18 December 2001): 15161–66.

Engelhardt, H., and J. Peters. "Structural Research on Surface Layers: A Focus on Stability, Surface Layer Homology Domains, and Surface Layer-cell Wall Interactions." *Journal of Structural Biology,* no. 124 (December 1998): 276–302.

Farrell P. G. et al., "Interferon Action: Two Distinct Pathways for Inhibition of Protein Synthesis by Double-stranded RNA." *Proceedings of the National Academy of Sciences* 75 (1978) 5896.

Ferris, F. G., W. S. Fyfe, and T. J. Beveridge. "Metallic Ion Binding by *Bacillus subtilis:* Implications for the Fossilization of Bacteria." *Geology,* no. 16 (February 1988): 149–52.

Finzi, D., et al. "Identification of a Reservoir for HIV-1 in Patients on Highly Active Antiretroviral Therapy." *Science,* no. 278 (November 1997): 1295–300.

———, et al. "Latent Infection of CD4+ T Cells Provides a Mechanism for Lifelong Persistence of HIV-1, Even in Patients on Effective Combination Therapy." *Nature Medicine,* no. 5 (May 1999): 512–17.

Frauenfelder, H., and H. C. Berg. "Physics and Biology." *Physics Today,* no. 2 (February 1994): 20–21.

Friedrich, M. J. "A Bit of Culture for Children: Probiotics May Improve Health and Fight Disease." *Journal of the American Medical Association,* no. 284 (September 2000): 1365–66.

Fuller, R. "Probiotics in Human Medicine." *Gut,* no. 32 (1991): 439–42.

Fuqua, W. C., et al. "Quorum Sensing in Bacteria: The LuxR-LuxI Family of Cell Density-responsive Transcriptional Regulators." *Journal of Bacteriology,* no. 176(1994): 269–75.

Gerhold, D., T. Rushmore, and C. T. Caskey. "DNA Chips: Promising Toys Have Become Powerful Tools." *Trends in Biochemical Science,* no. 24 (May 1999): 168–73.

Glaser, R., et al. "Stress-induced Modulation: Implications for Infectious Disease?" *Journal of the American Medical Association,* no. 281 (June 1999): 2268–70.

Goosney, D. L., D. G. Knoechel, and B. B. Finlay. "Enteropathogenic *E. coli, Salmonella,* and *Shigella*: Masters of Host Cytoskeletal Exploitation." *Emerging Infectious Diseases,* no. 5 (April-June 1999): 216–23.

Gorman, Christine. "Victory at Last for a Beseiged Virus Hunter." *Time* (November 22, 1993): 61.

Grebe, T. W., and J. Stock. "Bacterial Chemotaxis: The Five Sensors of a Bacterium." *Current Biology,* no. 8 (September 1998): R154-R157.

Green, Cornelia R., and Ira Gleiberman. "Brill-Zinsser: Still with Us." *The Journal of the American Medical Association* 264 (10 October 1990): 1811–12.

Griffith, J. S. "Self-replication and Scrapie." *Nature* 215 (1967): 1043–44.

Grossman, A., and R. Losick. "Extracellular Control of Spore Formation in *Bacillus subtilis.*" *Proceedings of the National Academy of Sciences,* no. 85 (1997): 4369–73.

Hancock, R. E. W., et al. "*Pseudomonas aeruginosa* Isolates from Patients with Cystic Fibrosis: A Class of Serum-sensitive, Non-typeable Strains Deficient in Lipopolysaccharide O Side Chain." *Infection and Immunity,* no. 42 (1983): 170–75.

Harris, J. D., and N. R. Lemoine. "Strategies for Targeted Gene Therapy." *Trends in Genetics,* no. 12 (1996): 400–04.

Henderson, Charles. "Vaccines for STDS: Possibility or Pipe Dream." *AIDS Weekly* (2 May 1994): 8.

Henderson, Randi. "Scientist Plays Many Roles." *Baltimore Sun* (October 13, 1991).

Henderson, S. O. "Candidiasis." *eMedicine Journal,* no. 3 (January 2002): 1–17.

Hilts, Philip J. "AIDS Advocates Are Angry at U. S, But Its Research Chief Wins Respect." *New York Times* (September 4, 1990): A14.

Hoehler, T. M., Bebout, B. M., Des Marais, D. J. "The Role of Microbial Mats in the Production of Reduced Gases on the Early Earth." *Nature* 412 (July 2001): 324–27.

Hunt, R. H. "Peptic Ulcer Disease: Defining the Treatment Strategies in the Era of *Helicobacter pylori.*" *American Journal of Gastroenterology,* no. 4 (Supplement 1997): 446–50.

Inglesby, T. V., et al. "Anthrax as a Biological Weapon." *Journal of the American Medical Association,* no. 281 (May 1999): 1735–45.

International Genome Sequencing Consortium. "Initial Sequencing and Analysis of the Human Genome." *Nature* 409 (2001): 860–921.

Jaenike, John. "Behind-the-Scenes Role of Parasites." *Natural History* (June 1994): 46–8.

Jeffords, J. M., and Tom Daschle. "Political Issues in the Genome Era," *Science* 291 (16 February 2001): 1249–50.

Jennings, V. M. "Review of Selected Adjuvants Used in Antibody Production." *ILAR Journal,* no. 37 (February 1995): 119–25.

Johnson, P., and D. A. Hopkinson. "Detection of ABO Blood Group Polymorphism by Denaturing Gradient Gel Electrophoresis." *Human Molecular Genetics* 1 (1992): 341–44.

Jordan, P., Fromme, P. et al. "Three-Dimensional Structure of Cyanobacterial Photosystem I at 2.5 Å Resolution." *Nature* 411 (June 2001): 909–17.

Joyce, L. "Special Report: Glassware, Plasticware Compete in Labs." *The Scientist,* no. 11 (May 1991): 23–7.

Kaiser, D., and R. Losick. "How and Why Bacteria Talk to Each Other." *Cell,* no. 73 (1993): 873–85.

Kessin, R. H., and M. M. van Lookeren Campagne. "The Development of a Social Amoeba." *American Scientist* 80 (1992): 556–65.

Kiecolt-Glaser, J. K., et al. "Chronic Stress Alters the Immune Response to Influenza Virus Vaccine in Older Adults." *Proceedings of the National Academy of Sciences,* no. 93 (1996): 3043–47.

Kiefer, D. M. "Chemistry Chronicles: Miracle Medicines." *Today's Chemist* 10, no. 6 (June 2001): 59–60.

Kiel, Frank W., and M. Yousouf Khan. "Brucellosis in Saudi Arabia." *Social Science and Medicine* 29 (1989): 999–1001.

Kirchhoff, L. V. "American Trypanosomiasis (Chagas' disease): A Tropical Disease Now in the United States." *New England Journal of Medicine,* no. 329 (August 1993): 639–44.

Krause, R. S. "Anaphylaxis." *eMedicine Journal,* no. 12 (December 2001): 1–22.

Kreeger, K. Y. "Genome Investigator Craig Venter Reflects on Turbulent Past and Future Ambitions." *The Scientist,* no. 9 (July 1995): 1, 10.

Kreft, J-U., G. Booth, and J. W. T. Wimpenny. "BacSim, a Simulator for Individual-based Modeling of Bacterial Colony Growth." *Microbiology,* no. 144 (1998): 3275–87.

Kump, Theresa. "Chicken Pox Survival Guide." *Parents' Magazine* 69 (May 1994): 29.

Lépine, Pierre. "Félix d'Hérelle (1873–1949)." *Annales de l'Institut Pasteur,* (1949): 457–60.

Lacy, D. B., and R. C. Stevens. "Unraveling the Structures and Modes of Action of Bacterial Toxins." *Current Opinion in Structural Biology,* no. 8 (1998): 778–84.

Lakhani, S. "Early Clinical Pathologists. Edward Jenner." *Journal of Clinical Pathology* 45 (1992): 756–58.

Lederberg, J. M., and E. M. Lederberg. "Replica Plating and Indirect Selection of Bacterial Mutants." *Journal of Bacteriology,* no. 63 (March 1952): 399–406.

Lemieux, B., A. Aharoni, and M. Schena. "Overview of DNA chip technology." *Molecular Breeding,* no. 4 (1998): 277–89.

Leparc. G. F. "Nucleic Acid Testing for Screening Donor Blood." *Infectious Medicine,* no. 17 (May 2000): 310–33.

Levin, G. V. "The Viking Labeled Release Experiment and Life on Mars. Instruments, Methods, and Missions for the Investigation of Extraterrestrial Microorganisms." *SPIE Proceedings,* no. 3111 (1997): 146–61.

Levin, N. A., and B. B. Wilson. "Cowpox Infection, Human." *eMedicine Journal,* no. 2 (December 2001): 1–8.

Levy, C. W., et. Al. "Molecular Basis of Triclosan Activity." *Nature,* no. 398 (1999): 383–84.

Li, X. P., Bjorkman, O., Shih, C., et al. "A Pigment-binding Protein Essential for Regulation of Photosynthetic Light Harvesting." *Nature* 403; (January 2000): 391–95.

Linder, R. "*Rhodococcus equi* and *Arcanobacterium haemolyticum*: Two Coryneform Bacteria Increasingly Recognized as Agents of Human Infection." *Emerging Infectious Diseases,* no. 3 (April-June 1997): 1–13.

Lockhart, D. J., and E. A. Winzeler. "Genomics, Gene Expressions, and DNA Arrays." *Nature* 405, no. 6788 (2000): 827–36.

Macnab, R. M., and D. E. Koshland, Jr. "The Gradient Sensing Mechanism in Bacterial Chemotaxis." *Proceedings of the National Academy of Sciences USA,* no. 69 (1972): 2509–12.

Madigan, M. T., and B. L. Marrs. "Extremophiles." *Scientific American* (April 1997).

Malin, M. C., and K. S. Edgett. "Evidence for Recent Groundwater Seepage and Surface Runoff on Mars." *Science,* no. 288 (2000): 2330–35.

Martinez, F. D. "The Coming-of-age of the Hygiene Hypothesis." *Respiratory Research,* no. 2 (March 2001): 129–32.

Martini, F, et al., "Human Brian Tumors and Simian Virus 40." *Journal of the National Cancer Institute,* no. 87 (September 1995): 1331a.

Mason, H. S., et al. "Immunogenicity of a Recombinant Bacterial Antigen Delivered in a Transgenic Potato." *Nature Medicine,* no. 4 (May 1998): 607–09.

Maxam, A., and W. Gilbert. "A New Method of Sequencing DNA." *Proceedings of the National Academy of Sciences of the United States of America* 74 (1998): 560–64.

Mazel, D., et al. "A Distinctive Class of Integron in the *Vibrio cholerae* Genome." *Science,* no. 280 (1998): 605–08.

McCluskie, M. J., et al. "CpG DNA is an Effective Oral Adjuvant to Protein Antigens in Mice." *Vaccine,* no, 19 (November 2000): 950–57.

Milius, S. "Red Snow, Green Snow." *Science News,* no. 157 (May 2000): 328–33.

Mirelman, D., S. Ankri, U. Katz, F. Padilla-Vaca, and R. Bracha. "Pathogenesis of *Entamoeba histolytica* Depends on the Concerted Action of Numerous Virulence Factors." *Archives in Medical Research,* no. 31 (2000): S214–S215.

Miyazawaa, Y., et al. "Immunomodulation by a Unicellular Green Algae (*Chlorella pyrenoidosa*) in Tumor Bearing Mice." *Journal of Ethnopharmacology,* no. 24 (1988): 135–46.

Montgomery, Paul L., "René Dubos, Scientist and Writer, Dead." *New York Times* (February 21, 1982): 32.

Murphy, F. A. "Emerging Zoonoses." *Emerging Infectious Diseases,* no. 4 (July-September 1998): 429–35.

Nataro, J. P., and J. B. Kaper. "Diarrheagenic *Escherichia coli*." *Clinical Microbiology Reviews,* no. 11 (January 1998): 142–201.

Nathanson, N. "Towards an AIDS Vaccine: the Role of Primate Models." *International Journal of STD AIDS,* no. 9 (January 1998): 3–7.

Nisbet, E. G., N. H. Sleep. "The Habitat and Nature of Early Life." *Nature* 409 (February 2001): 1083–91.

Nochimson, G. "Q Fever." *eMedicine Journal,* no. 3 (January 2002): 1–8.

O'Hern, Elizabeth M. "Alice Evans, Pioneer Microbiologist." *American Society for Microbiology News* (September 1973).

Oguma, K., et al. "Infant Botulism Due to *Clostridium botulinum* Type C Toxin." *Lancet,* no. 336(1990): 1449–50.

Old, L. J. "Immunotherapy for Cancer (Therapies of the Future)." *Scientific American,* no. 275 (September 1996):136–44.

Olle-Goig, Jaime E., and Jaume Canela-Soler. "An Outbreak of Brucella Melitensis. Infection by Airborne Transmission Among Laboratory Workers." *American Journal of Public Health* 77 (8 March 1987): 335–38.

Oprins, A., H. J. Geuze, and J. W. Slot. "Cryosubstitution Dehydration of Aldehyde-fixed Tissue: A Favorable Approach to Quantitative Immunocytochemistry." *Journal of Histochemistry and Cytochemistry,* no. 42 (1994): 497–503.

Orriss, G. D. "Animal Diseases of Public Health Importance." *Emerging Infectious Diseases,* no. 4 (October-December 1997): 497–502.

Parsonnet, J., et al. "*Helicobacter pylori* Infection and Gastric Lymphoma." *New England Journal of Medicine,* no. 330 (1994): 1267–71.

Perera, F. P., and I. B. Weinstein. "Molecular Epidemiology: Recent Advances and Future Directions." *Carcinogenesis* 21 (2000): 517–24.

Perry, R. D., and J. D. Fetherston. "Yersinia Pestis-Etiological Agent of Plague." *Clinical Reviews in Microbiology,* no. 10 (January 1997): 35–66.

Peters, C. J., and J. W. LeDuc. "An Introduction to Ebola: The Virus and the Disease." *The Journal of Infectious Diseases,* no. 179 (Supplement 1, February 1999): ix-xvi.

Pfennig, N. "Van Neil Remembered." *American Society for Microbiology News,* no. 53 (February 1987): 75–7.

Plotkin, Stanley A. "Vaccination in the 21st Century." *The Journal of Infectious Diseases* 168 (1993): 29–37.

———. "Vaccines for Chicken Pox and Cytomegalovirus: Recent Progress." *Science* 265 (2 September 1994): 1383.

Popescu, A., and R. J. Doyle. "The Gram Stain After More Than a Century." *Biotechnic and Histochemistry,* no. 71 (March 1996): 145–48.

Potera. C. "Studying Slime." *Environmental Health Perspectives,* no. 106 (December 1998): 1–5.

Pruisner, S. B. "Molecular Biology of Prion Diseases." *Science,* no. 252 (June 1991): 1515–22.

"Public-Sector Vaccination in Response to Measles." *Journal of the American Medical Association* 268, no. 8 (August 26, 1992): 963–64.

Razatos, A., Y. L. Ong, M. M. Sharma, and G. Georgiou. "Molecular Determinants of Bacterial Adhesion Monitored by Atomic Force Microscopy." *Proceedings of the National Academy of Sciences,* no. 95 (15 September 1998): 11059–64.

Reid, G., A. W. Bruce, and V. Smeianov. "The Role of *Lactobacilli* in Prevention of Urogenital and Intestinal Infections." *International Dairy Journal,* no. 8 (February 1998): 555–62.

Rillig, M. C., Field, C. B., Allen, M. F. "Soil Biota Responses to Long-term Atmospheric CO_2 Enrichment in Two California Annual Grasslands." *Oecologia* 119 (1999): 572–77.

Ritossa, F. M. "A New Puffing Pattern Induced by a Temperature Shock and DNP in *Drosophila.*" *Experimenta,* no. 18 (1962): 571–73.

Robinson, J. D. "Key Player Chronicles Fascinating Search for AIDS Viruses." *The Washington Post* (April 22, 1991): F1.

Rosenberg, S. A., et al. "Immunologic and Therapeutic Evaluation of a Synthetic Peptide Vaccine for the Treatment of Patients with Metastatic Melanoma." *Nature Medicine,* no. 4 (March 1998): 321–27.

Rossier, O., and N. P. Cianciotto. "Type II Protein Secretion Is a Subset of the PilD-dependent Processes that Promote Infection by *Legionella pneumophila.*" *Infection and Immunity,* no. 68 (2001): 2092–98.

Roth, J. A., et al. "Retrovirus Mediated Wild-type p53 Gene Transfer to Tumors of Patients with Lung Cancer." *Nature Medicine,* no. 2 (1996): 985–91.

Russell, Cristine. "Anthony S. Fauci: A Hard-Driving Leader of the Lab War on AIDS." *Washington Post* (November 3, 1986): A12–A13.

Sammons, Vivian O. "Blacks in Science and Medicine." *Hemisphere* (1990): 176.

Sanoff, Alvin P. "A Conversation With René Dubos." *U. S. News & World Report* (February 23, 1981): 72–3.

Sato, M., K. Machida, E. Arikado, et al. "Expression of Outer Membrane Proteins of *Escherichia coli* Growing at Acid pH." *Applied and Environmental Microbiology,* no 66 (March 2000): 943–47.

Schmeck, Harold M. Jr. "Dr. Jonas Salk, Whose Vaccine Turned Tide on Polio, Dies at 80" *New York Times* (24 June 1995).

Shizuya, H., et al. "A Bacterial Cloning System for Cloning Large Human DNA Fragments." *Proceedings of the National Academy of Sciences,* no. 89 (February 1992): 8794–97.

Shoemaker, D. D., et al. "Experimental Annotation of the Human Genome Using Microarray Technology." *Nature* 409, no. 6822 (2001): 922–27.

Shulaev, P., et al. "Airborne Signalling by Methyl Salicylate in Plant Pathogen Resistance." *Nature,* no. 385 (April 1997): 718–21.

Siegel, J. P., and R. T. Finley. "Alice Evans, 94, Bacteriologist, Dies." *Washington Post* (September 8, 1975): B4.

Sriskandan, S., and J. Cohen. "Gram-positive Sepsis: Mechanisms and Differences from Gram-negative Sepsis." *Infectious Diseases Clinicians of North America,* no. 13 (February 1999): 397–412.

St. Geme, J. W., III. "Bacterial Adhesins: Determinants of Microbial Colonization and Pathogenicity." *Advances in Pediatrics,* no. 44 (1997): 43–72.

Steinberg, J. P., et al. "Nosocomial and Community-acquired *Satphylococcus aureus* Bacteremias from 1980 to 1993: Impact of Intravascular Devices and Methicillin Resistance." *Clinical and Infectious Diseases,* no 23 (February 1996): 255–59.

Stephens, C. "Bacterial Sporulation: A Question of Commitment?" *Current Biology,* no. 8 (January 1998): R45–R48.

Steven Ashley. "It's Not Easy Being Green." *Scientific American* (April 2002): 20–1.

Surette, M. G., et al. "Quorum Sensing in *Escherichia coli, Salmonella typhymurium,* and *Vibrio harveyi*: A New Family of Genes Responsible for Autoinducer Production." *Proceedings of the National Academy of Sciences,* no. 96 (1999): 1639–44.

Taubenberger, J., et al. "Initial Genetic Characterization of the 1918 Spanish Influenza Virus." *Science,* no. 275 (May 1997): 1793–96.

Taubs, G. "TIGR's J. Craig Venter Takes Aim at the Big Questions." *Science Watch,* no. 8 (September/October 1997): 3–7.

Taylor, C. R., et al. "Strategies for Improving the Immunohistochemical Staining of Various Intranuclear Prognostic Markers in Formalin-paraffin Sections: Androgen Receptor, Estrogen Receptor, Progesterone Receptor, p53 Protein, Proliferating Cell Nuclear Antigen, and ki-67 as Revealed by Antigen Retrieval Techniques." *Human Pathology,* no. 25 (1994): 263–70.

Thomas, Stephen B., and Sandra Crouse Quinn. "The Tuskegee Syphilis Study, 1932–1972: Implications for HIV Education and AIDS Risk Education Programs in the Black Community." *The American Journal of Public Health.* (November 1991): 1498.

Tokunaga, T., et al. "Antitumor Activity of Deoxyribonucleic Acid Fraction from *Mycobacterium bovis* BCG: Isolation, Physcicochemical Charaterization, and Antitumor Activity." *Journal of the National Cancer Institute,* no. 75 (1984): 955–62.

Toleman, M., E. Aho, and M. Virji. "Expression of Pathogen-like Opa Adhesins in Commensal *Neisseria*: Genetic and Functional Analysis." *Cellular Microbiology,* no. 3 (2001): 33–44.

Tynes, Lee. "Tuberculosis: The Continuing Story." *The Journal of the American Medical Association* 270 (December 1, 1993): 2616.

Uchiyama, T. "Human T-cell Leukemia Virus Type I (HTLV-1) and Human Disease." *Annual Reviews of Immunology,* no. 15(January 1997): 15–37.

Van Neil, C. B. "On the Morphology and Physiology of the Purple and Green Sulfur Bacteria." *Archives fur Mikrobiologie,* no. 3 (1931): 1–112.

Vivas, E. I., and H. Goodrich-Blair. "*X. nematophilus* as a Model for Host Bacterium Interactions: *rpoS* Is Necessary for Mutualism with Nematodes." *Journal of Bacteriology,* no. 183 (2001): 4687–93.

Wade, Nicholas. "Method and Madness: The Vindication of Robert Gallo." *New York Times Magazine* (December 26, 1993) 12.

Waksman, Selman A. "Dr. René J. Dubos—A Tribute." *Journal of the American Medical Association* 174, no. 5 (October 1, 1960).

Walker, D. H., et. al. "Emerging Bacterial Zoonotic and Vector-Borne Diseases. Ecological and Epidemiological Factors." *Journal of the American Medical Association* 275 (1996): 463–69.

Walsby. A. E. "The Mechanical Properties of the *Microcystis* Gas Vesicle." *Journal of General Microbiology,* no. 137 (1991): 2401–08.

Wannamaker, L. "Rebecca Craighill Lancefield." *American Society for Microbiology News* 47 (1981): 555–58.

Watson, J. D., and F. H. C. Crick. "Molecular Structure of Nucleic Acids." *Nature* 171 (1953): 737–38.

———. "Genetical Implications of the Structure of Deoxyribonucleic Acid." *Nature* 171 (1953): 964–69.

Weinert, T. and , Hartwell, L. "The RAD9 Gene Controls the Cell Cycle Response to DNA Damage in *Saccharomyces cerevisiae*." *Science* 241 (1989) 317.

Weiss, D. S., J. C. Chen, J. M. Ghigo, et al. "Localization of Ftsl (PBP3) to the Septal Ring Requires its Membrane Anchor, the Z Ring, FtsA, FtsQ, and FtsL." *Journal of Bacteriology,* no. 181 (1999): 508–20.

Whitesides, M. D., and J. D. Oliver. "Resuscitation of *Vibrio vulnificus.* from the Viable but Nonculturable State." *Applied and Environmental Microbiology,* no. 63 (1997): 1002–05.

Whitman, Alden. "Schick, Who Devised Diphtheria Test, Dies." *New York Times* (Dec. 7, 1967): 1, 47.

Wilhems, A., S. R. Larter, I. Head, et al. "Biodegradation of Oil in Uplifted Basins Prevented by Deep-burial Sterilization." *Nature* 411 (June 2001): 1034–37.

Wong, B. S., D. R. Brown, M. S. Sy. "A Yin-yang Role for Metals in Prion Disease." *Panminerva Med* 43 (2001): 283–87.

Wright, Paul. "Brucellosis." *American Family Physician* 35 (May 1987): 155–59.

Yaspo, M. L. et al. "The DNA Sequence of Human Chromosome 21." *Nature* 6784 (May 2000): 311–19.

Zhaohui, Xu., J. D. Knafels, and K. Yoshino. "Crystal Structure of the Bacterial Protein Export Chaperone SecB." *Nature Structural Biology,* no. 7 (December 2000): 1172–77.

ZoBell, C. E. . "Bacteria as Geological Agents with Particular Reference to Petroleum." *Petroleum World,* no. 10 (January 1943): 30–43.

Zurer, Pamela S. "Food Irradiation: A Technology at a Turning Point." *Chemical & Engineering News* (May 5, 1986): 46–56.

Web Sites

Editor's Note: As the World Wide Web is constantly expanding, the URLs listed below were current as of June 15, 2002.

A Healthy Me. "Immunologic Therapies." 1999. <http://www.ahealthme.com/topic100587007?_requestid=32704> (February 22, 2002).

A Healthy Me. "Antiseptics." 1999. <http://www.ahealthme.com/topic/ntiseptic?_requestid=19185> (February 5, 2002).

A Healthy Me. "Immunoglobulin Deficiency Syndromes." 1999. <http://www.ahealthyme.com/topic/topic 100587006?_requestid=4018> (April 8, 2002).

ABC News Science. "Plankton Power." 1999. <http://abcnews.go.com/sections/science/DailyNews/plankton 990204.html> (February 6, 2002).

ABC News.com. "The Next Big Thing." 2001. <http://abc-news.go.com/sections/scitech/DailyNews/proteomics_ 010427.html> (February 13, 2002).

Access Excellence. "The collaboration of proteins during replication." @<http://www.accessexcellence.com/AB/GG/collaboration.html> (April 2, 2000).

AIDS.org. "New Drugs Against HIV: Immune Stimulators." 2001 <http://www.aids.org/FactSheets/404-new-drugs.html> (January 21, 2002).

AIDS.org. "New Drugs Against HIV: Reverse Transcriptase Inhibitors." 2001 <http://www.aids.org/FactSheets/402-new-drugs.html> (January 21, 2002).

Albert Einstein College of Medicine. "Microbiology Primer: Hemolysis." 2001 <http://gold.aecom.yu.edu/id/micro/hemolysis.htm> (February 21, 2002).

American Phytopathological Society. "The Irish Potato Famine and the Birth of Plant Pathology." 1998. <http://www.apsnet.org/on-line/feature/lateblit/chapter1/birthpp.htm> (3 February 2002).

American Society for Microbiology. "Careers in the Microbiological Sciences." 2000. <http://www.asmusa.org/edusrc/edu21.htm> (January 22, 2002).

American Type Culture Collection. "About ATCC." 2001. <http://www.atcc.org/ProgramsAndServices/About ATCC.cfm> (January 23, 2002).

Association of Schools of Public Health. "What is Public Health?" 2002. <http://www.asph.org/aa_section.cfm> (January 23, 2002).

Astrobiology.com. "Environmental Stress and the Search for Life on Mars." 1999. <http://www.astrobiology.com/asc2000/abstract.html> (January 31, 2002).

Australian Herpes Management Forum. "Varicella Zoster Virus (VSV)." 2001. <http://rpes.on.net/vzv/Deault.htm> (February 22, 2002).

Australian Institute of Medical Scientists. "Careers in Medical Laboratory Science." 2001. <http://www.aims.org.au/aims_org/careers.htm> (January 22, 2002).

Baby Bag On-line. "Tetanus from the Centers for Disease Control and Prevention." 1996. <http://www.babybag.com/articles/cdc_tetn.htm> (January 22, 2002).

"Bacteria Growth Requirements." <http://archive.food.gov.uk/hea/teachers/plainenglish/part2.html> (June 22, 2002)

Bacteria Museum. "Special Feature: Bacterial Diseases in History." 2002. <http://www.bacteriamuseum.org/niches/features/diseasehistory.html> (30 April 2002).

Bartleby.com. "Nuttall, George Henry Falkiner." 2001. <http://www.bartleby.com/65/nu/NuttallG.html> (9 February 2002).

"Basidomycetes." <http://wwwfac.wmdc.edu/HTMLpages/Academics/Biology/botf99/fungifromweb/basidomycetes.html>

BBC News. "Anthrax as a biological weapon." 2001. <http://news.bbc.co.uk/hi/emglish/health/newsid_159000 0/1590859.stm> (June 13, 2002).

BBC News. "Cold 'cure' comes one step closer." 1999. <http://news.bbc.co.uk/hi/english/health/newsid_526000/526904.htm> (January 25, 2002).

BBC News. "Q & A: Anthrax infection." 2001. <http://news.bbc.co.uk/hi/english/health/newsid_1580000/1580930.stm> (January 27, 2002).

Biological Research for Animals and People. "The Liver: Transplants and Medicines." 2001. <http://222.biorap.org/rg/rgptransmed.html> (May 20, 2002).

Biology Pages. "Histocompatibility Molecules." 2002. <http://www.ultranet.com/~jkimball/BiologyPages/H/HLA.html> (May 14, 2002).

Biology Pages. "The Complement System." 2002. <http://www.ultranet.com/~jkimball/BiologyPages/C/Complement.html> (May 15, 2002).

Biology Pages. "Viruses." 2002. <http://www.ultranet.com/~jkimball/BiologyPages/V/Viruses.html> (April 22, 2002).

Blakeslee, D. "Cytokines, Chemokines and Host Defense." JAMA HIV/AIDS Resource Center, <http://www.ama-assn.org/special/hiv/newsline/briefing/cyto.htm>. (June 15, 2002).

BSE Info Resource. "Creutzfeldt-Jacob Disease (CJD)." 2002. <http://www.bseinfo.org/resource/cjd_fact.htm> (January 21, 2002).

Building Better Health. "Immunosuppressant Drugs." 1999. <http://www.buildingbetterhealth.com/topic/immuno suppressant> (February 20, 2002).

California Polytechnic University. "Magnetotactic Bacteria at Cal Poly." 1996. <http://www.calpoly.edu/~rfrankelmtbcalpoly.html> (February 6, 2002).

Cambridge University. "George Frederick Nuttall." 1999. <http://www.path.cam.ac.uk/~schisto/History/Molteno_footnotes/Nuttall_footnote.html> (February 9, 2002).

Cambridge University. "Life cycle of Entamoeba histolytica. and the Clinical Manifestations of Infection in Humans." 1999. htpp://www-ermm.cbcu.cam.ac.uk/99000617h.htm> (February 14, 2002).

Cambridge University. "Molecules of Bacterial Cell Division." 2000. <http://www2.mrc-lmb.cam.ac.uk/groups/JYL/frame_mobcd.html> (February 6, 2002).

Canadian Shellfish Quality Resource. "Bacterial Indicators on Shellfish Water Quality." 2001. <http://www.shellfishquality.ca/indicators.htm> (February 20, 2002).

Carnegie Mellon University. "Bacterial Chemotaxis." 1999. <http://infor.bio.cmu.edu/Courses/03441/TermPapers/99 TermPapers/TwoCom/chemotaxis.html> (January 21, 2002).

Carnegie Mellon University. "Introduction to Bioluminescence." 1997. <http://info.bio.cmu.edu/Courses/03441/Termpapers/97TermPapers/lux/bioluminescence.html> (May 7, 2002).

Carnegie Mellon University. Overview of the Bacterial Cell Cycle." 1999. htpp://info.bio.cmu.edu/Courses/03441/TermPapers/99TermPapers/Caulo/intro.html> (February 7, 2002).

Center for Disease Control. "Update: Facts about Anthrax Testing and On-going Investigations in Florida, Nevada, New York, and Washington, D. C." 2001. <http://www.bt.cdc.gov/DocumentsApp/Anthrax/10162001PM/Updat e10162001PM.asp> (October 16, 2001).

Centers for Disease Control and Prevention. "About CDC." 2002. <http://www.cdc.gov/aboutcdc.htm> (May 14, 2002).

Centers for Disease Control. "CDC Dengue Fever Home Page." 2001. <http://www.cdc.gov/ncidod/dvbid/dengue/> (March 16, 2002).

Centers for Disease Control. "Ebola Hemorrhagic Fever." 2001. <http://www.cdc.gov/ncidod/dvrd/spb/mnpages/dispages/ebola.htm> (March 8, 2002).

Centers for Disease Control. "Group B Streptococcus. " 1998. <http://www.cdc.gov/ncidod/diseases/bacter/strep_b.htm> (March 18, 2002).

Centers for Disease Control. "Hand, Foot, and Mouth Disease." 2000. <http://www.cdc.gov/ncidod/dvrd/hfmd.htm> (February 21, 2002).

Centers for Disease Control. "Viral Gastroenteritis." 2000. htpp://www.cdc.gov/ncidod/dvrd/gastro.htm> (February 28, 2002).

Centers for Disease Control. "West Nile Virus." 2001. <http://www.cdc.gov/ncidod/dvbid/westnile/> (05 March 2002).

Centers for Disease Control. "Adhesins as Targets for Vaccine Development." 1999. <http://www.cdc.gov/ncidod/eid/vol5no3/wizeman.htm> (January 24, 2002).

Centers for Disease Control. "Anthrax." 2001. <http://www.cdc.gov/ncidod/dbmd/diseaseinfo/anthrax_t.htm> (January 27, 2002).

Centers for Disease Control. "Arenaviridae." 2001. <http://www.cdc.gov/ncidod/dvrd/spb/mnpages/dispages/arena.htm> (April 23, 2002).

Centers for Disease Control. "Biological Diseases/Agents Listing." 2001. <http://www.bt.cdc.gov/Agent/Agentlist.asp> (January 23, 2002).

Centers for Disease Control. "Biological Diseases/Agents Listing." 2001. <http://www.bt.cdc.gov/Agent/Agentlist.asp> (January 23, 2002).

Centers for Disease Control. "Biological Diseases/Agents Listing." 2001. <http://www.bt.cdc.gov/Agent/Agentlist.asp> (January 23, 2002).

Centers for Disease Control. "Botulism." 2001. <http://www.cdc.gov/ncidod/dbmd/diseaseinfo/botu-lism_g.htm> (March 20, 2002).

Centers for Disease Control. "Campylobacter Infections." 2001. <http://www.cdc.gov/ncidod/dbmd/diseaseinfo/campylobacter_g.htm> (January 24, 2002).

Centers for Disease Control. "Candidiasis." 2001. <http://www.cdc.gov/ncidod/dbmd/diseaseinfo/candidiasis_t.htm> (April 3, 2002).

Centers for Disease Control. "CDC Plague Home Page." 2001. <http://www.cdc.gov/ncidod/dvbid/plague/> (May 6, 2002).

Centers for Disease Control. "Chagas Disease." 1999. <http://www.cdc.gov/ncidod/dpd/parasites/chagsdisease/factsht_chags_disease.htm> (April 17, 2002).

Centers for Disease Control. "Epstein-Barr Virus and Infectious Mononucleosis." 1999. <http://www.cdc.gov/ncidod/diseases/ebv.htm> (January 26, 2002).

Centers for Disease Control. "Fact Sheet: Cryptosporidiosis." <http://www.cdc.gov/ncidod/dpd/parasites/cryptosporidiosis/factsht_cryptosporidiosis.htm> (February 6, 2002).

Centers for Disease Control. "Molds in the Environment." 2002. <http://www.cdc.gov/nceh/asthma_old/factsheets/molds/moldfacts.htm> (March 30, 2002).

Centers for Disease Control. "Q fever." 2001. <http://www.cdc.gov/ncidod/dvrd/qfever/> (March 30, 2002).

Centers for Disease Control. "Questions and Answers Regarding Bovine Spongiform Encephalopathy (BSE) and Creutzfeld-Jacob Disease (CJD)." 2001. <http://www.cdc.gov/ncidod/diseases/cjd/bse_cjd_qa.htm> (January 21, 2002).

Centers for Disease Control. "Six Common Misconceptions about Vaccination and How to Respond to Them." 2001. <http://www.cdc.gov/nip/publications/6mishome.htm> (January 30, 2002).

Centers for Disease Control. "Sterilization or Disinfection of Medial Devices: General Prinicples." 2000. <http://www.cdc.gov/ncidod/hip/Steile/Sterilgp.htm> (February 19, 2002).

Centers for Disease Control. "Viral Hemorrhagic Fevers." 2000. <http://www.cdc.gov/ncidod/dvrd/spb/mnpages/dispages/vhf.htm> (April 2, 2002).

Centers for Disease Control. "Yellow Fever: Disease and Vaccine." 2001. <http://www.cdc.gov/ncidod/dvbid/yellowfever/index.htm> (March 12, 2002).

Centers for Disease Control. "Zoonoses—Animals Can Make You Sick." 1992. <http://www.cdc.gov/niosh/nasd/doc2/as12600.html> (February 22, 2002).

City College of San Francisco. "Requirements for Microbial Growth." 1999. <http://www.ccsf.org/Departments/Biology/growth.htm> (January 31, 2002).

Colorado State University. "Microbial Life in the Digestive Tract." 1998. <http://arbl.cvmbs.colostate.edu/hbooks/pathphys/digestion/basics/gi_bugs.html> (April 27, 2002).

Columbia University. "Decontamination and Disinfection." 1999. <http://cpmcnet.columbia.edu/dept/ehs/decon.html> (February 19, 2002).

"Components of the Soil Biota." Soil Microbiology. <http://www.bsi.vt.edu/chagedor/biol_4684/microbes/SoilBiota.html> (June 15, 2002).

"Composting-Temperature." <http://www.trevolcottage.binternet.co.uk/Temperature.html> (June 15, 2002).

Cornell University. "Compost Microorganisms." 2000. <http://www.cfe.cornell.edu/compost/microorg.html> (February 8, 2002).

Corning.com. "General Guide for Cryogenically Storing Animal Cells." 2002. <http://www.corning.com/lifesciences/technical_information/cryogenic_storage/cryoanimalcc.asp> (January 26, 2002).

Dakota Wesleyan University. "Microbial Taxonomy." 1999. <http://www.dwu.edu/biology/Mullican/micrtaxon.htm> (February 7, 2002).

Davidson College. "Immunofluorescence Microscopy." 2000. <http://www.bio.davidson.edu/people/kabcrnd/seminar/indiv/msb/meth7.html> (March 12, 2002).

Daxor. "Personal Blood Service." 2000. <http://www.daxor.com/bbank.shtml> (May 15, 2002).

Defense Journal. "Anthrax as a Weapon of Terrorism and Difficulties Presented in Response to its Use." 1998. <http://www.defensejournal.com/dec98/anthrax.htm> (June 13, 2002).

Denis McCance et al. "Medical Virology." <http://www.urmc.rochester.edu/smd/mbi/med.html> (June15,2002).

Dermnet. "Bacteria in Acne." 2001. <http://www.dermnet.org.nz/dna.acne/acne.bac.html> (January 24, 2002).

National Museum of Natural History, Smithsonian Institution. Dept. of Botany "Dinophyta". <http://www.nmnh.si.edu/botany/projects/algae/Algd-Din.htm> (June 15, 2002).

Doctor Fungus. "Aspergillus spp. " 2001. <http://www.doctorfungus.org/thefungi/Aspergillus_spp.htm> (March 30, 2002).

Doctor Fungus. "Cryptococcosis." 2002. <http://www.doctorfungus.org/mycoses/human/crypto/Cryptococcosis.htm> (January 28, 2002).

Doctor Fungus. "Eye Infections." 2001. <http://www.doctorfungus.org/mycoses/human/other/eyeinfections.htm> (February 27, 2002).

Earth Observatory. "What are Phytoplankton?" 2000. <http://earthobservatory.nasa.gov:81/Library/Phytoplankton/> (February 6, 2002).

Ehendrick.org. "Bacteremia." 1999. <http://www.ehendrick.org/health/00039230.html> (March 22, 2002).

Engender Health. "Antiseptics and Disinfectants." 2002. <http://www.engenderhealth.org/ip/aseptic/atm5.htm> (February 5, 2002).

EPA United States Environmental Protection Agency. Oil Spill Program. "Biological Agents." <http://www.epa.gov/oilspill/bioagents.htm> (June 15, 2002).

e-Proteomics. "Information about Proteomics and techniques." 2001. <http://www.e-proteomics.net/tech.html> (February 13, 2002).

Expert Reviews in Molecular Medicine. "Life Cycle of *Entamoeba histolytica*. and the Clinical Manifestations of Infection in Humans." 1999. <http://www-ermm. cbcu.cam.ac.uk/99000617h.htm> (February 19, 2002).

Florida State University. "Antibody production-adjuvants." 1998. <http://www.fsu.edu/~FSULAR/adjuvant.html> (April 16, 2002).

Geocities.com. "Coryneform bacteria, Listeria and Erysipelothrix." 1999. <http://www.goecities.com/ SouthBeach/Port/3008/coryne.html> (January 23, 2002).

George Mason University. "American Type Culture Collection." 1996. <http://library.gmu.edu/collections/ atcc.html> (January 23, 2002).

Georgia Perimeter College. "Classification of Life." 1998. <http://www.gpc.peachnet.edu/~janderso/historic/ labman/nclassif.htm> (February 7, 2002).

Glasgow Caledonia University. "Dynamics of Bacterial Growth." 1998. <http://fhis.gcal.ac.uk/BIO/micro/ drjrattray/nutmicro/growth.html> (February 6, 2002).

Global-Flamework. "Comprehensive history of Lampworking." 1997. <http://www.global-flamework. com/history.htm> (March 23, 2002).

Harvard University. "Host-parasite Interactions: Normal Microbial Flora." 2000. <http://www.channing.harvard. edu/1b.htm> (February 2, 2002).

Harvard University. "Institute of Proteomics Research." 2000. <http://www.hip.harvard.edu/research.html> (February 13, 2002).

Harvard University. "U. S. Japan Expedition (1852–1854) and U. S. North Pacific Exploring Expedition (1853–1856)." 1998. <http://www.herbaria.harvard.edu/Libraries/ expinv/JAPAN.html> (February 3, 2002).

Health Canada. "Blue-green Algae (Cyanobacteria) and Their Toxins." 2001. <http://www.hc-sc.gc.ca/ehp/ehd/ catalogue/general/iyh/algae.htm> (March 28, 2002).

Health Square. "Salmonella Food Poisoning: What You Should Know." 2001. <http://www.healthsquare.com/ mc/fgmc0601.htm> (January 30, 2002).

HeliosHealth.com. "Acne causes." 2001. <http://www. helioshealth.com/shn/acne/causes.html> (January 24, 2002).

Hemophilia. "Blood-borne Infections." 2000. <http://www. shemphilia.org/resources/bbinfections.html> (February 12, 2002).

"Hepatitis B Virus (HBV)" 1999. <http://www.tulane.edu/ ~dmsander/WWW/335/HBV.html> (June 15, 2002).

Herpes.com. "Herpes Overview." 2001. <http://www.herpes. com/overview.shtml> (February 19, 2002).

Illinois Mycological Association. "Life Stages of Fungi." 2000. <http://www.ilmyco.gen.chicago.il.us/Terms/ mycel137.html> (February 7, 2002).

Indiana State University. "Hemolysis on Blood Agar." 2001. <http://www.indstate.edu/theme/micro/hemolys.html> (February 14, 2002).

Indiana State University. "Mechanisms of Bacterial Motility." 2000. <http://www.indstate.edu/theme/micro/flagella. html> (May 8, 2002).

Infection Control Education Institute. "Hand Hygiene and Hand Health: Important Links to Infection Prevention." 2001. <http://www.iceinstitute.com/on-line/OR22.html> (February 25, 2002).

Institute of Food Science and Technology. "Microbiological Food safety for Children and Vulnerable Groups." 2001. <http://www.ifst.org/hottop18.htm> (March 9, 2002).

University of California at Berkeley-Museum of Paleontology." Introduction to the Rhodophyta." <http://www.ucmp.berkeley.edu/protista/rhodophyta. html> (June 15, 2002).

Irish Agriculture and Food Development Authority. "Technological and economic benefits of biotechnology." 1999. <http://www.teagasc.ie/publications/agrifood1999/ paper07.htm> (3 April 2002).

Jane Nicklin. "Mycology Lecture Course." School of Biological and Chemical Sciences. Birkbeck College, University of London. <http://www~micro.le.ac.uk/224/ Mycology/3.html> (June 15, 2002).

Kansas State University. "Basic Biology of Cryptosporidium." 2001. <http://www.ksu.edu/parasitiology/basicbio> (February 6, 2002).

Kansas State University. "Taxonomic chronology of Cryptosporidium: some Historical Milestones (good or bad)." 2001. <http://www.ksu.edu/parasitology/ taxonomy> (February 6, 2002).

Kenneth Todar. "Nutrition and Growth of Bacteria." (2001). University of Wisconsin—Madison Department of Bacteriology. <http://www.bact.wisc.edu/Bact303/ NutritionandGrowth> (June 15, 2002).

Kids Health. "Adenovirus." 2001. <http://www.kidshealth. org/PageManager.jsp?dn=KidsHealth&lic=1&ps=107& cat_id=20043&article_set=22972> (January 31, 2002).

Kids Health. "Infectious Mononucleosis." 2001. <http://www.kidshealth.org/PageManager.jsp?dn= KidsHealth&lic=1&ps=107&cat_id=20028&article_set= 22788> (January 26, 2002).

Lawrence Livermore National Laboratory. "Crystallography 101." 2001. <http://www-structure.llnl.gov/Xray/ index_intro.html> (May 2, 2002).

"Lichen Planus Self-Help." Baylor College of Dentistry. <http://www.tambcd.edu/lichen> (June 15, 2002).

London School of Hygiene and Tropical Medicine. "Basic Information on Entamoeba." 1999. <http://www.lshtm.ac.uk/itd/units/pmbbu/enta/basics.htm> (February 19, 2002).

Long Island University. "Bacterial Reproduction, Growth and Preservation." 1997. <http://www.liunet.edu/cwis/bklyn/acadres/facdev/FacultyProjects/WebClass/micro-web/html-files/ChapterB-1.html> (February 6, 2002).

Louisiana State University. "Growth and Metabolism." 1996. <http://www.medschool.lsumc.edu/Micr./COURSES/DMIP/dmex06.htm> (February 1, 2002).

Macquarie University News. "Bacteria: the Path of Least Resistance." 2001. <http://www.pr.mq.edu.au/macquest/sciences8.htm> (January 24, 2002).

Medical Diagnostic Laboratories. "*Chlamydia pneumoniae.* and atherosclerosis." <http://www.mdlab.com/fees&serv/serv-athero.html> (January 31, 2002).

Medicine through Time. "Antiseptics." <http://www.bbc.co.uk/education/medicine/nonint/indust/as/inascs2.shtml> (February 5, 2002).

MediResource. "Eye Infections." 2001. <http://www/mediresource.net/canoe/health/PatientInfo.asp?DiseaseID=56> (February 27, 2002).

MedLine plus. "Serum sickness." 2002. <http://www.nlm.nih.gov/medlineplus/ency/article/000820.htm> (February 12, 2002).

Memorial University of Newfoundland. "Bacterial Conjugation. Historical Background." 2001. <http://www.mun.ca/biochem/courses/3107/Lectures/Topics/conjugation.html> (May 8, 2002).

Michael A. Pfaller, MD. "The Fungal Pathogen Shift in the United Sates: Patterns of Candida Species Infections Are Changing". Medscape CME circle. <http://www.medscape.com/viewarticle/413131_1> (June 15, 2002).

Michigan State University. "Disinfection." 2001. <http://www.orcbs.msu.edu/biological/ecp_01/disinfection.htm> (February 19, 2002).

Michigan State University. "History of Bergey's Manual." 2001. <http://www.cme.msu.edu/bergeys/history.html> (January 26, 2002).

Michigan State University. "Life Cycle." 1999. htpp://www.msu.edu/course/zol/316/ehisgut.htm> (February 19, 2002).

Michigan State University. "Magnetic Microbes." 2000. <http://commtechlab.msu.edu/sites/dld-me/curious/caOc96SC.html> (February 2, 2002).

Medscape. "The Stentor." 1994. <http://www.microscopy-uk.org.uk/mag/articles/stentor.html> (March 11, 2002).

Medscape. "Paramecium." 1999. <http://www.microscopy-uk.org.uk/mag/articles/param1.html> (April 9, 2002).

National Agricultural Laboratory. "Cryptosporidium: A Waterborne Pathogen." 1998. <http://www.nal.usda.gov/wqic/cornell.html> (February 6, 2002).

National Coalition for Adult Immunization. "Facts about Tetanus for Adults." 2001. <http://www.nfid.org/factsheets/tetanusadult.html> (January 22, 2002).

National Human Genome Research Institute. "Ethical, Legal and Social Implications of Human Genetic Research." (October 2000). <http://www.nhgri.nih.gov/ELSI/> (June 15,2002).

National Institute of Allergy and Infectious Disease. "The Common Cold." 2001. <http://www.niaid.nih.gov/factsheets/cold.htm> (January 22, 2002).

National Institute of Allergy and Infectious Diseases. "Facts about Shingles (Varicella-Zoster Virus)." 1999. <http://www.niaid.nih.gov/factsheets/shinglesFS.htm> (February 22, 2002).

National Institute of Allergy and Infectious Diseases. "Group A Streptococcal Infections." 1998. <http://www.niaid.nih.govfactsheets/strep.htm> (March 17, 2002).

National Institute of Allergy and Infectious Diseases. "Genital Herpes." 2001. <http://www.niaid.nih.gov/factsheets/stdherp.htm> (February 19, 2002).

National Institute of Child Health and Human Development. "What is Primary Human Immunodeficiency?" <http://www.nichd.nih.gov/publications/pubs/primaryimmunobooklet.htm> (June 15, 2002).

National Institutes of Health. "Antimicrobial Resistance: The NIH Response to a Growing Problem." 1999. <http://www.niaid.nih.gov/director/congress/1999/0225.htm> (January 24, 2002).

National Institutes of Health. "Atypical mycobacterial infection." 2002. <http://www.nlm.nih.gov/medlineplus/ency/article/000640.htm> (March 22, 2002).

National Institutes of Health. "Dental caries." 2001. <http://www.nlm.nih.gov/medlineplus/ency/article/001055.htm> (April 4, 2002).

National Institutes of Health. "NAIAD and Merck to Collaborate on HIV Vaccine Development." 2001. <http://www.nih.gov/news/pr/dec2001/niaid-20.htm> (January 14, 2002).

National Institutes of Health. "New Findings Explain T-cell Loss in HIV Infection." 2001. <http://www.nih.gov/newsroom/releases/tcellloss.htm> (January 21, 2002).

National Institutes of Health. "What is a latent virus?" 1999. <http://www.niaid.nih.gov/dir/labs/lir/hiv/packet3.htm> (April 27, 2002).

National Library of Medicine. "Introduction: Two Centuries of Health Promotion." 1998. <http://www.nlm.nih.gov/exhibition/phs_history/intro.html> (May 13, 2002).

National Louis University. "Electron Transport System and Chemiosmosis." 2000. <http://faculty.nl.edu/jste/electron_transport_system.htm> (March 22, 2002).

National Museum of Natural History, Dept. of Botany Smithsonian Institution. "Algae Division-*Phaeophyta*. " <http://www.nmnh.si.edu.botany/projects/algae/Algd-Pha.htm>#phaeo> (June 15, 2002).

Nature Genome Gateway. "Proteomics in action." 2002. <http://www.nture.com/genomics/post-genomics/action.html> (February 13, 2002).

New Scientist. "All Fall Down." 1998. <http://www.newscientist.com/nsplus/insight/bioterrorism/allfall.html> (June 14, 2002).

New York City Department of Health. "Poliomyelitis (Infantile Paralysis, Polio)." 2000. <http://www.nyc.gov/html>/doh/html>/imm/immpol.html> (February 12, 2002).

New York State Department of Health. "Amebiasis (amebic dysentery)." 1999. <http://www.health.stte.ny.us/nysdoh/consumer/commun.htm> (February 14, 2002).

New York State Department of Health. "Campylobacteriosis." 1999. <http://www.health.state.ny.us/nysdoh/consumer/camplo.htm> (January 24, 2002).

Northern Arizona University. "The Uses and Function of Agar; a review." 1997. <http://dana.ucc.nau.edu/~lmf2/algae97/reds/agar.html> (March 21, 2002).

Novartis Transplant. "History of Sandimmune(r) (cyclosporine, USP)." 2002. <http://www.novartis-transplant.com/history_sandimmune.html> (May 20, 2002).

O'Rourke, K. Journal of the American Veterinary Medical Association. "The Anthrax Detectives". 2001. <http://www.avma.org/onlnews/javma/doc01/s121501a.asp> (December 15, 2001).

Oak Ridge National Laboratory. "Potential Benefits of Human Genome Project Research." 1999. <http://www.ornl.gov/hgmis/project/benefits.html> (January 21, 2001).

Ohio State University. "Campylobacteriosis: a New Foodborne Illness." 1998. <http://ohioline.osu.edu/hyg-fact/5000/5565.html> (January 24, 2002).

Ohio State University. "The Carbon Cycle." 2000. <http://www.biosci.ohio-state.edu/~mgonzalez/Micro521/19.html> (April 10, 2002).

Oregon State University. "*E. coli*. Gene Regulation." 2000. <http://www.orst.edu/instruction/bb492/lectures/Regulation.html> (March 27, 2002).

Panix.com. "A Cole's Notes for the Imune System." 2001. <http://www.panix.com/~iayork/Immunology/vaccination.shtml> (January 30, 2002).

Pennsylvania State University. "Rumen Microbiology." 2000. <http://www3.das.psu.edu/dcn/catnut/422/part1/microbiol.html> (February 15, 2002).

Phage.org. "Bacterial Mechanisms of Pathogenicity." 1998. <http://www.phage.org/biol2060.htm> (February 21, 2002).

Phage.org. "Essential Concepts of Metabolism." 1999. <http://www.phage.org/blck05.htm> (February 8, 2002).

Phage.org. "Membrane Structure and Function." 1999. htpp://www.phage.org/campb108.htm> (February 8, 2002).

Phage.org. "Procaryote Extracellular Appendages." 1998. <http://www.phage.org/biol1084.htm> (January 26, 2002).

Physicians and Scientists for Responsible Application of Science and Technology. "How Are Genes Engineered?" 2001. <http://www.psrast.org/whisge.htm> (June 15, 2002).

Planned Parenthood. "Herpes: Questions and Answers." 2002. <http://www.plannedparenthood.org/STI-SAFESEX/herpes.htm> (February 19, 2002).

Queen's University. "Adenoviruses." 2001. <http://www.queensu.ca/micr/micr450/adeno.html> (January 31, 2002).

Queen's University. "RNA Tumor Viruses." 2000. <http://www.queensu.ca/micr/micr450/retro.html> (April 27, 2002).

Respiratory Reviews. "Can Handwashing Increase the Risk of Transmitting Infections?" 2000. <http://www.respiratoryreviews.com/aug00/rr_au00_handhyg. hml (February 2, 2002).

Roberts, G. University of Wisconsin—Madison. "Bacterial Genetics." 2000. <http://www.bact.wisc.edu/Microtex Book/BactGenetics/whydoit.html> (September 2000).

Ron Kennedy, MD. "Yeast Syndrome" The Doctor's Medical Library. <http://www.medical-library.net/sites/_yeast_syndrome.html> (June 15, 2002).

Salk Institute. "How to use the Coulter counter to count cells." 2000. <http://pingu.salk.edu/~sefton/Hyper_protocols/coulter.html> (April 30, 2002).

Salmonella Enteritidis Infection." National Center for Infectious Disease, Division of Bacterial and Mycotic Diseases, <http://www.cdc.gov/ncidod/index.htm>. (June 15, 2002).

Science Daily. "Slimy Bacteria Common Cause of Chronic Infections." 1999. <http://www.sciencedaily.com/releases/1999/05/990524040309.htm> (February 9, 2002).

Science.ca. "J. William (Bill) Costerton." 2001. <http://www.science.ca/scientists/scientistprofile.php?pID=143> (February 9, 2002).

Scientific American. "Antitoxin for Anthrax." 2001. <http://www.sciam.com/2001/1201issue/1201scicit4.html> (February 12, 2002).

Scientific American. "How to Rear a Plankton Menagerie." 2000. <http://www.sciam.com/2000/0800issue/0800amsci.html> (February 6, 2002).

Scientific American. "Researchers Decipher Final Component of Anthrax's Toxic Triad." 2002. <http://www.scientificamerican.com/news/012402/1.html> (January 27, 2002).

Scientific American. "Stopping Prions from Going Mad." 2000. htpp://www.sciam.com/explorations/2000/052900bse/> (March 30, 2002).

Scientific American. "The Artistry of Microorganisms." 1998. <http://www.sciam.com/1998/1098issue/1098levine.html> (February 1, 2002).

Scientific American. "What is a Prion?" 2000. <http://www.sciam.com/askexpert/medicine/medicine14.html> (March 30, 2002).

Society for Anaerobic Microbiology. "*Actinomyces.*—a Genus with Many Problems." 1999. <http://www.bms.ed.ac.uk/misc/sam/Articles/Article4.htm> (March 27, 2002).

Society for General Microbiology. "Careers in Microbiology." 1999. <http://www.socgenmicrobiol.org.uk/PA/edu_car/medinfo.htm> (January 22, 2002).

South African Museum. "Archaea (Archaebacteria)." 2001. <http://www.museums.org.za/bio/archaea> (February 15, 2002).

South Dakota State University. "Food Poisoning." 1999. <http://www.abs.sdstate.edu/flcs/foodsafety/menulist/doc/poison.htm> (January 30, 2002).

Southern Illinois University. "Immunoglobulins." 1997. <http://www.cehs.siu.edu/fix/medmicro/igs.htm> (February 28, 2002).

Southern Illinois University. "Histocompatibility." 1997. <http://www.cehs.siu.edu/fix/medmicro/mhc.htm> (May 14, 2002).

Stanford University. "Cowpox Virus." 2000. <http://www.stanford.edu/group/virus/pox/2000/cowpox_virus.html> (April 18, 2002).

Stanford University. "The Influenza Pandemic of 1918." 1997. <http://www.stanford.edu/group/virus/uda/> (March 24, 2002).

Stanford University. "What are Yeasts?" 1999. <http://genome-www.stanford.edu/Saccharomyces/VL-what_are_yeast.html> (April 28,2002).

State of Missouri. "History of Public Health Nursing." 2000. <http://www.health.state.mo.us/Publications/100-20.html> (May 13, 2002).

Steen-Hall Eye Institute. "Herpes Zoster (Shingles) Eye Infections." 2001. <http://www.steen-hall.com/zoster.html> (February 27, 2002).

Strange Horizons. "Living Lodestones." 2001. <http://www.strangehorizons.com/2001/20010702/living_lodestones.shtml> (February 2, 2002).

Sturtinova, V., J. Jakubovsky, and I. Hulan. "Pathophysiology: Principles of Disease." Slovak Academy of Sciences, 1995. <http://nic.savba.sk/logos/books/scientific/node32.html>. (June 15, 2002).

Tel Aviv University. "Adaptive Self-Organization during Growth of Bacterial Colonies." 1992. <http://star.tau.ac.il/~inon/publicationsself-org_abs.html> (February 1, 2002).

Texas A & M University. "Amino Acid Composition and Protein Sequencing." (April 28, 2001). <http://www.ntri.tamuk.edu/graduate/sequence.html>

Texas A & M University. "Bacterial Food Poisoning." 2001. <http://aggie-horticulture.tamu.edu/extension/poison.html> (January 30, 2002).

Texas A & M University. "Zooplankton." 1999. <http://www-ocean.tamu.edu/~wormuth/labhtml>/zooplankton.html> (February 6, 2002).

Texas A&M University. "Complement Fixation Tests (CF)." 2001. <http://vtpb-www.cvm.tamu.edu/vtpb/vet_micro/serology/cf/default.html> (April 17, 2002).

Texas Medical Center, Houston. "Coagulase Test." 1999. <http://medic.med.uth.tmc.edu/path/coag.htm> (February 14, 2002).

The Canadian Society for Aesthetic (Cosmetic) Plastic Surgery. "Botox." 2001. <http://www.csaps.ca/botox.htm> (March 20, 2002).

The Center for Biofilm Engineering. "CBE Director Bill Costerton." 1999. <http://www.erc.montana.edu/CBEssentials-SW/director's%20message/bill_costerton.htm> (February 20, 2002).

The Institute for Genomic Research. "About TIGR." 2002. <http://www.tigr.org/about/> (May 3, 2002).

The Institute for Genomic Research. "Life cycle of *Plasmodium falciparum.*" 1998. <http://www.tigr.org> (June 15, 2002).

The Internet Dermatology Society. "Biological Warfare and its Cutaneous Manifestations." 1995. <http://telemedicine.org/BioWar/biologic.htm> (May 10, 2002).

Ohio State University. "Wastewater Treatment Principles and Regulations." 1996. <http://ohioline.osu.edu/aex-fact/0768.html> (February 27, 2002).

The Royal College of Pathologists. "Medical Microbiology." 2002. <http://www.rcpath.org/recruitment/microbiology.html> (January 22, 2002).

University of Edinburgh. "*Bacillus thuringiensis..*" 2001. <http://helios.bto.ed.ac.uk/bto/microbes/bt.htm> (April 9, 2002).

University of Edinburgh. "The Microbial World: Themophilic Microorganisms." <http://helios.bto.ed.ac.uk/bto/microbes/thermo.htm> (February 8, 2002).

University of Texas at El Paso. "Infectious Waste Management." 1997. <http://www.utep.edu/eh&s/ppm/biosafety/mamagement.html> (February 26, 2002).

Tulane University. "Virus Replication." 1999. Htpp://www.tulane.edu/~dmsander/WWW/335/335 Replication.html> (February 20, 2002).

Tulane University. "Epidemiology of Infectious Disease." 1996. <http://www.tulane.edu/~dmsaunder/WWW/MBchB/10a.html> (May 13, 2002).

Tulane University. "Plant Viruses." 1999. htpp://www.tulane.edu/~dmsander/WWW/335/Plant.html> (April 17, 2002).

Tulane University. "Viral Classification and Replication: An Overview." 1999. <http://www.tulane.edu/~dmsander/WWW/224/Classification224.html> (April 27, 2002).

United States Department of Agriculture. "Classical Swine Fever." 1999. <http://www.aphis.usda.gov/oa/pubs/fscsf.html> (April 28, 2002).

United States Department of Agriculture. "United States Regulatory Agencies in Biotechnology." 1998. <http://www.aphis.udsa.gov/biotech/OECD/usregs.htm> (April 15, 2002).

United States Department of Energy. "Methane (Biogas) from Anaerobic Digestors." 2001. <http://www.eren.doe.gov/consumerinfo/refbriefs/ab5.html> (February 15, 2002).

United States Food and Drug Administration. "*Escherichia coli.* O157:H7." 2002. <http://vm.cfsan.fda.gov/~mow/chap15.htm> (March 4, 2002).

United States Food and Drug Administration. "*Giardia lamblia..*" 2002. <http://vm.cfsan.fda.gov/~mow/chap22.html> (March 5, 2002).

United States Public Health Service. "The History of the Commissioned Corps." 2001. <http://www.usphs.gov/html>/history.html> (May 13, 2002).

University Corporation for Atmospheric Research. "Bacteria Survives in Mars Environment." 2000. <http://www.windows.ucar.edu/tour/link=/headline_universe/mrs-bacteri.html> (February 15, 2002).

University Corporation for Atmospheric Research. "Bacteria Survives in Mars Environment." 2000. <http://www.windows.ucar.edu/tour/link=/headline_universe/mrs-bacteri.html> (February 15, 2002).

University of British Columbia. "General Characteristics of Acids and Bases." 2000. <http://www.science.ubc.ca/~chem/tutorials/pH/section0/content.html> (June 5, 2002).

University of British Columbia. "Porins of Gram-negative Bacteria." 2001. <http://www.cmdr.ubc.ca/bobh/porins.htm> (March 23, 2002).

University of Calgary. "Dinoflagellates." 1997. <http://www.geo.ucalgary.ca/~macrae/palynology/dinoflagellates/dinoflagellates.html> (February 20, 2002).

University of California at Berkeley. "Introduction to the Cyanobacteria." 2001. <http://www.ucmp.berkeley.edu/bacteria/cyanointro.html> (March 28, 2002).

University of California at Berkeley. "Bacillus Sporulation." 2000. <http://bark214-3.berkeley.edu/MCB113/lecture1.htm> (May 2, 2002).

University of California at Berkeley. "Bacteria: Life History and Ecology." 2000. <http://www.ucmp.berkeley.edu/bacteria/bacterialh.html> (February 8, 2002).

University Of California at Berkeley. "Introduction to the Xanthophyta." <http://www.ucmp.berkeley.edu/chromista/xanthophyta.html> (June 15, 2002).

University of California at San Diego. "Acne: what causes it?" 2000. <http://orpheus.ucsd.edu/shs/acne.html> (January 24, 2002).

University of Cape Town. "Adenovirus." 2000. <http://www.uct.ac.za/depts/mmi/stannard/adeno.html> (January 31, 2002).

University of Cape Town. "Kingdoms of Organisms." 2000. htpp://www.uct.ac.za/microbiology/tutorial/kingdom.htm> (February 7, 2002).

University of Cape Town. "Virus Origins." 2000. <http://www.uct.ac.za/microbiology/tutorial/virorig.html> (April 16, 2002).

University of Central Florida. "Bacterial/Viral Detection/Screening." 2000. <http://istf.ucf.edu/Tools/NCTs/living_systems/Bacterial-Viral_Detection-Screening/> (February 14, 2002).

University of Connecticut. "Topological Regulation of Bacterial Cell Division." 2001. <http://psel.uchc.edu/celldivision.html> (February 6, 2002).

University of Delaware. "Hydrothermal Vents." 1999. <http://www.ocean.udel.edu/deepsea/level-2/geology/vents.html> (April 3, 2002).

University of Florida. "*Entamoeba histolytica.*" 1999. <htpp://www.medinfo.ufl.edu/year2/mmid/bms5300/bugs/enthist.html> (February 19, 2002).

University of Goettingen. "*Clostridium tetani.*" 2002. <http://www.g21.bio.uni-goettingen.de/clostri.html> (January 22, 2002).

University of Guelph. "Pasteurization." 2001. <http://www.foodsci.uoguelph.ca/dairyedu/pasteurization.html> (April 11, 2002).

University of Guelph. "Research Answers Mysteries of Life 'Underground'." 2001. <http://www.uoguelph.ca/mediare/01-05-23/underground.html> (February 9, 2002).

University of Guelph. "They're Beating Bacteria: Vesicle Technology Overcomes Antibiotic Resistance." 1998. <http://www.uoguelph.ca/research/publications/health/pge42.html> (February 9, 2002).

University of Hamburg. "Improving Protein Solubility." 2001. <http://www.embl-heidelberg.de/ExternalInfo/geerlof/draft_frames/flowchart/exp_e_coli/Ecoli_solubility.html> (February 13, 2002).

University of Hamburg. "Plant Viruses and Viroids." 2001. <http://www.biologie.uni-hamburg.de/e35/35.htm> (April 27, 2002).

University of Illinois at Urbana-Champaign. "Bacterial Chromosome Structure." 2001. <http://www.life.uiuc.edu/micro/316/topics/chroms-genes-prots/chromosomes.html> (March 26, 2002).

University of Illinois at Urbana-Champaign. "Porins." 2001. <http://www.life.uiuc.edu/crofts/bioph354/bergman/kanal/porin/eporin.htm> (February 13, 2002).

University of Leeds. "Introduction to Dental Plaque." 2000. <http://www.dentistry.leeds.ac.uk/OROFACE/PAGES/micro/micro2.html> (March 21, 2002).

University of Leeds. "Nosocomial Infection." 2001. <http://www.bmb.leeds.ac.uk/mbiology/ug/ugteach/icu8/xinfect/intro.html> (April 5, 2002).

University of Leeds. "The Human Commensal Flora." 1996. <http://www.leeds.ac.uk/mbiology/ug/med/flora.html> (April 27, 2002).

University of Leicester. "Cyanobacteria." 2001. <http://www-micro.msb.le.ac.uk/video/Cyanobacteria.html> (February 20, 2002).

University of Leicester. "Biology of Plasmodium Parasites and Anopheles Mosquitoes." 1996. <http://www-micro.msb.le.ac.uk/224/Bradley/Biology.html> (March 27, 2002).

University of Leicester. "Virus Vectors and Gene Therapy: Problems, Promises and Prospects." 1998. <http://www-micro.msb.le.ac.uk/335/peel/peel1.html> (April 20, 2002).

University of Louisville. "Lab Safety: Fume Hoods." 1997. <http://www.louisville.edu/admin/dehs/lsfume.htm> (March 11, 2002).

University of Maryland. "Antibiotic Disk Susceptibilities (Kirby-Bauer Disk-Diffusion Method)." 2000. <http://www.life.umd.edu/classroom/bsci424/LabMaterialsMethods/AntibioticDisk.htm> (April 22, 2002).

University of Maryland. "Coagulase Test." 2000. <http://www.life.umd.edu/classroom/bsci424/LabMaterialsMethods/CoagulaseTest.htm> (February 13, 2002).

University of Minnesota-Duluth. "Membranes." 1997. <http://www.d.umn.edu/~sdowning/Membranes/lecturenotes.html> (February 8, 2002).

University of Nebraska-Lincoln. "Characteristics of Protists; Protozoa and Chromista." 2000. <http://plantpath.unl.edu/peartree/homer/sec.skp/protista.html> (February 7, 2002).

University of Pennsylvania. "Antimicrobial Susceptibility Testing: What Does it Mean?" <http://www.uphs.upenn.edu/bugdrug/antibiotic_manual/amt.html> (January 24, 2002).

University of Rochester. "Virology 7: Human Tumor Viruses." 1999. <http://www.urmc.rochester.edu/smd/mbi/med/lec7.html> (March 12, 2002).

University of South Carolina. "Antibody Formation." 2000. <http://www.med.sc.edu:85/mayer/Ab%20formation2000.htm> (February 1, 2002).

University of South Carolina. "Caulobacter crescentus. Overview." 1999. <http://www.cosm.sc.edu/caulobacter/cycle.html> (February 7, 2002).

University of Southern California. "Microbiology of Dental Plaque." 2000. <http://www.dent.ucla.edu/pic/members/microbio/mdphome.html> (March 21, 2002).

University of Southern Mississippi. "Chitin." 1999. <http://www.psrc.usm.edu/macrog/sea/chitin.htm> (April 23, 2002).

University of Texas at Galveston. "Xanthophyceae: the Class & its Genera". <http://www.bio.utexas.edu/research/utex/class/xanthophyceae.html> (June 15, 2002).

University of Texas. "Arenaviruses." 1996. <http://gsbs.utmb.edu/microbook/ch057.htm> (April 23, 2002).

University of Texas. "Bacterial Adhesion and Biofilm Formation." 2000. <http://www.che.utexas.edu/georgiou/Research/Bacterial_Adhesion.htm> (January 24, 2002).

University of Texas. "Haemophilus. ". 1995. <http://medic.med.uth.tmc.edu/path/00001504.htm> (March 27, 2002).

University of Toronto. "Enzyme Linked Immunosorbant Assay (ELISA)." 1999. <http://dragon.zoo.utoronto.ca/~jlm-gmf/T0401B/ELISA.html> (April 4, 2002).

University of Toronto. "Josef M. Penninger." 1999. <http://medbio.utoronto.ca/faculty/penninger.html> (February 15, 2002).

University of Toronto. "The Next Influenza Epidemic." 1997. htpp://www.utoronto.ca/kids/influenza.html> (May 8, 2002).

University of Virginia. "Plague and Public Health in Renaissance Europe." 1994. <http://www.iath.virginia.edu/osheim/plaguein.html> (May 13, 2002).

University of Washington. "An Historical Introduction to the MHC." 1996. <http://depts.washington.edu/rhwlab/dq/history.html> (May 15, 2002).

University of Wisconsin. *"Pseudomonas aeruginosa.."* 2002. <http://www.bact.wisc.edu/Bact330/lecturepseudomonas> (April 11, 2002).

University of Wisconsin. "Biotechnology in Yellowstone." 1994. <http://www.bact.wisc.edu/Bact303/b27> (April 16, 2002).

University of Wisconsin. "The Bacterial Flora of Humans." 2002. <http://www.bact.wisc.edu/Bact303/Bact303normalflora> (April 27, 2002).

University of Wisconsin. "The Cell Wall." 2002. <http://www.bact.wisc.edu/MicrtextBook/BacterialStructure/CellWall.html> (April 16, 2002).

University of Wisconsin. "The Control of Microbial Growth." 2000. <http://www.bact.wisc.edu/MicrotextBook/ControlGrowth/sterilization.html> (April 19, 2002).

University of Wisconsin. "The Diversity of metabolism in Prokaryotes." 2001. <http://www.bact.wisc.edu/Bact303/bact303metabolism> (May 9, 2002).

University of Wisconsin. "The Gram Negative Cell Wall." 2001. <http://www.bact.wisc.edu/microtextbook/BacterialStructure/MoreCellWall.html> (May 2, 2002).

University of Wisconsin-Madison. "Inclusions and Other Internal Structures." 2001. <http://www.bact.wisc.edu/microtextbook/bacterialstructure/Inclusions.html> (February 20, 2002).

University of Wisconsin-Madison. "Nutrition and Growth of Bacteria." 2001. <http://www.bact.wisc.edu/Bact303/NutritionandGrowth> (March 11, 2002).

University of Wisconsin-Madison. "Bacteria of Medical Importance." 2000. <http://www.bact.wisc.edu/microtextbook/disease/overview.html> (January 27, 2002).

University of Wisconsin-Madison. "Bacterial Resistance to Antibiotics." 1996. <http://www.bact.wisc.edu/Bact330/lecturebactres> (January 21, 2002).

University of Wisconsin-Madison. "Dilution Plating." 2001. <http://www.bact.wisc.edu/Bact102/102dil1.html> (January 26, 2002).

University of Wisconsin-Madison. "The Cell Wall." 2001. <http://www.bact.wisc.edu/MicrotextBook/BacterialStructure/CellWall.html> (January 24, 2002).

Utah State University. "Properties of Biofilms." 2000. <http://www.mth.utah.edu/~cogan/research/pper/node3.html> (February 6, 2002).

Vanderbilt University Medical Center. "Blastomycosis" <http://www.mc.vanderbilt.edu/peds/pidl/infect/index.htm> (June 15, 2002).

Virginia Polytechnic Institute. "An Overview of Hazard Analysis Critical Control Points (HACCP) and its Application to Animal production food Safety." 1999. <http://www.cvm.uiuc.edu/HACCP/Symposium/PIERSON.htm> (March 22, 2002).

VIRTUE Newsletter: Science. "Biofilm re-visited." 2000. <http://www.miljolare.no/virtue/newsletter/00_08/sci-jones/index.php> (February 8, 2002).

Washington University. "The Influenza Virus Hemagglutinin." 1999. <http://medicine.wustl.edu/~virology/influenza.htm> (March 29, 2002).

Web Health. "Benefits of Banking Umbilical Cord Blood." 2001. <http://jhhs.client.web-health.com/web-health/topics/WomensHealth/womenshealthsub/womenshealthpages/Pregnancy/umbilicalcordbanking.html> (May 15, 2002).

Whyfiles. "Brave New Biosphere." 1999. <http://whyfiles.org/022critters/hot_bact.html> (February 15, 2002).

Woodlands. "Why are Ticks and Tick Borne Infections Increasing?" 1997. <http://www.ctwoodlands.org/Summer/tick.html> (February 12, 2002).

World Federation for Culture Collections. "Cryopreservation of Bacteria with Special Reference to Anaerobes." 1989. <http://www.cbs.knaw.nl/publications/on-line/4cryopre.htm> (January 26, 2002).

World Health Organization. "Yellow Fever." 2001. <http://www.who.int/inf-fs/en/fact100.html> (March 11, 2002).

World Health Organization. "Bovine Spongiform Encephalopathy." 2000. <http://www.who.int/inf-fs/en/fact113.html> (January 21, 2002).

World Health Organization. "Cholera." 2000. <http://www.who.int/inf-fs/en/fact107.html> (April 30, 2002).

World Health Organization. "Dengue and Dengue Haemorrhagic Fever." 1998. <http://www.who.int/int-fs/cn/fact117.html> (March 16, 2002).

World Health Organization. "Leprosy: the Disease." 2000. <http://www.who.int/lep/disease/frmain.htm> (April 30, 2002).

World Health Organization. "Poliomyelitis." 2001. <http://www.who.int/inf-fs/en/fact114.html> (February 12, 2002).

World Health Organization. "The World Health Organization: 50 Years of International Public Health." 1998. <http://www.who.int/archives/who50/en/50years.htm> (May 15, 2002).

World Health Organization. "Tuberculosis." 2000. <http://www.who.int/inf-fs/en/fact104.html> (April 30, 2002).

World Water Day 2001. "Disease Fact Sheet: Campylobacteriosis." 2001. <http://www.worldwaterday. org/disease/campylo.html> (January 24, 2002).

Historical Chronology

Editor's note: This is a historical chronology principally devoted to marking milestones in human scientific achievement and is intended to provide a valuable reference that will enable readers to relate dates and events mentioned in the text to the larger scope of related scientific achievement. Although mention is made of epidemics and pandemics, it is beyond the scope of this chronology to provide a comprehensive listing of such events.

ca. 10000 B.C.

Neolithic Revolution: transition from a hunting-and-gathering mode of food production to farming and animal husbandry, that is, the domestication of plants and animals.

ca. 3500 B.C.

Sumerians describe methods of managing the date harvest.

ca. 700 B.C.

The use of anatomical models is established in India.

ca. 600 B.C.

Thales, the founder of the Ionian school of Greek philosophy, identifies water as the fundamental element of nature. Other Ionian philosophers construct different theories about the nature of the Universe and living beings.

ca. 500 B.C.

Alcmaeon, Pythagorean philosopher and naturalist, pursues anatomical research and concludes that humans are fundamentally different from animals. He also differentiates arteries from veins. His work establishes the foundations of comparative anatomy.

ca. 450 B.C.

Empedocles, Greek philosopher, asserts that the Universe and all living things are composed of four fundamental elements: earth, air, fire, and water.

ca. 430 B.C.

Plague of Athens caused by unknown infectious agent. One third of the population (increased by those fleeing the Spartan army) die.

ca. 400 B.C.

Hippocrates, Greek physician, establishes a school of medicine on the Aegean island of Cos. According to Hippocratic medical tradition, the four humors that make up the human body correspond to the four elements that make up the Universe. Hippocrates suggests using the developing chick egg as a model for embryology, and notes that offspring inherit traits from both parents.

ca. 400 B.C.

The Greek philosopher Democritus argues that atoms are the building blocks of the Universe and all living things. Democritus was an early advocate of the preformation theory of generation (embryology).

ca. 350 B.C.

The Greek philosopher Aristotle attempts to classify animals and describes various theories of generation, including sexual, asexual, and spontaneous generation. Aristotle argues that the male parent contributes "form" to the offspring and the female parent contributes "matter." He discusses preformation and epigenesis as possible theories of embryological development, but argues that development occurs by epigenesis.

ca. 50 B.C.

Lucretius proposes a materialistic, atomistic theory of nature in his poem *On the Nature of Things*. He favors the preformation theory of embryological development.

ca. A.D. 70
Roman author and naturalist Pliny the Elder (A.D. 23–79) writes his influential *Natural History*, a vast compilation combining observations of nature, scientific facts, and mythology. Naturalists will use his work as a reference book for centuries.

ca. 160 Bubonic plague (termed "barbarian boils") sweeps China.

ca. 166 Antonine plague in Rome (possibly smallpox or bubonic plague) eventually kills millions throughout the weakening Roman empire.

ca. 200 Galen, the preeminent medical authority of late Antiquity and the Middle Ages, creates a philosophy of medicine, anatomy, and physiology that remains virtually unchallenged until the sixteenth and seventeenth centuries. Galen argues that embryological development is epigenetic, although he disagrees with Aristotle about which organs are formed first and which are most important.

529 Byzantine Emperor Justinian closes the Academy in Athens that was founded by Plato and forbids pagan scientists and philosophers to teach. This causes an exodus of scientists to Persia.

ca. 980 Abu Al-Qasim Al-Zahravi (Abucasis) creates a system and method of human dissection along with the first formal specific surgical techniques.

ca. 1150
Hildegard of Bingen (1098–1179), Germanic author, publishes *The Book of Simple Medicine*, a treatise on the medicinal qualities of plants and minerals.

ca. 1267
Roger Bacon (1214–1292), English philosopher and scientist, asserts that natural phenomena should be studied empirically.

ca. 1275
William of Saliceto creates the first established record of a human dissection.

1348 The beginning of a three-year epidemic caused by *Yersinia pestis* that kills almost one-third of the population of urban Europe. In the aftermath of the epidemic, measures are introduced by the Italian government to improve public sanitation, marking the origin of public health.

1490 Leonardo da Vinci (1452–1519), Italian artist and scientist, describes patterns of capillary action.

1492 Venereal diseases, smallpox, and influenza brought by Columbus's expedition (and subsequent European explorers) to the New World. Millions of native peoples eventually die from these diseases because of a lack of prior exposure to stimulate immunity. In some regions, whole villages are wiped-out; and across broader regions, up to 95% of the native population dies as a result of exposure to these new pathogens.

ca. 1525
Paracelsus (1493–1541), Swiss physician and alchemist, uses mineral substances as medicines. Denying Galen's authority, Paracelsus teaches that life is a chemical process.

1542 Bubonic plague from China devastates Constantinople before advancing to repeatedly kill millions across Europe.

1543 Andreas Vesalius publishes his epoch-making treatise *The Fabric of the Human Body*. Vesalius generally accepts Galenic physiological doctrines and ideas about embryology, but corrects many of Galen's misconceptions regarding the human body. Vesalius is subsequently recognized as the founder of modern anatomy.

1546 Gerolamo Fracastoro (1478–1553) writes a treatise on contagious diseases that identifies and names syphilis. He presents a rudimentary concept of the germ theory of disease.

1568 Zacharias and Hans Janssen develop the first compound microscope. The innovation opens new opportunities for the study of structural detail.

1600 Girolamo Fabrizzi (Fabricus ab Aquapendente) publishes *De formato foetu* (On the formation of the fetus). The illustrations stir academic debate.

1604 German astronomer and mathematician Johannes Kepler (1571–1630) writes a treatise on optics.

1610 Jean Beguin (1550–1620) publishes the first textbook on chemistry.

1614 Italian physician Santorio Santorio (1561–1636) publishes studies on metabolism.

1628 William Harvey (1578–1657), English physician, publishes his *Anatomical Treatise on the Movement of the Heart and Blood*. This scientific classic presents the first accurate description of blood circulation, tracing the course of blood through the heart, arteries, and veins.

1651 Harvey publishes *On the Generation of Animals,*, a treatise on embryology in which Harvey asserts that all living things come from eggs. He argues that oviparous and viviparous generation are analogous, but maintains support for the Aristotelian doctrine that generation occurs by epigenesis.

1658 Dutch naturalist Jan Swammerdam publishes records of observations of red blood cells.

1660 Marcello Malpighi publishes his observations concerning vascular capillary beds and individual capillaries.

1664 René Descartes (1596–1650), French philosopher and mathematician, publicizes his idea of reflexive action. The assertion is included in a French edition of his posthumously published work on animal physiology. In his analysis Descartes applies his mechanistic philosophy to the analysis of animal behavior; he first uses the concept of reflex to denote any involuntary response the body makes when exposed to a stimulus.

1665 Robert Hooke publishes *Micrographia,* an account of observations made with the new instrument known as the microscope. Hooke presents his drawings of the tiny box-like structures found in cork and calls these tiny structures "cells." Although the cells he observes are not living, the name is retained. He also describes the streaming juices of live plant cells.

1668 Francesco Redi publishes *Experiments on the Generation of Insects*, in which he demonstrates that maggots develop from eggs laid by flies. His observations disprove the theory that maggots are spontaneously generated from rotting meats.

1669 Jan Swammerdam begins his pioneering work on the metamorphosis of insects and the anatomy of the mayfly. Swammerdam suggests that new individuals were embedded, or preformed, in their predecessors. Nicolas de Malebranche later reformulates Swammerdam's preformationist ideas into a more sophisticated philosophical doctrine that involves a series of embryos preexisting within each other like a nest of boxes.

1674 Antoni van Leeuwenhoek observes "animalcules" in lake water viewed through a ground glass lens. This observation of what will eventually be known as bacteria represents the start of the formal study of microbiology.

1683 Antoni van Leeuwenhoek discovers different types of minute organisms he refers to as "infusoria" in decomposing matter and stagnant water. He also describes protozoa and bacteria.

1700 Joseph Pitton de Tournefort presents an early version of the binomial method of classification, which is subsequently developed by Carl Linnaeus.

1727 Hales studies plant nutrition and measures water absorbed by plant roots and released by leaves. He argues that something in the air (carbon dioxide) is converted into food, and that light is a necessary element of this process.

1735 Carl Linnaeus publishes his *Systema Naturae, or The Three Kingdoms of Nature Systematically Proposed in Classes, Orders, Genera, and Species,*, a methodical and hierarchical classification of all living beings. He develops the binomial nomenclature for the classification of plants and animals. In this system, each type of living being is classified in terms of genus (denoting the group to which it belongs) and species (its particular, individual name). His classification of plants is primarily based on the characteristics of their reproductive organs.

1740 Abraham Trembley asserts that the fresh water hydra, or "polyp," appears to be an animal rather than a plant. When the hydra is cut into pieces, each part regenerates a complete new organism. These experiments raise many philosophical questions about the "organizing principle" in animals and the nature of development.

1746 Pierre-Louis Moreau de Maupertuis publishes *Venus Physique*. Maupertuis criticizes preformationist theories because offspring inherit characteristics of both parents. He proposes an adaptationist account of organic design. His theories suggests the existence of a mechanism for transmitting adaptations.

1748 Nollet describes osmosis.

1754 Pierre-Louis Moreau de Maupertuis suggests that species change over time, rather than remaining fixed.

1757 Albrecht von Haller (1757–1766) publishes the first volume of his eight-volume *Elements of Physiology of the Human Body*, subsequently to become a landmark in the history of modern physiology.

1759 Kaspar Friedrich Wolff publishes *Theory of Generation,* which argues that generation occurs by epigenesis (the gradual addition of parts). This book marks the beginning of modern embryology.

1762 Marcus Anton von Plenciz, Sr. suggests that all infectious diseases are caused by living organisms and that there is a particular organism for each disease.

1765 Abraham Trembley observes and publishes drawings of cell division in protozoans and algae.

1765 Lazzaro Spallanzani publishes his *Microscopical Observations.* Spallanzani's experiments refutes the theory of the spontaneous generation of infusoria.

1772 Joseph Priestley (1733–1804), an English theologian and chemist, discovers that plants give off oxygen.

1774 Antoine-Laurent Lavoisier (1743–1794), a French chemist, discovers that oxygen is consumed during respiration.

1779 Jan Ingenhousz (1739–1799), Dutch physician and plant physiologist, publishes his *Experiments upon Vegetables*. He shows that light is necessary for the production of oxygen, and that carbon dioxide is taken in by plants in the daytime and given off at night.

1780 Antoine-Laurent Lavoisier (1743–1794), French chemist, and Pierre-Simon Laplace (1749–1827), French astronomer and mathematician, collaborate to demonstrate that respiration is a form of combustion. Breathing, like combustion, liberates heat, carbon dioxide, and water.

1780 George Adams (1750–1795), English engineer, engineers the first microtome. This mechanical instrument cuts thin slices for examination under a microscope, thus replacing the imprecise procedure of cutting with a hand-held razor.

1789 Antoine-Laurent de Jussieu publishes his *Plant Genera,,* a widely acclaimed book that incorporates the Linnaean system of binomial nomenclature. This book comes to be regarded as the foundation of the natural system of botanical classification. Jussieu classifies plants on the basis of cotyledons, and divides all plants into acotyledons, monocotyledons, and dicotyledons.

1796 Edward Jenner (1749–1823) uses cowpox virus to develop a smallpox vaccine.

1796 Erasmus Darwin, grandfather of Charles Darwin and Francis Galton, publishes his *Zoonomia.* In this work, Darwin argues that evolutionary changes are brought about by the mechanism primarily associated with Jean-Baptiste Lamarck, i.e., the direct influence of the environment on the organism.

1797 Georges-Léopold-Chrétien-Frédéric Dagobert Cuvier establishes modern comparative zoology with the publication of his first book, *Basic Outline for a Natural History of Animals.* Cuvier studies the ways in which an animal's function and habits determine its form. He argues that form always followed function and that the reverse relationship did not occur.

1798 Government legislation is passed to establish hospitals in the United States devoted to the care of ill mariners. This initiative leads to the establishment of a Hygenic Laboratory that eventually grows to become the National Institutes of Health.

1800 Marie-François-Xavier Bichat publishes his first major work, *Treatise on Tissues,* which establishes histology as a new scientific discipline. Bichat distinguishes 21 kinds of tissue and relates particular diseases to particular tissues.

1802 Jean-Baptiste-Pierre-Antoine de Monet de Lamarck and Gottfried Reinhold Treviranus propose the term "biology" to denote a new general science of living beings that would supercede studies in natural history.

1802 John Dalton introduces modern atomic theory into the science of chemistry.

1809 Jean-Baptiste-Pierre-Antoine de Monet de Lamarck introduces the term "invertebrate" in his *Zoological Philosophy,,* which contains the first influential scientific theory of evolution. He attempts to classify organisms by function rather than by structure and is the first to use genealogical trees to show relationships among species.

1812 Kirchoff identifies catalysis and mechanisms of catalytic reactions.

1817 Georges-Léopold-Chrétien-Frédéric Dagobert Cuvier publishes his major work, *The Animal Kingdom,* which expands and improves Linnaeus's classification system. Cuvier groups related classes into a broader category called a phylum. He is also the first to extend this system of classification to fossils.

1818 William Charles Wells suggests the theory of natural selection in an essay dealing with human color variations. He notes that dark skinned people are more resistant to tropical diseases than lighter skinned people. Wells also calls attention to selection carried out by animal breeders. Jerome Lawrence, James Cowles Prichard, and others make similar suggestions, but do not develop their ideas into a coherent and convincing theory of evolution.

1820 First United States *Pharmacopoeia* is published.

1824 René–Joachim-Henri Dutrochet suggests that tissues are composed of living cells.

1826 James Cowles Prichard presents his views on evolution in the second edition of his book *Researches into the Physical History of Man* (first edition 1813). These ideas about evolution are suppressed in later editions.

1828 Friedrich Wöhler synthesizes urea. This is generally regarded as the first organic chemical produced in the laboratory, and an important step in disproving the idea that only living organisms can produce organic compounds. Work by Wöhler and others establish the foundations of organic chemistry and biochemistry.

1828 Karl Ernst von Baer publishes a book entitled *On the Developmental History of Animals* (2 volumes, 1828–1837), in which he demonstrates that embryological development follows essentially the same pattern in a wide variety of mammals. Early mammalian embryos are very similar, but they diverge at later stages of gestation. Von Baer's work establishes the modern field of comparative embryology.

1828 Robert Brown observes a small body within the cells of plant tissue and calls it the "nucleus." He also discovers what becomes known as "Brownian movement."

1831 Charles Robert Darwin begins his historic voyage on the H.M.S. *Beagle* (1831–1836). His observations during the voyage lead to his theory of evolution by means of natural selection.

1831 Patrick Matthew includes a discussion of evolution and natural selection in his book *On Naval Timber and Arboriculture.* Matthew later claims priority in the discovery of evolution by means of natural selection in an article published in 1860 in the journal *Gardeners' Chronicle.*

1832 The French physiologist Anselme Payen (1795–1871) isolates diastase from barley. Diastase catalyzes the conversion of starch into sugar, and is an example of the organic catalysts within living tissue that eventually come to be called enzymes.

1836 Félix Dujardin describes the "living jell" of the cytoplasm, which he calls "sarcode."

1836 Theodor Schwann carries out experiments that refute the theory of the spontaneous generation of infusoria. He also demonstrates that alcoholic fermentation depends on the action of living yeast cells. The same conclusion is reached independently by Charles Caignard de la Tour.

1837 French physiologist René–Joachim Dutrochet (1776–1847) publishes his research on plant physiology that includes pioneering work on osmosis. He is the first scientist to systematically investigate the process of osmosis, which he names, and to argue that chlorophyll is necessary for photosynthesis.

1838 Matthias Jakob Schleiden notes that the nucleus first described by Robert Brown is a characteristic of all plant cells. Schleiden describes plants as a community of cells and cell products. He helps establish cell theory and stimulates Theodor Schwann's recognition that animals are also composed of cells and cell products.

1839 Jan Evangelista Purkinje uses the term "protoplasm" to describe the substance within living cells.

1839 Theodore Schwann extends the theory of cells to include animals and helps establish the basic unity of the two great kingdoms of life. He publishes *Microscopical Researches into the Accordance in the Structure and Growth of Animals and Plants,* in which he asserts that all living things are made up of cells and that each cell contains certain essential components. He also coins the term "metabolism" to describe the overall chemical changes that take place in living tissues.

1840 Friedrich Gustav Jacob Henle publishes the first histology textbook, *General Anatomy.* This work includes the first modern discussion of the germ theory of communicable diseases.

1840 German chemist Justus von Liebig (1803–1873) shows that plants synthesize organic compounds from carbon dioxide in the air but take their nitrogenous compounds from the soil. He also states that ammonia (nitrogen) is needed for plant growth.

1840 Karl Bogislaus Reichert introduces the cell theory into the discipline of embryology. He proves that the segments observed in fertilized eggs develop into individual cells, and that organs develop from cells.

1842 Charles Robert Darwin writes out an abstract of his theory of evolution, but he does not plan to have this theory published until after his death.

1842 Theodor Ludwig Wilhelm Bischoff publishes the first textbook of comparative embryology, *Developmental History of Mammals and Man.*

1844 Robert Chambers anonymously publishes *Vestiges of the Natural History of Creation,* which advocates the theory of evolution. This controversial book becomes a best seller and introduces the general reading public to the theory of evolution.

1845 Karl Theodor Ernst von Siebold realizes that protozoa are single-celled organisms. He is the first scientist to define protozoa as organisms.

1847 A series of yellow fever epidemics sweeps the American Southern states. The epidemics recur every few years for more than 30 years.

1851 Hugo von Mohl publishes his *Basic Outline of the Anatomy and Physiology of the Plant Cell,* in which he proposes that new cells are created by cell division.

1854 Gregor Mendel begins to study 34 different strains of peas. He selects 22 kinds for further experiments. From 1856 to 1863, Mendel grows and tests over 28,000 plants and analyzes seven pairs of traits.

1855 Alfred Russell Wallace writes an essay entitled *On the Law Which has Regulated the Introduction of New Species* and sends it to Charles Darwin. Wallace's essay and one by Darwin are published in the 1858 *Proceedings of the Linnaean Society.*

1857 Louis Pasteur demonstrates that lactic acid fermentation is caused by a living organism. Between 1857 and 1880 he performs a series of experiments that refute the doctrine of spontaneous generation. He also introduces vaccines for fowl cholera, anthrax, and rabies, based on attenuated strains of viruses and bacteria.

1858   Charles Darwin and Alfred Russell Wallace agree to a joint presentation of their theory of evolution by natural selection.

1858   Rudolf Ludwig Carl Virchow publishes his landmark paper "Cellular Pathology," thus establishing the field of that name. Virchow asserts that all cells arise from preexisting cells (*Omnis cellula e cellula*). He argues that the cell is the ultimate locus of all disease.

1859   Charles Robert Darwin publishes his landmark book *On the Origin of Species by Means of Natural Selection*.

1860   Ernst Heinrich Haeckel describes the essential elements of modern zoological classification.

1860   Louis Pasteur carries out experiments that disprove the doctrine of spontaneous generation.

1860   Max Johann Sigismund Schultze describes the nature of protoplasm and shows that it is fundamentally the same for all life forms.

1863   Thomas Henry Huxley publishes *Evidence As to Man's Place in Nature*, which extends Darwin's theory of evolution to include humans. Huxley becomes the champion and defender of Darwinism in England.

1865   An epidemic of rinderpest kills 500,000 cattle in Great Britain. Government inquiries into the outbreak pave the way for the development of contemporary theories of epidemiology and the germ theory of disease.

1865   Gregor Mendel presents his work on hybridization of peas to the Natural History Society of Brno, Czechoslovakia. The paper is published in the 1866 issue of the Society's *Proceedings*. Mendel presents statistical evidence that hereditary factors are inherited from both parents in a series of papers on "Experiments on Plant Hybridization" published between 1866 and 1869. Although his experiments provide evidence of dominance, the laws of segregation, and independent assortment, his work is generally ignored until 1900.

1866   Ernst Heinrich Haeckel publishes his book *A General Morphology of Organisms*. Haeckel summarizes his ideas about evolution and embryology in his famous—though long-discredited—dictum "ontogeny recapitulates phylogeny" (or, the development of an individual organism follows the same stages as the development of its species). He suggests that the nucleus of a cell transmits hereditary information and introduces the term "ecology" to describe the study of living organisms and their interactions with other organisms and with their environment.

1866   The Austrian botanist and monk Johann Gregor Mendel (1822–1884) discovers the laws of heredity and writes the first of a series of papers on the subject (1866–1869). The papers formulate the laws of hybridization. Mendel's work is disregarded until 1900, when de Vries rediscovers it. Unbeknownst to both Darwin and Mendel, Mendelian laws provide the scientific framework for the concepts of gradual evolution and continuous variation.

1867   Robert Koch establishes the role of bacteria in anthrax, providing the final piece of evidence in support of the germ theory of disease. Koch goes on to formulate postulates that, when fulfilled, confirm bacteria or viruses as the cause of an infection.

1868   Charles Darwin publishes *The Variation of Animals and Plants under Domestication* (2 volumes).

1868   Thomas Henry Huxley introduces the term "protoplasm" to the general public in a lecture entitled "The Physical Basis of Life."

1869   Johann Friedrich Miescher discovers nuclein, a new chemical isolated from the nuclei of pus cells. Two years later he isolates nuclein from salmon sperm. This material comes to be known as nucleic acid.

1870   Thomas Huxley delivers a speech that introduces the terms biogenesis (life from life) and abiogenesis (life from non-life; spontaneous generation). The speech strongly supports Pasteur's claim to have refuted the concept of spontaneous generation.

1871   Charles Robert Darwin publishes *The Descent of Man, and Selection in Relation to Sex*. This work introduces the concept of sexual selection and expands his theory of evolution to include humans.

1871   Ferdinand Julius Cohn coins the term bacterium.

1872   Franz Anton Schneider observes and describes the behavior of nuclear filaments (chromosomes) during cell division in his study of the platyhelminth Mesostoma. His account is the first accurate description of the process of mitosis in animal cells.

1873   Camilo Golgi discovers that tissue samples can be stained with an inorganic dye (silver salts). Golgi uses this method to analyze the nervous system and characterizes the cells known as Golgi Type I and Golgi Type II cells and the "Golgi Apparatus." Golgi is subsequently awarded a Nobel Prize in 1906 for his studies of the nervous system.

1873   Franz Anton Schneider describes cell division in detail. His drawings include both the nucleus and chromosomal strands.

1873   Walther Flemming discovers chromosomes, observes mitosis, and suggests the modern interpretation of nuclear division.

1874 Wilhelm August Oscar Hertwig concludes that fertilization in both animals and plants consists of the physical union of the two nuclei contributed by the male and female parents. Hertwig subsequently carries out pioneering studies of reproduction of the sea urchin.

1875 Eduard Adolf Strasburger publishes *Cell-Formation and Cell-Division*, in which he describes nuclear division in plants. Strasburger accurately describes the process of mitosis and argues that new nuclei can only rise from the division of preexisting nuclei. His treatise helps establish cytology as a distinct branch of histology.

1875 Ferdinand Cohn publishes a classification of bacteria in which the genus name *Bacillus* is used for the first time.

1876 Edouard G. Balbiani observes the formation of chromosomes.

1876 Robert Koch publishes a paper on anthrax that implicates a bacterium as the cause of the disease, validating the germ theory of disease

1877 Robert Koch describes new techniques for fixing, staining, and photographing bacteria.

1877 Paul Erlich recognizes the existence of the mast cells of the immune system.

1877 Wilhelm Friedrich Kühne proposes the term enzyme (meaning "in yeast"). Kühne establishes the critical distinction between enzymes, or "ferments," and the microorganisms that produce them.

1878 Charles-Emanuel Sedillot introduces the term "microbe." The term becomes widely used as a term for a pathogenic bacterium.

1878 Joseph Lister publishes a paper describing the role of a bacterium he names *Bacterium lactis* in the souring of milk.

1878 Thomas Burrill demonstrates for the first time that a plant disease (pear blight) is caused by a bacterium (*Micrococcus amylophorous*).

1879 Albert Nisser identifies *Neiserria gonorrhoeoe* as the cause of gonorrhea.

1879 Walther Flemming describes and names chromatin, mitosis, and the chromosome threads. Fleming's drawings of the longitudinal splitting of chromosomes in eukaryotic cells provide the first accurate counts of chromosome numbers.

1880 C. L. Alphonse Laveran isolates malarial parasites in erythrocytes of infected people and demonstrates that the organism can replicate in the cells. He is awarded the 1907 Nobel Prize in Medicine or Physiology for this work.

1880 Louis Pasteur develops a method of weakening a microbial pathogen of chicken, and uses the term "attenuated" to describe the weakened microbe.

1880 The first issue of the journal Science is published by the American Association for the Advancement of Science.

1880 Walther Flemming, Eduard Strasburger, Edouard van Beneden, and others document the basic outlines of cell division and the distribution of chromosomes to the daughter cells.

1881 Eduard Strasburger coins the terms cytoplasm and nucleoplasm.

1881 Walther Flemming discovers the lampbrush chromosomes.

1882 Angelina Fannie and Walter Hesse in Koch's laboratory develop agar as a solid growth medium for microorganisms. Agar replaces gelatin as the solid growth medium of choice in microbiology.

1882 Edouard van Beneden outlines the principles of genetic continuity of chromosomes in eukaryotic cells and reports the occurrence of chromosome reduction during the formation of the germ cells.

1882 Pierre Émile Duclaux suggest that enzymes should be named by adding the suffix "ase" to the name of their substrate.

1882 The German bacteriologist Robert Koch (1843–1910) discovers the tubercle bacillus and enumerates "Koch's postulates," which define the classic method of preserving, documenting, and studying bacteria.

1882 Walther Flemming publishes *Cell Substance, Nucleus, and Cell Division*, in which he describes his observations of the longitudinal division of chromosomes in animal cells. Flemming observes chromosome threads in the dividing cells of salamander larvae.

1882 Wilhelm Roux offers a possible explanation for the function of mitosis.

1883 August F. Weismann begins work on his germplasm theory of inheritance. Between 1884 and 1888, Weismann formulates the germplasm theory that asserts that the germplasm was separate and distinct from the somatoplasm. He argues that the germplasm was continuous from generation to generation and that only changes in the germplasm were transmitted to further generations. Weismann proposes a theory of chromosome behavior during cell division and fertilization and predicts the occurrence of a reduction division (meiosis) in all sexual organisms.

1883 Edward Theodore Klebs and Frederick Loeffler independently discover *Corynebacterium diphtheriae*, the bacterium that causes diphtheria.

1883 Walther Flemming, Eduard Strasburger and Edouard Van Beneden demonstrate that, in eukaryotic cells, chromosome doubling occurs by a process of longitudinal splitting. Strasburger describes and names the prophase, metaphase, and anaphase stages of mitosis.

1883 Wilhelm Roux suggests that chromosomes carry the hereditary factors.

1884 Elie Metchnikoff discovers the antibacterial activity of white blood cells, which he calls "phagocytes," and formulates the theory of phagocytosis. He also develops the cellular theory of vaccination.

1884 Hans Christian J. Gram develops the Gram stain.

1884 Louis Pasteur and coworkers publish a paper entitled "A New Communication on Rabies." Pasteur proves that the causal agent of rabies can be attenuated and the weakened virus can be used as a vaccine to prevent the disease. This work serves as the basis of future work on virus attenuation, vaccine development, and the concept that variation is an inherent characteristic of viruses.

1884 Oscar Hertwig, Eduard Strasburger, Albrecht von Kölliker, and August Weismann independently report that the cell nucleus serves as the basis for inheritance.

1885 Francis Galton devise a new statistical tool, the correlation table.

1885 French chemist Louis Pasteur (1822–1895) inoculates a boy, Joseph Meister, against rabies. Meister had been bitten by an infected dog. The treatment saves his life. This is the first time Pasteur uses an attenuated germ on a human being.

1885 Paul Ehrlich proposes that certain chemicals such as arsenic are toxic to bacteria.

1885 Theodor Escherich identifies a bacterium inhabiting the human intestinal tract that he names *Bacterium coli* and shows that the bacterium causes infant diarrhea and gastroenteritis. The bacterium is subsequently named *Escherichia coli.*

1886 Adolf Mayer publishes the landmark article "Concerning the Mosaic Disease of Tobacco." This paper is considered the beginning of modern experimental work on plant viruses. Mayer assumes that the causal agent is a bacterium, though he is unable to isolate it.

1887 Julius Richard Petri develops a culture dish that has a lid to exclude airborne contaminants. The innovation is subsequently termed the Petri plate.

1888 Heinrich Wilhelm Gottfried Waldeyer coins the term "chromosome." Waldeyer also introduces the use of hematoxylin as a histological stain.

1888 Martinus Beijerinck uses a growth medium enriched with certain nutrients to isolate the bacterium *Rhizobium*, demonstrating that nutritionally tailored growth media are useful in bacterial isolation.

1888 The Institute Pasteur is formed in France.

1889 Richard Altmann develops a method of preparing nuclein that is apparently free of protein. He calls his protein-free nucleins "nucleic acids."

1889 Theodor Boveri and Jean-Louis-Léon Guignard establish the numerical equality of the paternal and maternal chromosomes at fertilization.

1891 Charles-Edouard Brown-Sequard suggests the concept of internal secretions (hormones).

1891 Paul Ehrlich proposes that antibodies are responsible for immunity.

1891 Robert Koch proposes the concept of delayed type hypersensitivity.

1892 August Weismann publishes his landmark treatise *The Germ Plasm: A Theory of Heredity*, which emphasizes the role of meiosis in the distribution of chromosomes during the formation of gametes.

1892 Dmitri Ivanowski demonstrates that filterable material causes tobacco mosaic disease. The infectious agent is subsequently showed to be the tobacco mosaic virus. Ivanowski's discovery creates the field of virology.

1892 George M. Sternberg publishes his *Practical Results of Bacteriological Researches*. Sternberg's realization that a specific antibody was produced after infection with vaccinia virus and that immune serum could neutralize the virus becomes the basis of virus serology. The neutralization test provides a technique for diagnosing viral infections, measuring the immune response, distinguishing antigenic similarities and differences among viruses, and conducting retrospective epidemiological surveys.

1893 William Bateson publishes *Materials for the Study of Variation*, which emphasizes the importance of discontinuous variations (the kinds of variation studied by Mendel).

1894 Alexandre Yersin isolates *Yersinia (Pasteurella) pestis*, the bacterium responsible for bubonic plague.

1894 Wilhelm Konrad Roentgen discovers x rays.

1897 John Jacob Abel (1857–1938), American physiologist and chemist, isolates epinephrine (adrenalin). This is the first hormone to be isolated.

1898   Carl Benda discovers and names mitochondria, the subcellular entities previously seen by Richard Altmann.

1898   Friedrich Loeffler and Paul Frosch publish their *Report on Foot-and-Mouth Disease*. They prove that this animal disease is caused by a filterable virus and suggests that similar agents might cause other diseases.

1898   Martin Wilhelm Beijerinck publishes his landmark paper "Concerning a Contagium Vivum Fluidum as Cause of the Spot Disease of Tobacco Leaves." Beijerinck thinks that the etiological agent, which could pass through a porcelain filter that removed known bacteria, might be a new type of invisible organism that reproduced within the cells of diseased plants. He realizes that a very small amount of the virus could infect many leaves and that the diseased leaves could infect others.

1898   The First International Congress of Genetics is held in London.

1899   A meeting to organize the Society of American Bacteriologists is held at Yale University. The society will later become the American Society for Microbiology.

1899   Jacques Loeb proves that it is possible to induce parthenogenesis in unfertilized sea urchin eggs by means of specific environmental changes.

1900   Carl Correns, Hugo de Vries, and Erich von Tschermak independently rediscover Mendel's laws of inheritance. Their publications mark the beginning of modern genetics. Using several plant species, de Vries and Correns perform breeding experiments that parallel Mendel's earlier studies and independently arrive at similar interpretations of their results. Therefore, upon reading Mendel's publication, they immediately recognized its significance. William Bateson describes the importance of Mendel's contribution in an address to the Royal Society of London.

1900   Hugo Marie de Vries describes the concept of genetic mutations in his book *Mutation Theory*. He uses the term mutation to describe sudden, spontaneous, drastic alterations in the hereditary material.

1900   Karl Landsteiner discovers the blood-agglutination phenomenon and the four major blood types in humans.

1900   Karl Pearson develops the chi-square test.

1900   Walter Reed demonstrates that Yellow Fever is caused by a virus transmitted by mosquitoes. This is the first demonstration of a viral cause of a human disease.

1900   Paul Erlich proposes the theory concerning the formation of antibodies by the immune system.

1901   Jules Bordet and Octave Gengou develop the complement fixation test.

1901   Theodor Boveri discovers that in order for sea urchin embryos to develop normally, they must have a full set of chromosomes. He concludes that the individual chromosomes must carry different hereditary determinants.

1901   William Bateson coins the terms genetics, F1 and F2 generations, allelomorph (later shortened to allele), homozygote, heterozygote, and epistasis.

1902   Carl Neuberg introduces the term biochemistry.

1903   Archibald Edward Garrod provides evidence that errors in genes caused several hereditary disorders in human beings. His 1909 book *The Inborn Errors of Metabolism* is the first treatise in biochemical genetics.

1903   Ruska develops a primitive electron microscope.

1903   Tiselius offers electrophoresis techniques that become the basis for the separation of biological molecules by charge, mass, and size.

1903   Walter S. Sutton publishes a paper in which he presents the chromosome theory of inheritance. The theory, which states that the hereditary factors are located in the chromosomes, is independently proposed by Theodor Boveri and is generally referred to as the Sutton-Boveri hypothesis.

1906   Viennese physician and immunological researcher Clemens von Pirquet (1874–1929) coins the term allergy to describe the immune reaction to certain compounds.

1909   Phoebus Aaron Theodore Levene (1869–1940), Russian-American chemist, discovers the chemical difference between DNA (deoxyribonucleic acid) and RNA (ribonucleic acid).

1909   Sigurd Orla-Jensen proposes that the physiological reactions of bacteria are primarily important in their classification.

1909   Wilhelm Ludwig Johannsen argues the necessity of distinguishing between the appearance of an organism and its genetic constitution. He invents the terms "gene" (carrier of heredity), "genotype" (an organism's genetic constitution), and "phenotype" (the appearance of the actual organism).

1911   Peyton Rous publishes the landmark paper "Transmission of a Malignant New Growth by Means of a Cell-Free Filtrate." His work provides the first rigorous proof of the experimental transmission of a solid tumor and suggests that a filterable virus is the causal agent.

1912 Casimir Funk (1884–1967), Polish-American biochemist, coins the term "vitamine." Since the dietary substances he discovers are in the amine group he calls all of them "life-amines" (using the Latin word *vita* for "life").

1912 The United States Public Health Service is established.

1912 Paul Ehrlich discovers a chemical cure for syphilis. This is the first chemotherapeutic agent for a bacterial disease.

1914 Frederick William Twort (1877–1950), English bacteriologist, and Felix H. D'Herelle (1873–1949), Canadian-Russian physician, independently discover bacteriophage.

1914 Thomas Hunt Morgan, Alfred Henry Sturtevant, Calvin Blackman Bridges, and Hermann Joseph Muller publish the classic treatise of modern genetics, *The Mechanism of Mendelian Heredity.*

1915 Frederick William Twort publishes the landmark paper "An Investigation of the Nature of Ultra-Microscopic Viruses." Twort notes the degeneration of bacterial colonies and suggests that the causative agent is an ultra-microscopic-filterable virus that multiplies true to type.

1915 Katherine K. Sanford isolates a single mammalian cell *in vitro* and allows it to propagate to form identical descendants. Her clone of mouse fibroblasts is called L929, because it took 929 attempts before a successful propagation was achieved. Sanford's work is an important step in establishing pure cell lines for biomedical research.

1916 Felix Hubert D'Herelle carries out further studies of the agent that destroys bacterial colonies and gives it the name "bacteriophage" (bacteria eating agent). D'Herelle and others unsuccessfully attempted to use bacteriophages as bactericidal therapeutic agents.

1917 D'Arcy Wentworth Thompson publishes *On Growth and Form,* which suggests that the evolution of one species into another occurs as a series of transformations involving the entire organism, rather than a succession of minor changes in parts of the body.

1918 Calvin B. Bridges discovers chromosomal duplications in *Drosophila.*

1918 More people are killed in a global influenza pandemic than soldiers die fighting World War I. By the end of 1918, approximately 25 million people die from a virulent strain of Spanish influenza.

1919 James Brown uses blood agar to study the destruction of blood cells by the bacterium *Streptococcus.* He observes three reactions that he designates alpha, beta, and gamma.

1919 The Health Organization of the League of Nations is established for the prevention and control of disease around the world.

1924 Albert Jan Kluyver publishes *Unity and Diversity in the Metabolism of Micro-organisms* He demonstrates that different microorganisms have common metabolic pathways of oxidation, fermentation, and synthesis of certain compounds. Kluyver also states that life on Earth depends on microbial activity.

1926 Bernard O. Dodge begins genetic studies on *Neurospora.*

1926 Thomas C. Vanterpool publishes a paper that clarifies the problem of "mixed infections" of plant viruses. His study of the condition known as "streak" or "winter blight" of tomatoes shows that it was the result of simultaneous infection of tomato plants by tomato mosaic virus and a potato mosaic virus.

1927 Hermann Joseph Muller induces artificial mutations in fruit flies by exposing them to x rays. His work proves that mutations result from some type of physical-chemical change. Muller goes on to write extensively about the danger of excessive x rays and the burden of deleterious mutations in human populations.

1927 Thomas Rivers publishes a paper that differentiates bacteria from viruses, establishing virology as a field of study that is distinct from bacteriology.

1928 Fred Griffith discovers that certain strains of pneumococci could undergo some kind of transmutation of type. After injecting mice with living R type pneumococci and heat-killed S type, Griffith is able to isolate living virulent bacteria from the infected mice. Griffith suggests that some unknown "principle" had transformed the harmless R strain of the pneumococcus to the virulent S strain.

1929 Francis O. Holmes introduces the technique of "local lesion" as a means of measuring the concentration of tobacco mosaic virus. The method becomes extremely important in virus purification.

1929 Frank M. Burnet and Margot McKie report critical insights into the phenomenon known as lysogeny (the inherited ability of bacteria to produce bacteriophage in the absence of infection). Burnet and McKie postulate that the presence of a "lytic unit" as a normal hereditary component of lysogenic bacteria. The "lytic unit" is proposed to be capable of liberating bacteriophage when it is activated by certain conditions. This concept is confirmed in the 1950s.

1929 Scottish biochemist Alexander Fleming (1881–1955) discovers penicillin. He observes that the mold *Penicillium notatum* inhibits the growth of some bacteria. This is the first anti-bacterial, and it opens a new era of "wonder drugs" to combat infection and disease.

1930 Curt Stern, and, independently, Harriet B. Creighton and Barbara McClintock, demonstrate cytological evidence of genetic crossing over between eukaryotic chromosomal strands.

1930 Max Theiler demonstrates the advantages of using mice as experimental animals for research on animal viruses. Theiler uses mice in his studies of the yellow fever virus.

1931 Phoebus A. Levene publishes a book that summarizes his work on the chemical nature of the nucleic acids. His analyses of nucleic acids seemed to support the hypothesis known as the tetranucleotide interpretation, which suggests that the four bases are present in equal amounts in DNAs from all sources. Perplexingly, this indicated that DNA is a highly repetitious polymer that is incapable of generating the diversity that would be an essential characteristic of the genetic material.

1932 William J. Elford and Christopher H. Andrewes develop methods of estimating the sizes of viruses by using a series of membranes as filters. Later studies prove that the viral sizes obtained by this method were comparable to those obtained by electron microscopy.

1934 John Marrack begins a series of studies that leads to the formation of the hypothesis governing the association between an antigen and the corresponding antibody.

1935 Wendall Meredith Stanley (1904–1971), American biochemist, discovers that viruses are partly protein-based. By purifying and crystallizing viruses, he enables scientists to identify the precise molecular structure and propagation modes of several viruses. Stanley wins the Nobel Prize in Chemistry in 1946.

1936 George P. Berry and Helen M. Dedrick report that the Shope virus could be "transformed" into Myxomatosis/Sanarelli virus. This virological curiosity was variously referred to as "transformation," "recombination," and "multiplicity of reactivation." Subsequent research suggests that it is the first example of genetic interaction between animal viruses, but some scientists warn that the phenomenon might indicate the danger of reactivation of virus particles in vaccines and in cancer research.

1936 Theodosius Dobzhansky publishes *Genetics and the Origin of Species,* a text eventually considered a classic in evolutionary genetics.

1937 Hans Adolf Krebs (1900–1981), German biochemist, describes and names the citric acid cycle.

1938 Emory L. Ellis and Max Delbrück perform studies on phage replication that mark the beginning of modern phage work. They introduce the "one-step growth" experiment, which demonstrates that after bacteriophages attack bacteria, replication of the virus occurs within the bacterial host during a "latent period," after which viral progeny are released in a "burst."

1939 Richard E. Shope reports that the swine influenza virus survived between epidemics in an intermediate host. This discovery is an important step in revealing the role of intermediate hosts in perpetuating specific diseases.

1939 Ernest Chain and H. W. Florey refine the purification of penicillin, making possible the mass production of the antibiotic.

1940 Ernest Chain and E. P. Abraham detail the inactivation of penicillin by a substance produced by *Escherichia coli.* This is the first bacterial compound known to produce resistance to an antibacterial agent.

1940 Helmuth Ruska obtains the first electron microscopic image of a virus.

1941 George W. Beadle and Edward L. Tatum publish their classic study on biochemical genetics entitled *Genetic Control of Biochemical Reactions in Neurospora.* Beadle and Tatum irradiate red bread mold *Neurospora* and prove that genes produce their effects by regulating particular enzymes. This work leads to the one gene–one enzyme theory.

1941 Lipmann describes and identifies the biochemical and physiological role of high energy phosphates (e.g., adenosine triphosphate; ATP).

1942 Jules Freund and Katherine McDermott identify adjuvants (e.g., paraffin oil) that act to boost antibody production.

1942 Salvador E. Luria and Max Delbrück demonstrate statistically that inheritance of genetic characteristics in bacteria follows the principles of genetic inheritance proposed by Charles Darwin. For their work the two (along with Alfred Day Hershey) are awarded the 1969 Nobel Prize in Medicine or Physiology.

1942 Salvador E. Luria and Thomas F. Anderson publish the first electron micrographs of bacterial viruses. The *Escherichia coli* bacteriophage appears to have a round, or polyhedral head and a thin tail.

1942 Selman Waksman suggests that the word "antibiotics" be used to identify antimicrobial compounds that are made by bacteria.

1944 New techniques and instruments, such as partition chromatography on paper strips and the photoelectric ultraviolet spectrophotometer, stimulate the development of biochemistry after World War II. New methodologies make it possible to isolate, purify, and identify many important biochemical substances, including the purines, pyrimidines, nucleosides, and nucleotides derived from nucleic acids.

1944 Oswald T. Avery, Colin M. MacLeod, and Maclyn McCarty publish a landmark paper on the pneumococcus transforming principle. The paper is entitled "Studies on the chemical nature of the substance inducing transformation of pneumococcal types." Avery suggests that the transforming principle seems to be deoxyribonucleic acid (DNA), but contemporary ideas about the structure of nucleic acids suggest that DNA does not possess the biological specificity of the hypothetical genetic material.

1944 Salvador E. Luria and Alfred Day Hershey prove that mutations occur in bacterial viruses, and they develop methods to distinguish the mutations from other alterations.

1945 Joshua Lederberg and Edward L. Tatum demonstrate genetic recombination in bacteria.

1945 Max Delbrück organizes the first session of the phage course at Cold Spring Harbor Laboratory. The widely influential phage course, which is subsequently taught for 26 consecutive years, serves as the training center for the first two generations of molecular biologists

1946 James B. Sumner, John H. Northrop, and Wendell M. Stanley receive the Nobel Prize in Chemistry for their independent work on the purification and crystallization of enzymes and viral proteins.

1946 Joshua Lederberg and Edward L. Tatum demonstrate that genetic recombination occurs in bacteria as the result of sexual mating. Lederberg and Tatum announce their discovery at the 1946 Cold Spring Harbor Symposium on Microbial Genetics, an event that becomes recognized as a landmark in the development of molecular biology.

1946 Max Delbrück and W. T. Bailey, Jr. publish a paper entitled "Induced Mutations in Bacterial Viruses." Despite some confusion about the nature of the phenomenon in question, this paper establishes the fact that genetic recombinations occur during mixed infections with bacterial viruses. Alfred Hershey and R. Rotman make the discovery of genetic recombination in bacteriophage simultaneously and independently. Hershey and his colleagues prove that this phenomenon can be used for genetic analyses. They construct a genetic map of phage particles and show that phage genes can be arranged in a linear fashion.

1947 Joshua Lederberg and Norton Zinder, and, independently, Bernard D. Davis, develop the penicillin-selection technique for isolating biochemically deficient bacterial mutants.

1948 Barbara McClintock publishes her research on transposable regulatory elements ("jumping genes") in maize. Her work was not appreciated until similar phenomena were discovered in bacteria and fruit flies in the 1960s and 1970s. McClintock was awarded the Nobel Prize in Medicine or Physiology in 1983.

1948 World Health Organization is formed. The WHO subsequently becomes the principle international organization managing public health related issues on a global scale. Headquartered in Geneva, the WHO becomes, by 2002, an organization of more than 190 member countries. The organization contributes to international public health in areas including disease prevention and control, promotion of good health, addressing disease outbreaks, initiatives to eliminate diseases (e.g., vaccination programs), and development of treatment and prevention standards.

1949 John F. Ender, Thomas H. Weller, and Frederick C. Robbins publish "Cultivation of Polio Viruses in Cultures of Human Embryonic Tissues." The report is a landmark in establishing techniques for the cultivation of poliovirus in cultures on non-neural tissue and for further virus research. The technique leads to the polio vaccine and other advances in virology.

1949 The role of mitochondria is finally revealed. These slender filaments within the cell, which participate in protein synthesis and lipid metabolism, are the cell's source of energy.

1949 Macfarlane Burnet and his colleagues begin studies that lead to the immunological tolerance hypothesis and the clonal selection theory. Burnet receives the 1960 Nobel Prize in Physiology or Medicine for this research.

1950 British physician Douglas Bevis demonstrates that amniocentesis could be used to test fetuses for Rh-factor incompatibility.

1950 Erwin Chargaff demonstrates that the Tetranucleotide Theory is incorrect and that DNA is more complex than the model developed by Phoebus A. Levene. Chargaff proves that the nucleic acids are not monotonous polymers. Chargaff also discovers interesting regularities in the base composition of DNA; these findings are later known as "Chargaff's rules." Chargaff discovers a one-to-one ratio of adenine to thymine and guanine to cytosine in DNA samples from a variety of organisms.

1950   Robert Hungate develops the roll-tube culture technique, which is the first technique that allows anaerobic bacteria to be grown in culture.

1950   Ruth Sager's work on the algae *Chlamydomonas* proves that cytoplasmic genes exist and that they can undergo mutation. She shows that such genes can be mapped on a "cytoplasmic chromosome." Confirmation is provided when other researchers report similar findings in yeast and *Neurospora,*. Subsequently the DNA is shown to be associated with cytoplasmic organelles.

1951   Esther M. Lederberg discovers a lysogenic strain of *Escherichia coli* K12 and isolates a new bacteriophage, called lambda.

1951   Rosalind Franklin obtains sharp x-ray diffraction photographs of deoxyribonucleic acid.

1952   Alfred Hershey and Martha Chase publish their landmark paper "Independent Functions of Viral Protein and Nucleic Acid in Growth of Bacteriophage." The famous "blender experiment" suggests that DNA is the genetic material. When bacteria are infected by a virus, at least 80% of the viral DNA enters the cell and at least 80% of the viral protein remains outside.

1952   James T. Park and Jack L. Strominger demonstrate that penicillin blocks the synthesis of the peptidoglycan of bacteria. This represents the first demonstration of the action of a natural antibiotic.

1952   Joshua Lederberg and Norton Zinder report the discovery of a phenomenon they call "transduction." Lederberg and Zinder prove that transduction in *Salmonella* is caused by phage particles that occasionally carry assorted host genes into new hosts (i.e., bacteriophage particles serve as the vectors of genetic exchange). The discovery of transduction is announced at Cold Spring Harbor in 1951. The next year, Zinder and Lederberg publish their results in a paper entitled "Genetic Exchange in Salmonella. New mechanism for the heritable transfer of genetic traits from one bacterial strain to another."

1952   Joshua Lederberg coins the term "plasmid" to describe genetic material that is capable of replicating but is not part of the chromosome.

1952   Karl Maramorosch demonstrates that some viruses can multiply in both plants and insects. This work leads to new questions about the origins of viruses.

1952   Lederberg and Ester Lederberg develop the replica plating method that allows for the rapid screening of large numbers of genetic markers. They use the technique to demonstrate that resistance to antibacterial agents such as antibiotics and viruses is not induced by the presence of the antibacterial agent.

1952   Renato Dulbecco develops a practical method for studying animal viruses in cell cultures. His so-called plaque method is comparable to that used in studies of bacterial viruses, and the method proves to be important in genetic studies of viruses. These methods are described in his paper "Production of Plaques in Monolayer Tissue Cultures by Single Particles of an Animal Virus."

1952   William Hayes isolates a strain of *E. coli* that produces recombinants thousands of times more frequently than previously observed. The new strain of K12 is named Hfr (high-frequency recombination) Hayes.

1953   James D. Watson and Francis H. C. Crick publish two landmark papers in the journal *Nature*, "Molecular structure of nucleic acids: a structure for deoxyribose nucleic acid" and "Genetical implications of the structure of deoxyribonucleic acid." Watson and Crick propose a double helical model for DNA and call attention to the genetic implications of their model. Their model is based, in part, on the x-ray crystallographic work of Rosalind Franklin and the biochemical work of Erwin Chargaff. Their model explains how the genetic material is transmitted.

1953   Jonas Salk begins testing a polio vaccine comprised of a mixture of killed viruses.

1954   Seymour Benzer deduces the fine structure of the rII region of the bacteriophage T4 of *Escherichia coli*, and coins the terms cistron, recon, and muton.

1955   François Jacob and Elie L. Wollman determine the mechanism of the transmission of genetic information during bacterial mating. Jacob and Wollman use a blender to interrupt the mating process and then determine the sequence of genetic transfer between bacterial cells.

1955   Fred L. Schaffer and Carlton E. Schwerdt report on their successful crystallization of the polio virus. Their achievement is the first successful crystallization of an animal virus.

1955   Heinz Fraenkel-Conrat and Robley C. Williams prove that tobacco mosaic virus can be reconstituted from its nucleic acid and protein subunits. The reconstituted particles exhibit normal morphology and infectivity.

1956   Alfred Gierer and Gerhard Schramm demonstrate that naked RNA from tobacco mosaic virus is infectious. Subsequently, infectious RNA preparations are obtained for certain animal viruses.

1956   Arthur Kornberg demonstrates the existence of DNA polymerase in *Escherichia coli*.

1956   Joe Hin Tijo and Albert Levan prove that the number of chromosomes in a human cell is 46, not 48, as had been argued since the early 1920s.

1957   Alick Isaacs and Jean Lindenmann discover and publish their pioneering report on interferon, a protein produced by interaction between a virus and an infected cell that can interfere with the multiplication of viruses.

1957   François Jacob and Elie L. Wollman demonstrate that the single linkage group of *Escherichia coli* is circular; they suggest that the different linkage groups found in different Hfr strains are the results of different insertion points of a factor in the circular linkage group, which determines the rupture of the circle.

1957   Francis Crick proposes that during protein formation each amino acid is carried to the template by an adapter molecule containing nucleotides and that the adapter is the part that actually fits on the RNA template. Later research demonstrates the existence of transfer RNA.

1957   The World Health Organization advances the oral polio vaccine developed by Albert Sabin as a safer alternative to the Salk vaccine.

1958   Frederick Sanger is awarded the Nobel Prize in chemistry for his work on the structure of proteins, especially for determining the primary sequence of insulin.

1958   George W. Beadle, Edward L. Tatum, and Joshua Lederberg are awarded the Nobel Prize in Medicine or Physiology. Beadle and Tatum are honored for their work in *Neurospora* that led to the one gene–one enzyme theory. Lederberg is honored for discoveries concerning genetic recombination and the organization of the genetic material of bacteria.

1958   Matthew Meselson and Frank W. Stahl publish their landmark paper "The replication of DNA in Escherichia coli," which demonstrates that the replication of DNA follows the semiconservative model.

1959   Arthur Kornberg and Severo Ochoa are awarded the Nobel Prize in Medicine or Physiology for their discovery of enzymes that produce artificial DNA and RNA.

1959   Robert L. Sinsheimer reports that bacteriophage ØX174, which infects *Escherichia coli*, contains a single-stranded DNA molecule, rather than the expected double stranded DNA. This provides the first example of a single-stranded DNA genome.

1959   Sydney Brenner and Robert W. Horne publish a paper entitled

The two researchers develop a method for studying the architecture of viruses at the molecular level using the electron microscope.

1959   English biochemist Rodney Porter begins studies that lead to the discovery of the structure of antibodies. Porter receives the 1972 Nobel Prize in Physiology or Medicine for this research.

1961   François Jacob and Jacques Monod publish *Genetic regulatory mechanisms in the synthesis of proteins*, a paper that describes the role of messenger RNA and proposes the operon theory as the mechanism of genetic control of protein synthesis.

1961   Francis Crick, Sydney Brenner, and others propose that a molecule called transfer RNA uses a three-base code in the manufacture of proteins.

1961   Marshall Warren Nirenberg synthesizes a polypeptide using an artificial messenger RNA (a synthetic RNA containing only the base uracil) in a cell-free protein-synthesizing system. The resulting polypeptide contains only the amino acid phenylalanine, indicating that UUU was the codon for phenylalanine. This important step in deciphering the genetic code is described in the landmark paper by Nirenberg and J. Heinrich Matthaei, "The Dependence of Cell-Free Synthesis in E. coli upon Naturally Occurring or Synthetic Polyribonucleotides." This work establishes the messenger concept and a system that could be used to work out the relationship between the sequence of nucleotides in the genetic material and amino acids in the gene product.

1961   French pathologist Jacques Miller discovers the role of the thymus in cellular immunity.

1961   Noel Warner establishes the physiological distinction between the cellular and humoral immune responses.

1962   James D. Watson, Francis Crick, and Maurice Wilkins are awarded the Nobel Prize in Medicine or Physiology for their work in elucidating the structure of DNA.

1963   Ruth Sager discovers DNA in chloroplasts. Boris Ephrussi discovers DNA in mitochondria.

1964   Barbara Bain publishes a classic account of her work on the mixed leukocyte culture (MLC) system that is critical in determining donor-recipient matches for organ or bone marrow transplantation. Bain shows that the MLC phenomenon is caused by complex genetic differences between individuals.

1965   François Jacob, André Lwoff, and Jacques Monod are awarded the Nobel Prize in Medicine or Physiology for their discoveries concerning genetic control of enzymes and virus synthesis.

1966 Bruce Ames develops a test to screen for compounds that cause mutations, including those that are cancer causing. The so-called Ames test utilizes the bacterium *Salmonella typhimurium*.

1966 Marshall Nirenberg and Har Gobind Khorana lead teams that decipher the genetic code. All of the 64 possible triplet combinations of the four bases (the codons) and their associated amino acids are determined and described.

1967 Charles T. Caskey, Richard E. Marshall, and Marshall Warren Nirenberg suggest that there is a universal genetic code shared by all life forms.

1967 Charles Yanofsky demonstrates that the sequence of codons in a gene determines the sequence of amino acids in a protein.

1967 Thomas Brock discovers the heat-loving bacterium *Thermus aquaticus* from a hot spring in Yellowstone National Park. The bacterium yields the enzyme that becomes the basis of the DNA polymerase reaction.

1968 Lynne Margulis proposes that mitochondria and chloroplasts in eukaryotic cells originated from bacterial symbiosis.

1968 Mark Steven Ptashne and Walter Gilbert independently identify the bacteriophage genes that are the repressors of the lac operon.

1968 Werner Arber discovers that bacteria defend themselves against viruses by producing DNA-cutting enzymes. These enzymes quickly become important tools for molecular biologists.

1969 Julius Adler discovers protein receptors in bacteria that function in the detection of chemical attractants and repellents. The so-called chemoreceptors are critical for the directed movement of bacteria that comes to be known as chemotaxis.

1969 Max Delbrück, Alfred D. Hershey, and Salvador E. Luria are awarded the Nobel Prize in Medicine or Physiology for their discoveries concerning the replication mechanism and the genetic structure of viruses.

1969 Stanford Moore and William H. Stein determine the sequence of the 124-amino-acid chain of the enzyme ribonuclease.

1970 Hamilton Smith and Kent Wilcox isolate the first restriction enzyme, HindII, an enzyme that cuts DNA molecules at specific recognition sites.

1970 Har Gobind Khorana announce the synthesis of the first wholly artificial gene. Khorana and his coworkers synthesize the gene that codes for alanine transfer RNA in yeast.

1970 Howard Martin Temin and David Baltimore independently discover reverse transcriptase in viruses. Reverse transcriptase is an enzyme that catalyzes the transcription of RNA into DNA.

1971 Christian B. Anfinsen, Stanford Moore, and William H. Stein are awarded the Nobel Prize in chemistry. Anfinsen is cited for his work on ribonuclease, especially concerning the connection between the amino acid sequence and the biologically active conformation. Moore and Stein are cited for their contribution to the understanding of the connection between chemical structure and catalytic activity of the active center of the ribonuclease molecule.

1972 Paul Berg and Herbert Boyer produce the first recombinant DNA molecules.

1972 Recombinant technology emerges as one of the most powerful techniques of molecular biology. Scientists are able to splice together pieces of DNA to form recombinant genes. As the potential uses—therapeutic and industrial—became increasingly clear, scientists and venture capitalists establish biotechnology companies.

1973 Annie Chang and Stanley Cohen show that a recombinant DNA molecule can be maintained and replicated in *Escherichia coli*.

1973 Concerns about the possible hazards posed by recombinant DNA technologies, especially work with tumor viruses, leads to the establishment of a meeting at Asilomar, California. The proceedings of this meeting are subsequently published by the Cold Spring Harbor Laboratory as a book entitled *Biohazards in Biological Research*.

1973 Herbert Wayne Boyer and Stanley H. Cohen create recombinant genes by cutting DNA molecules with restriction enzymes. These experiments mark the beginning of genetic engineering.

1973 Joseph Sambrook and coworkers refine DNA electrophoresis by using agarose gel and staining with ethidium bromide.

1974 Peter Doherty and Rolf Zinkernagel discover the basis of immune determination of self and non-self.

1975 César Milstein and George Kohler create monoclonal antibodies.

1975 David Baltimore, Renato Dulbecco, and Howard Temin share the Nobel Prize in Medicine or Physiology for their discoveries concerning the interaction between tumor viruses and the genetic material of the cell and the discovery of reverse transcriptase.

1976 First outbreak of Ebola virus observed in Zaire. There are more than 300 cases and a 90% death rate.

1976 Michael J. Bishop, Harold Elliot Varmus, and coworkers obtain definitive evidence that confirms the oncogene hypothesis. They discover that normal genes can malfunction and cause cells to become cancerous.

1977 Carl R. Woese and George E. Fox publish an account of the discovery of a third major branch of living beings, the Archaea. Woese suggests that an rRNA database could be used to generate phylogenetic trees.

1977 The last reported smallpox case is recorded. Ultimately, the World Health Organization (WHO) declares the disease eradicated.

1977 Frederick Sanger develops the chain termination (dideoxy) method for sequencing DNA, and uses the method to sequence the genome of a microorganism.

1977 Holger Jannasch demonstrates that heat-loving bacteria found at hydrothermal vents are the basis of an ecosystem that exists in the absence of light.

1977 Philip Allen Sharp and Richard John Roberts independently discover that the DNA making up a particular gene could be present in the genome as several separate segments. Although both Roberts and Sharp use a common cold–causing virus, called adenovirus, as their model system, researchers later find "split genes" in higher organisms, including humans. Sharp and Roberts are subsequently awarded the Nobel Prize in Medicine or Physiology in 1993 for the discovery of split genes.

1980 Paul Berg, Walter Gilbert, and Frederick Sanger share the Nobel Prize in Chemistry. Berg is honored for his fundamental studies of the biochemistry of nucleic acids, with particular regard to recombinant-DNA. Gilbert and Sanger are honored for their contributions to the sequencing of nucleic acids. This is Sanger's second Nobel Prize.

1980 Researchers successfully introduce a human gene, which codes for the protein interferon, into a bacterium.

1980 The United States Supreme Court rules that a living organism developed by General Electric (a microbe used to clean up an oil spill) can be patented.

1981 Karl Illmensee clones baby mice.

1982 The United States Food and Drug Administration approves the first genetically engineered drug, a form of human insulin produced by bacteria.

1983 O157:H7 is identified as a human pathogen.

1983 Andrew W. Murray and Jack William Szostak create the first artificial chromosome.

1983 Luc Montagnier and Robert Gallo discover the human immunodeficiency virus that is believed to cause acquired immunodeficiency syndrome (AIDS).

1984 Steen A. Willadsen successfully clones a sheep.

1984 The United States Department of Energy (DOE), Office of Health and Environmental Research, U.S. Department of Energy (OHER, now Office of Biological and Environmental Research), and the International Commission for Protection Against Environmental Mutagens and Carcinogens (ICPEMC) cosponsor the Alta, Utah, conference highlighting the growing role of recombinant DNA technologies. OTA incorporates the proceedings of the meeting into a report acknowledging the value of deciphering the human genome.

1985 Alec Jeffreys develops "genetic fingerprinting," a method of using DNA polymorphisms (unique sequences of DNA) to identify individuals. The method, which is subsequently used in paternity, immigration, and murder cases, is generally referred to as "DNA fingerprinting."

1985 Elizabeth Blackburn and Carol Greider discover the enzyme telomerase, an unusual RNA-containing DNA polymerase that can add to the telomeres (specialized structures found at the ends of chromosomal DNA). Telomeres appear to protect the integrity of the chromosome. Most normal somatic cells lack telomerase, but cancer cells have telomerase activity, which might explain their ability to multiply indefinitely.

1985 Kary Mullis, who was working at Cetus Corporation, develops the polymerase chain reaction (PCR), a new method of amplifying DNA. This technique quickly becomes one of the most powerful tools of molecular biology. Cetus patents PCR and sells the patent to Hoffman-LaRoche, Inc. in 1991.

1985 Japanese molecular biologist Susuma Tonegawa discovers the genes that code for immunoglobulins. He receives the 1986 Nobel Prize in Physiology or Medicine for this discovery.

1985 American molecular biologist and physician Leroy Hood leads a team that discovers the genes that code for the T cell receptor.

1986 The United States Food and Drug Administration approves the first genetically engineered human vaccine for hepatitis B.

1987 Maynard Olson creates and names yeast artificial chromosomes (YACs), which provided a technique to clone long segments of DNA.

1987 The United States Congress charters a Department of Energy advisory committee, The Health and Environmental Research Advisory Committee (HERAC), which recommends a 15–year, multidisciplinary, scientific, and technological undertaking to map and sequence the human genome. DOE designates multidisciplinary human genome centers. National Institute of General Medical Sciences at the National Institutes of Health (NIH NIGMS) begin funding genome projects.

1988 The Human Genome Organization (HUGO) is established by scientists in order to coordinate international efforts to sequence the human genome.

1989 Cells from one embryo are used to produce seven cloned calves.

1989 James D. Watson is appointed head of the National Center for Human Genome Research. The agency is created to oversee the $3 billion budgeted for the American plan to map and sequence the entire human DNA by 2005.

1989 Sidney Altman and Thomas R. Cech are awarded the Nobel Prize in chemistry for their discovery of ribozymes (RNA molecules with catalytic activity). Cech proves that RNA could function as a biocatalyst as well as an information carrier.

1990 Michael R. Blaese and French W. Anderson conduct the first gene replacement therapy experiment on a four-year-old girl with adenosine deaminase (ADA) deficiency, an immune-system disorder. T cells from the patient are isolated and exposed to retroviruses containing an RNA copy of a normal ADA gene. The treated cells are returned to her body where they help restore some degree of function to her immune system.

1990 Research and development begins for the efficient production of more stable, large-insert bacterial artificial chromosomes (BACs).

1991 The Genome Database, a human chromosome mapping data repository, is established.

1992 Craig Venter establishes The Institute for Genomic Research (TIGR) in Rockville, Maryland. TIGR later sequences the genome of *Haemophilus influenzae* and many other bacterial genomes.

1992 Francis Collins replaces James Watson as head of the National Center for Human Genome Research at the National Institutes of Health. Watson had clashed with Craig Venter, then at NIH, over the patenting of DNA fragments known as "expressed sequence tags."

1992 Guidelines for data release and resource sharing related to the Human Genome Project are announced by the United States Department of Energy and National Institutes of Health.

1993 Hanta virus emerged in the United States in a 1993 outbreak on a "Four Corners" area (the juncture of Utah, Colorado, New Mexico, Arizona) Native American reservation. The resulting Hanta pulmonary syndrome (HPS) had a 43% mortality rate.

1993 French Gépnéthon makes mega-YACs available to the genome community.

1993 George Washington University researchers clone human embryos and nurture them in a Petri dish for several days. The project provokes protests from many ethicists, politicians, and other critics of genetic engineering.

1994 DOE announce the establishment of the Microbial Genome Project as a spin-off of the Human Genome Project.

1994 Geneticists determine that DNA-repair enzymes perform several vital functions, including preserving genetic information and protecting the cell from cancer.

1994 The 5-year goal for genetic-mapping is achieved one year ahead of schedule.

1994 The Human Genome Project Information Web site is made available to researchers and the public.

1995 Peter Funch and Reinhardt Moberg Kristensen create a new phylum, Cycliophora, for a novel invertebrate called *Symbion pandora*, which is found living in the mouths of Norwegian lobsters.

1995 Researchers at Duke University Medical Center report that they have transplanted hearts from genetically altered pigs into baboons. All three transgenic pig hearts survive at least a few hours, suggesting that xenotransplants (cross-species organ transplantation) might be possible.

1995 The genome of the bacterium *Haemophilus influenzae* is sequenced.

1995 The sequence of *Mycoplasma genitalium* is completed. *Mycoplasma genitalium*, regarded as the smallest known bacterium, is considered a model of the minimum number of genes needed for independent existence.

1996 International participants in the genome project meet in Bermuda and agree to formalize the conditions of data access. The agreement, known as the "Bermuda Principles," calls for the release of sequence data into public databases within 24 hours.

1996 Scientists report further evidence that individuals with two mutant copies of the CC-CLR-5 gene are generally resistant to HIV infection.

1996 The sequence of the *Methanococcus jannaschii* genome provides further evidence of the existence of third major branch of life on earth.

1996 William R. Bishai and co-workers report that SigF, a gene in the tuberculosis bacterium, enables the bacterium to enter a dormant stage.

1997 Ian Wilmut of the Roslin Institute in Edinburgh, Scotland, announces the birth of a lamb called Dolly, the first mammal cloned from an adult cell (a cell in a pregnant ewe's mammary gland).

1997 The DNA sequence of *Escherichia coli* is completed.

1997 The National Center for Human Genome Research (NCHGR) at the National Institutes of Health becomes the National Human Genome Research Institute (NHGRI).

1997 William Jacobs and Barry Bloom create a biological entity that combines the characteristics of a bacterial virus and a plasmid (a DNA structure that functions and replicates independently of the chromosomes). This entity is capable of triggering mutations in *Mycobacterium tuberculosis*.

1998 Craig Venter forms a company (later named Celera), and predicts that the company would decode the entire human genome within three years. Celera plans to use a "whole genome shotgun" method, which would assemble the genome without using maps. Venter says that his company would not follow the Bermuda principles concerning data release.

1998 DOE funds bacterial artificial chromosome and sequencing projects.

1998 Dolly, the first cloned sheep, gives birth to a lamb that had been conceived by a natural mating with a Welsh Mountain ram. Researches said the birth of Bonnie proved that Dolly was a fully normal and healthy animal.

1998 Immunologist Ellen Heber-Katz, researcher at the Wistar Institute in Philadelphia, reports than a strain of laboratory mice can regenerate tissue in their ears, closing holes that scientists had created for identification purposes. This discovery reopens the discussion on possible regeneration in humans.

1998 The genome of the *Mycobacterium tuberculosis* bacterium is sequenced.

1998 Two research teams succeed in growing embryonic stem cells.

1999 The public genome project responds to Craig Venter's challenge with plans to produce a draft genome sequence by 2000. Most of the sequencing is done in five centers, known as the "G5": the Whitehead Institute for Biomedical Research in Cambridge, Massachusetts; the Sanger Centre near Cambridge, United Kingdom; Baylor College of Medicine in Houston, Texas; Washington University in St. Louis, Missouri; the DOE's Joint Genome Institute (JGI) in Walnut Creek, California.

2000 On June 26, 2000, leaders of the public genome project and Celera announce the completion of a working draft of the entire human genome sequence. Ari Patrinos of the DOE helps mediate disputes between the two groups so that a fairly amicable joint announcement could be presented at the White House in Washington, DC.

2001 The complete draft sequence of the human genome is published. The public sequence data is published in the British journal *Nature* and the Celera sequence is published in the American journal *Science*.

2001 United States President George Bush announces the United States will allow and support limited forms of stem cell growth and research.

2001 In the aftermath of the September 11 terrorist attacks on the United States, a number of deaths result from the deliberate release of the bacterial agent of anthrax.

2001 Advanced Cell Technology announces that its researchers have created cloned human embryos that grew to the six-cell stage.

2002 In the aftermath of the September 11, 2001 terrorist attacks on the United States, the United States Government dramatically increases funding to programs concerned with research on microorganisms and other agents that could potentially be used in bioterrorist attacks.

2002 Traces of biological and chemical weapon agents are found in Uzbekistan on a military base used by U.S. troops fighting in Afghanistan. Early analysis dates and attributes the source of the contamination to former Soviet Union biological and chemical weapons programs that utilized the base.

2002 The planned destruction of stocks of smallpox causing Variola virus at the two remaining depositories in the US and Russia is delayed over fears that large scale production of vaccine might be needed in the event of a bioterrorist action.

GENERAL INDEX

A

Abbé, Ernst, **1:1,** 2:388
Abel, John Jacob, 2:650
Abraham, E.P., 2:653
Accutane, 1:2
Acid-loving bacteria, 1:211
Acidity, pH, 2:433
aCL. *See* Anticardiolipin antibodies
Acne, microbial basis of, **1:1–2,** 1:2
        See also Microbial flora of the skin
Acquired immunity, 2:361–362
Acquired resistance, 1:47
Acrasiomycota, 2:518
Acridine orange, **1:2–3,** 1:24
Actinomyces, **1:3,** 1:132
Actinomyces infection, 1:3
Actinomycosis, 1:3
Activated sludge process, 1:218
Active immunity, 1:288–290
Active transport, 1:109
Acyclovir, 1:116, 1:184, 2:572, 2:573
ADA deficiency, 1:297
Adams, George, 2:646
Adenosine triphosphate (ATP), 2:392, 2:484–485
Adenoviruses, **1:3–4,** 1:4, 2:579, 2:580, 2:581, 2:584
Adickes, Franz, 1:178
Adjuvant, **1:4–5,** 2:567–568
Adjuvant therapy, 1:116
Adler, Julius, 2:657
Aedes aegypti, 1:153
Aedes albopictus, 1:153
Aerobes, **1:5**
        activated sludge process, 1:218
        Azotobacter, 1:41
        electron transport system, 1:182
        photosynthetic microorganisms, 2:437
        wastewater treatment, 1:218
Aerobic respiration, 2:484–485
Aerolysin, 1:189
Aeromonas hydrophila, exotoxin, 1:189

Aflatoxin, 2:394, 2:395
AFM. *See* Atomic force microscope
African sleeping sickness, 2:462
African swine fever, 2:536
African trypanosomiasis, 2:462
Agammaglobulinemia, 1:293, 1:301
Agar and agarose, **1:5–7,** 1:6, 1:23, 1:255, 2:473
Agar diffusion, **1:7,** 1:7
Agar diffusion assay, 1:7
Agaropectin, 1:6
Agarose, 1:6
Agrobacterium, 1:354
Agrobacterium tumefaciens, 2:442
AIDS, **1:7–10,** 1:296, 2:512
        animal models of infection, 1:19
        antiviral drugs, 1:33
        Elion, Gertrude Belle, 1:183–185
        epidemics, 1:196–198
        human T-cell leukemia virus (HTLV), 1:281
        Kaposi's sarcoma, 1:267, 1:314
        mycobacteria, atypical, 2:407
        mycoplasma infections, 2:408
        pneumonia with, 2:445
        as public health issue, 1:19–22, 2:467
        recent advances in, 2:401, 2:486, 2:493–494
        retroviruses, 2:486–487
        seroconversion, 2:508
        treatment for, 2:487
        vaccine, 1:9, 2:513, 2:570–571
        See also Human immunodeficiency virus
AIDS, recent advances in research and treatment, 2:401
        retroviruses, 2:486–487
        RNA tumor viruses, 2:493–494
Alcmaeon, 2:643
Alcohol, as disinfectant, 1:159
Alcoholic beverages, fermentation, 1:217
Aldehyde compounds, as disinfectant, 1:159
Alexander, Hattie Elizabeth, **1:10**
Alexandrium, 2:481
Alexin, 1:287
Algae, 2:387, 2:460

photosynthetic microorganisms, 2:437
xanthophylls, 2:605
Avery, Oswald Theodore, **1:39–41,** 1:114, 1:167, 1:274, 1:337, 2:359, 2:367, 2:382, 2:654
Avihepadnavirus, 1:264
Axial filaments, 1:48, 1:52, 2:525
Azidothymidine (AZT), 1:8, 1:116, 1:183
Azotobacter, **1:41**
AZT, 1:8, 1:116, 1:183

B

B cells (B lymphocytes), **1:43,** 1:288, 1:291, 1:293, 2:539
Epstein-Barr virus, 1:201
immune system, 1:287–288
B lymphocyte deficiency, 1:293
Babesia, 2:464, 2:526
Babesiosis, 1:82
BAC. *See* Bacterial artificial chromosome
Bacillariophyta, 2:460
Bacillary dysentery, 1:168, 2:514
Bacillus anthracis
anthrax, 1:19–21, 1:*20*
biological warfare, 1:70
surface layers, 1:53
Bacillus Calmette-Guerin, 1:286
Bacillus stearothermophilus, 1:160, 2:405
Bacillus subtilis
colony, 1:129
sporulation, 2:527
thermal death, 2:546
Bacillus thuringiensis, **1:43–44,** 1:*44*
Bacon, Roger, 2:644
Bacteremia, 1:44, 1:45
Bacteremic, **1:44–45,** 2:435
Bacteria
acid-loving bacteria, 1:211
Actinomyces, 1:3
adaptation, 1:46–47
aerobes, 1:5
alkaline-loving bacteria, 1:211
anaerobes and anaerobic infection, **1:16–17**
appendages, 1:47–48, 1:52, 1:67
asexual generation and reproduction, 1:35–36
attractants and repellents, 1:37
autotrophic bacteria, 1:39, 1:115
Azotobacter, 1:41
bacterial kingdoms, 1:51
bioluminescence, 1:72–73, 1:354
Caulobacter crescentus, 1:101
chemoautotrophic and chemolithotrophic bacteria, 1:115–116
cloroxybacteria, 2:436
colony and colony formation, 1:129–130
contamination, 1:135–136
coryneform bacteria, 1:136–137, 1:157
Coulter counter, 1:137–138
cryoprotection, 1:141–142
cyanobacteria, 1:82–83
DNA, 1:161
electron transport system, 1:182
Enterobacteriaceae, 1:187–188
environmental contamination, 1:136–137
episomes, plasmids, insertion sequences, and transposons, 1:200

Eubacteria, 1:203
evolutionary origin, 1:208–209
extremophiles, 1:211–212
fossilization of bacteria, 1:228
Francisella tularensis, 2:557
germ theory of disease, 1:28, 1:246–247, 1:273
gliding bacteria, 1:52, 1:249
growth and division, 1:49–51
Haemophilus, 1:257
halophilic bacteria, 1:211
indicator species, 1:308
invasiveness and intracellular infection, 1:315
"iron" bacteria, 1:115, 2:514
lactic acid bacteria, 1:336
Lactobacillus, 1:336–337
luminescent bacteria, 1:354
magnetotactic bacteria, 2:360–361
mesophilic bacteria, 1:50, 1:276
methane oxidizing and producing bacteria, 1:101, 2:378–379
microbial flora of the oral cavity, dental caries, 2:379–380
microbial flora of the skin, 2:380
microbial flora of the stomach and gastrointestinal tract, 2:380–381
movement of, 1:52
nitrogen-fixing bacteria, 2:410
nosocomial infection, 2:411–412
Pasteurella, 2:426
photosynthetic, 2:436, 2:437
plankton and planktonic bacteria, 2:440–441
plaque, 1:17, 1:67, 2:387, 2:442
probiotics, 2:450
protein export, 2:453–454
protoplasts and spheroplasts, 2:462
Pseudomonas, 2:465–466
psychrophilic bacteria, 2:466
purple non-sulfur bacteria, 2:436
radiation-resistant bacteria, 2:478–479, 2:532
Salmonella, 2:503–504
sensitivity to temperature and pH ranges, 2:404, 2:433
sheathed bacteria, 2:514
Shigella, 2:514–515
spirochetes, 1:48, 1:52, 2:384, 2:385, 2:525–526
staphylococci and staphylococci infections, **2:529–530**
streptococci and streptococcal infections, **2:533–535**
surface layers, 1:53
thermophilic bacteria, 1:133, 1:211
transposons, 1:126, 1:200, 2:554
ultrastructure, 1:53–54
viable but nonculturable bacteria, 2:577
Bacteria and bacterial infection, **1:45–46,** 1:*46*
See also Bacteria; Bacterial infection
Bacterial adaptation, **1:46–47**
antibiotic resistance, 1:47
biofilms, 1:67–68
heat shock response, 1:261
luminescent bacteria, 1:354
sensitivity to temperature and pH ranges, 2:404–405, 2:433
sporulation, 2:527
viable but nonculturable bacteria, 2:577
Bacterial appendages, **1:47–48**
bacterial movement, 1:52
biofilms, 1:67
sheathed bacteria, 2:514

Chancroid, 2:512

Chang, Annie, 2:657

Chaperones, **1:113–114,** 1:261, 2:429, 2:582

Chargaff, Erwin, 2:595, 2:654

Charophyceae, 1:119

Chase, Martha Cowles, **1:114,** 1:269, 2:655

Chediak-Higashi syndrome (CHS), 1:297

Chemical mutagenesis, **1:114–115,** 1:161–164

    See also Mutations and mutagenesis

Chemoautotrophic and chemolithotrophic bacteria, **1:115–116,** 2:451

    carbon cycle, 1:101

    extremophiles, 1:211–212

    hydrothermal vents, 1:282–283

    methane oxidizing and producing bacteria, 2:378–379

    photosynthetic microorganisms, 2:437

    sulfur cycle, 2:536

    Winogradsky column, 2:601

Chemotaxis, 1:47

    See also Bacterial movement

Chemotherapy, **1:116–117,** 2:416

Chermann, Jean-Claude, 2:400

Chiasmata, 1:105

Chickenpox, 2:572–573, 2:573

Childbed fever, 2:535

Chitin, **1:117–118,** 1:232

Chlamydia infection, 2:512

    eye infections, 1:213

    pneumonia, 1:118

Chlamydia pneumoniae, 1:118

Chlamydia psittaci, 1:118, 2:445

Chlamydia trachomatis, 1:118, 1:123

Chlamydial pneumonia, **1:118**

Chlamydomonas, 2:460

Chlamydomonas nivalis, 2:522

Chloramphenicol, typhoid, 2:560

Chlordexidine, as disinfectant, 1:159

Chlorella, 1:119

Chlorination, **1:119–120**

    cysts, 1:119

    wastewater treatment, 2:590

Chloroflexus auranticus, 1:249

Chlorophyceae, 1:119

Chlorophyll, **1:119**

    Chlorophyta, 1:119–120

    chloroplasts, 1:82, 1:120, 1:155

    protozoans, 2:462

Chlorophyta, **1:119–120,** 2:460

    lichens, 1:348, 2:407, 2:411

Chloroplasts, 1:82, **1:120,** 1:155, 2:436

Chlortetracycline, 1:116

Cholera, 1:193, 1:196, 1:327

Cholera toxin, 1:189

Chondrus, 2:488

Chorioretinitis, 1:212

Chromatium spp., 2:409

Chromatography, 1:64

Chromosome number defects, 1:121

Chromosomes, **1:120–123,** 2:550

    See also Chromosomes, eukaryotic; Chromosomes, Prokaryotic

Chromosomes, eukaryotic, **1:120–122,** 2:387, 2:412

    polymerase chain reaction (PCR), 2:446–447

    recombinant DNA molecules, 2:480–481

Chromosomes, prokaryotic, **1:122–123**

    bacteriophages and bacteriophage typing, 1:55–56

    polymerase chain reaction (PCR), 2:446–447

    recombinant DNA molecules, 2:480–481

    yeast artificial chromosome (YAC), 2:610–611

Chronic bacterial disease, **1:123–124**

    ear infections, 1:172

    helicobacteriosis, 1:262

Chronic fatigue syndrome, mycoplasma, 2:408

Chronic gastritis, 1:262

Chronic granulomatous disease (CGD), 1:297

Chronic hepatitis, 1:264, 1:314

Chronic myelogenous leukemia (CML), 2:415, 2:416

Chrysochromulina polylepis, 2:482

CHS. *See* Chediak-Higashi syndrome

Chyrids, 1:232

Chytridiomycetes, 1:284, 2:407

cI protein, 1:356

Ciguatera, 1:157

Ciliates, 2:459

Ciliopa, 2:459

Ciprofloxacin, 2:467

Citric acid cycle, 2:484

CJD disease, **1:89–93**

    ethical issues and socio-economic impact, 1:90–92

    research advances, 1:92–93

    See also BSE and CJD disease

Cladina alpestris, 1:349

Cladistics, 2:438

Cladocera, 2:616

Class A pipette, 2:439

Class B pipette, 2:439

Class I antigens, 2:554

Class I MHC genes, 2:361

Class I viruses, 2:577

Class II MHC genes, 2:361

Class II antigens, 2:554

Class II viruses, 2:577

Class III MHC genes, 2:361

Class III viruses, 2:577

Class IV viruses, 2:577

Class V viruses, 2:577

Class VI viruses, 2:577

Clinical microbiology. *See* Microbiology, clinical

Clonal deletion, 2:539

Clonal selection theory, 1:302

Cloning: applications to biological problems, **1:124,** 1:230, 2:412, 2:658, 2:660

    embryo cloning, 1:75

    molecular cloning, 1:75

    plasmids, 1:200, 2:442–443

    positional cloning, 1:75

    shotgun cloning, 1:49, 1:242, 2:515

    therapeutic cloning, 1:124

    yeast artificial chromosome (YAC), 2:610–611

Cloroxybacteria, 2:436

Clostridium. *See* Botulism

Clostridium baratii, 1:84, 1:85

Clostridium botulinum, 1:16, 1:84–85, 2:576

Clostridium butyricum, 1:101

Clostridium difficile, 2:465

Clostridium perfringens, thermal death, 2:546

Clostridium tetani, 2:543

Club fungi, 1:232

Cryptosporidium muris, 1:143
Cryptosporidium parvum, 1:143, 1:236, 1:315, 2:526
Crystallography, proteins, 2:452, *2:453*
CTLs. *See* Cytotoxic T-lymphocytes
Culture, 1:*144,* **1:144–145,** 1:335–336
    defined, 1:49
    dilution theory and techniques, 1:156
    genetic identification of microorganisms, 1:240–241
    planktonic bacteria, 2:441
Curing, 1:224
Cuvier, Georges, 2:646
Cyanobacteria, 1:82–83, 1:203, 2:436
    chlorophyll, 1:119
    chloroplast, 1:120
    evolution of, 1:208
    fossils, 1:228
    gas vacuoles, 1:235
Cyclops, 2:616
Cyclosporin, 1:84, 1:307
Cystoseira osmundacea, 1:323
Cysts
    chlorination, 1:119
    Giardia, 1:249
    protozoa, 2:423
Cytogenetics. *See* Molecular biology and molecular genetics
Cytokines, 1:104, 1:105, **1:145,** 1:291, 1:306, 1:313–314, 2:539
Cytokinesis, 1:107–108, 1:244
Cytomegalovirus, 1:33
Cytoplasm, eukaryotic, **1:145–146,** 1:*146*
Cytoplasm, prokaryotic, **1:146–147,** 2:551–553
Cytotoxic T-lymphocytes (CTLs), 2:539

D

D. immitis, 2:423
da Vinci, Leonardo, 2:644
Dalton, John, 2:646
Daraprim, 1:184
DARPA. *See* Defense Advanced Research Project
Darwin, Charles Robert, **1:150–151,** 2:647, 2:648
Darwin, Erasmus, 2:646
Dausset, Jean, 1:288
Davaine, C.J., 1:326
Davies, J.A.V., 2:538
Davies, Julian E., **1:151–152**
Davis, Bernard D., 2:654
Dawkins, Richard, 2:507
de Baillou, Guillaume, 2:402
de Broglie, Louis Victor, **1:152–153,** 1:179, 2:388, 2:496
de Jussieu, Antoine-Laurent, 2:646
de Maupertuis, Pierre-Moreau, 2:645
de Tournefort, Joseph Pitton, 2:645
de Vries, Hugo, 2:651
Dedrick, Helen M., 2:653
Defects of cellular immunity. *See* Immunodeficiency disease syndromes
Defense Advanced Research Project (DARPA), 1:77
Dehydration, 1:223
Deinococcus, 1:54, 2:532
Deinococcus radiodurans, 2:404
Deisenhofer, Johann, 2:436
Delayed immunity, 1:288–290
Delbrück, Max, 1:55, 1:268, 1:269, 1:321, 2:594, 2:653, 2:654, 2:657
Deletion mutations, 2:405, 2:406

Democritus, 2:643
Dendrogram, 2:383–384
Dengue fever, **1:153–154,** 1:263, 2:499
Denitrification, 2:411
Dental caries, **2:379–380**
Dental plaque, 1:17, 1:67, 2:387, 2:442
Deoxyribonucleic acid. *See* DNA
Dermatomes, 2:574
Dermatomycoses, 2:517
Descartes, René, 2:645
Desiccation, **1:154**
Desulfovibrio hydrocarbonoclasticus, 2:432
Detection of mutants. *See* Laboratory techniques in microbiology
d'Hérelle, Félix, 1:55, **1:149–150,** 1:356, 2:652
Diaptomus, 2:616
Diarrhea
    Cryptosporidium parvum, 1:143, 1:236, 1:315
    enterobacterial infection, 1:188
    gastroenteritis, 1:236
    giardiasis, 1:249
    pseudomembranous colitis, 2:465
    See also Dysentery; Gastroenteritis
Diarrhetic shellfish poisoning, 2:482
Diatomic nitrogen, 2:410
Diatoms, **1:154–155,** 2:421, 2:460, 2:*461,* 2:462, 2:482
Diauxy, 2:398
Dictyostelium, **1:155**
Dictyostelium discoideum, 1:130, 1:155, 2:518
Didanoside, 1:8
Diffusion, cell membrane transport, 1:109–110
DiGeorge syndrome, 1:294, 1:297
Dilution plating, 1:156
Dilution theory and techniques, **1:156**
Dinitrogen-fixing symbioses, 2:411
Dinoflagellates, **1:156–157,** 1:*181,* 2:460, 2:470
    bioluminescence, 1:73
    diarrhetic shellfish poisoning, 2:482
    red tide, 1:156–157, 2:460, 2:481–482
Dinophysis, 2:481
Diphtheria, **1:157–158**
    Behring, Emil von, 1:58–59, 1:178
    coryneform bacteria, 1:136–137
    history of, 1:59
    Loeffler, Friedrich, 1:353
    Schick, Bela, 2:505–506
Diphtheria toxin, 1:189
Directional selection, 2:506
Directly Observed Therapy (DOT), 2:557
Disease outbreaks. *See* Epidemics and pandemics
Disinfection and disinfectants, **1:158–160**
    antiseptics, 1:31–32
    chlorination, 1:118–119
    contamination, 1:134
    disposal of infectious microorganisms, 1:160–161
    HACCP, 1:259–260
    hygiene, 1:283–284
    wastewater treatment, 2:590
Disposal of infectious microorganisms, 1:*160,* **1:160–161,** 2:590
Distemper, 2:575
DNA, **1:161–164,** 1:*162,* 1:*163,* 2:486, 2:550
    acridine orange and, 1:2, 1:3
    adenoviruses, 1:3
    agarose, 1:7

E

psychrophilic bacteria, 2:466
radiation-resistant bacteria, 2:478–479
sensitivity to pH and temperature, 2:404–405
sulfur cycle, 2:536
taq enzyme, 2:540–541
thermophiles, 1:211
See also Mutants: enhanced tolerance or sensitivity to temperature and pH ranges
Eye infections, 1:33, **1:212–213**

F

F genes, 1:133
F-pili, 1:48
Fabaceae, 2:411
Fabrizzi, Girolamo, 2:644
Facilitated diffusion, 1:109
  See also Cell membrane transport
Fairy shrimp, 2:616
Famciclovir, 1:33
Fannie, Angelina, 2:649
Fansidar, 1:184
Farber, Sidney, 1:116
Fatal familial insomnia (FFI), 1:90, 2:520
Fauci, Anthony S., **1:215–216**
Feather boa kelp, 1:323
Feldman, Harry Alfred, **1:216–217,** 1:252
Feline leukemia, 2:487
Feline leukemia virus (FELV), 2:487, 2:575
Fermentation, 1:174, 1:*217*, **1:217–218,** 2:377
  carbon cycle, 1:100–101
  defined, 1:224
  mold, 2:394–395
  wine making, 2:599–601
Fertility. *See* Reproductive immunology
Fertility genes (F genes), 1:133
FFI. *See* Fatal familial insomnia
FGF. *See* Fibroblastic growth factor
Fibrinolysin, 1:125
Fibroblastic growth factor (FGF), 1:104, 1:106
Field ion microscope, 1:180
Filiariasis, 2:423
Filoviruses, 1:172–173, 1:263
Filtration, 1:54, 2:532
FimH, 1:23
Finger, Ernest, 1:339
Finlay, Carlos, 2:545
Firefly, bioluminescence, 1:73
Fischer, Emil, 1:192, 1:339
FISH. *See* Fluorescence *in situ* hybridization
Flagella, 1:48, 1:52
Flagellates, 2:459
Flagellin, 1:48
Flash pasteurization, 2:426–427
Flaviviridae, 2:536
Flaviviruses, 1:263, 2:585
Fleas, 2:423
Fleming, Alexander, 1:112, 1:116, **1:218–219,** 1:*219,* 1:274, 1:276, 2:427, 2:*428,* 2:604, 2:648, 2:653
Flemming, Walther, 2:649, 2:650
Flesh-eating disease, 2:534
Flexner, Simon, 2:494
Florey, Howard Walter, 1:112, 1:116, **1:219–220,** 1:276, 2:427, 2:653

Flu
  epidemics and pandemics, 1:193–194, 1:312
  Great Flu Epidemic of 1918, 1:220–221
  hemagglutinin(HA) and neuraminidase (NA), 1:262–263
  See also Influenza
Flukes, 2:423
Fluorescein isothiocyanate, 1:286
Fluorescence *in situ* hybridization (FISH), **1:221–222,** 2:415
Fluorescence microscopy, acridine orange and, 1:2–3
Fluorescent dyes, 1:65, **1:222**
  acridine orange, 1:2–3, 1:24
  antibiotic resistance tests, 1:23–24
  See also Biochemical analysis; Laboratory techniques in immunology; Laboratory techniques in microbiology
Fluorescent probes, 2:415
Folic acid, 1:116
Foliose lichens, 1:348–349
Folliculitis, 2:516
Food additives, 1:225
Food preservation, **1:222–225**
  Appert, Nicolas François, 1:33–34
  enzymes, 1:192–194
  mold, 2:394–395
  pasteurization, 1:54, 1:246, 1:272, 2:426–427, 2:532, 2:569
  Salmonella, 2:503–505
  yeast, infectious, 2:612–613
Food safety, **1:225–226,** 1:*226*
  Appert, Nicolas François, 1:33–34
  Campylobacter jejuni, 1:99–100
  dinoflagellates, 1:157
  E. coli O157:H7 infection, 1:171
  enzymes, 1:192–194
  food preservation, 1:222–225
  HACCP, 1:259–260
  mold, 2:394–395
  pasteurization, 1:54, 1:246, 1:272, 2:426–427, 2:532, 2:569
  Salmonella, 2:503–504
  Shigella, 2:514–515
  toxoplasmosis, 2:548
  yeast, 2:612–613
Foodborne illnesses, 1:225, 1:226
  paralytic shellfish poisoning, 1:157, 2:482
  Salmonella, 2:503–504, 2:558
  staphylococci, 2:530
Foot-and-mouth disease, 1:*227,* **1:227–228,** 1:354
Forensic identification of microorganisms. *See* Genetic identification of microorganisms
Formaldehyde, as disinfectant, 1:159
Fossilization of bacteria, **1:228**
  diatoms, 1:154–155
  photosynthetic microorganisms, 2:437
  See also Evolutionary origin of bacteria and viruses
Fox, George E., 2:658
Fracastoro, Gerolamo, 1:273, 2:644
Fraenkel-Conrat, Heinz, 2:655
Frameshift mutations, 2:405
Francisella tularensis, 2:557
Franek, Frantisek, 1:176
Franklin, Rosalind Elsie, 1:162, 2:595, 2:598, 2:655
Freeze-drying, 1:223
Freezing, 1:224
Frerichs, Friedrich von, 1:177
Freund, Jules, 2:653

Freund's Complete Adjuvant, 1:5
Friedewald, W.F., 2:495
Friend, Charlotte, 1:228–229, 1:*229*
Friend virus, 1:229
Frosch, Paul, 1:227, 1:354, 2:651
Fructose lichens, 1:349
Frustules, 1:155
Fucalean alga, 1:323
Fucoxanthin, 2:460
Fuligo septica, 2:519
Fume hood, **1:229–230,** 1:284
Funch, Peter, 2:659
Fungal genetics, **1:230–231**
    See also Microbial genetics
Fungal infection
    candidiasis, 1:100, 2:516–517, 2:609, 2:612
    eye infections, 1:213
    fungicides, 1:232
    infection control, 1:310–311
    skin, 2:517
    thrush, 1:261, 2:546–547
Fungi, 1:*231*, **1:231–232,** 2:387
    aerobes, 1:5
    Armillaria ostoyae, 1:35
    basidomycetes, 1:57
    Berkeley, Rev. M.J., 1:62–63
    candidiasis, 1:100
    chitin, 1:117–118
    colony and colony formation, 1:129–130
    cryoprotection, 1:141–142
    cryptococci and cryptococcosis, 1:142–143
    hyphae, 1:284
    lichens, 1:348–349, 2:407, 2:411
    mesophilic, 2:376
    mycelia, 1:230, 1:231, 2:394, 2:406
    Saccharomyces cerevisiae, 2:501
    sensitivity to temperature and pH ranges, 2:404
    Sick Building Syndrome, 2:408
    See also Fungal genetics; Fungal infection; Fungicides; Mold; Mycology
Fungicides, 1:158–160, **1:232**
Funk, Casimir, 2:652
Furious rabies, 2:476–477
Furth, Jacob, 1:229

G

Galen, 2:644
Gallagher, Robert E., 1:234
Gallo, Robert C., 1:7, **1:233–235,** 2:401, 2:487, 2:658
Gambierdiscus toxicus, 1:*181*
Gamma globulins, 1:250
Gamma hemolysis, 1:80
Gamma radiation, 2:479
Ganciclovir, 1:33
Ganders, 2:465
Garrod, Archibald Edward, 1:192, 2:651
Gas gangrene, 1:16
Gas vacuoles and gas vesicles, **1:235**
Gasohol, 1:218
Gastritis, chronic, 1:262
Gastroenteritis, 1:236
    adenoviruses, 1:3

    campylobacteriosis, 1:99–100
    Enterobacteriaceae, 1:187–188
    rotavirus, 1:236
    Sporozoa, 2:526
    See also Microbial flora of the stomach and gastrointestinal tract
Gastrointestinal tract. *See* Microbial flora of the stomach and gastrointestinal tract
GBS. *See* Guillain-Barre syndrome
Gel electrophoresis, 1:122, 1:242
Gelactose, 1:6
Gelidiuim, 2:488
Gelidium comeum, 1:6
Gene, **1:236–238,** 2:489
    Berg, Paul, 1:60–62
    oncogene, 1:104, 1:243, 2:415, 2:558
    restriction enzymes, 2:485
    See also Genetic identification of microorganisms; Genotype and phenotype; Mutations and mutagenesis
Gene amplification
    restriction enzymes, 2:485
    yeast artificial chromosome (YAC), 2:610–611
Gene chips. *See* DNA chips and microarrays
Gene flow, 1:207
Gene splicing, 1:85
Gene therapy, 1:60–62, 2:510, 2:578–579
Genetic code, 1:162, **1:238–240,** 1:*239,* 2:550
    Berg, Paul, 1:60–62
    gene, 1:237–238
    genotype and phenotype, 1:245–246
    operon, 1:237, 1:354, 2:398, 2:416
    proteins, 1:15
    restriction enzymes, 2:485
Genetic diseases, 1:121
Genetic diversity, conjugation, 1:133
Genetic drift, 1:207–208
Genetic engineering, 1:75, 1:134
Genetic identification of microorganisms, **1:240–241**
    bioterrorism, 1:77
    gene, 1:237–238
    genetic code, 1:239–240
    genotype and phenotype, 1:245–246
    microbial taxonomy, 2:383–384
    restriction enzymes, 2:485
    See also DNA; Microbial genetics
Genetic mapping, 1:*241,* **1:241–242**
    gene, 1:237–238
    The Institute for Genomic Research (TIGR), 2:544
    restriction enzymes, 2:485, 2:*485*
Genetic regulation of eukaryotic cells, **1:106–108, 1:242–244**
    cell cycle, 1:106–108
    DNA, 1:161–164
    recombinant DNA molecules, 2:480–481
    restriction enzymes, 2:485
    RNA, 2:488–492
    See also Cell cycle (eukaryotic), genetic regulation of
Genetic regulation of prokaryotic cells, **1:244–245**
    bacteriophages and bacteriophage typing, 1:55–56
    cell cycle, 1:108–109
    DNA, 1:161–164
    recombinant DNA molecules, 2:480–481
    transcription, 2:548–549
    translation, 2:551–553
    See also Cell cycle (prokaryotic), genetic regulation of

H

Hand-foot-mouth disease, **1:258**

Hand washing, 1:283, 1:*283*

Hansen, Christian, 2:609

Hansen's disease. *See* Leprosy

Hansma, Paul, 1:37

Hantavirus and Hanta disease, 1:198, **1:258–259**, 2:659

Hantavirus pulmonary syndrome (HPS), 1:258, 1:259, 1:263

Hantzsch, Arthur, 1:339

Hartwell, Lee, 2:611

Harvey, William, 1:246, 2:644

Hata, Sahachiro, 2:538

HAV. *See* Hepatitis and hepatitis viruses

Hay fever, 1:10, 1:*11*

Hayes, William, 1:133, 2:655

Hazard Analysis and Critical Control Points Program (HACCP),
    1:259–260

Hazen, Elizabeth, **1:260–261**

HBV. *See* Hepatitis and hepatitis viruses

HCV. *See* Hepatitis and hepatitis viruses

HDV. *See* Hepatitis and hepatitis viruses

Health Alert Network (HAN), 1:79

Hearst, John, 1:102

Heart disease, *Chlamydia trachomatis*, 1:123

Heartworm, 2:423

Heat, bacteriocidal methods, 1:54

Heat shock proteins, 1:113, 1:261

Heat shock response, 1:47, **1:261**

Heating, for food preservation, 1:224

Heatley, Norman, 2:427

Heavy mutagenesis, 2:406

Heber-Katz, Ellen, 2:660

Heidelberger, Charles, 1:116

Heidelberger, Michael, 1:287

Helicobacter pylori, 1:262, 2:366, 2:381, 2:386

Helicobacteriosis, **1:262**

Helminths, 2:423, 2:597

Helper T cells, 1:288

Hemagglutinin (HA) and neuraminidase (NA), **1:262–263**

Hemolysis and hemolytic reactions, 1:80

Hemophiliacs, blood borne infection, 1:82

Hemophilus. See Haemophilus

Hemorrhagic colitis, 1:171

Hemorrhagic fever with renal syndrome (HFRS), 1:258, 1:259

Hemorrhagic fevers and diseases, 1:80–82, **1:263–264**
    arenavirus, 1:34–35
    dengue fever, 1:153–154, 1:263, 2:499
    Ebola virus, 1:172–173
    epidemics, 1:197
    hantavirus and Hanta disease, 1:258–259
    as public health issue, 2:467

Henle, Friedrich Gustav, 2:647

HEPA filter. *See* Fume hood

Hepadnaviruses, 1:264, **1:264**, 2:584

Hepatitis and hepatitis viruses, **1:264–267**, 1:*265*, 2:513
    chronic, 1:264, 1:314, 2:558
    hepatitis A virus (HAV), 1:264, 2:580
    hepatitis B virus (HBV), 1:264, 1:265–266, 2:508, 2:558, 2:584
    hepatitis C virus (HCV), 1:264, 1:266–267, 2:508
    hepatitis D virus (HDV), 1:267
    hepatitis E virus (HEV), 1:264, 1:267
    hepatitis G virus (HGV), 1:267
    seroconversion, 2:508
    vaccine, 1:265, 2:513

Herpes and herpes virus, **1:267–268,** 1:340, 2:513, 2:581, 2:584
    blood borne infection, 1:82
    chemotherapeutic agent, 1:116
    Epstein-Barr virus, 1:82, 1:201, 1:267, 2:399, 2:584
    herpes zoster virus, 1:212
    HHV4, 1:267
    HHV5, 1:267
    HHV6, 1:267
    HHV7, 1:267
    HHV8, 1:267
    HSV-1 (HHV1), 1:267
    HSV-2 (HHV2), 1:267

Herpes zoster virus (HZV), 1:212

Herpetosiphon, 1:249

Hershey, Alfred Day, 1:114, **1:268–270**, 2:654, 2:655, 2:657

Hertwig, Wilhelm, 2:649, 2:650

Hesse, Walter, 2:649

Heterokaryon, 1:230

Heterotrophic bacteria, 1:203, 1:255, 1:*270*, **1:270**

HEV. *See* Hepatitis and hepatitis viruses

Hfr strains, *Escherichia coli,* 1:133

HFRS. *See* Hemorrhagic fever with renal syndrome

HGV. *See* Hepatitis and hepatitis viruses

HHV. *See* Herpes and herpes virus

High efficiency particulate air filter. *See* Fume hood

Highly Active Anti-Retroviral Therapy (HAART), 1:9

Hildegard of Bingen, 2:644

Hillier, James, 1:180

Hinshelwood, Cyril, 1:86

Hinton, William A., 2:538

Hippocrates, 2:643

Histamine, 1:11, 1:16, **1:270–271**

Histocompatibility, **1:271**, 1:280

History of development of antibiotics, 1:116, 1:*276*, **1:276–277**
    Fleming, Alexander, **1:218–219**
    germ theory of disease, 1:28, 1:246–247, 1:273
    nosocomial infections, 2:411–412
    penicillin, 2:427, 2:511
    sulfa drugs, 2:535

History of immunology, **1:271–273**
    Avery, Oswald Theodore, 1:39–41
    historical chronology, 2:643–660
    Koch's postulates, 1:247, 1:274, 1:327, 1:328, 1:353
    measles, 2:368–369
    mumps, 2:402–403
    Schick, Bela, 2:505–506

History of microbiology, **1:273–274,** 1:*274*
    DNA, 1:161–163
    fermentation, 1:217–218
    food preservation, 1:222–225
    food safety, 1:224–225
    germ theory of disease, 1:28, 1:246–247, 1:273
    historical chronology, 2:643–660
    Koch's postulates, 1:247, 1:274, 1:327, 1:328, 1:353

History of public health, **1:274–276,** 1:*275*
    Centers for Disease Control (CDC), 1:110–112
    chemotherapy, 1:116–117
    food preservation, 1:222–225
    germ theory of disease, 1:28, 1:246–247, 1:273
    gonorrhea, 1:251
    Koch's postulates, 1:217, 1:247, 1:274, 1:328, 1:353
    measles, 2:368–369
    mumps, 2:402–403

I

General Index

history of, 1:271–273
immune system, 1:287–288
immunosuppressant drugs, 1:306–307
interferons, 1:313–314
measles, 2:368–369
nutritional aspects, **1:305**
phagocyte and phagocytosis, 2:434–435
radioisotopes, 2:479–480
Schick, Bela, 2:506
transplantation genetics and immunology, 2:553–554
vaccine, 2:568–572
See also Antibody and antigen; Antibody-antigen, biochemical and molecular reactions; Immune system; Immunity; Immunochemistry; Immunogenetics; Immunologic therapies; Laboratory techniques in immunology; Reproductive immunology
Immunology, nutritional aspects, **1:305**
Immunomodulation, **1:305–306**
Immunosuppressant drugs, 1:306–307
    Borel, Jean-François, 1:84
    thrush, 2:546–547
    transplantation genetics and immunology, 2:553–554
In vitro and *in vivo* research, **1:307–308**
Incineration
    disposal of infectious microorganisms, 1:161
Indicator species, **1:308,** 2:616–617
Indirect Coombs' test, 2:488
Industrial microbiology. *See* Economic uses and benefits of microorganisms
Infection
    animal models of infection, 1:*18,* **1:18–19**
    anti-adhesion, 1:23–24
    bacteremia, 1:44
    chemotherapy, 1:116–117
    complement, 1:131
    complications of, 1:312–313
    defined, 1:309
    germ theory of disease, 1:28, 1:246–247, 1:273
    immune system, 1:287–288
    intracellular, 1:315
    invasiveness, 1:315
    microbial flora of the oral cavity, dental caries, 2:379–380
    microbial flora of the skin, 2:380
    microbial flora of the stomach and gastrointestinal tract, 2:380–381
    nosocomial infection, 2:411–412
    pertussis, 2:429–430
    phagocyte and phagocytosis, 2:434–435
    prions, 2:449
    skin infections, 2:516–517
    sulfa drugs, 2:535
    symptoms, 1:312
    See also Bacterial infection; Fungal infection; Infection and resistance; Infection control; Viral infection
Infection and resistance, **1:308–310,** 1:*309*
    invasiveness and intracellular infection, 1:315
    See also Bacterial infection; Fungal infection; Infection control; Viral infection
Infection control, **1:310–311,** 1:*311*
    antiseptics, 1:31–32
    chlorination, 1:119–120
    hygiene, 1:310–311
    microbial flora of the oral cavity, dental caries, 2:379–380

microbial flora of the skin, 2:380
microbial flora of the stomach and gastrointestinal tract, 2:380–381
Pasteur, Louis, 2:424–426
steam pressure sterilizer, 2:530–531
sterilization, 1:31, 1:154, 1:158, 2:530, 2:531–532, 2:546
See also Epidemiology; Infection; Infection and resistance
Infection hypothesis, 1:31
Infectious mononucleosis, 1:201, **2:399**
Inflammation, **1:311,** 1:*311*
    autoimmunity, 1:38
    histamine and, 1:16
    phagocyte and phagocytosis, 2:434–435
Influenza, **1:311–313,** 1:*312*
    epidemics, 1:193–194, 1:196–198, 1:312
    Great Flu Epidemic of 1918, 1:193, 1:220–221
    history of, 1:193
Influenza virus, 1:262, 1:312, 1:*312,* 2:570
Ingenhousz, Jan, 2:645
Inhalation anthrax, 1:70, 1:76
Inherent resistance, 1:47
Inoculating loop, 1:335
Insecticides, *Bacillus thuringiensis,* 1:43–44, 1:*44*
Insertion mutations, 2:405, 2:406
Insertion sequences, 1:200, 2:486
The Institute for Genomic Research (TIGR), 1:49, **2:544**
Insulin-like growth factor (IGF), 1:104, 1:106
Interferon actions, **1:313,** 2:568–572
Interferon-alpha, 1:314
Interferon-gamma, 1:314
Interferon-tau, 1:314
Interferons, 1:313, **1:313–314,** 2:568–572
Interleukin-2, 1:233, 1:234
Intermediate yellow fever, 2:613
Interphase, 1:103, 1:243
Intracellular infection, 1:315
Introns, 2:457
Invasiveness and intracellular infection, **1:315**
    immune system, 1:287–288
    virus replication, 2:581–582
Iridovirisae, 2:536
Irish potato famine, 1:231
"Iron" bacteria, 1:115, 2:514
Isaacs, Alick, 1:314, 2:656
Isayev, Vasily Isayevich, 2:432
Iso-Sensitest agar, 1:23
Isoelectric focusing (IEF), 1:183
Isotypes and allotypes, **1:315–316**
Ivanovsky, Dmitri Iosifovich, **1:316,** 2:528, 2:650

J

Jacob, François, 1:87, 1:141, **1:317–319,** 1:*318,* 2:375, 2:381, 2:398, 2:655, 2:656
Jacobs, William, 2:660
Jannasch, Holger Windekilde, 1:283, **1:319,** 2:658
Janssen, Hans, 2:644
Janssen, Zacharias, 2:644
Japanese B encephalitis, 2:499
JC papovirus, 2:519
Jeffreys, Alex, 2:658
Jenner, Edward, 1:28, 1:32, 1:196, 1:246, 1:271, 1:272, 1:274, 1:287, 1:292, 1:303, **1:319–321,** 1:*320,* 2:521, 2:569, 2:584, 2:646

Jerne, Niels D., **1:321–322,** 2:392
Jock itch, 2:517
Johannsen, Wilhelm, 1:237, 2:651
Johnsen, C.D., 1:252
Johnson, Claude D., 2:402
Johnson, Irving S., 1:116
Johnson, William Arthur, 1:331
"Jumping genes," 2:555
Jungle yellow fever, 2:613
Junin virus, 1:34, 1:35
Justinian, 2:644

K

Kahn, Reuben Leon, 2:538
Kaposi's sarcoma, 1:267, 1:314
Karstroem, Henning, 2:398
Karyotype analysis, 1:121, 2:415
Kearns-Sayre syndrome, 2:393
Kelp and kelp forests, 1:6, **1:323–324,** 2:421, 2:460
Kendall, Edward, 1:287
Keratitis, 1:212
Keratoconjunctivitis, 1:3
Khorana, Har Gobind, **1:324–325,** 2:657
Killer T cells, 1:288
Kinetochores, 1:244
Kirby-Bauer disk-diffusion assay, 1:7
"Kissing bugs," 1:111
"Kissing disease." *See* Mononucleosis, infectious
Kitasato, Shibasaburo, 1:59, 1:272, 1:287, **1:325**
Klebs, Edward Theodore, 2:650
Klebsiella, ultrastructure of, 1:52
Klebsiella infection, 1:188
Kluyver, Albert Jan, **1:325–326,** 2:409, 2:652
Knoll, Max, 1:179–180, 2:496
Knoop, Franz, 1:330
Koch, Robert, 1:59, 1:177, 1:252, 1:272, 1:273, 1:274, 1:325, **1:326–328,** 1:327, 1:353, 2:648, 2:649, 2:650
　　agar, 1:6
　　anthrax, 1:19, 1:247, 1:326
　　cholera, 1:327
　　Pfeiffer, Richard, 2:432
　　tuberculosis, 1:327, 2:555
Koch's postulates, 1:247, 1:274, 1:327, **1:328,** 1:353
Kohl, 1:31
Köhler, Georges, 1:28, 1:30, 1:321, **1:328–329,** 2:392, 2:657
Kolletschka, Jakob, 2:508
Koplik's sports, 2:368
Kornberg, Arthur, 1:324, 2:655, 2:656
Kossel, Albrecht, 1:162, 2:489
Kovalevsky, Alexander, 2:377
Krebs, Hans Adolf, 1:192, **1:329–331,** 2:653
Krebs cycle, **1:331–332,** 2:392–393
Kristensen, Reinhardt Mobert, 2:659
Kühne, Wilhelm Friedrich, 2:649
Kunkel, Henry, 1:175, 1:176
Kuru, 1:90
Kyasanur Forest disease, 1:263

L

L-forms, 2:462
Laboratory techniques in immunology, **1:333–334,** 1:334, 2:439

contamination, 1:133–135
disposal of infectious microorganisms, 1:160–161
electrophoresis, 1:182–183, 1:333
ELISA, 1:190–191, 1:333–334
enzyme-linked immunosorbant assay (ELISA), 1:190–191
epidemiological tools, 1:199–200
fluorescence *in situ* hybridization (FISH), 1:221–222, 2:415
growth and growth media, 1:254–255, 1:335–336
immune complex test, 1:285–286
immunoelectrophoresis, 1:298, 1:333
Koch's postulates, 1:247, 1:274, 1:327, 1:328, 1:353
monoclonal antibodies, 1:334
pipette, 2:438–439
protein crystallography, 2:452
Pyrex, 2:468–469
recombinant DNA molecules, 2:480–481
spectroscopy, 2:524–525
in vitro and *in vivo* research, 1:307–308
See also Biochemical analysis techniques; Immunological analysis techniques; Microscope and microscopy
Laboratory techniques in microbiology, 1:335, **1:335–336,** 2:439
acridine orange and, 1:2–3, 1:24
agar and agarose, 1:5–7
agar diffusion, 1:7
antibodies, 1:27
bacteriophages and bacteriophage typing, 1:55–56
blood agar, hemolysis, and hemolytic reactions, 1:80
buffer, 1:95–96
conjugation, 1:133–134
contamination, 1:133–135
Coulter counter, 1:137–138
culture, 1:144–145
dilution theory and techniques, 1:156
disposal of infectious microorganisms, 1:160–161
electron microscopic examination of microorganisms, 1:180–181
epidemiological tools, 1:199–200
fluorescence *in situ* hybridization (FISH), 1:221–222, 2:415
germ theory of disease, 1:28, 1:246–247, 1:273
Gram staining, 1:253–254
growth and growth media, 1:254–255, 1:335–336
Koch's postulates, 1:247, 1:274, 1:327, 1:328, 1:353
Petri, Richard Julius, 2:430–431
pipette, 2:438–439
polymerase chain reaction (PCR), 2:446–447
protein crystallography, 2:452
Pyrex, 2:468–469
radioisotopes, 2:479–480
recombinant DNA molecules, 2:480–481
spectrophotometer, 2:523–524
spectroscopy, 2:524–525
steam pressure sterilizer, 2:530–531
sterilization, 2:531–532
thermal death, 2:546
in vitro and *in vivo* research, 1:307–308
See also Biochemical analysis techniques; Microscope and microscopy
LAC. *See* Lupus anticoagulant
Lactic acid bacteria, **1:336,** 2:381
Lactobacillus, 1:23, **1:336–337**
Lactobacillus acidophilus, 1:174, 1:337, 2:450
Lactobacillus bulgaricus, 1:337
Lactobacillus GG, 1:337, 2:450
LAD. *See* Leukocyte adhesion defect

WORLD OF MICROBIOLOGY AND IMMUNOLOGY General Index

clinical, 2:384–387
historical chronology, 2:643–660
history of, 1:273–274
medical training and careers in microbiology, 2:371–373
petroleum microbiology, 2:431–432
proteomics, 2:457–458
radioisotopes, 2:479–480
in vitro and *in vivo* research, 1:307–308
See also History of microbiology; Laboratory techniques in microbiology; Marine microbiology; Microscope and microscopy; Qualitative and quantitative analysis in microbiology; Quality control in microbiology; Veterinary microbiology
Microbiology, clinical, **2:384–387**, 2:*385*, 2:*386*
Microcystin, 1:82
Microcystis aeruginosa, 1:82
Microorganisms, **2:387**
attractants and repellents, 1:37
biogeochemical cycles, 1:68–69
carbon cycle, 1:100–101
nitrogen cycle, 2:410–411
oxygen cycle, 2:418–419
sulfur cycle, 2:536
See also Bacteria; Bacterial infection; Fungal infection; Fungi; Genetic identification of microorganisms; Microbial symbiosis; Microbial taxonomy; Microscope and microscopy; Viral infection; Viruses and responses to viral infection
Micropipettes, 2:439
Microscope and microscopy, 1:335, **2:388–389**, 2:*389*
Abbe, Ernst, 1:1
atomic force microscope, 1:36–37
bacterial ultrastructure, 1:53–54
electron microscope, 1:179–180
electron microscopic examination of microorganisms, 1:180–181
epifluorescence microscopy, 1:222
field ion microscope, 1:180
fluorescent dyes, 1:222
immunofluorescence microscopy, 1:299
light microscope, 2:388, 2:*389*
negative staining, 1:181
scanning confocal microscope, 2:473
scanning electron microscopy (SEM), 1:180, 2:388
scanning tunneling microscope (STM), 2:388
spectroscopy, 2:524–525
transmission electron microscope (TEM), 1:*179*, 1:179–181, 2:388
See also Dyes; Laboratory techniques in microbiology
Microwave spectroscopy, 2:524
Miescher, Johann, 1:161, 2:488, 2:648
Miller, Jacques, 2:656
Miller, Stanley L., 1:351, 2:389, **2:390–391**
Miller-Urey experiment, **2:389–390**, 2:403, 2:563
Milstein, César, 1:28, 1:30, 1:321, **2:391–392**, 2:*392*, 2:657
Milstein-Köhler technique, 1:30
Missense mutations, 2:405
Mitchell, Peter, 1:182
Mites, 2:423
Mitochondria and cellular energy, **2:392–393**
disorders of, 2:393
Krebs cycle, 1:331–332
mitochondrial DNA, 2:393
mitochondrial inheritance, 2:393–394
Mitochondrial DNA, **2:393**

mitochondria and cellular energy, 2:392–393
mitochondrial inheritance, 2:393–394
See also Mutations and mutagenesis
Mitochondrial encephalomyopathy, lactic acidosis and strokelike episodes (MELAS), 2:393
Mitochondrial EVE, 2:394
Mitochondrial inheritance, **2:393–394**
Miller-Urey experiment, 2:389–390, 2:403
mitochondria and cellular energy, 2:392–393
mitochondrial DNA, 2:393
See also Mutations and mutagenesis
Mitosis, 1:103–104, 1:*104*
eukaryotes, 1:106–107, 1:121, 1:243–244
MMR. *See* Measles, mumps, and rubella (MMR) vaccine
Moist heat sterilization, 2:532
Mold, **2:394–395**
colony and colony formation, 1:129–130
Dictyostelium discoideum, 1:155
eye infections, 1:213
Neurospora crassa, 2:409–410
Sick Building Syndrome, 2:408
slime molds, 1:155, 2:461, 2:518–519
See also Mycology
Molecular biology and molecular genetics, **2:395–397**, 2:*396*
amino acid chemistry, 1:14–16, 1:*15*
Asilomar conference, 1:36
bacterial artificial chromosome (BAC), 1:48–49
bacterial ultrastructure, 1:53–54
fluorescence *in situ* hybridization (FISH), 1:221–222, 2:415
gene, 1:237–238
mitochondrial inheritance, 2:393–394
oncogene, 2:415
phenotype and phenotypic variation, 2:435
plasmids, 1:200, 2:442–443
polymerase chain reaction (PCR), 2:446–447
protein crystallography, 2:452
protein export, 2:453–454
proteomics, 2:457–458
radiation mutagenesis, 2:477–478
restriction enzymes, 2:485
transduction, 2:549
transformation, 2:549–550
transgenics, 2:550–551
translation, 2:551–553
in vitro and *in vivo* research, 1:307–308
See also Mutations and mutagenesis
Molecular chaperones, 1:113
Molecular cloning, 1:75
Molecular rotational resonance spectroscopy, 2:524
Möllendorff, Wilhelm von, 1:330
Monera, 2:450
Monoclonal antibodies, 1:28, **1:29–30**, 1:304, 1:334
Monod, Jacques Lucien, 1:138, 1:141, 1:318, 2:381, **2:397–399**, 2:656
Mononucleosis, infectious, 1:201, **2:399**
Monovalent antiserum, 1:32
Montagnier, Luc, 1:7, 1:233, 1:234, **2:399–401**, 2:*400*, 2:658
Montague, Mary Wortley, 1:246, **2:401–402**, 2:569
Moore, Ruth Ella, **2:402**
Moore, Stanford, 2:657
Morgan, Thomas Hunt, 1:161, 1:237, 1:241, 2:398, 2:652
Mosquitoes, as carriers of disease, 2:423
Mössbauer, Rudolf, 2:525
Mössbauer effect, 2:525

Mössbauer spectroscopy, 2:525
Most probable number method, 1:156
Motility, 1:52, 1:249, 2:473
    See also Bacterial movement
Mouth. *See* Microbial flora of the oral cavity, dental caries
mRNA. *See* Messenger RNA
MRSA. *See* Methicillin-resistant *Staphylococcus aureus*
Mucor, 2:394
Mucus-associated lymphoid tissue (MALT), 1:290
Muller, Erwin Wilhelm, 1:180
Muller, Hermann Joseph, 2:652
Mullis, Kary, 2:658
Multidrug-resistant tuberculosis (MDR TB), 2:556
Multiplex PCR, 1:240–241
Mumps, **2:402–403**
Mumps virus, 2:402
Murchison meteorite, **2:403**
Murein. *See* Peptidoglycan
Murine typhus, 2:560
Murray, Andrew W., 2:658
Murray, Robert, **2:403–404,** 2:478
Mushrooms, 1:57, 1:117, 1:232
Mutants: enhanced tolerance or sensitivity to temperature and pH ranges, **2:404–405,** 2:433
Mutations and mutagenesis, 1:207, 2:384, **2:405–406**
    chemical mutagenesis, 1:114–115
    hemagglutinin(HA) and neuraminidase (NA), 1:262–263
    immunogenetics, 1:28, 1:299–300
    mutants: enhanced tolerance or sensitivity to temperature and pH ranges, 2:404–405, 2:433
    oncogene research, 2:415–416
    proteins, 1:15
    radiation and, 2:477–478
    See also Microbial genetics
Mutualism, 2:382, 2:383
Mycelium, 1:230, 1:231, 2:394, **2:406**
Mycobacterial infections, atypical, **2:406–407**
Mycobacterium avium, 1:347
Mycobacterium leprae, 1:108, 1:346–348
Mycobacterium tuberculosis, 1:123, 2:555, 2:660
Mycology, **2:407–408**
    See also Fungal genetics; Fungal infection; Fungi; Fungicides; Lichens; Mold; Yeast
Mycoplasma, 1:52, 2:576
Mycoplasma fermentans, 2:408
Mycoplasma genitalium, 2:408, 2:659
Mycoplasma infections, **2:408**
Mycoplasma pneumoniae, 2:408
Mycorrhizae, 1:57
Mycotoxins, 2:394, 2:395
Myeloma, 1:304
Myoclonus epilepsy with ragged red fibers (MERFF), 2:393
Mysidacea, 2:616
Myxobacteria, 1:249
Myxoma virus, 2:507
Myxomycota, 2:518

N

N protein, 2:433
Nageli, Carl Wilhelm von, 1:255
"Naked" DNA, 1:10
National Center for Human Genome Research (NCHGR), 2:660

National Electronic Data Surveillance System (NEDSS), 1:79
National Human Genome Research Institute (NHGRI), 2:660
National Pharmaceutical Stockpile Program (NPS), 1:78
Natural resistance, 1:47
Natural selection, 1:208, 2:506–507
NCHGR. *See* National Center for Human Genome Research
Necrotizing enterocolitis, 1:188
Necrotizing fasciitis, 2:534
NEDSS. *See* National Electronic Data Surveillance System
Negative staining, 1:181
Neisser, Albert, 1:251
Neiserria, eye infections, 1:213
Neiserria gonorrheae, 1:48
Neisseria meningitides, 1:22, 1:195
Nematodes, 2:423
Nereocystis leutkeana, 1:323
Neuberg, Carl, 2:651
Neuraminidase (NA), 1:263
Neuroritinitis, 1:212
Neurospora, **2:409–410**
Neurospora crassa, 1:230, 2:409, 2:541
Neurotoxins
    Clostridium tetani, 2:543
    Pyrrophyta, 2:470
Neurotransmitters, 1:16
Neva, Franklin Allen, 2:424, 2:597
NHGRI. *See* National Human Genome Research Institute
Nicolle, Charles-Jean-Henri, 2:402
Nicolson, G.L., 2:373
Nikaido, Hiroshi, 2:447
Nirenberg, Marshall Warren, 1:141, 1:238, 2:656, 2:657
Nisser, Albert, 2:649
Nitrate, 2:410, 2:411
Nitrifying bacteria, 1:115
Nitrobacter, 1:115, 2:411
Nitrogen cycle in microorganisms, **2:410–411**
    Azotobacter, 1:41
    biogeochemical cycles, 1:68–69
Nitrogen fixation, *Azotobacter,* 1:41
Nitrogen-fixing bacteria, 2:410
Nitrogenase, 2:410
Nitrosomonas, 1:115, 2:411
Nitzchia occidentalis, 2:482
NMR. *See* Nuclear magnetic resonance
Noctiluca, 1:156
Non-culturable bacteria. *See* Viable but non-culturable bacteria
Non-specific immunity. *See* Immunity, active, passive and delayed
Nonsense mutations, 2:405
Nontyphoidal *Salmonella* infection, 1:188
Nori, 2:488
North Asian tick typhus, 2:493
Northern blotting, 1:183
Northrop, John N., 1:192, 2:654
Norwalk virus, gastroenteritis, 1:236
Nosocomial infections, **2:411–412,** 2:*412*
Notobiotic animals. *See* Animal models of infection
Novotny, Ergo, 2:*453*
NPS. *See* National Pharmaceutical Stockpile Program
Nuclear magnetic resonance (NMR), 2:524
Nucleic acids, 1:238–240, 2:488
    See also DNA; RNA
Nuclein, 2:489
Nucleolus, 2:412

Peptidoglycan, 1:25, 1:51, 2:427, 2:428, **2:429**
Peptostreptococcus, 1:16
Periplasm, 1:51, **2:429**, 2:453
Perlmann, Gertrude, 1:338
Perry, Seymour, 1:233
Pertussis, **2:429–430**
Pesticide resistance, 2:506
Pestivirus, 2:536
Petri, Richard Julius, **2:430–431**, 2:650
Petri dish (Petri plate), 1:335, 2:430
Petroleum microbiology, **2:431–432,** 2:488
Petroleum spills, bioremediation, 1:73
Pettenkoffer, Max Josef von, 1:252, 1:255
Pfeiffer, Richard Friedrich Johannes, 1:83, 1:287, **2:432–433**
Pfeifferella, 2:432
Pfeiffer's agar, 2:432
Pfeiffer's phenomenon, 2:432
pH, 1:95–96, **2:433**
pH sensitivity. *See* Mutants: enhanced tolerance or sensitivity to temperature and pH ranges
Phaeophyta, 1:323–324, 2:421, **2:421,** 2:460
Phage genetics, **2:433–434**
   radiation mutagenesis, 2:477–478
   See also Bacteriophage and bacteriophage typing
Phage therapy, **2:434**
   See also Bacteriophage and bacteriophage typing
Phagocyte and phagocytosis, 1:5, **2:434–435**
Phagocyte defects. *See* Immunodeficiency disease syndromes
Phagocytosis, 1:5, 1:109, 2:434
   bacterial surface layers, 1:53
   defined, 1:291
   opsonization, 2:416–417
Phase G0, 1:103
Phenol oxidase, 1:142–143
Phenotype and phenotypic variation, 1:101, 1:208, 1:245, **2:435**
   See also Genotype and phenotype
Phi X 174, 2:516
Phosphodiester, 1:120
Phosphoglycerides, 2:435
Phospholipids, 1:52, **2:435**
Photoautotrophic organisms, 1:39, 1:255, 2:451
Photobacterium fischeri, 2:474
Photoisomerization, 2:437
Photosynthesis, **2:436–437,** 2:451
   Chlorophyta, 1:119–120
   chloroplast, 1:120
   photosynthetic microorganisms, 2:437
   Pyrrophyta, 2:470
Photosynthetic microorganisms, **2:437**
   blue-green algae, 1:82–83, 1:119, 1:120, 1:154, 1:203, 1:228, 1:235, 2:436
   Chlorophyta, 1:119–120, 1:348, 2:407, 2:411, 2:460
   gas vacuoles and gas vesicles, 1:235
   Phaeophyta, 1:323–324, 2:421, 2:460
   Pyrrophyta, 2:470
   soil formation, involvement of microorganisms, 2:523
   xanthophylls, 2:605
   Xanthophyta, 2:605–606
   See also Algae
Photosystem I, 2:605
Photosystem II, 2:605
Phycobilins, 2:460, 2:488
Phycobiont, 1:348

Phycocyanin, 1:82
Phycoerythrin, 1:82
Phylogenetic tree, 2:384
Phylogeny, **2:437–438**
Physarum polycephalum, 2:519
Phytophthora infestans, 1:231
Phytoplankton, 2:440
Picornaviruses, 2:580
"Pigging," 2:432
Pili, 1:48, 1:52, 1:133
Pilin, 1:48
Pilobolus, 2:394
"Pink eye," 1:3
Pinocytosis, 1:109
Pipette, **2:438–439,** 2:*439*
Pirosky, Ignacio, 2:391
Pittman, Margaret, **2:440**
Plague, bubonic. *See* Bubonic plague
Plankton and planktonic bacteria, **2:440–441,** 2:616–617
   diatoms, 1:154–155
   photosynthetic microorganisms, 2:437
   red tide, 1:156–157, 2:460, 2:481–482
   See also Zooplankton
Planktonic bacteria, 2:441
Plant alkaloids, chemotherapeutic, 1:117
Plant viruses, 2:441, **2:441–442,** 2:547
Plantar warts, 2:516
Plaque, 1:17, 1:67, 2:387, **2:442**
Plaque assay, 2:434
Plasmids, 1:108, 1:200, 1:230, **2:442–443,** 2:*443,* 2:550
   bacterial artificial chromosome (BAC), 1:48–49
   recombinant DNA molecules, 2:480–481
Plasmodial slime molds, 2:518, 2:519
Plasmodium, 2:363, **2:443–444,** 2:461, 2:463, 2:526
Plasmodium falciparum, 2:363, 2:443, 2:444
Plasmodium malariae, 2:363, 2:443
Plasmodium ovale, 2:363, 2:443
Plasmodium vivax, 2:363, 2:443, 2:444
Platelet-derived growth factor (PDGF), 1:104, 1:106
Pliny the Elder, 2:644
PML. *See* Progressive multifocal leukoencephalopathy
Pneumocystis carinii, 2:445, 2:526
Pneumonia, bacterial and viral, **2:444–445**
   chlamydial pneumonia, 1:118
   defined, 1:17
   Legionnaires' disease, 1:344–346
   Pneumocystis carinii, 2:445, 2:526
   walking pneumonia, 1:118
Podospora anserine, 1:230
Pol I, 2:491
Pol II, 2:491
Polaromonas vacuolata, 1:211
Polio vaccine, 1:186, 2:499, 2:570
Poliomyelitis and polio, **2:445–446**
   Center for Disease Control (CDC), 1:111
   Sabin, Albert, 2:499–501
   Salk, Jonas, 2:501–503
   vaccine, 1:186, 2:499, 2:570
Poliovirus, 2:446
Pollens, allergies, 1:10
Pollution, bioremediation, 1:73–74
Polymerase chain reaction (PCR), 1:240, **2:446–447**
   Actinomyces, 1:3

Syphilis, **2:537–538**
    epidemic, 1:251
    Wasserman test, 1:83, 2:589–590
Szostak, Jack William, 2:658

T

T-8 lymphocytes, 2:593
T-8 suppressor cells, 2:540
T-cell growth factor, 1:234
T-cell leukemia virus. *See* Human T-cell leukemia virus
T cell receptor (TCR), 2:539
T cells (T lymphocytes), 1:288, 1:291, 1:303, **2:539–540**
    AIDS, 1:9
    allergies, 1:10–11
    immune synapse, 1:286–287
    immune system, 1:287–288
T delayed hypersensitivity cells, 1:292
T4 phage, 1:55
T phages, 2:577
T suppresser cells, 1:292
Taiwan acute respiratory agent, 1:118
Tamoxifen, 1:116
Tapeworms, 2:423
Taq enzyme, 2:*540*, **2:540–541**
Tatum, Edward Lawrie, 1:175, 1:274, 1:341, 2:382, **2:540–541**, 2:653, 2:654, 2:656
Taxol, 1:116, 2:438
Taxonomy. *See* Microbial taxonomy
Taxus brevifolia, 2:438
Taxus cuspidata, 2:438
TCR. *See* T cell receptor
Teissier, Georges, 2:398
Teliomycetes, 1:57
Telomeres, 1:123
Telophase, 1:103, 1:107, 1:244
TEM. *See* Transmission electron microscope
Temin, Howard, 1:56, 2:657
Temperate phages, 2:433
Temperature sensitivity. *See* Mutants: enhanced tolerance or sensitivity to temperature and pH ranges
Terrorism. *See* Bioterrorism
Tetanolysin, 2:543
Tetanospasmin, 2:543
Tetanus and tetanus immunization, **2:543**
    antiserum, 1:32
    vaccine, 2:543
Tetanus toxoid, 2:543
Tetracyclines, 1:116, 1:118
Tetrad, 1:105
Thales, 2:643
The Institute for Genomic Research (TIGR), 1:48, **2:544**
Theiler, Max, **2:544–546**, 2:653
Therapeutic cloning, 1:124
Thermal death, **2:546**
Thermal death point, 2:546
Thermophilic bacteria, 1:133, 1:211
Thermophilic fungi, composting, 1:133
Thermotolerant bacteria. *See* Extremophiles
Thermus aquaticus, 1:88, 1:211, 2:540
Thiobacillus ferroxidans, 1:101, 1:115, 2:536
Thiobacillus prosperus, 2:536
Thiobacillus thiooxidans, 1:115, 2:536

Thiosarcina rosea, 2:409
Thiotrix, 1:115, 2:536
Thompson, D'Arcy Wentworth, 2:652
Thrush, 1:261, **2:546–547**
Thylakoid sacs, 1:120
"Thyphoid Mary," 2:559
Thyrotricin, 1:116
Ticks, 1:82, 2:423
Tiger mosquito, 1:153
TIGR. *See* The Institute for Genomic Research
Tijo, Joe Hin, 2:656
Tinea capitis, 2:517
Tinea corporis, 2:517
Tinea cruris, 2:517
Tiselium, Arne, 1:183
Tiselius, 2:651
Tobacco mosaic virus (TMV), 2:441, 2:528, **2:547**, 2:582
    Beijerinck, Martinus Willem, 1:59–60, 1:316
    Ivanovsky, Dmitri Iosifovich, 1:316
Todd, Alexander, 1:324, 2:489
Togaviruses, 2:580
Tonegawa, Susuma, 2:658
Torovirus, 1:129
Toxic shock syndrome, 2:529, 2:534, **2:547–548**
Toxins. *See* Enterotoxin and exotoxin
Toxoid, 1:32
Toxoplasma gondii, 2:548
Toxoplasmosis, 2:526, **2:548**
Tracking diseases with technology. *See* Epidemiology, tracking diseases with technology
Transcription, 1:238, 1:261, 2:486, 2:489, **2:548–549**, 2:*549*
Transduction, **2:549**
Transfer RNA (tRNA), 2:489, 2:491, 2:551
Transformation, 2:462, **2:549–550**
Transgenics, **2:550–551**
    biodegradable substances, 1:66–67
Transient hypogammaglobulinemia, 1:301
Transitions, 2:555
Translation, 1:33, 2:548, **2:551–553**, 2:*552*
Transmembrane proteins, 1:109
Transmission electron microscope (TEM), 1:*179*, 1:179–180, 2:388
Transmission of pathogens, **2:553**, 2:*553*
    blood borne infections, 1:80–82
    food safety, 1:225–226
    hygiene, 1:283–284
Transplantation genetics and immunology, **2:553–554**
    cloning, 1:124
    history of, 1:307
    immunosuppressant drugs, 1:306–307
    major histocompatibility complex (MHC), 2:361–363
Transport proteins, 1:109
Transposable elements, 2:485–486
Transposase, 2:485–486
Transposition, 2:485–486, **2:554–555**
Transposons, 1:126, 1:200, 2:554, 2:555
Trematodes, 2:423
Trembley, Abraham, 2:645
Treponema. *See* Syphilis
Treponema pallidum, 1:52, 2:526, 2:589
Treviranus, Gottfried Reinhold, 2:646
Triatomines, 1:111
Trichinella spiralis, 2:423, 2:597
Trichonymphs, 2:462

enterotoxin, 1:189
sensitivity to temperature and pH ranges, 2:404
Vibrio fischeri, 1:354
Vibrio furnisii, 1:118
Vibrio parahaemolyticus, 1:47
Vinblastine, 1:117
Vincristine, 1:117
Vinograd, Jerome, 2:375
Viral classification, 2:579
Viral epidemics. *See* Epidemics and pandemics; Epidemics, viral
Viral gastroenteritis, 1:236
Viral genetics, 2:438, **2:577–578**
    Asilomar conference, 1:36
    bacteriophages and bacteriophage typing, 1:55–56
    latent viruses and disease, 1:340–341
    lysogeny, 1:356–357
    oncogene, 2:415
    phage genetics, 2:433–434
    phage therapy, 2:434
    phylogeny, 2:437–438
    plant viruses, 2:441–442
    radiation mutagenesis, 2:477–478
    retroviruses, 2:486–487
    RNA tumor viruses, 2:493–494
    slow viruses, 2:519–520
    transduction, 2:439
    See also Microbial genetics; Viral vectors in gene therapy
Viral infection
    AIDS, 1:7–9
    antiviral drugs, 1:33
    arenavirus, 1:34–35
    blood borne infections, 1:80–82
    cats, 2:575
    Centers for Disease Control (CDC), 1:110–112
    chickenpox, 2:572–573
    common cold, 1:127–128
    dogs, 2:575
    enterovirusinfection, 1:189–190
    environmental contamination, 1:136–137
    epidemics, 1:193–194, 1:196–198
    eye infections, 1:212–213
    gastroenteritis, 1:236
    hand-foot-mouth disease, 1:258
    hantavirus and Hanta disease, 1:258–259
    hemorrhagic fevers and diseases, 1:263–264
    hepatitis, 1:264–267
    human immunodeficiency virus, 1:279–280
    immune system, 1:287–288
    infection and resistance, 1:308–310
    infection control, 1:310–311
    invasiveness and intracellular infection, 1:315
    latent viruses, 1:340–341
    Lichen planus, 1:348
    measles, 2:368–369
    meningitis, 2:374–375
    mononucleosis, 2:399
    mumps, 2:402–403
    pneumonia, 2:444–445
    poliomyelitis and polio, 2:445–446
    rabies, 2:475–477
    retroviruses, 2:486–487
    rheumatic fever, 2:532
    sexually transmitted diseases (STDs), 2:510–514
    skin infections, 2:516–517
    slow viral infection, 2:519
    smallpox, 1:76, 1:196, 2:520–522, 2:568–572
    strep throat, 2:532
    swine fever, 2:536–537
    T cells (T lymphocytes), 2:539–540
    transduction, 2:439
    varicella, 2:572–573
    varicella zoster virus, 2:573–574
    variola virus, 2:520–521, 2:574
    West Nile virus, 2:597–598
    yellow fever, 2:613–614
    See also Plant viruses
Viral infections
    chemotherapy, 1:116–117
    cowpox, 1:138
    transmission of pathogens, 2:553
Viral pneumonia, 2:444–445
Viral vectors in gene therapy, **2:578–579**
    phage therapy, 2:434
    retroviruses, 2:486–487
Virchow, Rudolf, 1:247, 2:648
Virology, viral classification, types of viruses, **2:579–581**
    Centers for Disease Control (CDC), 1:110–112
    epidemics, 1:196–198
    latent viruses and disease, 1:340–341
    oncogene, 2:415
    plant viruses, 2:441–442
    See also Viral genetics; Viral infection; Viral vectors in gene therapy; Virus replication; Viruses and responses to viral infection
Virus replication, **2:581–582**, 2:582
    bacteriophages and bacteriophage typing, 1:55–56
    Beijerinck, Martinus Willem, 1:59–60
    herpes and herpes virus, 1:267–268
    interferons, 1:313–314
    lysogeny, 1:356–357
    oncogene, 2:415
    retroviruses, 2:486–487
Viruses, **2:582–585**
    adenoviruses, 1:3–4, 2:581, 2:584
    AIDS, 1:7–9
    Andes virus, 1:259
    antiviral drugs, 1:33
    arenavirus, 1:34–35
    Arenaviruses, 1:34–35, 1:263
    Asfivirus, 2:536
    Bayou virus, 1:259
    Birnaviruses, 2:580
    Black Creek Canal virus, 1:259
    Blue River virus, 1:259
    Bunyavirus group, 1:263
    cauliflower mosaic virus (CMV), 2:515
    Centers for Disease Control (CDC), 1:110–112
    classification of, 2:577, 2:579
    cold viruses, 1:128–129
    common cold, 1:127–128
    contamination, 1:135–136
    Coronavirus, 1:129, 2:575
    Coxsackie virus group, 1:258
    Ebola virus, 1:81, 1:*81*, 1:172–173, 1:*173*, 1:264, 2:585, 2:657
    enterovirus infections, 1:189–190
    epadnaviruses, 1:264

W

X

Y

Z